Better Homes and Gardens®

NEW FAMILY MEDICAL GUIDE

Edited by

Edwin Kiester, Jr.

Illustrations by

Kelly Solis-Navarro
and
Evanell Towne
Based in part on illustrations
conceived and created by
Paul Zuckerman

© Copyright 1989 by Meredith Corporation,
Des Moines, Iowa. All Rights Reserved.
Printed in China
Fourth Edition. Printing Number and Year: 10 9 8 7 6   97 96 95 94
Library of Congress Catalog Card Number: 80-68457
ISBN: 0-696-00345-7 (hard cover)
ISBN: 0-696-00346-5 (trade paperback)

FOREWORD

When the Better Homes and Gardens® *Family Medical Guide* was first published in the early 1960s, tuberculosis was a major cause of illness and death. Children routinely endured the discomforts of measles and mumps, and heart disease was rampant. At the same time, it was the age of medical miracles. In the most dramatic example, polio vaccine in a single stroke had virtually eradicated one of the most feared of all diseases.

Health-conscious Americans needed a reliable and authoritative guide through this maze of old problems and new solutions. The eminent science writer and editor, Donald G. Cooley, enlisted a nationally recognized corps of medical specialists from prominent hospitals and universities to provide it. Specially commissioned artwork was researched and executed by the distinguished medical illustrator, Paul Zuckerman. The contributors to the Better Homes and Gardens® *Family Medical Guide* were assigned one simple objective: to explain in lucid, everyday terms and with clear illustrations how the body works, what can go wrong, and how to repair it.

How well they succeeded can be measured. The *Family Medical Guide* quickly became a best-seller and has sold millions of copies.

In the 1990s, the picture of American health and sickness is vastly different. Tuberculosis is rare.

Immunizations have almost wiped out the classic childhood diseases. Yet new afflictions have risen ominously to overshadow those of the past. Acquired immune deficiency syndrome (AIDS), unknown when previous editions were printed, has claimed thousands of lives. Meanwhile, as Americans live longer, chronic illnesses, rather than acute episodes, are the main burden of care.

Patterns of treatment have changed, too. Hospital stays are shorter; more care is provided outside hospitals; people are given (and accept) more responsibility for their own care. The emphasis is on maintaining health and preventing illness rather than cure.

The Better Homes and Gardens® *New Family Medical Guide,* as revised for the 1990s, seeks to meet these new needs. Aimed at a different generation with different concerns, it encompasses the best of today's knowledge in both word and picture. But in a larger sense this edition is unchanged. The broader goal is better health for all Americans.

Throughout its history, the roster of contributors to the *Family Medical Guide* has read like a who's who of medicine. Many past contributors have retired or passed on after a lifetime of accomplishment; it no longer is possible to list all their names. The equally distinguished contributors to this edition appear, along with those who provided counsel and review.

ACKNOWLEDGMENTS

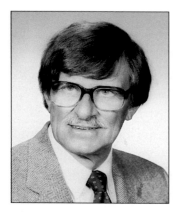

Edwin Kiester, Jr., editor of the Better Homes and Gardens® Family Medical Guide, *is co-author with Sally Valente Kiester of the* Better Homes and Gardens® New Baby Book *and the* Better Homes and Gardens® Eating Healthy Cook Book. *His articles on health, medicine, science, and other topics have appeared in many magazines.*

Contributors

Fred Ayvazian, M.D., Chief, Pulmonary Section, Veterans Administration Medical Center, East Orange, New Jersey; Professor of Medicine, College of Medicine and Dentistry of New Jersey; Professor of Clinical Medicine, New York University Medical Center, New York City.

Robert A. Bagramian, D.D.S., Dr. P.H., Professor and Chairman of Community Dentistry, School of Dentistry, and Professor of Dental Public Health, School of Public Health, University of Michigan.

Arthur E. Baue, M.D., Donald Guthrie Professor and Chairman, Department of Surgery, Yale University School of Medicine; Chief of Surgery, The Yale-New Haven Hospital, New Haven, Connecticut.

Philip W. Brickner, M.D., F.A.C.P., Director, Department of Community Medicine, St. Vincent's Hospital and Medical Center of New York; Associate Professor of Clinical Medicine, New York Medical College.

William D. Carey, M.D., Staff Physician, Cleveland Clinic Foundation; Member, American Association for the Study of Liver Disease, American Society of Gastrointestinal Endoscopy, and American Gastroenterological Asssociation.

William H. Crosby, M.D., F.A.C.P., Colonel, Medical Corps, United States Army. Department of Hematology, Walter Reed Army Institute of Research; Professor of Medicine, Uniformed Services University; Clinical Professor of Medicine, George Washington University.

Michael Eliastam, M.D., M.P.P., Assistant Professor of Medicine and Surgery, Stanford University School of Medicine; Director of Emergency Services, Stanford University Hospital, Palo Alto, California.

Richard G. Farmer, M.D., F.A.C.P., Chairman, Division of Medicine, and Head, Department of Gastroenterology, Cleveland Clinic Foundation; Past President, American College of Gastroenterology; Member, National Commission on Digestive Diseases.

Robert D. Fazzaro, M.D., Director, Respiratory Therapy Services, Millville (New Jersey) Hospital.

Daniel X. Freedman, M.D., Louis Block Professor of Biological Sciences, and Chairman, Department of Psychiatry, Pritzker School of Medicine, University of Chicago; President, American Psychiatric Association, 1981–82.

Richard R. Gacek, M.D., F.A.C.S., Professor and Chairman, Department of Otolaryngology and Communication Sciences, State University Hospital, Upstate Medical Center, Syracuse, New York; Research Adjunct Professor, Institute for Sensory Research, Syracuse University; Lecturer in Otolaryngology, Harvard Medical School.

Harlan R. Giles, M.D., Professor and Associate Chairman, Department of Obstetrics and Gynecology, and Director, Maternal Fetal Medicine and Genetics, Texas Tech University School of Medicine.

Robert J. Haggerty, M.D., President, William T. Grant Foundation; Clinical Professor of Pediatrics, Cornell University Medical College; Editor, *Pediatrics in Review.* Former Professor and Chairman, Deparment of Pediatrics, School of Medicine and Dentistry, University of Rochester; former Roger I. Lee Professor and Chairman, Department of Health Services, Harvard School of Public Health.

J. Timothy Hesla, Assistant Director, Institute of Nutrition, University of North Carolina. Member, Society for Nutrition Education; Past President, North Carolina Council on Food and Nutrition.

Howard N. Jacobson, M.D., Director, Institute of Nutrition, University of North Carolina; former Member, Food and Nutrition Board and Committee on Recommended Dietary Allowances, National Research Council/National Academy of Sciences.

A. Everette James, Jr., Sc.M., J.D., M.D., Professor and Chairman, Department of Medical Imaging and Radiological Sciences; Professor of Medical Administration; Lecturer in Legal Medicine; Senior Research Associate, Institute for Public Policy, Vanderbilt University School of Medicine.

Sylvia C. Johnson, M.D., Dermatologist, Group Health Cooperative, Seattle; Assistant Professor of Medicine (Dermatology), Clinical Faculty, University of Washington School of Medicine.

Michael M. Kaback, M.D., Professor, Departments of Pediatrics and Medicine, UCLA School of Medicine; Associate Chief, Division of Medical Genetics, Harbor-UCLA Medical Center; Director, Prenatal Diagnosis and Genetic Counseling Center, Harbor-UCLA Medical Center, Los Angeles.

Edward H. Kass, M.D., Ph.D., William Ellery Channing Professor of Medicine and Director, Channing Laboratory, Harvard Medical School and Peter Bent Brigham Hospital, Boston.

Warren A. Katz, M.D., F.A.C.P., Clinical Professor of Medicine and Chief, Division of Rheumatology, Medical College of Pennsylvania; Acting Director of Rheumatology, Moss Rehabilitation Hospital (Arthritis Center), Philadelphia, and Attending Physician, Albert Einstein Medical Center, Philadelphia.

Peter F. Kohler, M.D., Professor of Medicine and Head, Division of Clinical Immunology, University of Colorado Health Sciences Center, Denver; Consultant, Veterans Administration Hospital, Denver.

Calvin M. Kunin, M.D., F.A.C.P., Professor and Chairman, Department of Medicine, Ohio State University College of Medicine; Chief, Veterans Administration Outpatient Clinic, Columbus, Ohio.

Herbert G. Langford, M.D., Professor of Medicine and Physiology, and Chief, Endocrinology and Hypertension Section, University of Mississippi Medical Center, Jackson, Mississippi.

Donald B. Lucas, M.D., Professor of Orthopaedic Surgery and Chairman Emeritus, Department of Orthopaedic Surgery, School of Medicine, University of California, San Francisco.

Richard L. Masland, M.D.H., Houston Merritt Professor Emeritus, Department of Neurology, College of Physicians and Surgeons, Columbia University; former Executive Director, National Commission for the Control of Epilepsy and Its Consequences; former Director, National Institute of Neurological Diseases and Blindness, National Institutes of Health.

John Stirling Meyer, M.D., Chief, Cerebrovascular Research, Veterans Administration Medical Center, Houston; Professor of Neurology, Baylor College of Medicine; former Member, Advisory Council, National Institute of Neurological and Communicative Diseases and Stroke; Chairman, Stroke Committee, President's Commission on Heart Disease, Cancer, and Stroke; Diplomate, American Board of Neurology and Psychiatry, Inc.

Gerald P. Murphy, M.D., D.Sc., Professor of Surgery, State University of New York at Buffalo; Director, Roswell Park Memorial Institute, Buffalo.

William L. Proudfit, M.D., Clinical Emeritus Consultant, Cleveland Clinic Foundation; former Head, Department of Clinical Cardiology, Cleveland Clinic Foundation.

Aldo A. Rossini, M.D., Associate Professor of Medicine and Director of Diabetes and Metabolism, Division of Endocrinology and Metabolism, University of Massachusetts Medical Center, Worcester, Massachusetts.

Gloria E. Sarto, M.D., Ph.D., Professor and Assistant Chairman, Department of Obstetrics and Gynecology, Northwestern University Medical School and Prentice Women's and Maternity Center of Northwestern Memorial Hospital, Chicago.

Clark T. Sawin, M.D., Professor of Medicine, Tufts University School of Medicine; Chief, Endocrine-Diabetes Section, Veterans Administration Medical Center, Boston.

Michael B. Shimkin, M.D., Professor Emeritus of Community Medicine and Oncology, School of Medicine, University of California at San Diego.

Lester F. Soyka, M.D., F.A.A.P., Professor of Pharmacology and Pediatrics and Chairman, Department of Pharmacology, University of Vermont College of Medicine; Chairman, Section of Clinical Pharmacology and Therapeutics, American Academy of Pediatrics.

William J. Spanos, Jr., M.D., Assistant Professor of Radiotherapy and Assistant Radiotherapist, University of Texas System Cancer Center, and Assistant Professor, University of Texas Medical School.

Bruce E. Spivey, M.D., Professional Chairman, Department of Ophthalmology, Pacific Medical Center, San Francisco; President, Pacific Medical Center, San Francisco; Executive Vice President, American Academy of Ophtalmology.

Patti Tighe, M.D., Associate Professor and Director of Education, Department of Psychiatry, Pritzker School of Medicine, University of Chicago.

James F. Toole, M.D., L.L.B., Professor of Neurology and Chairman of Department of Neurology, Bowman-Gray School of Medicine, Wake Forest University; Member, Advisory Council, National Institute of Neurological Diseases and Stroke.

Julia A. Walsh, M.D., Associate in Medicine, Harvard Medical School and Peter Bent Brigham Hospital, Boston.

Jess R. Young, M.D., Head, Department of Peripheral Vascular Disease, Cleveland Clinic Foundation.

Consultants

Special thanks to Keith B. Taylor, M.D., George DeForest Barnett Professor of Medicine, Stanford University School of Medicine, for his help with this project. Thanks to the following members of the faculty of the Stanford University School of Medicine for review and consultation on this edition of the book:

Elizabeth A. Abel, M.D. (Dermatology)
Thomas E. Davis, M.D. (Oncology)
Willard E. Fee, Jr., M.D. (Ear, Nose & Throat)
Robert Ginsburg, M.D. (Peripheral Vascular Disorders)
Stuart B. Goodman, M.D. (Orthopedic Surgery)
Robert Kessler, M.D. (Urology)
Fredric B. Kraemer, M.D. (Diabetes)
Stephen J. Peroutka, M.D., Ph. D. (Neurology)
Thomas A. Raffin, M.D. (Respiratory)
C. Peter Rosenbaum, M.D. (Psychiatry)
Peter A. Rudd, M.D. (Hypertension)
Eugene Sandberg, M.D. (Gynecology & Obstetrics)
Gary K. Schoolnik, M.D. (Infectious Disease)
John Sper Schroeder, M.D. (Cardiology)
Frank E. Stockdale, M.D., Ph.D. (Oncology)
Robert S. Swenson, M.D. (Nephrology)
Abba I. Terr, M.D. (Allergy)
Ernesto Zatarain, M.D. (Arthritis)

Also:

R. Hewlett Lee, M.D., Palo Alto Medical Foundation (Surgery), Palo Alto, California.
Steven D. Johnson, PA-C, Palo Alto Medical Foundation (Home Care/Geriatrics), Palo Alto, California.
Antonio C. Ragadio, Jr., D.D.S., San Francisco.

CONTENTS

CHAPTER 1

A PREVENTIVE APPROACH TO HEALTH

Good health begins with awareness of your body. You need to sense how your body usually functions so that you can detect variations from normal. Many of these differences are unimportant in themselves. You only need to be aware of them so that you can detect change. Your physician should be alerted to such changes so that he or she can help you recognize significant ones.

It also is important to be aware of your medical history. The illnesses of earlier years may have a bearing on your health today. Keep a thorough record and make certain that your doctor has the information. As you know, certain diseases are family connected. Therefore, a family health history, concerning your grandparents, parents, siblings, and other close relatives, is valuable. Maintain an accurate record of this material for your doctor.

A TIMETABLE FOR CHECKUPS*

AGE IN YEARS	BIRTH	10	20	30	40	50	60	70	80

EYE DISEASE
Eye examination *(at birth)*
Eye examination *(at age 3 or 4)*
Eye examination *(every 2 to 4 years, 12 to 20)*
Eye examination *(at age 40)*
Eye examination *(every 2 or 3 years after 55)*

BREAST CANCER
Self-examination *(monthly after 20)*
Baseline mammogram *(once between 35 and 39)*
Mammogram *(every 1 to 2 years from 40 to 49)*
Mammogram *(annually after 50)*
Physical examination *(every 3 years, 20 to 40)*
Physical examination *(annually after 40)*

COLON-RECTAL CANCER
Digital rectal examination *(annually after 40)*
Stool blood slide test *(annually after 50)*
Proctosigmoidoscopy
  (annually for 2 years starting at 40)
Proctosigmoidoscopy
  (every 3 to 5 years after 2 normal exams)

UTERINE CANCER
Pap test *(annually for 3 years after 20)*
Pap test
  (at physician's discretion after 3 normal exams)

OVARIAN CANCER
Pelvic examination *(annually after 40)*

PROSTATE CANCER
Rectal examination *(annually after 40)*

HYPERTENSION
Blood pressure measurement *(at least every
  2½ years in persons with normal blood pressure)*

HEART DISEASE
Electrocardiogram
  (at 20, 40, and 60 in asymptomatic persons)
Plasma lipids *(every 5 years, 20 to 60)*
Cholesterol and triglycerides *(optimal after 60)*

LUNG CANCER
Baseline chest X ray *(at 40)*

DIABETES MELLITUS
Fasting glucose test *(every 5 years, 20 to 60)*
Fasting glucose test *(every 2½ years, 61 to 75)*

MEDICAL EXAMINATION
General exam *(every 5 years, 20 to 60)*
General exam *(every 2½ years, 61 to 75)*
General exam *(annually, after 75)*

NUTRITION AND VITAMINS

The foods we eat and the liquids we drink contain the building blocks for the construction and maintenance of a healthy body. Chapter 21, "Nutrition," explains the essentials of nutrition, such as what nutrients are present in what foods and how the body uses them. Here we will discuss the importance of nutrition in keeping healthy.

Healthy adults who eat a normal American diet almost invariably are well-nourished. That normal diet contains ample vitamins, making supplementary vitamins unnecessary. Obviously, there are special needs for infants and children, pregnant women and nursing mothers, and people who are ill. These require advice from a physician.

Basic nutrition. The appropriate amounts of proteins, carbohydrates, fats, vitamins, and trace elements, all in sufficient quantity, are present in any prudent diet. All these elements are needed, as Chapter 21 explains. Sometimes people who are misguided adopt diets that overemphasize one element or another. The Food and Nutrition Board of the National Research Council has concluded: "We are aware of no convincing evidence of unique health benefits accruing from consumption of a large excess of any one nutrient."

Any claims that excessive amounts of foods or vitamins will cure diseases are likely to be wrong, and should be looked at with skepticism.

Calories are the fuel that the machinery of the body needs to operate. If we take in too few calories we lose weight, and if we continue to do so, the result is illness and starvation. Consuming too many calories, on the other hand, produces obesity and may lead to disease. The balance is not difficult to maintain. Use of a simple bathroom scale is sufficient.

What ideal weight should we strive for? Guidelines published by the U.S. Department of Agriculture are shown in a chart in Chapter 21, "Nutrition," but they are only a rough measure. There is no need to seek compulsively to remain within these figures.

An average woman engaged in a normal amount of physical activity needs about 2,000 calories daily. Men, because they have larger frames, require about 2,700. This rough guide varies widely, depending on age and energy expenditure. Active, growing teenagers need more calories, and sedentary elderly people need fewer.

Proteins are the materials used by the body to form most of the molecules needed in biological activity. Growth and development of the individual, virtually all biological functions, and the basic structure of all cells require protein. The quality and amount of protein we eat, therefore, is of major importance. The bulk of protein in the American diet comes from meat, fish, eggs, milk, and milk products. Other food sources are certain fruits, nuts, beans, vegetables, and grains. At least one-third of daily protein intake should be derived from animal sources, including eggs and dairy products, although protein needs can be met by scrupulously following a careful vegetarian diet. Less than 15 percent of the calories in a proper diet should be protein.

Carbohydrates. Almost half of the calories in the typical American diet come from carbohydrates, found in grains and root vegetables. Sugar is a pure carbohydrate. By and large, carbohydrates are inexpensive, are easily digested, and serve as a major source of energy for all bodily activity. Potatoes, bread, pasta, and certain root vegetables are good examples. Many carbohydrates in the American diet, however, come from soft drinks, candy, and snack foods.

Fats contain basic materials essential to good health. They are found widely in the food chain and contribute about 35 percent of the calories in the diets of most Americans. Fats are stored in the body and serve as a reservoir to be drawn upon when needed. They are carriers of fat-soluble vitamins. They provide much of the taste and flavor in our foods, as well as improving its texture.

As discussed in Chapter 5, "The Heart and Circulation," cholesterol is a natural substance synthesized by the body but also is found in certain foods of animal origin, especially meats, shellfish, and egg yolks. It is essential for cell membranes and for the manufacture of certain hormones. But high levels of cholesterol in the blood are considered a risk factor for heart disease. Government-backed studies have shown that reducing cholesterol reduces the risk of heart attack. The exact relationship between dietary cholesterol and blood cholesterol is complex and controversial. The government has recommended that Americans cut back on eggs, cheese, and other sources of cholesterol, and couple this diet with exercise, which also appears to lower cholesterol. The body can synthesize all the cholesterol it needs, so the dietary change is not harmful.

For persons with elevated cholesterol, drug treatment, as explained in Chapter 5, "The Heart and Circulation," sometimes is recommended.

Because cholesterol and saturated fat often are found in food together, adult Americans are advised to restrict saturated (mostly animal) fat to 10 percent of calories and all fats to 30 percent.

Vitamins are naturally occurring chemical compounds that are necessary for proper functioning of the body. Quantities required are small and are obtained easily from the foods we eat. Only in peculiar conditions of illness, bizarre diets, or the special needs of infancy, childhood, pregnancy, and lactation are vitamin supplements required.

If vitamin pills and capsules are eaten by people on normal diets, the substances are simply wasted, excreted in the stool and urine. Indeed, certain vitamins taken in excess can cause physical symptoms and illness.

EXERCISE

Keeping your body fit pays off with increased vigor and appetite for life. We should value exercise for the pleasure it provides, the companionship it may offer, and the calories it can lose for us. Also, repeated studies have shown that persons who remain physically active have fewer illnesses and less time lost from work than those who do not. However, exercise in itself does not prolong life, and it may shorten life if we use bad judgment.

For people who are not in shape when the exercise program starts, the key element is a gradual increase in effort. The muscles, tendons, and joints of mature adults usually have lost some of youth's flexibility. Unless they are slowly brought into shape, injury can result from sudden use. Beyond this, sudden maximum effort by the untrained body places a strenuous demand on the heart. It may not be able to pump blood fast enough to meet the body's demands, or satisfy its own need for blood through the coronary arteries.

Good judgment dictates a graduated exercise program. Walking and swimming are excellent forms of exercise to start with, and safe (assuming you know how to swim). Pace and time should be slowly increased to the point of maximum satisfaction. Roughly an hour of vigorous activity a day for average adults is a reasonable goal.

Exercise is beneficial for all body components. The heart and lungs are stimulated by a properly planned program to function at a more efficient level. Muscles, joints, and even bones become stronger.

It is important to note that physical activity need not consist of an organized exercise program. Simple chores like gardening or housework also contribute to physical activity. The key point is to avoid a sedentary life-style.

As other chapters in this book explain, exercise also plays a role in countering the effects of many illnesses. Arthritis patients, for instance, are encouraged to exercise to prevent disability.

REST AND SLEEP

No one knows how much sleep the human body requires. Elaborate experiments have shown that, removed from the stimulus of the clock or the sun, people still sleep about eight hours out of 24. But whether this amount is learned behavior or biologically dictated is not known.

We do know that regular amounts of restful sleep are as important for good health as food and exercise. Experiments also have shown that when people are kept awake for long periods, they lose their capacity to perform simple tasks. We all know from experience that we do not think as clearly when sleepy. We also know that chronically fatigued people are more vulnerable to illness. The body-building mechanisms of sleep may be related to the levels of certain chemicals and hormones, which have been demonstrated to vary with the clock.

Adequate rest is obviously important in maintaining normal health. Persistent attempts to work excessive hours are self-defeating. An exhausted mind and a tired body cannot carry out first-quality tasks.

STRESS AND EMOTIONS

Psychological stability is essential to health. We put ourselves at risk when we place excessive emotional stress upon ourselves. Although it is true that we achieve nothing in life unless we make rigorous demands on our abilities and use our skills and experience fully, it is equally true that there are limits to the pressures we can tolerate.

Preventing psychological breakdown requires a realistic assessment of our abilities and the nature of the tasks we face. To maintain equilibrium demands that each of us have a good level of self-understanding and the willingness to seek professional counseling when we need it.

Forging and maintaining healthy relationships is an important part of emotional health. This includes relationships with coworkers, neighbors, schoolmates and relatives and family. A network of relationships is particularly important for the health of older people. Isolated elders have more illnesses, and they die sooner.

SMOKING, DRUGS, AND ALCOHOL

Although the term "drug abuse" has been part of our everyday language, the more accurate term is "substance abuse."

Smoking

Cigarette smoking is hazardous. Evidence of the hazards continues to grow.

● Cigarette smokers have substantially higher rates of death and disability than their nonsmoking counterparts. They die earlier and have more days of disability than comparable nonsmokers.

● A substantial number of early deaths and excess disability cases would not have occurred if those affected had never smoked.

● Pregnant women who smoke give birth to babies of low birth weight.

The most common type of lung cancer occurs most frequently in cigarette smokers. Cigarette smoking, indeed, is almost wholly responsible for the increase in the incidence of lung cancer, especially among young women. Emphysema and chronic bronchitis, two forms of potentially disabling lung disease, are clearly made worse by smoking. Coronary disease also is associated with cigarette smoking. One theory is that the carbon monoxide that enters the bloodstream and heart damages the heart muscle and coronary arteries.

Pipe or cigar smokers face lesser risks, according to careful studies. Pipe smokers face a small increased incidence of cancer of the mouth and throat. However, there are definite risks of oral cancer by users of smokeless tobacco (snuff).

Effects on others. Smokers also harm those around them. Careful studies have shown higher incidence of respiratory illness, including bronchogenic cancer, among families of smokers. "Passive smoking" also causes eye and throat irritation to others. Thus, airlines have sharply restricted smoking in flight, and many restaurants, office buildings, and other public places have established "no smoking" areas. Nonsmokers who are ill with heart or lung disease can be made sicker by inhaling smoke-filled air.

Stopping Smoking

The decision to stop smoking is a tough challenge for any confirmed smoker, and fully deserves support. Fortunately, many community agencies now offer "smoke-outs" and "smoke-ender" programs that help smokers to quit. These usually can be found in local newspapers or the Yellow Pages. Hospitals and health maintenance organizations offer help, too. The health benefits of quitting are vast. Within five years, the former smoker's risks of cancer or heart disease are the same as if he or she had never smoked. These benefits occur even if the person has been a heavy smoker for many years. Many smokers gain weight after quitting, however, and must be on guard against the health hazard of obesity.

The Use of Drugs

Drugs that alter mood have been taken since man has been able to put hand to mouth. Because the human capacity for self-delusion about the value and safety of drugs is so widespread, and because with money and determination people can obtain whatever they wish, we must assume that drug abuse will remain a problem in our society.

What is abuse? Drug abuse is nonmedical use of drugs for the purpose of altering the user's mood, producing novel experiences, or changing the user's perception of himself or herself and the world. Generally, drugs are sought for their effect on the psyche. Physical effects also may occur, however. These range from virtually unnoticeable increases in heart rate and blood pressure after taking stimulants to extreme changes in the consciousness level—and perhaps death—from overdose of depressants.

Classification of Drugs

One way to classify drugs is by their major effect, although there are numerous areas of overlap. The confusion is magnified when people take several drugs simultaneously.

Narcotics relieve pain, but can be abused for the highly pleasurable sensation. Taking any narcotic carries the risk of addiction. Addiction means that withdrawal from the drug (stopping its use) produces discomfort and sometimes an uncontrollable compulsion to take more. Drugs such as morphine, Demerol, and codeine are of great value for their painkilling effects, but of great risk when abused. Opium and heroin originally were used for pain, but now their use is entirely illegal.

Methadone is supplied legally to heroin addicts in organized programs designed to wean them away from the more hazardous drug. The results vary, but one unfortunate consequence has been the appearance of methadone on the illegal market. Another legitimate use of methadone, when mixed with other approved drugs, is the control of certain kinds of pain in cancer patients.

Sedatives. Substances used to depress brain function include barbiturates and other sleep inducers, tranquilizers, inhalants such as gasoline and glue, and alcohol, discussed at length elsewhere in this chapter.

This diverse group has important elements in common:
- Addiction potential.
- Withdrawal symptoms physically more dangerous than those associated with narcotics.
- Production of calmness followed by sleep, and by death from failure to breathe when taken in excessive amounts.
- Increased hazard when mixed, especially the combination of alcohol and other sedatives. The effect of each is multiplied significantly, and can be life-threatening.

Some of these drugs are taken for their initial excitatory effect. Sniffing glue, for instance, produces a brief jag, but then somnolence. Alcohol, although it loosens inhibitions, also depresses bodily functions.

Tranquilizers (benzodiazepines) are among the leading prescription drugs and include chlordiazepoxide (Librium) and diazepam (Valium). But they also are among the most abused. Prescribed for their calming effect, they can create marked physical dependency with long-term, high-dose use. Abrupt withdrawal can even cause convulsive seizures. Tranquilizers are extremely valuable substances, but they should be used with caution.

Stimulants. Amphetamines and cocaine once were in vogue for treatment of physical disorders. Cocaine was used as a local anesthetic in the care of eye diseases, and amphetamines were used to suppress appetite in obese people. When abused, a common effect is a rapid onset of euphoria and grandiose thinking. The immediate danger is a potential for aggressive, violent behavior.

Amphetamines still are available by prescription, for specific medical purposes, but cocaine is illegal in all states and most other nations. In its powder form, for inhaling, and as "crack," which can be smoked, its use has become widespread. Long-term effects of its use, including damage to the respiratory system, can be devastating.

Hallucinogens. A vast number of substances cause hallucinations. These include marijuana and similar drugs, LSD, and a group of abused substances with names that shift and change as fads come and go.

Marijuana causes feelings of relaxation and ease, similar to alcohol intoxication. Emotions are enhanced and all seems more profound.

Carefully controlled scientific studies have shown that heavy smoking of marijuana distorts perceptions and interferes moderately with fine hand coordination. It apparently hampers immediate memory and intellectual function, and decreases levels of male sex hormone. The question of damage to future children of users remains unclear. It is certain that use of marijuana by pregnant women poses a risk to the fetus.

Treatment of Drug Abuse

Certain early warning signs can alert parents or friends to drug use.

(1) Physical evidence of drug availability. The individual may almost deliberately leave drugs around the house or in his or her room, clothes, or school locker, perhaps unconsciously wanting to be discovered.

(2) Specific signs of particular drugs are easily recognizable if one is able to accept the fact that one's child, friend, or companion is using drugs.

● *Alcohol:* odor on the breath, or the inappropriate use of breath mints or candy, garrulous talking, loud speech, excited and then sedated behavior, oversleeping in the morning.

● *Marijuana:* the distinctive odor after smoking, the presence of fragments of dried leaves in the clothing, giggling, bloodshot eyes, skipping from subject to subject when talking.

● *Amphetamine:* excitation, hyperactivity, depression, inappropriate fits of temper, difficulty concentrating, belligerent attitude.

● *Barbiturates and other hypnotic-sedative:* excitation, users are unsteady on their feet, clumsy, and appear to have ingested alcohol.

● *Cocaine:* produces excitability, hyperactivity, and aggressiveness, but these indications may wear off quickly and not be discernible to others.

(3) It should be general policy to discuss from time to time the use of drugs with children by gently probing about drug use among their friends, classmates, and other children in the neighborhood. The child or teenager who talks very much about drugs, or not at all about drug use, and is embarrassed or expresses an overly vigorous denial when asked about personal experimentation with drugs, is highly suspect.

(4) Poor school performance, especially inability to get assignments done on time, sloppy work, deterioration in handwriting, tardiness, and unexplained absences.

(5) A general lack of motivation and withdrawal from academic and extracurricular activities, particularly by an individual who previously has engaged in them.

(6) The individual who is frequently out of the house, particularly when his or her friends are members of the community suspected of drug use.

(7) A deterioration in appearance, unkempt and untidy clothing, and generally poor personal hygiene.

(8) A new group of friends unknown to parents or withdrawal from old friendships.

Drug abuse can be hidden easily and the possibility of drug use should not be dismissed because of a lack of signs.

LSD causes a marked change in the user's sense of the surrounding world. The user experiences feelings of unreality and other delusions. Poor judgment follows.

The common psychosis of LSD use, with delusions, usually lasts up to 48 hours. It abates spontaneously, but occasionally an episode can last for weeks. More severe episodes of psychosis with homicidal or suicidal behavior have occurred rarely.

The most well-known hazard is the so-called "bad trip," manifested by uncontrollable fear and panic, with a belief that insanity is impending.

Other drugs used for hallucinogenic effects include several chemical structures known by their initials (DMT, DET, DOM). Others are peyote and mescaline, obtained from cactus, and medications such as atropine and scopolamine, which in proper dosage can be taken safely for clinical purposes, but are abused for their side effects.

Beyond the ability to cause hallucinations, all these substances accelerate the heart rate, increase blood pressure, and diminish appetite.

Complications of injection. Beyond the physical and psychological effects, specific diseases and health problems may result from the injection of drugs. Puncturing the skin may allow bacteria to enter the body. Because drug users do not always observe sterile technique, infection is commonplace. The consequences range in severity from abscess formation, which is painful but treatable, to potentially fatal diseases such as tetanus and bacterial endocarditis (inflammation of the lining of the heart). The most widely publicized of these is acquired immune deficiency syndrome (AIDS), which is most commonly contracted when infected intravenous drug users exchange needles, as explained in Chapter 32, "Infectious Disease."

Certain forms of hepatitis, a virus disease of the liver, also are transmitted by shared needles or syringes.

In addition, veins used as injection sites may become inflamed and allow clotted blood to deposit. Clots can break off as solid matter (emboli), flow through the bloodstream into the heart, and plug a blood vessel in the lung. Obviously, this can be life-threatening.

Alcohol

Drinking of alcohol is a common social custom in the Western world, including the United States. Drinking has long been associated with festive occasions. When misused, however, alcohol can produce personal and social consequences of grave import. We all realize the potential damage of alcohol abuse, but often we fail to grapple effectively with this issue in our lives. It is vital that we each preserve for ourselves full opportunity to make intelligent and educated choices about the use of alcohol.

Who is an alcoholic? Is excessive drinking a disease or is it the result of a moral defect? This remains a hotly debated issue. In any case, we must define the term "alcoholism" before we can obtain a genuine understanding of the problem, which may lead to treatment and cure.

Anyone who repeatedly drinks alcoholic beverages to the point of loss of control is an alcoholic. This definition covers a wide range of people, including skid-row derelicts, housewives, blue collar workers, executives, and elected officials. It may well include friends, family members, and you.

There appears to be a genetic component to alcoholism. Epidemiologic studies indicate that Irish and Swedish males, whether they reside in their native country or emigrate to the United States, have the highest rates of alcoholism. Animal studies also show that certain strains have a preference for alcohol-containing solutions, indicating alcoholism may have a genetic, biochemically determined basis.

How many alcoholics? About 7 percent of the people in the U.S. are considered problem drinkers, and some 100,000 people die in this country yearly from alcohol-related causes.

There are roughly 10 million adult Americans with a drinking problem, including about 2 million women. The adolescents who drink too much number several million and their numbers are said to be increasing.

Consequences of Drinking

The abuse of alcohol and other drugs appears closely related to stress levels in our society. Drinking, in turn, leads to many problems. The most apparent are disease, injuries, suicides, and violence to others, including murder.

Injury. Because drinking causes loss of judgment, people injure themselves more easily when drunk than sober. This is a major issue in industry, and applies particularly to drivers. The toll of injury and death from automobile accidents has become so high that many states have cracked down on drinking drivers, who are believed to account for well over half of all automobile fatalities. Community agencies have set up "dial-a-ride" services for such occasions as New Year's Eve, and have urged partygoers to choose a "designated driver" who will remain sober and shuttle others home. In addition, agencies have campaigned for stricter control of alcohol advertising.

Suicide. There is a high suicide rate among alcoholics compared to the general population. The reasons are unclear, but either depression leads to drinking and ends in self-destruction, or alcoholism itself creates suicidal wishes.

Violence to others. Investigation of people who commit major criminal acts against others shows a high incidence of alcoholism. Murder, assault, rape, and child beating in significant proportions are included. The loss of personal control caused by drinking is in part responsible.

Level of Alcohol Use And Risks to Fetus

"Regular" Social Drinking
(2 or more drinks daily)

 Intrauterine growth retardation
 Increased risk of birth defects
 Behavioral effects in the
  newborn and infant
 Increased risk of stillbirth
 Decreased placental weight

"Binge" Drinking
(5 or more drinks on occasion)

 Structural brain abnormalities

Very Heavy Drinking
(a quart of alcohol daily)

 Fetal alcohol syndrome

Disease. Alcohol can damage major organs. The liver is a key target. Alcohol can cause fatty changes that enlarge the liver, sometimes leading to scarring of the organ. This condition is called cirrhosis and can result in jaundice, bleeding, and death (see Chapter 8, "The Digestive System").

Heart disease is also a major consequence of alcoholism. A poisoning effect takes place in the heart muscle, resulting in disordered heart action. A different and more common cardiac problem, coronary artery disease, also is more frequent among alcoholics.

Cancer occurs more commonly among heavy drinkers than in the general population. Malignancies of the esophagus, stomach, liver, and lungs increase. Alcohol also can damage the brain. Loss of memory and ability to concentrate is common among alcoholics.

Drinking in pregnancy. Ingestion of alcohol by a pregnant woman causes a measurable risk to the fetus. The full-blown fetal alcohol syndrome causes poor growth of the fetus and the newborn. Abnormalities of head and face structure, joint, limb, and heart abnormalities, and mental deficiency are part of the picture. This syndrome has caused some states to require warning posters where alcohol is sold.

Drinking presents a danger to the pregnant woman, too. The combination of a few drinks and the swaybacked posture of pregnancy may make her unsteady, leading to the possibility of a dangerous fall. However, it now appears that concerns about dangers to infants as a result of drinking by nursing mothers have been exaggerated.

Treatment of Alcohol Problems

Help is available for the treatment of alcoholism. The prerequisite is motivation on the part of the alcoholic to stop drinking.

Hospitals and clinics. A growing number of hospitals, clinics, and freestanding services now offer alcoholism recovery programs. These institutions operate on an inpatient basis. During an extended period of residence, the alcoholic patient is provided a combination of group therapy, counseling, physical and medical care, and dietary assistance. Many of these programs are provided by corporations and other employers for their employees. The cost may be underwritten by health insurance. In addition, many hospitals now have established services to diagnose and treat alcoholics while they are being treated for other medical problems.

Professional counseling. Psychologists, psychiatrists, pastors, and other professionally trained therapists may be an asset to alcoholics. This is likely when drinking is a result of personal strain that can be relieved by counseling. The counseling process may include family members.

Federal and state programs. Through the Veterans Administration (VA) and state mental hospitals, thousands of people with drinking problems receive help each year. At the VA, eligible veterans get treatment for acute episodes of drinking and long-term follow-up counseling, both without charge. At the state hospital level, the bulk of care is simple confinement, but some institutions provide group therapy and educational resources.

Alcoholics Anonymous (AA) is the single most effective alcoholism recovery program in terms of numbers of people who have been helped to stop drinking. AA defines itself as a "worldwide fellowship of men and women who help each other maintain sobriety and who offer to share their recovery experience freely with others who may have a drinking problem."

Who Is an Alcoholic?

Identifying who is an alcoholic and who is a social drinker remains controversial because of overlap in the behaviors and because of the derogatory implications of the word "alcoholic." Society still is debating whether alcoholism is a medical illness, social disease, or moral handicap. The National Council on Alcoholism has developed extensive, precise criteria to establish the diagnosis of alcoholism. In brief, the major criteria include:

- Physiological dependency as demonstrated by evidence of a withdrawal syndrome—tremors, hallucinations, seizures, or delirium tremens (DTs).
- Evidence of tolerance for the effects of alcohol. One example is a blood alcohol concentration of more than 150 milligrams per deciliter without gross evidence of intoxication. Another is the daily consumption of a fifth of a gallon of whiskey or the equivalent amount of wine or beer.
- Medical findings indicating a major alcohol-associated illness.
- Drinking despite strong medical and social recommendations, or the patient's own recognition of loss of control over alcohol consumption.

Of great importance is the recognition of early signs of alcoholism: gulping drinks; surreptitious drinking; early morning drinking; medical absences from work for a variety of reasons; shifting from one alcoholic beverage to another; preference for drinking companions, bars, and taverns; a loss of interest in activities not directly associated with drinking; drinking more than the peer group; unexplained changes in family, social, and business relationships; complaints about spouse, job, and friends; major family disruptions; loss or frequent change of jobs; and financial difficulties.

YOUR PHYSICIAN

As part of a sound health program, it is important to have a physician or established health service that knows you and your situation. Although medical care can be obtained on a walk-in basis, having a regular physician can achieve these goals:
- A coordinated program of patient and family education on how to stay healthy and fit.
- Application of preventive medical techniques, including immunizations and regular examination according to the schedules listed in specialty chapters in this book.
- Maintenance of ongoing health history and medical records in one place.
- Family counseling.
- Regular physical assessment.
- Availability during acute illness.
- Treatment as needed.

Finding a doctor. We all want a physician who is both competent and responsive. Word of mouth from trustworthy friends and relatives is a likely basis for referral. Another useful source of information is the local hospital or medical society. Health insurance programs often provide lists of recommended physicians, including specialists.

Health maintenance organizations (HMOs) make it an objective to keep people healthy and treat them when sick. Hospital outpatient departments serve the needs of many people.

When to see the doctor. Routine visits to the physician's office should be planned to meet the age and health status of each person. Pregnant women, for instance, and healthy infants require regular appointments for assessment.

During childhood, adolescence, and adulthood, when most people are healthy, a base-touching visit to the doctor should be scheduled on a regular basis, with contact frequent enough to allow doctor and patient to know each other.

When to seek medical help. Minor symptoms, such as those of the common cold, should not require a doctor. On the other hand, if the patient already is chronically ill, new symptoms should be viewed with concern.

Some parts of the body are especially vulnerable. A quick call to the doctor is important after a head injury, eye damage, or other accidents. As described in Chapter 35, "Emergency," many communities have a paramedical service to handle emergency cases. A doctor or paramedical service also should be called for chest pain, which may indicate a heart attack, and for marked shortness of breath.

The general rule: When in doubt, call. If no paramedical service is available in your community, a hospital emergency room or walk-in clinic should be sought.

The value of asking questions. The basic knowledge of the human body, through standard educational opportunities, is available to all of us. However, when more complex issues arise, such as those related to fertility, pregnancy, lactation, care of infant and child, or diagnosis and treatment of disease, asking questions of your doctor is the key to understanding.

Common areas of confusion concern diet, medications, and preparations for medical tests. Unless you understand the instructions, everybody's effort is wasted, and prospects for good health are diminished. Don't hesitate to ask, and be certain that you understand what you are told.

Patient rights and responsibilities. You have a right to understand every aspect of treatment and diagnosis, in order to care for yourself properly. Your doctor should cooperate happily with you in providing such information. Most doctors prefer working with well-informed patients because the likelihood of successful treatment is enhanced. Statements of patients' rights are provided by many hospitals and supported by insurance programs, which often insist that a second opinion be provided before a procedure is undertaken.

Be open and frank with your doctor. If medications and treatment are prescribed, if advice about health habits is offered, it is useless to pretend that you will cooperate if you have no such intention. Medical care is of value only if you carry out your part intelligently and consistently.

It also is your responsibility to avoid obvious risks to health. You have yourself to blame, for instance, if you are injured in an automobile accident while not wearing a seat belt. Similar obvious tasks include safetyproofing the house if infants or young children are present. Stairs should be protected by gates, medication enclosed in proper containers, cleaning materials and other potentially poisonous substances kept out of reach of children. Safetyproofing tips are provided in Chapter 35, "Emergency."

Monitoring your own health. An annual physical examination is expensive and seldom necessary. However, you should have certain tests at regular intervals, such as the Pap smear for uterine cancer in women. A recommended schedule of checkups by the American Cancer Society and American Heart Association is included in this chapter. Recommendations for other tests are included in individual chapters.

Immunizations for children (and in some cases, for adults) are important. A schedule recommended by the American Academy of Pediatrics is included in Chapter 29, "Taking Care of Your Child."

Self-tests are simple and readily available. Blood pressure, for instance, may be measured at home (or, often in shopping centers or at health fairs). An important measure of health is a simple bathroom scale, which may disclose weight gain leading to obesity, or weight loss that could reveal undiagnosed illness.

Finally, every home should be equipped with first-aid supplies, as identified in Chapter 35, "Emergency."

MEDICATIONS

Prescription and nonprescription drugs have great potential for both good and harm. The instructions of the prescribing physician should be understood and followed with care. By all means, ask questions if you are uncertain about any aspect of drug treatment.

Side effects and drug allergies. Make sure that your doctor knows your history of problems with medications, including allergic reactions, before prescriptions are written. It is sensible to carry with you a record of allergies and other side effects from previous treatments. When seeing a new doctor, one of the first points is to enter this information on your new medical record. This is the best way to avoid inadvertent use of medicines that are wrong for you.

Medication control. Medicine containers should be labeled clearly with the name of the drug, the patient, the doctor, the dosage, and the frequency. This information may be useful if questions arise later.

Drugs can become outdated, so ask the pharmacist to date the label if he or she does not automatically do so.

Drug interactions. When a person is taking more than one prescription or nonprescription drug (sometimes prescribed unknowingly by different doctors), the possibility exists that the drugs will cancel each other, or, equally seriously, interact with potentially harmful effects. This is a particular problem in older persons, who take up or excrete drugs more slowly. You should always inform a physician of all drugs you are taking, including those for other conditions.

Safety precautions. When people take more than one medication, the possibility of error exists. If a patient has poor vision or is mentally confused by illness, even greater potential for harm arises. Drug containers should have large, easy-to-read labels, or color coding. It may help to place daily doses in separate glasses or receptacles and use check-off lists. If necessary, medication should be taken under supervision.

Sleeping pills, sedatives, and tranquilizers. The tendency to feel that there is a pill to solve every problem has led many of us to depend on sedatives, tranquilizers, and similar drugs. Our bodies and minds are structured to survive the stress of daily life without the use of chemicals. In an important sense, the use of drugs that obliterate our direct connection with reality is a weak way of avoiding important issues. Problems are not solved, merely avoided temporarily.

These drugs can be dangerous. Dependency, even addiction, may occur. Overdoses may cause death, particularly if taken with alcohol, when even small amounts can be fatal.

Under ordinary circumstances these drugs should be avoided, and certainly never used without a physician's advice. Under unusual and temporary circumstances, or during illness, there may be a reason for them. Basically, it pays to remember that nature is on your side. You can solve the problem, you can sleep, and you can do so without being drugged.

HOSPITALIZATION
AND HEALTH INSURANCE

Hospital and health insurance is a rapidly changing field, but being prepared for the financial costs of illness is an important part of a preventive approach to health. This is particularly true at a time of escalating hospital and medical costs. Still, many persons are without insurance because they cannot afford it or through sheer neglect.

Although many health insurance plans are wholly or partly financed by employers, often a choice of plans is available. Health maintenance organizations (HMOs) take full responsibility for keeping insured persons well, in addition to treating them if they become ill. Other plans require that you use the services of specified doctors or hospitals, in return for a lower premium. A program also may specify that you pay a portion of your bill, or specify a deductible amount per patient or family. It is important to tailor your coverage to your own needs.

Medicare. This is federally funded comprehensive health insurance under the sponsorship of the social security system. It is available to almost all people over the age of 65, and to persons totally and permanently disabled. Part A of Medicare covers the hospital costs of a semiprivate room. Part B covers physicians' fees and has some other benefits. Be certain to obtain both parts when you apply. Medicare clients pay a monthly premium and for their first day's hospitalization.

Medicaid. This form of health insurance, sponsored by most states, is available to people whose income places them below established levels, which may vary among states. Most people eligible for welfare benefits also may obtain Medicaid coverage. Check with your local welfare office.

General rules. Obtain copies of your insurance papers and read them carefully. Understand the benefits you are entitled to; be aware of the exclusions and of the deductible provisions that may apply. If in doubt, ask questions. After you become ill, it is too late to make changes.

CHAPTER 2

TESTS AND PROCEDURES

This past half-century has seen remarkable progress in prevention and treatment of human disease, and in our knowledge of what causes many diseases. Part of this success has been due to technical advances. Diagnostics, that part of medicine devoted to the uncovering and identifying of disease, has been an essential part of the progress. Doctors say, "Diagnosis is part of treatment." When therapies were few, and often ineffective, diagnosis was largely an intellectual exercise for the physician. Today, the physician's insights are backed up by increasingly sophisticated equipment, tests, and procedures that have greatly increased the amount of information on which a diagnosis can be built. The application of basic principles of physics, utilizing sound waves, X rays, fiber optics and lasers, radiation from radioactive materials, and more recently, high-energy magnetic fields, has created the means for vastly enhancing diagnostic accuracy. And the more accurate the diagnosis, the more effective the treatment.

Two examples of these new tools are familiar. The computer has enormously enhanced the reach of some diagnostic techniques. The miniaturized television camera enables us to look into confined areas and project the image for many persons to see—and even to videotape for further consultation and review. Many diagnostic techniques have been further developed to provide means of treatment. The therapeutic applications of X rays, radioactive emissions, lasers, and ultrasound now are firmly established.

Some of these methods and machines are applied to special organs or systems. Measuring blood pressure or the electrical activity associated with the beating of the heart (electrocardiograph), or the capacity of the lungs to exchange oxygen and carbon dioxide, is done using equipment designed for studying that one system or organ.

By contrast, many diagnostic techniques utilize X rays and other forms of radiation, supersonic sound, lasers, and fiber optics in ways that are applicable to many or all organs or systems.

DIAGNOSTIC PROCEDURES

Biopsy

Examination of pieces of tissue taken from the skin, gastrointestinal tract, or internal organs as deep seated as the bone marrow, liver, pancreas, and brain provides an important means of diagnosing disease. Sampling tissue is termed biopsy, meaning literally "viewing life," and is done by a number of different "invasive" methods. The simplest biopsy uses a scalpel, surgical scissors, or circular punches to cut out a small piece of skin, which then is put in a fixative to prevent changes, and processed in a surgical pathology department. Very thin slices are mounted on glass slides and examined under a microscope. This technique often is used to diagnose possible cancers of the skin as well as the breast, but also may be used to diagnose rashes and other lesions.

Specifically designed, long, hollow needles are used to take very small cores of tissue from internal organs such as the liver or kidney. Because these organs are large and their positions relatively fixed, the technique is simple. A preliminary anesthetic is injected, and the needle is introduced through the skin. There is little discomfort because the deeper structures are not supplied by nerves that sense pain. Very thin needles reduce the risk of damage to blood vessels or other structures.

If the target organ is small, or if tissue is required from a specific area of the liver, the biopsy needle is guided by special X-ray or ultrasound imaging. Biopsies of the gastrointestinal tract and the bronchial tree of the lungs are obtained by passing a flexible, lighted tube called an endoscope, which can be fitted with tiny forceps to obtain the needed tissue. Brain biopsies, used to diagnose Alzheimer's disease, for instance, are done by neurosurgeons through access holes drilled in the skull.

Fiber-Optic Instruments

Until the mid-1960s, looking into organs such as the stomach, large bowel, lungs, and bladder could be done only by using rigid tubes. Great ingenuity was applied to their design, using systems of magnifying lenses and special lights and mirrors to provide a clear view of structures at the end of the tube. Flexibility, essential in traversing winding or angled natural passages such as those in the intestine, was limited by a fundamental property of light; it needs mirrors to go around corners.

Fiber optics, using strands of glass so fine that they are highly flexible, has revolutionized this field. These pencil-thin devices use an inner circular core of glass of low optical density surrounded by a sheath of glass of higher optical density. Light traveling along the inner core in either direction becomes trapped, as if it were being reflected inward by a continuous mirror. Using bundles of fibers, it is possible to build instruments of different lengths and diameters, and of remarkable flexibility. High-intensity light passes down the fiber bundle, and the cavity then can be observed through an eyepiece or its image projected on a television screen. Hand controls move wires in the outer sheaths of the endoscope, and make it possible to change the direction of the tips of the instrument as much as 180 degrees.

Endoscopes can readily be passed into the esophagus, stomach, and duodenum, using local anesthesia in the patient's throat. The colon, and even the small intestine, can be examined by similar instruments via the rectum. Suitably modified endoscopes can be introduced into the trachea and bronchi of the lungs, the urinary bladder, and the peritoneal cavity, and through blood vessels, even

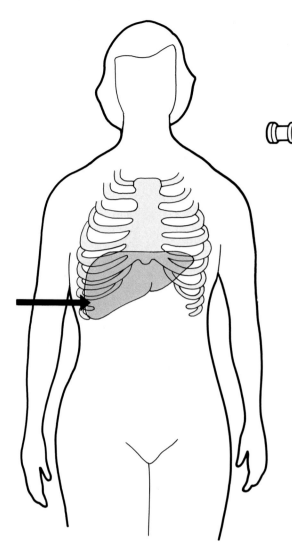

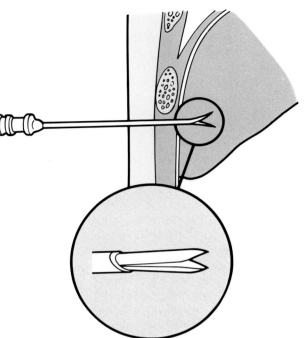

LIVER BIOPSY
Tissue obtained directly from the liver for examination under a microscope can give important information about some forms of liver disease. The left drawing shows that the liver is accessible through the space between the ribs. In the drawing above, a special needle has been inserted into the liver tissue. The needle's forcepslike tip can grasp a small piece of tissue and withdraw it through the hollow handle.

into the interior of the heart. Thus, the surfaces of virtually every hollow organ of the body can be seen with the eye. Moreover, the endoscope can be fitted with small cutting forceps to obtain tissue, or with wire snares or cauterizing devices to remove growths. These techniques have eliminated abdominal surgery for thousands of persons with stomach lesions or polyps of the colon, some of which might otherwise have become cancerous.

Bleeding ulcers of the stomach and duodenum, or bleeding from tiny vessels on the surface of the colon, also can be treated by an endoscopic method. A device called a thermocoagulator is passed through the endoscope to the site of bleeding and an intense, very localized electric current is used to seal off the vessels and halt the flow.

Fiber-optic channels also are ideal for transmitting laser beams, with their intense heat. In fact, laser technology would have been a nonstarter in medicine without fiber optics. It is possible to apply laser energy to superficial layers, without damage to underlying ones—another means of arresting bleeding.

Fiber-optic endoscopy also is used in a different way to treat varices of the esophagus, which resemble varicose veins in the legs and occur in patients with advanced cirrhosis of the liver. Varices pose a serious threat to life because of their tendency to bleed without warning. By injecting a

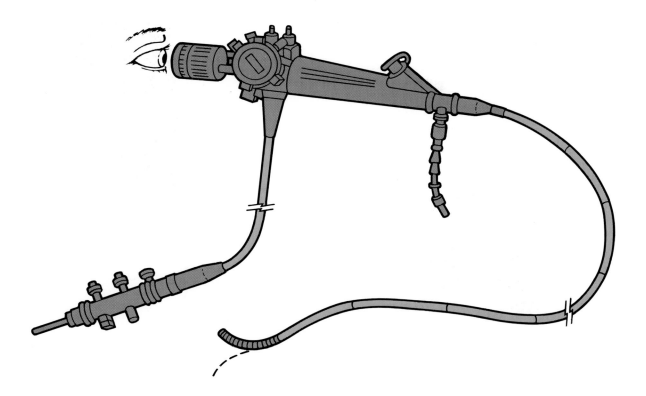

SEEING THE INSIDE
Fiber-optic scopes, which allow light to bend around corners, are used by many specialists to examine organs of the body otherwise hidden from sight. Above, the eyepiece can be moved, refocused, or magnified using the control handle below. The flexible tip can be moved 180 degrees to permit close scrutiny of interior surfaces. It also can be fitted with cutting blades, lasers, or other devices to permit retrieval of tissue, halt hemorrhaging, or cut away growths.

clotting solution via a cannula fitted into the endoscope, bleeding can be stopped and the risk of subsequent bleeding episodes reduced.

Diagnostic X Rays

One of the most valuable and widely used diagnostic tools in medicine also has the longest history and record of achievement. Wilhelm Roentgen, a professor of physics at the University of Wurzburg, in Germany, discovered X rays in 1895 while passing electric currents through sealed glass tubes from which most of the air had been evacuated. X rays are streams of electrons, which if sufficiently energetic, will pass through solids.

They are part of the spectrum of electromagnetic radiation, to which radio waves, heat, infrared, visible light, and ultraviolet rays also belong. The medical application requires a source of X rays and a surface sensitive to X rays on the opposite side of the body. Rays are directly focused on the body part to be examined, to avoid radiation of surrounding tissues or overexposure of radiologists or technicians.

The sensitive surface, or fluoroscopic screen, is very similar to a television screen. It is coated with chemicals that emit visible light when exposed to X rays, converting very short wavelength rays to longer wavelength visible light. Alternatively, a photographic film can be used, or X-ray motion pictures taken. The radiologist can even record important parts of the examination on videotape for playback.

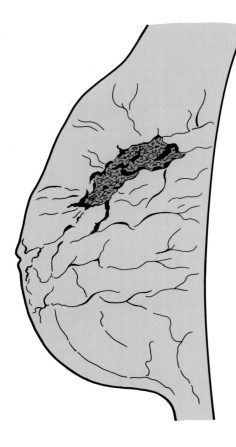
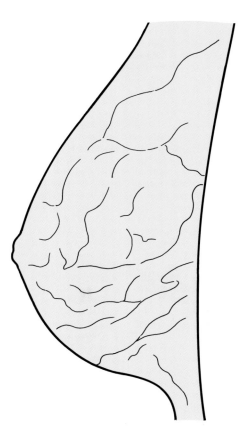

A WOMAN'S BEST FRIEND
Mammography, a highly sophisticated form of X ray, can detect early breast abnormalities too small to be felt even by a trained specialist. The drawing above right shows the structure of a normal breast; the dark shadow in the drawing above left discloses intraductal growth. Although the abnormality above is large, those as small as 1 millimeter in diameter can be found, making early treatment possible.

Although many persons are understandably concerned about the hazards of radiation exposure, modern equipment (especially the use of proper shielding) and increased sensitivity of fluoroscopy screens and films have markedly reduced the doses of radiation received during an examination. In general, exposure in a standard examination is less than that to which we are constantly exposed from natural sources.

However, it is important to avoid or minimize irradiation of the male or female reproductive organs, so that irreversible genetic damage is not caused; and to be careful during pregnancy because radiation may cause damage to the unborn child. For these reasons, gonads are shielded, usually by use of a lead apron, and no X rays are taken of women of childbearing age if there is any possibility of an early pregnancy.

X rays penetrate the tissues of the body to different degrees. Bones, containing minerals such as calcium, are the least penetrable; soft tissues and air-containing cavities, such as the lungs, are the most penetrable. These differences make it possible to picture bone fractures or the condition of the teeth, changes in the lungs, the size or shape of the

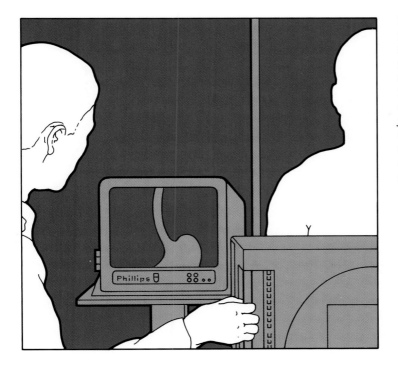

UPPER GI SERIES
To inspect the digestive system, the radiologist relies on a contrast material that will absorb X rays, creating an image of the organs it passes through. The patient swallows barium while the doctor watches the progress by using a fluoroscope. The upper GI series allows the doctor to observe the structure of the affected organs and how they work. It often is used in patients suspected of having an ulcer or a tumor.

heart, or the presence or absence of gas in the intestine, for instance. Comparisons of X rays at different times can detect change, or in the case of fractures, help to monitor healing.

Mammography, the standard X-ray examination of female breasts, has been shown to be the most effective way of diagnosing breast cancer. Several X rays are taken of each breast, with the breast gently flattened against the photographic plate. Small tumors or cysts, which cannot be felt by the hand, may be revealed; mammography is so sensitive that more than 90 percent of such tumors are detectable. The American Cancer Society recommends one baseline mammogram for women between 35 and 40 years of age, every other year for those between 40 and 50 years of age, and once a year for those over 50 years of age.

Contrast media. The ability of X rays to provide information is greatly increased by the use of chemicals that do not transmit X rays; they are said to be X-ray opaque. In the gastrointestinal tract, barium sulfate is the chemical most often used. Barium is an insoluble heavy metal that is virtually impervious to X rays. When suspended in resins, barium can be consumed in a liquid form and followed by X ray as it passes through the gastrointestinal tract. The resulting visualization or film can provide important information about the contours of the surface of the esophagus, stomach, duodenum, and small bowel, or the functioning of these organs. Barium also can be injected by a catheter into the large bowel via the rectum (barium enema) for inspection of large bowel function and frequently the last part of the small bowel.

Iodine-containing dyes also are X-ray opaque. They can be injected into blood vessels to outline their walls, a technique called angiography, or into the cavities of the heart. This technique is extremely important in the diagnosis of coronary artery disease, especially in locating arterial blockage, and is described in detail in Chapter 5, "The Heart and Circulation." Some of these dyes have special properties, so that when injected into the blood, or ingested and absorbed, they are concentrated in the bile formed by the liver, and stored in the gall bladder. This allows X rays of the gall bladder and bile ducts, and may provide evidence of the presence of gallstones, tumors, or narrowed segments that can obstruct normal bile flow. Some iodine-containing dyes are concentrated by the kidneys, where they provide information about kidney function, and the urine-collecting tubules and bladder; a diseased kidney, or one with a defective

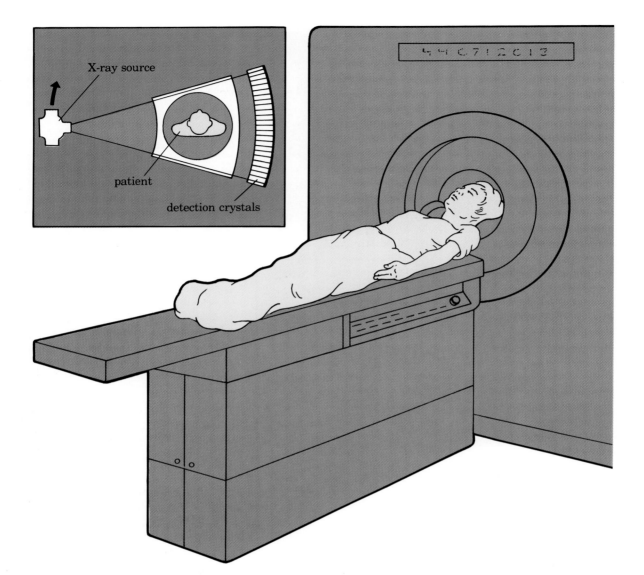

THE CT SCAN

Computerized tomography (CT scan) has vastly increased doctors' ability to see inside the body. The method is widely used, for purposes as diverse as studying lymph-node enlargement and diagnosing kidney abnormalities. As in the drawing above, the patient moves into a tunnellike area and a series of X-ray pictures are taken from many different angles. These images then are analyzed by computer, producing a remarkably detailed series of "cuts" through the target organ.

blood supply, will fail to concentrate radiopaque dye normally. Similarly, the capacity of the liver and spleen to concentrate specific iodine-containing compounds can be assessed. Other special tests involve instilling an iodine-containing oil into the trachea and bronchi of the lungs (bronchography). Iodine-containing emulsions can be injected by lumbar puncture into the spinal canal, and by tilting the patient head-down and then head-up, the material, which is heavier than the cerebro-spinal fluid, will move with gravity and demonstrate abnormalities in the canal, such as tumors or prolapsed intervertebral disks (myelography).

Tomography and Computerized Tomography ("CT scans"). In some special instances, it was found that a better image of a localized abnormality, such as a suspected lung tumor or tuberculous lesion, could be obtained by taking X-ray pictures at different angles, while keeping the lesion in focus. Surrounding tissues then are blurred and the lesion shows up as a succession of sharp images. This technique, termed tomography, has proved especially valuable for X-raying the skull, particularly structures around the ear.

Tomography has led to the Nobel prize-winning development of computerized tomography (CT). This technique involves taking large numbers of X-ray pictures of the same segment of the body, then analyzing the images by computer. The result is a remarkably detailed series of "cuts" through the body or head, permitting detection of abnormalities in the liver, spleen, and walls of the gastrointestinal tract; tumors, abscesses, or cysts in the pancreas, lungs, kidneys, brain, or pelvis; and enlarged lymph glands. Use of appropriate contrast media can enhance the information enormously.

Endoscopic retrograde cholangiopancreatography. The development of fiber-optic endoscopic instruments has made it possible not only to examine the areas beyond the stomach, but also to insert a fine tube into the biliary and pancreatic ducts, and inject radiopaque dye in a retrograde fashion, outlining the biliary tract and the pancreatic ductular system, and thus obtain information on their functions.

Obstructions due to gallstones or tumors thus can be defined, as can chronic inflammation of the pancreas, or pancreatitis.

If the biliary obstruction blocks dye from running back toward the liver, a needle can be passed through the anesthetized abdominal wall to inject dye into bile ducts, permitting an X-ray picture of the biliary system in the liver or from the liver to the gallbladder and duodenum. This is called percutaneous transhepatic cholangiography.

Radioactive Isotopes and Nuclear Scanning

Most chemical elements possess unstable, radioactive isotopes that give off so-called alpha, beta, or gamma rays, or some mixture of them. The ranges of alpha and beta rays are very short and easily blocked, but gamma rays penetrate tissues, particularly soft tissues, with ease. Thus, accumulations of gamma-emitting radioisotopes in the body may be detected, using sensitive "gamma cameras."

The rate of loss of radioactivity by a radioisotope is expressed in half-lives: the length of time in which an isotope loses half of its radioactivity. This may range from fractions of a second to hundreds of years. Radioisotopes with a long half-life are unsuitable for use in humans because over time they can produce significant amounts of radiation damage. For clinical use, an isotope should have a short half-life, preferably in minutes or hours, should emit gamma radiation sufficiently powerful to be detected by a camera outside the body, and should produce as little beta and alpha radiation as possible. Radioactive isotopes of iodine, iron, and indium are used most often in diagnostics.

Radioactive iodine, injected intravenously, may provide information about the size and activity of the thyroid gland. The iodine is rapidly incorporated into thyroid hormones and can be detected by a gamma camera. Most radioisotopes, however, are used as "tags"—combined by a chemical reaction to some biological molecule present in the body fluids or to the surfaces of red or white blood cells or blood platelets, or to some nonbiological molecule that is taken up by specific cells. For instance, the dye rose bengal can be tagged with radioiodine and injected intravenously; it is picked up or concentrated specifically by the cells of the liver. The gamma camera picture will show whether the liver contains areas that do not take up the dye, which might indicate such abnormalities as metastatic tumors, or cysts or abscesses.

In other cases, a patient's own white blood cells may be labeled with radioindium; the cells are reinjected into the circulation, and the gamma

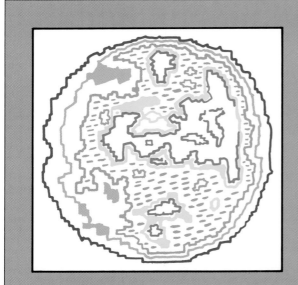

The Brain at Work

The remarkable computerized technique called positron emission transaxial tomography (PETT) allows doctors to visualize the metabolic processes of the brain. Glucose and other substances are "tagged" with radioactive isotopes and tracked as they move through the brain. The historic pictures here show for the first time what happens during the aura of a classic migraine attack. Different colors represent different volumes of blood flow. During the attack (left), blood flow is markedly reduced on one side of the brain, bringing on the hallucinations and disorientation that are the main feature of classic migraines.

camera can disclose whether they concentrate in an area of inflammation or pus formation. Or the patient's own red cells may be labeled and reinjected to search for bleeding in the gastrointestinal tract, which will appear as an accumulation of radioactive material in the hollow spaces of the stomach or small or large bowel.

Other Uses of Radioisotopes

Some radioisotopes are used to label various biologically active substances so that their behavior in the body can be measured. An example is vitamin B_{12}. Its molecule contains an atom of cobalt. Thus, the molecule can be made radioactive by introducing a radioactive cobalt isotope. The labeled vitamin, in very small amounts, is taken by mouth and its absorption and excretion from the body can be measured, using very sensitive detectors of radioactivity.

Positron Emission Transaxial Tomography (PETT)

The technique of computerized tomography can be applied to nuclear scanning, and provide information about metabolic processes in tissues. Currently, the brain is the organ that has been studied most often. Selected substances such as glucose, some fatty acids, and neurotransmitters are labeled with radioactive isotopes, and injected intravenously. They cross from the circulation into the brain, where they are used in different processes. Scintillation (gamma) cameras record the patterns of the substances' distribution, which then are assembled by computer and presented, often in contrasting colors. Normal and abnormal tissues in the brain process the isotopes differently and thus produce different images. The remarkable sensitivity of the technique makes it possible to chart metabolic activities within the brain during reading, solving mathematical problems, and recollecting past experiences. The potential for this technique is mind-boggling.

Magnetic Resonance Imaging (MRI)

Previously termed nuclear magnetic resonance, this technique involves the use of an enormous magnet. No radiation or contrast medium is involved. The powerful magnetic field in which the patient lies, as in a small tunnel, aligns the protons of atoms present in body tissues. Brief pulses of external radio waves then set the aligned protons flipping back and forth. As the protons move, they radiate minute pulses of energy at different rates, according to tissue type, water content, and whether the tissue is normal or injured by disease. The energetic pulses are received by sensitive electronic detectors and converted into electrical energy, which is amplified and analyzed and enhanced by computer. Pictures of the brain and spinal cord are even more detailed and informative than those obtained by CT scan, and the same is becoming true of the liver and heart.

Diagnostic Ultrasound

A major advance in diagnostic technique utilizes sound waves of very high frequency, which cannot be detected by the human ear. Such waves penetrate tissues, but some tissues will reflect them more than others. The sound source is combined with a sensitive microphone, which picks up the pattern of reflected sounds and converts them to a visual display on a television screen. The amount and accuracy of information about the heart, liver, gallbladder, biliary tree and pancreas, and other structures improves year by year, and the technique has the merit of being noninvasive and harmless to body structures. A particularly valuable application is in pregnancy, where it is used to define the state of the fetus. The technique is so sensitive that it can detect the sex of the fetus within a few weeks of gestation.

THERAPEUTIC TECHNIQUES

Many of the technical advances that have been applied very successfully in diagnosis also have important applications in treatment. As noted above, dilated veins or varices in the esophagus, and bleeding in the stomach, duodenum or colon, or urinary bladder can be treated successfully with fiber-optic methods.

Recent advances in instrumentation successfully mitigate or cure diseases in the biliary tract. Instruments with wires at the tip can be fitted into a gastroduodenoscope; an electric current then is passed down the instrument to form an electrocautery. This method can open a narrowed or tight sphincter at the ampulla of Vater, promote the flow of bile or pancreatic secretions, and permit the passage of small gallstones or sludge. Wire cages attached to the ends of flexible wires can be passed into the common bile duct by the same route and used to snare gallstones missed during gallbladder surgery. The technique may obviate a second abdominal operation.

In patients with cancer of the bile ducts, a semirigid plastic tube, called a stent, can be introduced from the duodenum by the same route to maintain bile drainage. This is relatively painless, does not require general anesthesia, and may give elderly persons who cannot undergo surgery added months or even years of comfortable life.

Radiotherapy

X rays are capable of killing cells in their path. The damage done depends on the nature of the irradiated tissue—most cancerous cells are more susceptible to ionizing radiation than is normal tissue—and the energy and duration of the X rays. This makes X rays a powerful tool in destroying or inhibiting the growth of cancers in the body. Focusing devices allow precise, restricted application of X rays to very superficial areas—the skin, for instance—or very deep lesions in the bone or in the tissues in between.

Some malignant tumors are much more sensitive to X-ray irradiation than others, but this is not always predictable. X-ray treatment of cancers must be assessed on an individual basis, and its continuation is determined by early response.

Preliminaries to radiotherapy include very careful definition of the tumor to be irradiated. The target area must be marked indelibly to guide positioning, and X-ray-impermeable screens used to block all rays except those focused on the tumor.

Radioactive implants sometimes make it possible to focus a higher local concentration of ionizing radiation than can be achieved by X rays alone.

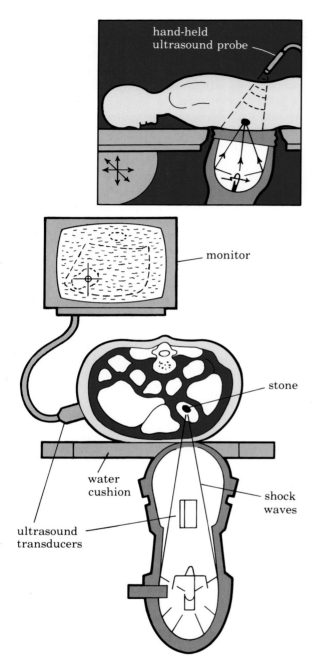

monitor

stone

water cushion

shock waves

ultrasound transducers

SHOCKING THE STONES

Lithotripsy is a high-tech way to dissolve kidney and bladder stones and gallstones without surgery. As shown in the treatment for gallstones above, the patient lies on a table above a bath of warm water, and high-energy sound waves are beamed through the water. The TV monitor allows the beams to be focused directly on the stones. Powerful pulses of sound are emitted by the reflector, which causes the stones to disintegrate and be flushed away.

Radioisotopes of cobalt and of indium are used most frequently. Radium and radon, a radioactive gas produced during the decay of radium, also are used. The radioactive material is sealed in small hollow tubes and inserted in or near malignant tumors.

A very new and exciting area of development is the use of radioisotopes linked to antibodies to an antigen present in a cancer. Theoretically, the material will "home" in to the tumor selectively, carrying a high concentration of the isotope, which will kill or inhibit the tumor cells.

To date, the problem has been to define specific antigens in various tumors, so that antibodies will home to the tumor and nowhere else. The greatest achievement so far is the production of monoclonal antibodies, which may provide an effective carrier of a tumor-destructive radioisotope.

Therapeutic Application of Lasers

Highly energetic laser beams have tremendous destructive power. They can be used to cut tissue with very little bleeding. Lasers are being used increasingly for various forms of surgery, especially in combination with fiber-optic endoscopy. An esophagus obstructed by a surgically inoperable tumor, for instance, can be "reamed" out by laser surgery, thus ensuring extra months of normal life.

Lasers also are used for microsurgery, because the laser beam can be focused in three dimensions with great precision onto very tiny areas. Overgrowth of very small blood vessels in the retina of the eye, a result of diabetes mellitus that impairs vision, can be treated effectively by laser. Detachment of the retina from the wall of the eyeball also can be treated by "spot welding" the tissues using minute bursts of heat.

Lithotripsy

Ultrasound waves of high energy can disintegrate solid matter. This capability has been used to treat stones in the kidneys, urinary tract, and gallbladder as a substitute for surgery. The technique, called lithotripsy, applies powerful pulses of sound, or shock waves, using high-voltage electrical sparks, like bolts of lightning outside the body. The sound waves are focused through water, which transmits them better than air, through the body to the stone. Repeated shocks are required to disintegrate the stone.

LABORATORY MEDICINE

The examination of the blood and other tissues of the body, and of the urine, stools, and expired air are essential parts of the diagnostic workup of many diseases. Following the course of these diseases and providing information necessary for monitoring treatment with drugs also are essential.

The range of tests done in modern clinical laboratories is vast and is continuously enlarging. It is of the greatest importance that results be accurate and reproducible, and that errors of collection, testing, and reporting be kept to a minimum. In the past 20 years automation and the computer have significantly reduced the drudgery and risks of error.

Examination of the Blood

The contents of the blood reflect changes of function of most organs or systems of the body, because the blood provides the principal means of supplying the tissues with nutrients and oxygen, and of removing the waste products. The two parts of the blood are the blood cells and platelets and the liquid component called plasma.

Plasma, like whole blood, changes from a liquid to a jellylike mass when bleeding occurs following injury, or when blood is withdrawn from the body. This is due to a process termed clotting or coagulation. Blood clotting is essential for controlling and terminating blood loss after external or internal bodily injury. In simple terms, it is affected by the conversion of some proteins, normally present in solution in plasma, into a lattice of molecules of a protein called fibrin. This insoluble substance is termed a clot. Clot formation leaves a fluid called blood serum, which has the same contents as plasma minus the clot-forming proteins.

Abnormalities of mechanisms involved in blood clotting are responsible for some diseases in which spontaneous bleeding or prolonged bleeding after injury occurs. The best known is hemophilia.

Blood Culture

When bacterial or viral infection is suspected as a cause of illness, or in patients who have persistent or intermittent fever for which no cause can be found, samples of blood are drawn and cultured in a laboratory. Any living microorganisms present in the blood will multiply and can be identified. Tests of their sensitivity to antibiotics may provide important indicators for treatment.

Some disease-producing parasites, such as those causing malaria, cannot be cultured, but can be identified in appropriately stained red blood cells spread on glass slides (a blood smear or film).

Blood Counts

Counts of the various types of blood cells, subgroups, and blood platelets may provide valuable diagnostic information. These techniques are described in Chapter 7, "The Blood."

Blood Chemistry

Proteins, salts, enzymes, and hormones are estimated from serum. Specific chemical reactions for most of these components result in a colored end product. The quality and intensity of the color can be measured accurately in a device called a spectrophotometer. Modern laboratories use automated equipment for the majority of these tests.

Radioimmunoassay

The amount of any specific hormone present in serum is an indicator of how much is being produced by the synthesizing (endocrine) gland. Examples are the thyroid, adrenal, and pituitary glands. The amounts usually are extremely small, many in the range of a few million-millionths of a gram in a milliliter of serum. They can be measured, however, by a remarkable technique called radioimmunoassay. The method can be applied to the measurement of any hormone (or drug) to which a specific antibody can be produced, including such substances as cocaine or anabolic steroids. The substance is first labeled with a radioactive isotope. Radioimmunoassay measures the difference in amount of labeled hormone binding with the specific antibody in the patient's serum. Any hormone naturally present in the patient's serum will compete with the radioactive substances for binding sites on the antibody, thus reducing the amount of radioactive material bound to the antibody. By measuring the reduction, an estimate can be derived of the amount of hormone in the patient's serum. Radioimmunoassay is widely used to monitor hormone and medication levels, and gives precise readings even when the substances are present in very small amounts.

Serological Tests

Estimations of the amounts and types of antibodies to bacteria and viruses present in serum can provide information about the nature and course of current infections. On this basis, appropriate treatment can be planned. Serological tests also provide information about past infections, and whether the subject is likely to be immune to subsequent exposure.

Examination of the Urine

The urine of a subject in good health may vary greatly in color, depending on time of day, fluid consumption, and how much body water has been lost through the lungs, skin, and intestinal tract. Urine should contain only a trace of protein, rare white and red blood cells, and no blood sugar. In various kidney diseases there will be increased amounts of protein and often large numbers of red and white blood cells in the urine.

In uncontrolled or poorly controlled diabetes mellitus, blood sugar spills over into the urine. Consequent sweetness of the urine was the quality by which physicians centuries ago diagnosed diabetes mellitus (mellitus means sweet). Today the sugar is detected by a chemical reaction, which is the basis for the tests that patients with diabetes mellitus use to test their own urine.

Examination of the Stools

Many infections of the lower gastrointestinal tract are accompanied by diarrhea. Diarrhea persisting for more than two to three days should be investigated by examination of the stools for the presence of white blood cells, which may indicate infection with pathogenic (disease-causing) bacteria, or more usually, traces of blood, indicating inflammation and ulceration. The stools also should be examined for protozoa, such as amoebae and giardia, which can be seen under the microscope, or samples may be cultured with the presence of different nutrients and substances that inhibit the growth of some bacteria, thus allowing others to grow.

Examination of the stools for blood also is done using special chemically treated detector cards, which change color in the presence of small amounts of blood. Positive tests indicate bleeding into the gastrointestinal tract, for which it is important to find the cause, which may be an ulcer, a polyp, or cancer.

When a person is losing weight despite regular food intake, failure to absorb calories and other nutrients from the small intestine is suspected, indicating disease of the small bowel or other organs of digestion, such as the pancreas or biliary system.

The standard test for such malabsorption is to measure the amount of fat present in the stool by chemical means. All stools passed in a period of 72 hours must be collected, and the subject must eat a diet containing about 4 ounces (100 grams) of total fat per day. In patients with malabsorption, the amount of stool fat is significantly increased.

Direct visual examination of some of the cavities of the body can be made by using narrow-bore rigid tubes that are introduced into the cavity through a small incision in the anesthetized skin and tissues deep in the skin. These tubes are provided with illuminating devices. When applied to the abdominal cavity, the procedure is termed peritoneoscopy and laparoscopy, and it permits limited viewing of the surface of the abdominal cavity, termed the peritoneum, and of organs, especially the liver. Laparoscopy also is used for inspection and treatment of the female reproductive organs.

The cavity of large joints may be inspected, using an arthroscope, and the linings of chest and lungs using a pleuroscope. Some minor surgical procedures may be performed, and small tissue samples obtained, for diagnostic purposes. Fibrous tissue binding loops of bowel together, termed adhesions, which may follow surgery, may be divided through the laparoscope, and fragments of cartilage, behaving as foreign bodies, may be removed from joints through the arthroscope.

Samples of blood usually are obtained from a suitable vein in the arm by venipuncture. A tourniquet is applied to the arm above the site of sampling to impede blood flow. The skin is cleansed with an alcohol swab, and a hollow, sharp, pointed and beveled needle is inserted into the vein. Blood is withdrawn into either a syringe or a tube.

When blood counts or estimates of one of the contents of blood plasma are to be done, the blood is immediately treated to prevent clotting. The usual anticoagulants are heparin or a chemical that binds the calcium in the blood, thus preventing its essential role in blood clotting.

WHAT BLOOD TESTS MEAN

	HIGH LEVEL	LOW LEVEL
ELECTROLYTES		
Sodium	Dehydration	Protracted vomiting, heat exhaustion, some liver and kidney diseases
Potassium	Dehydration	Overuse of some diuretics, diarrhea
Calcium	Parathyroid disease	Failure of intestinal absorption
Magnesium	Overdosage	Severe chronic diarrhea, alcoholism
Chloride		Protracted vomiting
ORGANIC WASTE PRODUCTS		
Urea	Kidney failure	Severe liver disease
Creatinine	Kidney failure	
PROTEINS		
Albumin		Severe kidney and liver disease, starvation
Globulin	Chronic infection, some immune disorders	
OTHER PROTEINS		
Glucose	Diabetes mellitus	Hypoglycemia
LIPIDS		
Cholesterol	Familial, excessive animal fat, constipation, obstructive jaundice	
Triglycerides	Excessive calorie consumption, including alcohol	Starvation
LIVER ENZYMES		
Transaminase	Liver disease	
Alkaline phosphatase	Obstructive biliary disease	

CHAPTER 3

PAIN

Pain is an important symptom of illness—sometimes the most important symptom—but it is not fully understood. Only recently, for instance, have scientists identified the endorphins, substances within the brain that modulate pain. Even this discovery was serendipitous, because scientists were studying the effects of illegal drugs that suppress pain.

Moreover, pain is individual and resists measurement. One person may stoically endure a toothache that would send another frantically to a dentist. Pain also can be fleeting or intermittent, difficult to pin down or even to describe. Sometimes pain occurs far from where it originates, as in sciatica—pain in the leg caused by nerve compression in the spine.

Finally, although pain is primarily a clue to illness (often, the body's way of notifying us of an illness), it often is so severe and debilitating that it causes harmful effects of its own. The disability of arthritis often occurs because an arthritic, trying to prevent pain, fails to use an afflicted joint or limb. Thus, pain control has become a specialty in itself. Pain control clinics now operate in many major hospitals.

PAIN RELIEF

Anesthesia

Anesthetics are used to desensitize the body or part of the body, thus allowing surgical procedures that once would have been too painful for a patient to tolerate. Anesthetics also put the body or body part "to sleep," eliminating involuntary movement that could handicap the procedure.

Not surprisingly, the principle of anesthesia was first demonstrated by a dentist. H. G. Wells, D.D.S, in 1845 showed how inhalation of nitrous oxide (laughing gas) could overcome pain during dental or surgical operations. Since then, anesthesia has been widely developed and improved. Anesthesiology, the administration of anesthetics, now is a recognized medical specialty.

Anesthetics are broadly divided into two types. General anesthetics anesthetize the entire body so that the patient "sleeps" through the entire procedure and "wakes up" when it has been completed. Local anesthetics block pain in a particular region of the body, so that the patient remains conscious but has no sensation in the anesthetized area. Some anesthetics are classed as regional, because an entire region of the body may be anesthetized. A "spinal block," for instance, eliminates all sensation below the waist.

General anesthesia is used for abdominal surgery and many other procedures in which the body is opened. It is less commonly used for operations for which it once was commonplace, such as childbirth or eye surgery. Although overwhelmingly safe, general anesthesia carries a certain degree of risk. It also requires a period of hospital recovery. Thus, operations such as cataract surgery now are done under local anesthesia on an ambulatory basis.

General anesthesia is administered in two ways. The traditional method is inhalation of various gases, including nitrous oxide, ether, halothane, and ethane. Injection of anesthetic directly into the vein now is preferred in many cases. Rapidly acting sodium pentothal and other barbiturates are the most commonly used.

The local anesthetic with which most persons are familiar is probably novocaine and its derivatives. The staple of dental practice, it is injected directly into the area to be desensitized. Both its duration and its spread are limited. The novocaine family sometimes is used for athletic injuries. The effects of these short-term "locals" usually wear off in a few hours.

Longer lasting anesthetics are another reason many operations can be performed on an outpatient basis or patients can be discharged more quickly after surgery. These anesthetics continue to reduce pain in the operative site, while permitting the patient to return home for recuperation.

Analgesics

The most common pain medications can be bought over the counter and probably are found in every family's medicine chest. Aspirin has been a mainstay of pain relief for 100 years even though its method of operation still is not fully understood. Apparently, aspirin reduces pain by acting on blood platelets, which are involved in inflammation. For this reason, it is a mainstay in arthritis and recently has been found valuable, when taken according to a specific regimen, in forestalling heart attacks. Aspirin's most common uses, however, are for headache, dental pain, and symptomatic relief in flu. The standard dosage is 325 milligrams, but it also is available in extra-strength and children's dosages. (However, aspirin should not be given to children with chicken pox or flu symptoms, because of possible complications described in Chapter 29, "Taking Care of Your Child.")

Acetaminophen has the same pain-relieving qualities as aspirin and frequently is preferred by those who do not tolerate aspirin well. (It does not offer heart-attack protection, however.) Marketed under several names, it is available in tablet, capsule, or liquid form for children.

Ibuprofen, also marketed under several names, is one of a class of medications defined as nonsteroidal anti-inflammatory drugs. It also is used for arthritis pain relief.

Prescription Pain Medication

Codeine, a relative of morphine, often is prescribed in combination with other analgesics, such as aspirin and acetaminophen. The combination is available without prescription in some other countries but must be prescribed in the U.S. because codeine is addictive. However, addiction is very slow to develop. Codeine and its combinations usually are prescribed for dental pain, pain of sports injury, and other forms of mild pain. It also is used as a cough suppressant. Doctors frequently prescribe codeine because it can reach effective blood levels when taken by mouth.

Meperidine (Demerol) is a synthetic, orally effective compound that possesses essentially the same properties as morphine. It often is prescribed postoperatively. Meperidine is a frequently abused drug. Drugs closely related to meperidine are alphaprodine (Nisentil), frequently used by anesthesiologists, and diphenoxylate, used to control diarrhea.

Propoxyphene (Darvon) is derived from methadone, a drug used to rehabilitate heroin addicts but also an abused drug, as described in Chapter 1, "A Preventive Approach to Health." Darvon is one of the most widely prescribed pain-reducing drugs; its potency is estimated to be somewhere between that of aspirin and codeine. It often has been used by athletes wishing to continue to perform in spite of pain.

Because of its potential for abuse, particularly in combination with other drugs, propoxyphene is listed in Schedule IV of the Controlled Substances Act, meaning that it may cause limited physical or pseudological dependence, but still may be prescribed by physicians. A package insert warns that propoxyphene can threaten life when used in combination with alcohol, tranquilizers, and sedatives.

Morphine is the earliest and still most effective medication for continuing, severe pain. It is commonly prescribed for pain relief for patients in the terminal stages of cancer. Obtained from opium, the dry juice of the poppy plant, morphine elevates the pain threshold and alters the user's reaction to pain. Morphine appears to achieve its effects through interaction with the brain's own pain-modulating substances, the endorphins, and may be chemically related to them. Morphine can be highly addictive (although the addiction can be reversed) but is rarely abused. The usual dose for a patient in pain is $1/100$ gram twice a day, but tolerance builds rapidly. Addicts have been known to take as much as four grams a day.

CHAPTER 4

MEDICAL GENETICS

We all begin life with our future partially programmed. In every cell of our bodies, we carry specialized material called genes, a legacy from each of our parents. These genes determine our body build, the color of our eyes, and whether our hair is curly or straight. They contribute to our intelligence, too.

Genes have an important impact on lifelong health. Genetics, the study of the genes and their role in the development of organisms, is a rapidly expanding area of research, and not all the answers are known. It is suspected, for instance, that genes partially determine not only how our cells develop but when they wear out. Heredity may explain why members of one family develop cataracts, diabetes, or arthritis at age 60, while members of another family are not afflicted until 90. Our genes probably play some part in cancer, heart disease, perhaps even susceptibility to the common cold.

Although medical genetics concerns itself with hereditary influences throughout life, this chapter addresses itself to conditions present at birth or evident shortly afterward that affect the health and welfare of the child.

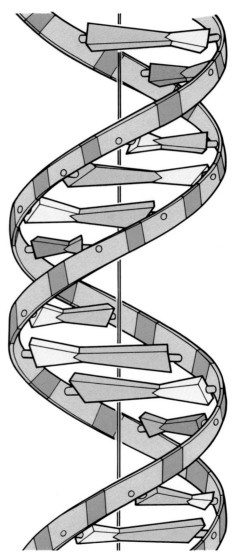

THE DOUBLE HELIX OF HEREDITY
The long molecule of DNA (deoxyribonucleic acid) that contains the human genetic code resembles a spiral stairway. The sides or rails are chains of sugar (ribose) and phosphate molecules. The steps or rungs are built of molecules of thymine, cytosine, adenine, and guanine repeated thousands of times in different sequences.

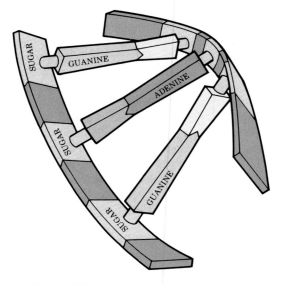

A CLOSE-UP OF DNA
The DNA "ladder" shows distinctive features. Guanine always links with cytosine, thymine with adenine, to form "rungs" attached to sugar-phosphate chains, but in different sequences of bases encoded with genetic information.

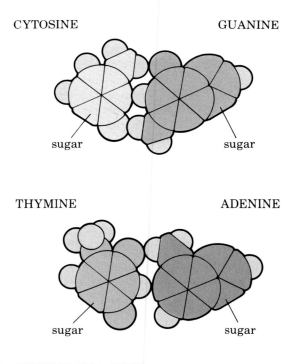

CYTOSINE   GUANINE

sugar   sugar

THYMINE   ADENINE

sugar   sugar

SCHEME OF A GENE
Pairs of DNA bases compose the structure of the molecule. A gene is thought to be a tiny segment of DNA in which a cluster of several base pairs activates a process of heredity, singly or in conjunction with other genes.

GENETICS AND INFANCY

Every parent wonders before a child is born, "Will my baby be normal?" But fewer than 2 percent of babies are born with any kind of defect, and most of those are trifling and easily corrected. Thus, relatively few couples have the slightest reason to undergo exhaustive tests and genetic studies to assess the potential liabilities of offspring. However, there is reasonable cause for concern if a couple already has borne an infant with a birth defect, or if an obviously hereditary trait recurs in direct bloodlines. In addition, there are times when, because of parental age, ethnic background, or certain reproductive problems, consultation with a physician can be helpful.

Often, the conversation itself is enough. For example, the doctor can assure the unaffected brother of a person with classic hemophilia, a hereditary inability of the blood to clot, that he cannot transmit the disease to his offspring. The doctor can assure a couple that cerebral palsy due to premature birth or birth injury is not hereditary. Diagnosis and treatment of the most frequent forms of congenital disease are within the physician's area of competence. The small number of patients who need special help can be referred to genetic counselors and specialists.

About 3,000 disorders, too many and too rare to be enumerated, have been identified as hereditary. But there still are great gaps in knowledge. Medical geneticists cannot give hard and fast answers to every question. Sometimes answers are immensely consoling, sometimes qualified. Often, risks can be stated only in rather cold terms of mathematical odds. But in almost every instance, a more informed basis can be reached upon which decisions about having children can be made.

Congenital or Hereditary

A congenital abnormality is one that is present at birth. It is not necessarily hereditary, which means not necessarily transmitted by germ cells of the parents.

Accidental birth defects fall into this class. They include defects caused by birth injury, infections of the mother with German measles or toxoplasmosis during pregnancy, or exposure of the mother during early pregnancy to drugs, alcohol, toxins, or radiation. Cerebral palsy, some forms of epilepsy, and certain types of retardation usually have an accidental cause.

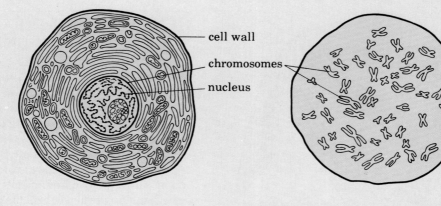

cell wall

chromosomes

nucleus

normal male karyotype

1 2 3
— A —
4 5
— B —

6 7 8 9 10 11 12 X —
— C — X

13 14 15 16 17 18
— D — — E —

19 20 21 22
— F — — G — Y

normal female karyotype

1 2 3
— A —
4 5
— B —

6 7 8 9 10 11 12 X
— C —

13 14 15 16 17 18
— D — — E —

19 20 21 22
— F — — G — Y

CHROMOSOMES

Chromosomes determine the heredity of every organism. The "package" of chromosomes of any organism, when analyzed, is called its karyotype. Top drawings show delicate filaments in every cell nucleus (left) that contract, segment, and form "arms," as in the close-up at right. Center drawings show normal human karyotypes, each of which contains 23 pairs of chromosomes. The 23rd pair of chromosomes determines sex. The drawing at left shows a normal male karyotype, containing a large X chromosome in the 23rd pair, and a small Y chromosome. The right drawing of a normal female karyotype has two large X chromosomes. The lower drawing shows a "banded" karyotype of a normal male. When the chromosomes are prepared and chemically stained, they can be seen under a microscope. Each pair has a unique pattern of staining (banding).

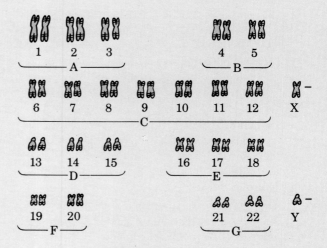

"banded" karyotype

Hereditary birth defects are transmitted by parental germ cells. Mathematical odds for or against repetition usually can be calculated.

Many birth defects are thought to result from extremely complex interactions of genes and environment. The more complex the genetics of a particular defect (cleft palate, heart abnormalities), the less likely it is to be repeated. Parents of a baby with a cleft palate can be assured that odds are more than 25 to 1 against another baby with the same condition. That calculates to a less than 5 percent risk, only slightly greater than the overall risk for all birth defects combined in the general baby population.

Family susceptibility. A third category includes diseases that are not strictly hereditary but appear to have a hereditary component. They involve an inborn susceptibility or predisposition that may be triggered into full-blown disease if the person is exposed to certain factors in the environment. These are the diseases we usually mean when we refer to those that "run in families." Geneticists sometimes speak of the "two-hit" theory, meaning that the person is "hit" at birth with a susceptible gene, but no disease will develop until a second "hit" occurs. Thus, diabetes tends to recur in families, but a middle-aged person who is genetically predisposed to diabetes may never develop the disease if he or she stays physically fit and eats a well-balanced diet.

In the future, medical genetics may play a greater role in preventive medicine by informing us early of hereditary vulnerabilities against which medical defenses may be built. Moreover, research advances in genetic engineering and gene therapy portend a future where gene replacement may be possible for selected disorders.

GENETIC BLUEPRINTS

All of the directions for the structure and functioning of our bodies are contained in our genes, which are carried in our chromosomes. Both are composed primarily of structural protein and DNA (deoxyribonucleic acid). These are molecules of heredity, so heredity basically is a chemical phenomenon.

Chromosomes are the threadlike particles in the nucleus of every cell. When stained and prepared, they can be seen under a microscope. Human beings normally have 46 chromosomes, comprised of 23 pairs. One chromosome in each pair comes from the mother through the egg cell. The other chromosome of each pair comes from the sperm of the father. At conception, the two sets combine into a single cell, which develops into the new human being.

Heredity is enclosed within the DNA of each chromosome. Long DNA molecules consist of two intertwining chains coiled around a common axis, something like a spiral ladder, with thousands of connecting "rungs" or steps. The rungs are built of four rather simple chemical units, repeated thousands upon thousands of times in different sequences along the length of the chain. The "double helix" is illustrated in this chapter.

A gene is a very small cluster of these units, constituting the rungs and sides of a particular tiny portion of the long DNA molecule. Each gene or gene combination is a unit of heredity, specifying a particular trait, such as whether an organism has blue or brown eyes. Collectively, genes determine whether an organism will have the organs and functions of a mouse or a man.

How can an infinitesimal group of molecules have such omnipotence? The "one gene, one enzyme" concept holds that a gene directs the assembly of an enzyme, which is a chemical catalyst essential for some body process. If a gene is defective, its associated enzyme is defective or lacking. The effect may be harmless and not apparent, or it may impose a derangement of some body process.

Gene-containing DNA imprints the genetic code upon a slightly different nucleic acid, RNA (ribonucleic acid). Forms of RNA direct the cell to manufacture specific enzymes and other proteins by linking amino-acid building blocks (at least 22 different types) in inviolable sequences. A seemingly insignificant error, such as a "wrong" amino acid in a chain of many hundreds, may have far-flung effects.

How Traits Are Inherited

One of the 23 pairs of human chromosomes constitutes the sex chromosomes, designated XX in the female and XY in the male. The other 22 pairs are called autosomes and are identical in male and female. Sexual reproduction makes human variation possible by drawing upon the unique traits of parents in random ways. Whether a fetus is male or female is a matter of chance, depending on whether a sperm carrying an X or Y fertilizes an egg. If a sperm with a Y chromosome unites with a maternal X (the female sex chromosome is always X), the offspring will be XY and male. An X-carrying sperm produces a female.

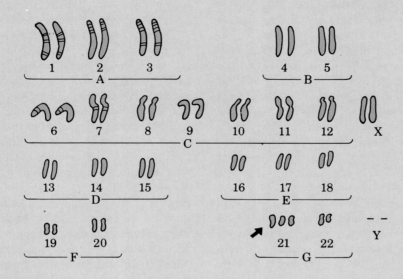

DOWN SYNDROME

The chromosome arrangement of a female infant shows the extra chromosome characteristic of Down syndrome, or mongolism, a form of retardation. The extra bit of genetic material is in position 21, and is known as Trisomy 21 (arrow). Banding, in which each chromosome stains in a unique way, allows specific identification of the extra chromosome as a 21.

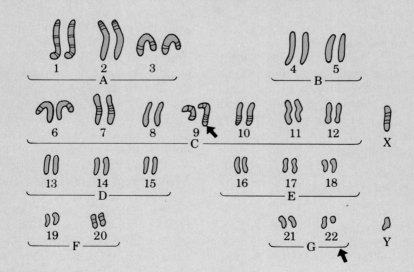

TRANSLOCATION

When a pair of chromosomes carries an extra part from another chromosome, the phenomenon is called translocation. Above, a portion of chromosome 22 has been "translocated" to chromosome 9. The male with this arrangement is a victim of chronic myelogenous leukemia. Previously, it was believed the condition was caused by the absence of one of the 22 chromosomes. Banding techniques enabled researchers to discover the true cause, the transfer of materials as indicated by arrows.

Some traits appear to be determined multigenically, which means two or more genes in combination influence whether they recur. There are other complexities and unknowns, but in general, a single gene influences a single trait. In common genetic language, genes (and the traits they shape) are thought of as "recessive" or "dominant."

One might think of a recessive gene as "weak," unable to generate its specific enzyme, producing too little of it, or an abnormal molecule. But if it is paired with a normal gene, the latter takes over the job of influencing that particular trait and no abnormal symptoms appear. However, if recessive genes are transmitted from both parents—a "double dose"—the disorder appears in the offspring. If only one parent has a recessive gene, he or she is a carrier, but offspring will be normal. Carriers of such recessive traits are completely unaffected and their carrier state has implications only for their children. In fact, every human being is estimated to carry five or six recessive traits among their 50,000 to 100,000 individual genes.

In the case of a dominant gene, the "dose" transmitted from one parent overrides the effects of a normal matching gene from the other parent and thus appears in the offspring.

Most inherited metabolic diseases are transmitted recessively. The most common in the United States are sickle-cell disease and cystic fibrosis, a disease of young people in which the mucous glands are defective (see Chapter 10, "The Lungs").

Dominant hereditary disorders include Huntington's disease, a progressive disorder of the nervous system, and achondroplasia, the most common form of dwarfism. Certain birth defects and some forms of stomach ulcers also are transmitted as dominant traits in specific families.

Conditions such as hemophilia (the so-called "bleeder's disease"), color-vision deficiency or "color blindness," and certain forms of muscular dystrophy are sex-linked. The trait is determined by the X chromosomes received from the mother, who is a carrier but is not affected by the diseases herself. Each son of the carrier mother has a 50 percent chance of being affected, and each daughter has a 50 percent chance of being a carrier.

Members of a family with sex-linked or recessive disorders should know that both parents of an affected child are invariably normal. Each is a carrier, so the child receives the recessive gene in a double dose. Usually, both partners are completely unaware that they are carriers. Generations may have passed without the disorder appearing in their families.

Fortunately, relatively simple tests often can be performed to determine whether other family members carry the recessive trait. These tests can be invaluable in allaying anxieties about their own reproduction or aiding those "at risk."

Genetic Disorders In Ethnic Groups

More than 100 recognized genetic disorders occur predominantly in specific population groups. This is easily understood because, over the centuries, people of ethnic, religious, racial, or national backgrounds have tended to marry and reproduce with individuals of the same ancestry. Because each of us carries a few recessive traits, certain genes have tended to become "inbred" within certain population groups. Double doses of recessive genes thus are much more likely to occur. None of these disorders are absolutely restricted to a particular group. Tay-Sachs disease in infants of European Jewish ancestry, sickle-cell anemia in American blacks, and betathalassemia (another serious blood disorder) in persons of Mediterranean heritage are among the best known examples of such disorders in the United States.

Recent technological developments make it possible to determine the carriers of such traits by simple blood tests. In this way, two persons of Jewish ancestry, for example, can learn if they are carriers for the Tay-Sachs gene. If neither partner or only one carries the gene, there is no risk to their offspring. In about one of 750 Jewish couples, however, both are carriers. Through genetic counseling, these couples can be helped to have only unaffected children, if they choose. Similar capabilities are available for sickle-cell anemia and thalassemia, and soon may be possible for cystic fibrosis as well.

What the Odds Mean

If a child has a recessively transmitted disease, chances that a subsequent child of the same parents will have the disease are 1 in 4. Looked at positively, this means a 75 percent chance that the next child will be healthy. If a disorder is dominantly transmitted, there is a 50 percent chance that each child will be affected.

A sex-linked disorder carries its own odds. The chances are 50-50 that a son will be affected. The disease-free son cannot transmit the disease to his children. Likewise, chances are 50-50 that a daughter will carry the gene, making her offspring vulnerable although she herself is not affected.

Daughters who do not inherit the gene are not carriers and neither their sons nor daughters will be affected.

No matter what the odds on paper, it is quite possible that a given hereditary defect of either type will appear in none of the children of a couple, or in very rare instances, in all of them. If a coin is tossed and comes down heads, chances that the next toss will come down tails are not increased. They are still 50-50. Each toss is "a whole new ball game."

DIAGNOSIS AND COUNSEL

If supposed hereditary disease or birth defects are a cause for worry, the first step is accurate diagnosis. Rare and complex hereditary conditions require careful detective work, detailed knowledge of genetics, and exacting discrimination.

Newborn Screening

In most states, a newborn screening test for treatable hereditary disorders (involving only a tiny blood sample) is mandatory. Early diagnosis can lead to simple lifesaving treatment. The list includes such metabolic disorders as phenylketonuria (PKU), methylmalonic acidemia (an inability to break down certain amino acids), and galactosemia (an inborn error of milk-sugar metabolism), in which the tiny body is unable to metabolize certain substances that then accumulate and can cause mental retardation or death. Relatively simple dietary or replacement therapies can offset the disease's effects before damage is done.

Hypothyroidism, which stems from a deficiency of thyroid hormone and which is a major cause of mental and growth retardation, also can be treated effectively if detected early. A screening test for hypothyroidism has been adopted in some states.

Fetal Diagnosis

A rapidly increasing number of tests and studies help greatly to evaluate the developing fetus, often quite early in pregnancy, and to establish the facts as a sound basis for counseling. This new area of medical genetics, called prenatal diagnosis, can be very valuable in certain pregnancies.

Ultrasound, described in Chapter 2, "Tests and Procedures," uses high-frequency sound waves to obtain a visual-echo image of the fetus within the uterus from early stages of development, thus revealing characteristics of the fetal anatomy. This is particularly important when conditions such as hydrocephalus (fluid accumulation in the brain) or severe dwarfing disorders are suspected.

Ultrasound also helps determine a multiple birth, the stage of fetal development, and the placement of the placenta within the uterus.

Amniocentesis is the withdrawal of a sample of amniotic fluid in which the fetus "swims." The fluid contains fetal cells, which can be grown in culture, and other products, which can be studied for evidence of certain birth defects. About 100 genetic diseases now can be diagnosed in this way.

The procedure is a relatively simple one, usually undertaken about the 16th week of pregnancy. Guided by ultrasound, a very thin needle is inserted through the mother's abdominal wall into the uterine cavity. Only a small amount of the fluid is needed, which is rapidly replaced. Analyzing the sample takes about two weeks. Many specialists consider amniocentesis particularly important if the mother is of advanced reproductive age (over age 35) because older women face a much greater risk of giving birth to an infant with Down syndrome (formerly called mongolism).

Chorionic villus sampling (CVS) is a new, safe, and accurate method of fetal diagnosis. Performed at eight to 11 weeks of pregnancy, CVS utilizes tiny samples of placental tissue, which genetically are identical to the fetus, to determine the chromosomal and genetic constitution.

Sex of the fetus also is readily determined by these methods, and this knowledge can have more than mere curiosity value. For instance, Duchenne muscular dystrophy, the most common form, is a genetic disease that afflicts only males. If the fetus is female, the baby will not have muscular dystrophy. When a son has been affected, such information can greatly allay a family's anxiety.

AFP, a blood protein present throughout fetal development, has been shown to be dramatically elevated when the formation of the brain or spinal cord of the fetus somehow has been interrupted early in development. The problem can be detected by testing for AFP levels in the amniotic fluid. The AFP test often is recommended for families that in the past have had children with abnormalities, or where other family members have been affected. Recently, it has become possible to measure the AFP factor in the mother's blood in early pregnancy to determine whether she is at increased risk for such a defect in her fetus, even when there has been no prior history. Applied to all pregnant women, such a screening test could greatly increase the detection rate of such defects during fetal life.

Chromosome studies. A number of birth defects can be diagnosed by identifying abnormalities of structure or number of chromosomes, using the amniotic fluid. These defects are not hereditary but "developmental" or environmental, because some unknown disturbs the fusion of normal parental chromosomes in the fertilized egg.

The most common chromosomal birth defect diagnosed by amniocentesis cell studies is Down syndrome. The affected child has abnormal features, mental retardation, and abnormalities of many systems of the body. An extra chromosome in position 21, as illustrated in this chapter, is responsible. The abnormality is caused by a defect in separation of chromosomes called nondisjunction. The parents almost always have normal chromosomes, so the defect is not truly hereditary. Chances that a subsequent child will be normal are quite good, except that the risks of bearing a Down syndrome child, regardless of family history, go up sharply after maternal age 35.

A different, quite rare form of Down syndrome affects infants of young as well as older mothers. This form also has a distinctive chromosome abnormality. One pair of chromosomes carries an extra part from another chromosome, a phenomenon called translocation. This form of the disorder may be hereditary. One of the parents can carry the chromosomal rearrangement in a "balanced form" and not be affected by it. If the mother carries the rearrangement, there is an 8 to 12 percent chance that each of her children will have Down syndrome. If the father carries the rearrangement, the risk is about 2 to 5 percent with each pregnancy.

Differences in two seemingly identical diseases underline the importance of fine discrimination when doing genetic studies. In addition, such chromosome rearrangements may lead to increased spontaneous pregnancy losses. Families in which three or more pregnancies have been lost spontaneously may benefit from chromosome tests in order to rule out a chromosomal rearrangement in a parent.

Pedigrees

Accurate interpretation of genetic factors may require that facts be obtained by pedigree studies, detailed investigations of the health histories of blood relatives through parents, siblings, cousins, aunts, grandparents, and beyond. Pedigrees can give insight into patterns of inheritance of a trait and give a basis for prediction. It is essential that this information be accurate. This is not always easy if relatives live at great distances or if records in their communities are sketchy. Nonetheless, health professionals trained in medical genetics can be skilled in overcoming these difficulties and obtaining accurate genetic information.

TREATMENT

An increasing number of genetic disorders can be treated. Approaches include modification of diet or hormone replacement to prevent mental retardation and offset certain metabolic errors. Children with cystic fibrosis may have fewer symptoms when treated with pancreatic enzymes and mist inhalations. Hemophilia can be treated by victims themselves with home transfusions of the needed clotting factor. Unfortunately, however, effective therapies or cures are not available for many hereditary disorders.

If tests performed in early pregnancy reveal that the fetus is afflicted with a serious and untreatable hereditary disorder, the parents then have a choice, strictly their own, of terminating pregnancy or of completing pregnancy and having the child with the abnormal condition. For many families, the opportunity to have fetal testing performed has provided an option that has enabled them to have children unaffected with the condition for which they were at risk—children who otherwise might not have been conceived or born.

Genetic diseases vary in implications and handicaps. Many developmental birth defects have no known genetic basis. Not a few worries about supposed hereditary traits arise from misconceptions. Medical counsel can bring the facts to light. There is reason to hope that genetic disease may someday be treated and cured by "gene therapy."

WHERE TO SEEK HELP

The first source of help is the family physician. If he or she recognizes that special skills are needed, patients can be referred to reliable laboratory and counseling centers. Another type of service is a birth defects treatment center, usually established in a teaching hospital or in affiliation with the medical school of a university. Few communities are far away from laboratory and counseling services in large towns and cities. A list of the names and addresses of genetic counseling services is available from the medical department of the National Foundation-March of Dimes, P.O. Box 2000, White Plains, NY 10602.

CHAPTER 5

THE HEART AND CIRCULATION

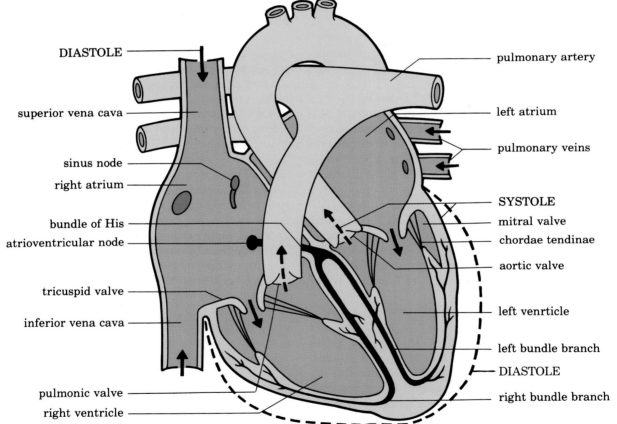

DIASTOLE

superior vena cava

sinus node

right atrium

bundle of His

atrioventricular node

tricuspid valve

inferior vena cava

pulmonic valve

right ventricle

pulmonary artery

left atrium

pulmonary veins

SYSTOLE

mitral valve

chordae tendinae

aortic valve

left venrticle

left bundle branch

DIASTOLE

right bundle branch

ANATOMY OF THE HEART

The heart is divided into four compartments. The right atrium and ventricle constitute the pulmonary circulation; the left atrium and ventricle, the systemic circulation. Blood returning from the body collects in the right atrium, and pours downward into the right ventricle, which pumps it through the pulmonary artery to the lungs for oxygenation. The oxygenated blood returns to the left atrium, then moves to the left ventricle to be pumped

throughout the body. Four valves (arrows) open and close between the chambers and vessels to permit blood flow. The conduction system (right and left bundle branches, bundle of His, nodes) carries electrical impulses that trigger and control the heart's activity. The dashed line shows how the heart relaxes and contracts during the two phases of the heartbeat, called diastole and systole.

The human heart is a large mass of hollow muscle spelled L-I-F-E. As a pump that propels oxygen-carrying blood to every cell of the body, it is literally the "heart" of our existence. Not surprisingly then, it is a remarkably strong and resilient organ that neither works itself to death nor wears out in the literal sense. Nonetheless, diseases of the heart are by far the leading cause of death in industrialized society.

EXAMINING THE HEART

The illustration *opposite* shows the basic anatomy of the heart.

Symptoms. The symptoms of an illness usually are the reason for seeking medical care. In problems of the heart, symptoms also may be the principal diagnostic clues. Some heart symptoms are highly specific and may indicate disease when all diagnostic examinations are normal.

The principal symptoms of heart disease are pounding of the heart (palpitation), shortness of breath (dyspnea), swelling of the legs (edema), fainting (syncope), and pain. Coughing, spitting up blood, and weakness also may occur. None of these symptoms occurs only in heart disease. Shortness of breath, for example, is more frequently caused by a condition not related to the heart. "Shortness of breath" is also difficult to define. Many normal people consider themselves short of breath but are able to ascend a flight of stairs without resting, and feel no need to pause for breath when walking on the street. Others have shortness of breath at rest, often accompanied by light-headedness and numbness of the arms and legs. This is hyperventilation syndrome, a sign of nervous tension resulting in unconscious over-breathing.

Swelling of the legs is common in people in good health, especially in hot weather, but it may be a sign of heart failure. In those cases, shortness of breath almost always accompanies the swelling.

Fainting in heart disease usually occurs with little or no warning, so that the person often injures himself when he falls. Many other conditions can cause sudden fainting, however. Fainting followed by weakness, sweating, and nausea usually stems from nervous tension.

Chest pains are the symptoms most persons associate with heart disease, but these, too, may have many other explanations. Dull aching or sharp pains in the left side of the chest are rarely caused by heart disease. Pain lasting more than 15 minutes usually is caused by some other condition. Occasionally, momentary severe chest pains may result from premature contractions of the heart, but these are of no serious significance.

On the other hand, pain precipitated by walking and relieved in a few minutes by rest is characteristic of angina pectoris (meaning "strangling in the chest"), and usually stems from heart disease, especially disease of the coronary arteries. The pain strikes anywhere in the upper half of the body, but most commonly is felt in the center of the chest. Use of the arms or a strong emotion often precipitates the pain, and cold weather or eating may bring it on more quickly. Dreams sometimes initiate chest pains, or pain may occur when the individual first lies down at night. Mild shortness of breath, nausea, and sweating may accompany the pain.

Listening to the heart. When a doctor listens to the heartbeat, he or she often gets important clues to heart disease. The sounds are better heard than described. Medical students learn to recognize them from tapes, not books. It usually is said that the normal adult heart makes paired sounds described as a noise like "lubb-dupp." The thudding "lubb" represents the closing of the mitral and tricuspid valves and the beginning of the ventricular contraction. The higher-pitched "dupp" represents the clicking shut of the aortic and pulmonic valves. A third sound of any sort may indicate heart disease.

Heart noises include swishing, whooshing, clicking, crackling, and even breathing sounds. They may be harsh and noticeable or faint. Some are classified as murmurs, prolonged noises occupying a part of the heart cycle, but murmurs also may be heard in normal people. Loud systolic murmurs, occurring during the contraction phase, usually indicate heart disease, but softer murmurs often are normal and are almost universal in children. Diastolic murmurs, occurring during the resting phase, always indicate heart disease, although it may not be serious. Rubbing sounds over

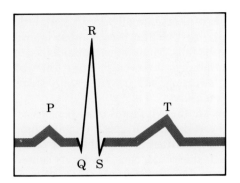

THE ELECTROCARDIOGRAM
The path of electrical impulse through the heart can be traced by an electrocardiogram, or ECG. The waves and spikes are given alphabetical designations. Above, the P wave represents electrical stimulation of the atrium. The QRS complex shows the spread of electrical activity through the ventricles. The T wave is the recovery of the ventricle after stimulation.

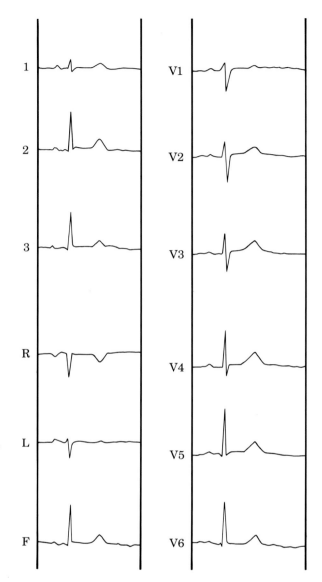

the heart may be a sign of inflammation of the pericardium, or pericarditis. Crackling sounds over the lower part of the lungs in the back may indicate congestion, a clue to inefficient action of the heart.

Besides these extraneous noises, the heartbeat may be rapid and irregular, but this seldom is a specific sign of heart disease.

The electrocardiogram. If heart disease is suspected, an electrocardiogram may be performed in the doctor's office to record electrical activity within the heart muscle. With the person lying down or resting in a chair, a set of electrodes, or "leads," are affixed to several parts of the body and attached to a machine, where moving pens trace the electrical rhythm on a moving strip of paper. The leads to the arms and legs are identified as 1, 2, 3, R, L, and F; those to the chest are usually V-1 to V-6. Positioning is important because limb leads are most useful in diagnosing irregularities of heart rhythm and certain types of heart attacks, while the chest leads are more helpful in diagnosing problems of enlargement of the heart and other types of heart attacks.

The line traced by the movements of the pen follows a readily interpreted pattern. The sharp spikes and smoother curves of the electrocardiogram are named for letters of the alphabet from P to T. The P wave is a small deflection representing

NORMAL HEART WAVES
To measure the heart's electrical activity, five to 10 wires are attached to small metal plates (electrodes) at various points on the body. The number of contact points depends on whether the combinations of wires are recorded simultaneously or in sequence. The wires from the arms and legs are designated 1, 2, 3, R, L, and F. Those on the chest are V-1 through V-6. Each lead produces a distinctive tracing. The normal patterns are shown above.

aortic valve (open)   mitral valve (open)

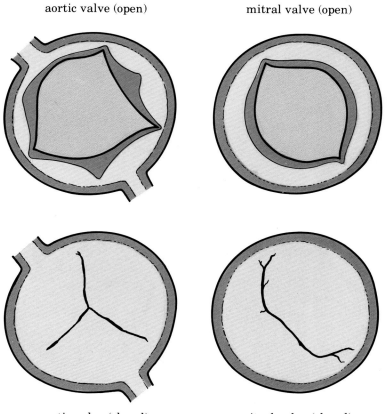

aortic valve (closed)   mitral valve (closed)

HOW THE VALVES WORK
Seen from above, the valves between the heart's upper and lower chambers look like this. The aortic valve, opening to the general circulation, has three cusps or leaflets that fold back to allow the blood to enter, then form a tight seal against backflow. The mitral valve, which controls flow on the heart's left side, has only two cusps that form a curved-line junction.

the electrical activity of the upper chambers of the heart (atria). Although there are two chambers, there is only one wave because the electrical events occur simultaneously in the two chambers. If the rhythm is abnormal, the P wave is abnormal, either in shape or frequency. The first downward deflection after the P wave is called the Q wave, the first upward wave is the R wave, and the downward deflection following the R wave is an S wave. Sometimes, this group of three is called the QRS complex. It represents electrical transmission through the ventricles. The usually smaller rounded wave after the QRS complex is the T wave. Abnormalities of the QRS complex are more specific than those of the T wave.

The electrocardiogram, often referred to as ECG or EKG, may be normal even though heart disease is present. Because it records only the heart's electrical activity, it may be essential in diagnosing disturbances of the heart rhythm, and it provides important clues to other conditions, but is not infallible in disclosing heart disease.

An office electrocardiogram, moreover, records electrical activity only during the brief period of examination. Sometimes a fleeting, intermittent disturbance of heart rhythm is suspected, yet cannot be captured by ordinary means. In such cases, a continuous tape recording of the electrocardiogram for 12 to 24 hours may be required. To achieve this, a person may wear a miniature recording device as he or she goes about daily activity. Or a disturbance may be suspected only when the heart is stressed. Then an ECG may be taken during and after exercise performed on a two-step staircase, a calibrated bicycle, or a treadmill.

X ray of the chest is most useful in determining the size of the heart, or in showing enlargement of one or more chambers, which gives a clue to the presence or severity of certain anatomical defects. The X ray also will show the lungs and arteries supplying the lungs, and disclose congestion or increased circulation.

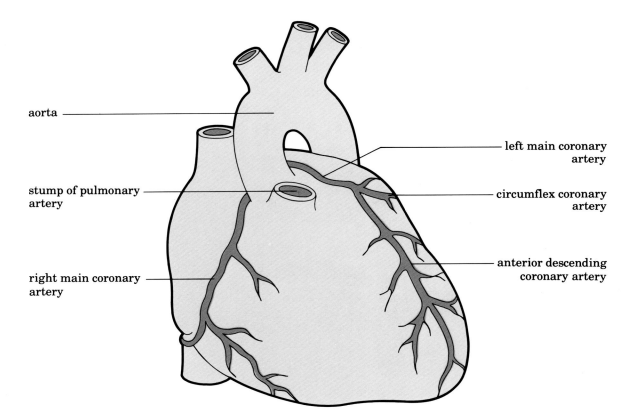

aorta

stump of pulmonary artery

right main coronary artery

left main coronary artery

circumflex coronary artery

anterior descending coronary artery

CORONARY ARTERIES

The heart's own blood supply is received via the coronary arteries, so called because they are said to resemble a crown. The right main coronary artery supplies the right ventricle and part of the left ventricle. The left main coronary artery has two large branches, *the anterior descending artery and the circumflex artery, which circles around the back of the heart. Consequently, it is often said that there are three coronary arteries. In this drawing, the pulmonary artery has been cut away to show the left main coronary artery.*

The echocardiogram is a painless test using sound waves to gain information about the interior of the heart. A blunt probe that emits a sound wave is applied to the surface of the chest over the heart. The echocardiograph measures the time required for the wave to strike a portion of the heart and be reflected back to the probe. Sometimes a movable probe or several probes are used. Fluid in the sac around the heart (pericardial fluids), valve defects, abnormalities during contraction, and variations in chamber size or wall thickness can be disclosed by this method.

Radioactive substances also are used to investigate coronary disease. The amount of material taken up by the heart muscle or passed through the chambers may be measured. Sometimes this method is combined with electrocardiographic exercise testing.

Catheterization. For some conditions, only catheterization of the heart will yield the information needed for proper treatment, especially when surgery is required. Catheterization means insertion of a tiny flexible tube through the circulation to obtain an accurate "road map" of blood flow. It is particularly important for repair of most congenital heart defects, in valve problems, or in surgical treatment of coronary artery disease.

Either or both sides of the heart may be catheterized, depending on the problem. The procedure is carried out with local anesthesia, and the patient is unaware of the passage of the flexible catheter through the circulation. A small incision is made in the arm or groin, and the catheter is inserted or threaded over a wire that has been inserted through the skin into a vessel. If a vein is used, the right side of the heart is studied. If an artery is used, the left side of the heart is investigated. Pressures in the various chambers may be measured, the pressure waves in the chambers recorded, the output (the amount of blood pumped) of the heart determined, and photographs of the chambers or coronary arteries obtained. The risk of this procedure is slight, and the importance of the information it produces usually outweighs that risk.

Other clues to heart disease. Besides the symptoms above, there are two other serious conditions common to several types of heart disease.

Congestive heart failure occurs when the heart's output is not enough to meet the demands of the body. Sometimes the output may be normal, but the demands, excessive. This occurs in such unusual conditions as toxic thyroid, thiamine chloride deficiency (vitamin B_1), and abnormal connections between a major artery and a vein. More commonly, congestive heart failure occurs because the heart pumps inadequately as a result of disease in the muscle or pericardium, or because of narrowing of a valve.

In all of these conditions, the body retains sodium (salt), which causes retention of excess water. The fluid accumulates most obviously in the lungs and in the legs. Shortness of breath occurs because of the fluid, and the person may be unable to lie down, or may awaken with acute breathing difficulty, usually relieved by sitting up for 5 to 15 minutes. Sometimes the shortness of breath persists longer at night and is accompanied by wheezing and cough, a condition known as cardiac asthma. These are signs of serious heart disease and are indications for intensive treatment. Response to treatment usually is good. Sodium in the form of salt or baking soda is restricted, and a drug called digitalis or a derivative is given. Diuretics (drugs to promote the loss of fluids) are prescribed.

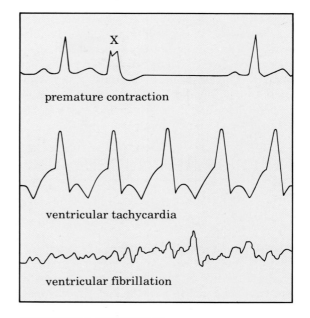

ABNORMAL RHYTHMS
Three types of disturbed ventricular rhythms produce these distinctive electrocardiogram tracings. The top line depicts premature contraction of a ventricle (marked X), a common abnormality sometimes described as "skipping a beat." In ventricular tachycardia (center line), the heart rate is rapid and the rhythm is slightly irregular. The width of the QRS complex is increased. The bottom line shows ventricular fibrillation, a very serious abnormality. It is characterized by irregular and extremely rapid contractions, and is fatal unless corrected quickly.

In severe cases, medication to relax the blood vessels and lower the blood pressure may be used. It is important to determine the cause of congestive heart failure and to correct the cause if possible.

Blood clots are another serious complication of several types of heart disease. A clot (thrombus) tends to form in the heart if blood flow in a chamber is extraordinarily sluggish or if the endocardium or valves are inflamed. This may result from narrowing of the mitral valve associated with irregularity of heartbeat. Or it may stem from bacterial infection of a valve, severe impairment of pumping action, acute damage to the endocardium as a result of a heart attack, or a bulge (aneurysm) of the left ventricle resulting from a previous heart attack. Clots in the heart may break off and flow to any part of the body where they may lodge in smaller arteries and obstruct circulation, causing damage or even death. Such a clot is called an embolus. The most serious are those going to the brain, though often the clots are small and cause no permanent disability. Anticoagulants and surgery offer protection against recurrences.

TYPES OF HEART DISEASE

Heart disease may be classified in several ways, but a common method is by cause.

Abnormalities of Rhythm

Abnormalities of the heart rhythm (arrhythmias) are common. In fact, the majority of apparently healthy people have a type of rhythm disturbance called premature contraction, although few are aware of it. Some persons have only occasional irregularity, but others have periods in which every other beat is premature. A spot in an atrium or ventricle discharges electrically without waiting for the impulse to be received from the sinus node. There is a pause following this discharge, then normal rhythm is restored. Some people are aware of the irregularity and say that their heart "stops," or "turns flip-flops," or "skips." Occasionally, a momentary sharp pain may be experienced. Treatment seldom is required, but drugs may be prescribed if symptoms are bothersome.

Atrial paroxysmal tachycardia is an irregularity in which the atria beat about 180 times a minute, two to three times the normal rate. The ventricles respond to each beat. The rhythm is regular. Attacks begin and end abruptly, lasting for a few seconds to hours. Attacks occur more commonly in young people than in the elderly and often disappear in middle or old age. Sweating, weakness, and palpitation may accompany the attacks. Sometimes the attacks may be stopped by forceful breath-holding, voluntary gagging, immersing the face in ice-cold water for 30 seconds, or pressing on a nerve center near the angle of the jaw. Occasionally, medical treatment is required, and may be needed to prevent frequent episodes.

Atrial flutter is marked by an atrial rate of about 300 beats per minute. The ventricles respond to alternate atrial contractions, so the pulse rate is about 150 per minute and usually is regular. Drugs can be used to slow the ventricular rate

until the attack ends. Electric shock across the chest during brief anesthesia will end an attack.

Atrial fibrillation. Rheumatic disease of the mitral valve is likely to cause extremely rapid and incomplete contractions of the atria. Fibrillation starts suddenly, although the patient may not be aware of it. The rate is variable, usually 120 to 160 beats per minute, and the rhythm is irregular. The rate can be controlled by drugs. Electric shock may be used to restore normal rhythm.

Ventricular tachycardia usually is associated with organic heart disease. A small area in one ventricle starts beating spontaneously at a rapid rate, with slightly irregular rhythm. The atrial rhythm does not change. The output of blood from the heart may decrease severely. Marked weakness, sweating, and even fainting may occur if the rate is rapid. Some attacks end spontaneously, but often drug treatment or an electric shock is required to end them.

A large family of drugs now exists to suppress ventricular tachycardias. Often, the cardiologist will induce tachycardia in a catheterization laboratory, then prescribe the specific drug that best suppresses it. This method has made possible the successful management of many tachycardias, even in the presence of serious heart disease.

Ventricular fibrillation usually is fatal unless stopped by treatment in a matter of minutes. Although there is electrical activity in the ventricles, the contraction of the heart is uncoordinated and the aortic valve does not open. The flow of blood stops and unconsciousness occurs in five to eight seconds. External massage of the heart accompanied by mouth-to-mouth breathing will maintain circulation temporarily, and external electric shock will restore normal rhythm in many cases. Organic heart disease usually is responsible, so the outlook may not be good unless the basic problem can be corrected.

Ventricular asystole is similar to ventricular fibrillation, except there is no electrical activity in the ventricle, so the beat stops. Occasionally, a vigorous blow over the heart will restore beating. External heart massage and artificial respiration may maintain life until normal rhythm can be restored. Sometimes, a temporary electrical pacemaker may be used and a permanent unit installed later if the response has been good.

Heart block occurs when transmission of the electrical impulse from the atrium to the ventricles through the conduction system is partially or completely blocked. In partial block, some impulses are transmitted, and others are not. Sometimes, alternate beats are blocked, causing a slow heart rate, or there may be a total block of all impulses so that the atria and ventricles beat at different rates, the ventricle at about half the normal rate. This is called complete heart block, and it is a serious abnormality. The rate of ventricle contractions can be increased with drugs, but much more effectively with an artificial pacemaker.

Bundle branch block is sometimes confused with complete heart block. In this condition, however, the impulse from the atrium reaches the bundle of His normally, but transmission through one of the bundle branches is blocked. The impulse that starts contraction of the ventricles is transmitted throughout the heart but more directly to one ventricle than to the other. People who have bundle branch blocks often live normal life spans without disability. Occasionally, the block may progress to complete heart block.

Treatment of arrhythmias. There are three important methods used for treating critical heartbeat irregularities.

External resuscitation, also called cardiopulmonary resuscitation, often is used by trained lay persons and paramedical personnel. It is described in Chapter 35, "Emergency."

Electric shock treatment usually stops ventricular fibrillation. Large metal paddles are applied to the skin of the chest and a strong shock is passed through the heart. The heart muscle reacts by contracting uniformly, and normal rhythm is restored. Shock also may be used to stabilize less serious rhythm abnormalities. Electric shock is less risky and more effective than drug treatment in many instances.

An artificial pacemaker is a miniature electrical device installed within the body to stimulate the heart to beat rhythmically. Some pacemakers are developed for specific purposes, but the common type operates at a fixed rate, which usually is adjustable. The pacemaker may stimulate continually or only when the heart rate falls below a certain level. The impulse is transmitted through wires contained in a small tube, the tip of which is wedged into the right ventricle. The generating portion of the unit is buried under the skin of the chest or abdomen. Sometimes, a wire is attached to the surface of the heart for stimulation.

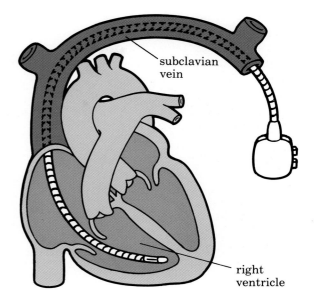

THE PACEMAKER
A battery-powered electrical device called a pacemaker can be implanted in the chest to regulate an erratic heart to beat rhythmically. The generating unit is implanted in the chest, and impulses are transmitted via wires to the right ventricle. Some pacemakers can be left in place up to 10 years, and some may be recharged without removing them.

Originally, the batteries of permanent units lasted a year or two, but improvements have resulted in an estimated battery life of 10 years. Some pacemakers need not be removed for recharging. Complete heart block is the most common reason for installing a pacemaker.

Congenital Heart Disease

Heart defects present at birth are of two general types: cyanotic ("blue babies") and noncyanotic. The noncyanotic types are more common, and most can be corrected surgically.

Septal defects are holes in the wall (septum) separating the right and left side of the heart. Normally, the fetus has an opening between the atria so that blood can pass between them without circulating through the lungs, because fetal lungs contain no air. This opening, called the foramen

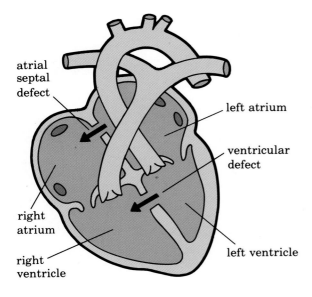

atrial
septal
defect

left atrium

ventricular
defect

right
atrium

right
ventricle

left ventricle

HEART DEFECTS
*Two types of congenital heart defects
are shown here, although they seldom
occur together. The arrow at top
indicates an atrial septal defect, or
opening in the wall separating the right
and left atria, which allows oxygenated
and unoxygenated blood to mix. An
opening is normal in the fetus, but
usually closes at birth. The lower arrow
shows a ventricular defect, which causes
abnormal flow out of the left ventricle.
Small defects may close naturally.
Others can be corrected surgically.*

ovale, normally closes at birth. Defects in the up-per septum often are small and cause no complica-tions throughout life. If they are large, however, a considerable amount of blood may be transferred from the left to the right atrium because the pres-sure is slightly higher in the left. That means the right side of the heart must pump several times as much blood as the left. The vessels of the lungs en-large to accommodate the additional blood flow. Eventually, the high blood flow through the lungs may cause changes in the structure and function of the vessels and blood pressure may rise. Irrevers-ible changes in the vessels may develop. The treat-ment is surgical. Small defects are closed by

stitches and larger ones eliminated by sewing a patch of synthetic material over the hole. The risk of the operation is minimal.

A defect in the lower atrial septum is less com-mon than in the upper portion and often is associ-ated with an abnormality of the mitral valve. It may be accompanied by a loud murmur. These defects also can be closed, although closure is more difficult. Often, the mitral valve must be repaired or replaced.

The ventricular septum also may have defects, which allow blood to flow from the left to the right ventricle because of the left's higher pressure. Usu-ally, a loud, characteristic murmur discloses the abnormal opening. An unusually large defect may cause heart failure in infancy or childhood, but often it is well tolerated. Some of these holes close spontaneously as a child develops. If not, or if serious problems arise early in childhood, surgical closure can be done at low risk. The technique is similar to that for septal defects between the atria.

Pulmonic stenosis, narrowing of the pulmonic valve, is the most common important congenital valve defect of the heart. This valve lies at the outflow of the right ventricle and normally has three cusps. The cusps are fused in pulmonic ste-nosis, with only a small central opening for blood to flow to the lungs. The valve may be opened relatively simply, with little risk and good results. Sometimes, the muscular tissue just below the pul-monic valve narrows the outflow track of the right ventricle. This, too, may be treated surgically, but the procedure is more difficult.

"Blue babies" most commonly are victims of a condition called tetralogy of Fallot, named for the French physician who first described it. Tetralogy means there are four defects but only two are essential to understanding the condition: pulmonic stenosis and interventricular septal defect. If pul-monic stenosis is severe, the pressure in the right ventricle may exceed that in the left, so blood flows from right to left. The blood in the right ventricle has not been circulated to the lungs, so it is "blue." If the flow is large, the skin and lips have a bluish tinge.

Recent advances in surgery make it possible to do a total correction of tetralogy of Fallot in one operation with excellent results.

Patent ductus arteriosus is not a true congeni-tal heart defect but a condition of the arteries. The ductus arteriosus is a vessel through which blood passes from the pulmonary artery to the aorta, the body's main artery, in the fetus before birth. Nor-mally, it closes soon after birth, but sometimes it remains open, allowing blood to pass from the aorta to the pulmonary artery because of the higher pressure in the aorta. This leakage puts an added burden on the heart. Cutting the ductus and sewing the two ends together is a relatively simple surgical treatment that repairs the problem.

Coarctation of the aorta also is a congenital arterial defect. The aorta is narrowed severely or completely closed just beyond the beginning of the artery that supplies the left arm. Blood may reach the lower part of the body by way of collateral arteries, which reroute the blood from vessels in and about the neck through the various connecting arteries until it finally empties into the aorta in the lower chest or abdomen. If the involved portion of the aorta is large and the two cut ends cannot be sewed together directly, the narrowed area of the aorta can be removed and a fabric graft used to bring the two ends together.

Rheumatic Heart Disease

Rheumatic fever is an inflammation resulting from a bacterial infection of the throat by an organism called the hemolytic streptococcus. It is related to scarlet fever, the kidney disorder called Bright's disease or glomerulonephritis, and other conditions caused by delayed reaction to a particular kind of "strep" infection. Symptoms usually begin about two weeks after the initial illness and last several weeks or months. They often include fever plus joint pain and swelling, but may be so mild that the condition is not recognized. The heart is affected in about half of the cases, sometimes seriously and even fatally. The victim, usually a child, generally recovers from the acute attack, but recurrences are frequent.

Rheumatic fever was once common and widely feared in the United States. The incidence began to decrease in the 1930s and has continued to decline. It still is common in less developed countries.

Rheumatic heart disease develops during rheumatic fever, but often causes no symptoms for a decade or more. In at least half of the cases, the person cannot recall the earlier episode. The disease deforms the valves by scarring them, so the heart must work harder to pump blood. The valves on the left side of the heart are affected more frequently than those on the right.

Various combinations of valve defects occur in rheumatic heart disease, and characteristic murmurs are generated by each. In mitral valve disease, atrial fibrillation is a common complication. If the disease is severe, shortness of breath and congestive heart failure may occur. Fainting, pain, and shortness of breath also may strike those with aortic stenosis. Congestive heart failure is a common complication of any form of rheumatic heart disease.

If all rheumatic fever could be prevented, rheumatic heart disease would be eliminated. Similarly, if streptococcal infections were prevented or treated immediately, rheumatic fever would not be a problem. Unfortunately, many streptococcal infections may cause only mild symptoms difficult to notice, and even severe sore throats in children are not always treated aggressively. Rheumatic fever itself also must be treated properly. After an attack, oral penicillin may be administered regularly for years to prevent recurrences.

If rheumatic heart disease has caused severe symptoms, surgery may be necessary. Often, catheterization of the heart is required before the operation, especially in middle-aged and elderly persons, who constitute the majority of symptomatic patients today.

Often, calcium is deposited in a scarred valve that has been damaged by rheumatic heart disease. The hardened mineral prevents the valve from opening and closing normally. In rare cases, the valve will function quite well if the calcium is removed and the valve is opened surgically, but usually the affected valve must be replaced with an artificial substitute (see Chapter 33, "Understanding Your Operation").

Early valve operations were done by touch, and only mitral stenosis could be treated well. Even then, the results were only fair. Later, it became possible to replace temporarily the pumping function of the heart with a heart-lung machine. This device receives "blue blood" from the veins, passes it through oxygenators, and returns it to the arterial side of the circulation. The heart thus can be opened and operated on under direct vision while the heart-lung machine does the heart's work.

Open-heart surgery has brought vast benefits. In mitral stenosis, the valve can be opened under direct vision more effectively than in the days when the finger was used blindly, and valve replacements can only be performed with a heart-lung machine. Formerly, a great deal of blood was required for the heart-lung machine, but now only a pint or two may be necessary, sometimes none.

Although surgery to open valves remains common, the method often used today is balloon angioplasty, described in detail below, in which a

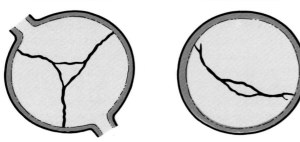

aortic stenosis   mitral stenosis

VALVE DISEASE
When the aortic or mitral valves become diseased, scar tissue prevents them from opening or closing normally. At left, aortic stenosis has fused the valve except for a small central portion, shown in the open position. At right, scar tissue has formed along the leaflets of the mitral valve so that only a small area, as shown, can open to permit blood flow.

catheter with a tiny balloon is threaded through a leg artery into the heart. The balloon is then suddenly inflated, forcing the valve open.

The development of artificial prosthetic valves also has been a great advance. There are two general types. One is made of plastic and metal and the other of human or animal tissue, often combined with a supportive artificial skeleton. The most commonly used valves are taken from pigs, giving them the name porcine valves. Although these valves tend to deteriorate after about seven years, they are preferred because they produce fewer complications. Plastic valves may be a ball or disk seated in a ring and enclosed in a cage. The great advantage of tissue valves is that "blood thinners" (anticoagulants) that prevent development of clots around the valves are required for only a short time after operation.

Most often, a single valve is replaced, but sometimes two or three valves are required. Recovery is rapid and long-term results are usually good.

Nonrheumatic Valve Disease

Besides rheumatic valvular disease, there are several other types of valve problems, grouped as nonrheumatic defects.

Prolapse (ballooning) of the mitral valve is the most common. The valve closes properly but reopens during the middle of the contraction phase.

By this point, most of the blood has been pumped out of the left ventricle, so little blood leaks into the left atrium. In mild cases, there is no leak; although the valve balloons, it does not reopen. When the valve balloons, a distinct "click" often is heard.

The anatomy of the mitral valve includes small threads of tissue called chordae tendineae, which connect to the muscular wall of the left ventricle. For reasons unknown, these threads sometimes degenerate and rupture, causing severe mitral insufficiency. This condition is relatively rare, and surgical treatment is required.

The normal valve tissue is thin but strong. In rare instances, however, it degenerates and thins further. The valves enlarge and sometimes tear. Either the mitral or aortic valve may be affected, and replacement is required.

Aortic stenosis is mentioned under rheumatic heart disease, but more commonly is nonrheumatic. Often it is congenital, in which case the valve has two leaflets instead of three. Symptoms are the same as in rheumatic aortic stenosis: shortness of breath, fainting, pain, and eventual congestive heart failure. Sometimes, the original defect is mild, but calcium deposits gradually build up in the valve and further narrow the opening. Most cardiologists believe that there also is a form of nonrheumatic, noncongenital aortic stenosis, because aortic stenosis often occurs in middle-aged people who have not had a murmur early in life.

Diseases of the Heart Muscle

The muscle of the heart (myocardium) is responsible for the pumping action. If the entire muscle is severely diseased, the force of contraction is decreased and heart failure results. There are several causes of heart muscle damage.

Viral infections sometimes damage the heart muscle. The damage may be difficult to diagnose because the cardiac manifestations may be delayed for days or weeks after the fever of the original illness has subsided, or the symptoms may have been so mild that they are not recalled at a later date. There is no specific treatment other than the measures used to treat congestive heart failure. Permanent damage, even death, may result.

Defects of metabolism. Normally, the heart extracts oxygen and nutrients from the blood supplied to it and uses them to provide the energy needed for contractions. This is a complex chemical process, and it is suspected that the chemical reactions in some way go awry. The usual symptom is congestive heart failure, and sometimes there are rhythm irregularities. There may be periods of symptoms separated by long intervals in which the heart seems perfectly healthy. With effective treatment, patients may survive for many years.

Hypertension (high blood pressure) puts a strain on the heart because of the increased work demand. Hypertension is discussed in detail in Chapter 8.

Subaortic stenosis, which means narrowing under the aortic valve, is a peculiar heart ailment that mimics rheumatic valvular disease yet is different. The left side of the wall (septum) between the ventricles enlarges, narrowing the channel through which blood must flow to reach the aortic valve. Usually, there is an abnormality of the mitral valve as well. Treatment with beta-blocking drugs to decrease the strength of contraction of the heart muscle can be helpful. An operation is rarely required. The cause of subaortic stenosis is unknown. Some think it is a congenital defect that often goes unrecognized until adult life.

ARTERIOSCLEROTIC
HEART DISEASE

Arteriosclerosis, popularly known as hardening of the arteries, is universal with advancing age. It is not known whether the thickening and hardening of the arterial walls and the loss of their elasticity represents a natural phenomenon or is the result of diseases. Under certain conditions, arteriosclerosis may occur even in childhood, and there is evidence that the process begins early in life.

Arteriosclerosis does no harm if the process does not decrease the inside diameter of the arteries. In the form called atherosclerosis, the lining membrane (intima) of one or more arteries becomes thickened, and a fatty substance called cholesterol is deposited. As deposits build up, blood must pass through a tube smaller than normal. A clot may form in the narrowed opening and stop blood flow completely.

None of the arteries are spared from the arteriosclerotic process (see Chapter 6, "Blood Vessel Disorders," and Chapter 13, "Stroke"). Common targets, however, are the coronary arteries controlling the blood supply to the heart. Disease of these arteries is widespread in Western society. It is the leading cause of death in the United States and most of Europe. Symptoms arise when the narrowed arteries choke off the blood flow to the heart muscle.

Although the basic features of coronary arteriosclerosis are well known, the explanation for them is still debated despite a great deal of research. The fat (cholesterol) deposited in the lining membrane (intima) may be accompanied by clumps of blood platelets (necessary for normal clotting of the blood). Many cardiologists think that the primary problem is a defect in fat metabolism that leaves fats that accumulate in the lining membrane. About half of the people who have coronary disease show abnormal amounts of fat in the blood. Other cardiologists think that deposits of blood platelets or occasionally blood clots come first and that fats later invade the affected areas. A recent theory is that the problem does not start in the lining membrane but in the middle wall of the artery. The muscle cells in the middle wall migrate into the lining membrane, where they degenerate. Fat then is deposited in the degenerated cells. More understanding of the mechanism of arteriosclerosis is necessary if effective prevention and treatment are to be expected.

The risk factors. Statistically, certain circumstances increase the chances that a person will develop coronary arteriosclerosis. Risk factors are not synonymous with causes of coronary artery disease. They are simply characteristics found in large population samples that are associated with increased likelihood of developing the disease.

● *Age* is the most obvious risk factor. Coronary disease is more common in the elderly, and is diagnosed most frequently between the ages of 45 and 55.

● *Heredity.* If one of your parents had coronary disease before age 50, your risk is significantly increased.

● *Being male.* Men are more likely to be affected than women before the age of 50, but the risks are about even after age 60.

● *Obesity.* Distribution of excess weight (abdominal girth, or "pot belly") may be more important than amount. Physically active people appear less likely to develop coronary disease than those who are sedentary.

● *Smoking.* Avoiding cigarettes may be the single most important step toward preventing coronary disease. The increase in smoking among young women may be one explanation for increased coronary disease in females.

● *Stress.* Some believe that the Type A personality—the conscientious, compulsive "doer"—

strongly increases the likelihood of coronary disease, but others are less sure.

● *High blood pressure* (hypertension) is definitely associated with coronary disease as well as other disease of the blood vessels. So is diabetes (see Chapter 19, "Diabetes Mellitus"), especially when it is acquired early in life.

● *Cholesterol.* The higher the level of cholesterol in the blood, the greater the risk of heart disease. Although some persons still differ with that statement, repeated government studies substantiate it and have shown that lowering cholesterol levels reduces that risk. Accordingly, the government has recommended that persons with cholesterol readings greater than 200 milligrams per deciliter of blood (200 mg/dl) take steps to reduce it. That applies to half the U.S. population, and 95 percent of adult men.

Cholesterol is a natural substance manufactured in the body and vital for cell membranes and hormones. It also is found in many foods, especially eggs and meats. Normally, the body makes all the cholesterol it needs, and excess taken in by diet is excreted. However, it also may accumulate in the blood and in blood vessels.

Cholesterol may be lowered by diet or drugs. A new family of drugs has been successful in cholesterol reduction and is recommended for persons with cholesterol levels above 240 mg/dl—about one in four adults. Drug treatment, however, is expensive and lifelong. For others, the government recommends a diet in which less than 30 percent of calories come from saturated fat—mainly animal fat. The recommended diet calls for not more than six ounces daily of lean meat, fish, or chicken; low-fat dairy products; no butter; and not more than four eggs a week.

Cholesterol combines with proteins for transport in the blood and thus is found in two forms. High-density lipoproteins (HDL) appear to exert a protective effect against heart disease. Low-density lipoproteins (LDL) are the bad guys that appear to accumulate in arterial walls. Some doctors believe the balance between HDL and LDL may be more important than total cholesterol. Exercise appears to reduce "bad" LDL and increase "good" HDL.

The so-called coronary risk factors do not fully explain the occurrence of the disease. Certainly, no risk factor has been shown to be a direct cause of disease. Protecting against heart disease is an important part of a preventive approach to health, and is covered in Chapter 1, "Prevention."

Symptoms of Coronary Disease

In chronic coronary disease, angina pectoris (chest pain) is the most common symptom.

The chest pain of angina pectoris results when the work demanded of the heart is greater than the blood flow that can be delivered through the coronary arteries. Usually, this occurs because the work load is increased by exertion or emotional upset. Sometimes, the work load is unchanged and the inadequate flow is caused by a spasm that clamps down one or more arteries.

Walking is the most common activity to bring on the feelings of pain, pressure, tightness, and burning that characterize angina. The amount of exercise required to cause distress may remain the same for years or may increase with the passage of time. Improvement may stem from the development of small arteries (collateral vessels) which detour or reroute blood from one artery or part of an artery to another. These small arteries exist from birth but may increase in size in the presence of disease. In other cases of angina, the ability to walk is impaired progressively. Pain may come even at rest.

Heart Attack

The medical term for the common heart attack is myocardial infarction. This means death of heart muscle. Coronary thrombosis (blood clot) often is used to designate the same condition, but the two are not synonymous. Myocardial infarction occurs without coronary thrombosis, and coronary thrombosis occurs without myocardial infarction. Sometimes, a heart attack is spoken of as "a coronary." This is poor English as well as poor medicine.

Myocardial infarction is caused by a clot superimposed on plaque in a narrowed coronary artery. The result is an abrupt drop in blood flow. The drop may be so severe that a portion of heart muscle dies. Chest pain similar to that experienced with angina pectoris is the typical symptom, but usually is more severe, is not ordinarily precipitated by walking, and is prolonged for hours unless relieved by medication. The pain often is felt in the left arm and shoulder as well and may be accompanied by nausea, vomiting, sweating, and loss of consciousness.

Sometimes, there is only mild pain or none at all, and other symptoms are evidence of the heart attack. A large number of heart attacks are "si-

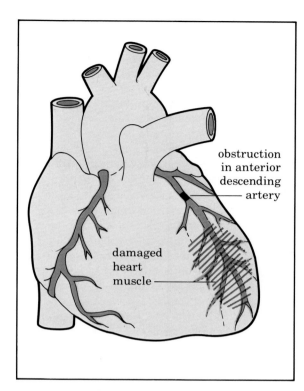

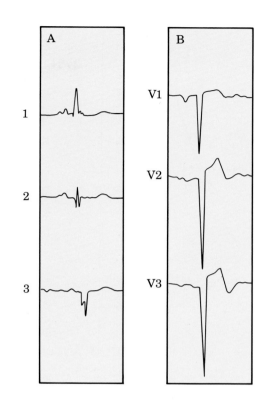

HEART ATTACK

The common heart attack, or myocardial infarction, occurs when one of the coronary arteries becomes blocked, usually by a blood clot lodged in a narrowed section of the artery. The blood supply is reduced or closed off and the heart muscle that depends on it is damaged or dies. The outlook for the victim depends on the amount of damage and its location. The accompanying electrocardiogram recorded during the attack shows a typical pattern when compared to the normal tracing on page 46. Drawing A shows damage to the bottom wall of the heart; drawing B, to the front wall. Some infarctions can be reversed by injection of a clot-dissolving substance.

lent," meaning that there is neither pain nor symptoms and damage is discovered only later. About one in four heart attacks fall into this category.

If it were possible to predict an impending heart attack, early treatment might prevent serious damage. Unfortunately, there are no reliable early warning signs. The appearance of pain not relieved by rest or nitroglycerin (if the drug is available) usually is the first symptom, but this is commonly a sign that the attack is taking place rather than a warning sign of something yet to come.

The initial symptoms of myocardial infarction often may be so vague that they are ignored or rationalized. Pain in the chest may be written off as indigestion, and perspiration blamed on mild fever or a warm day. Although speed is important in obtaining treatment, studies have shown that the average patient delays at least three hours after symptoms begin before seeking aid, and longer if the symptoms begin at night.

When myocardial infarction occurs, it is an emergency. Many persons die within minutes, before reaching a hospital or medical aid.

For those who do reach medical care within four hours, it is possible to dissolve the clot and reverse the heart attack. This lifesaving procedure uses one of several clot-dissolving substances—usually streptokinase, a naturally occurring substance, or tissue plasminogen activator (TPA), produced by techniques of genetic engineering. The drug is inserted into the blocked artery via the

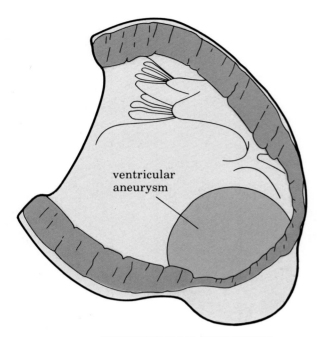

VENTRICULAR ANEURYSM

A ventricular aneurysm is a dome-shaped ballooning of the heart wall. It may develop after a heart attack if a large area of heart muscle has been damaged, as shown in this cross section. Paradoxically, the aneurysm may be stronger than the rest of the heart wall because it is composed of scar tissue. However, the heart may have to work harder because it pumps blood into the balloon-shaped area, and heart failure can result.

catheterization method. Results are swift, usually reversing symptoms within minutes. The treatment has reduced death rates for those reaching the hospital by 20 to 30 percent.

If these methods fail, emergency bypass surgery, described below, or balloon angioplasty also may reverse the attack.

In addition to heart muscle damage, blood pressure may decrease markedly during a heart attack, plunging the person into a state of shock. This is a serious complication, and the victim has a poor outlook. Sometimes, a balloon assist device is used to increase and maintain blood pressure. A catheter tube on which a deflated balloon is mounted is threaded through an artery, usually in the leg, and passed into the aorta, the body's main artery. The balloon can be inflated and deflated alternately to help the pumping of the heart. Inflation of the balloon is timed by the electrocardiogram to occur during the resting phase of the heart cycle, so that the natural and artificial pumps do not compete. Blood pressure often rises markedly and may be maintained at a satisfactory level for hours or days. Unless the heart's total pumping ability is severely impaired, the patient is gradually "weaned" from the balloon pump.

After recovery from an acute heart attack, a scar forms in the region of dead muscle. If the scar is not extensive, the total pumping action of the heart returns to normal, which is the usual outcome. However, damage may be widespread or there may be scars from previous attacks, so that the heart does not function efficiently as a pump. Heart failure may result. Or, when a large area is damaged, the wall of the heart may bulge, especially during contraction, assuming a dome-shaped appearance called ventricular aneurysm. In acute myocardial infarction, the thin wall of the heart may rupture, but ventricular aneurysms do not rupture because an aneurysm is composed of a strong scar, sometimes lined by blood clots. However, a large aneurysm reduces the heart's blood output because some blood is pumped into the bulge instead of out through the aortic valve. The result may be congestive heart failure. Some aneurysms are removed surgically.

Coronary Insufficiency

Coronary insufficiency causes more prolonged pain than angina pectoris, yet produces no evidence of damage to the heart muscle as in myocardial infarction. The patient usually has typical angina pectoris as well. The prolonged pains usually occur without any apparent cause, lasting for 15 minutes to hours. Sometimes one or more of these pains may strike just before a myocardial infarction ("heart attack"), but more frequently infarction does not follow.

Treating Coronary Artery Disease

The treatment of chronic coronary artery disease aims to decrease the work of the heart and increase the coronary circulation. Neither of these objectives attacks the basic problem, the narrowing or total obstruction of one or more arteries. An ideal treatment would restore the lining membrane of the coronary arteries to normal but no such approach has been developed. Future possibilities are promising because coronary arteriography has shown that severely obstructed areas occasionally tend to return to normal.

A class of drugs known as beta-blocking agents decreases the work of the heart by impairing the strength of contraction, slowing the pulse rate, and sometimes decreasing the blood pressure. The demand for coronary blood flow diminishes, so the reduced supply provided by the narrowed arteries may be sufficient. Angina may improve markedly or even disappear. Control of hypertension also can improve symptoms by decreasing demand.

Other drugs known as calcium blockers also have been successful in treating symptoms by lowering the heart's work load. Limiting physical activity or the speed of activity can do the same. Regular exercise is important, but repeatedly precipitating angina by exertion should be avoided. With regular exercise, it is possible to increase the amount of exercise performed before symptoms occur. This benefit appears to result from improvement in the efficiency of the skeletal muscles rather than from any direct effect on the heart.

Drugs called vasodilators (blood vessel expanders) are used to increase the coronary circulation. The best known is nitroglycerin, which usually relieves angina after a minute or two when placed under the tongue. Nitroglycerin also lowers blood pressure. The drug is destroyed rapidly in the body so that the effect dissipates in about 15 minutes. Because of its fast action and short-term effect, it sometimes is used before performance of an activity likely to precipitate pain, such as hurrying or sexual intercourse. But the short duration of effectiveness is a disadvantage, so longer-lasting drugs in combination with beta or calcium blockers often are used instead.

Few people are severely disabled by angina, although they may be inconvenienced. Some of the anxiety of angina patients stems from the realization that coronary disease is serious and angina serves as a recurrent reminder of the danger.

Coronary disease tends to be episodic rather than relentlessly progressive. A person may have angina for five years and then experience a myocardial infarction. After that, the angina may disappear or persist for 10 years, when another infarction may occur. Several years later, a third infarction may cause death. Another patient may die suddenly at the first sign of heart disease. Still another may have an infarction and live for 30 years without further problems. Statistically, a person who has suffered one infarction faces a greater risk of a second, but the statistic has little meaning in individual cases.

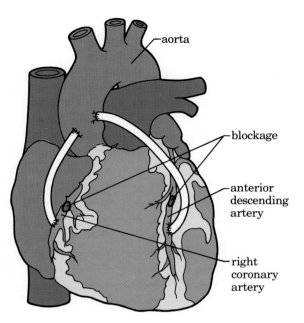

BYPASSING A BLOCK
The coronary bypass graft has become one of the most commonly performed operations. The two most common types use the saphenous vein from the leg or an internal mammary artery to detour blood flow around a blockage in a coronary artery. The graft at left shunts blood from the aorta to the right coronary artery; at right, to the anterior descending artery. Sometimes multiple grafts are performed.

Coronary Bypass Operations

The coronary bypass operation has become one of the most widely performed operations, with hundreds of thousands of bypasses each year. Its value remains controversial, however.

The most common bypass operation involves removing a vein from the leg and using a segment or several segments of the vein as conduits between the aorta and one or more of the coronary arteries. The grafts are inserted to bypass the narrowed area of the artery. If the graft remains open, which

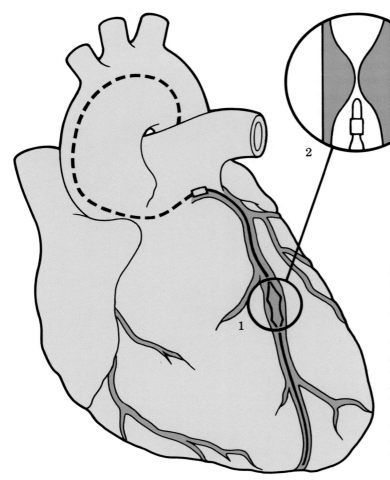

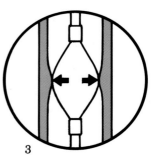

CORONARY ANGIOPLASTY
The technique of balloon angioplasty uses a child's toy to open narrowed coronary arteries. A tiny, sausage-shaped balloon is attached to a catheter, which is inserted into an artery in the groin and advanced until it reaches the area of the artery that has been narrowed by cardiovascular plaque. In drawing 2 above, the catheter has reached the blockage in the left anterior descending artery. The balloon then is moved into place in the narrowed section (drawing 3). Inflation of the balloon squeezes the plaque into the walls of the artery, or breaks it up, to reopen the channel. In 75 percent of cases, the channel remains open. Angioplasty sometimes is successfully performed during heart attack, and also is used to open blocked vessels elsewhere in the body.

it does in about 85 to 90 percent of cases, a normal blood flow may reach each artery grafted.

Another bypass technique, the internal mammary artery graft, connects one of the arteries inside the chest to a coronary artery. This operation is more difficult, but these vessels stay open more often. The left anterior descending artery is most feasible for this type of graft. Often, this operation is combined with a vein graft for other arteries.

In some cases, multiple grafts may be performed. Properly performed bypass surgery brings relief of angina, and therefore better quality of life, in properly selected patients. It is uncertain whether life is prolonged. The outlook seems better for patients at highest risk, those who have obstructions of the left main coronary artery or the three principal coronary arteries.

Bypass surgery does not cure coronary disease, but it does deal with the effects. Fortunately, narrowing of the coronary arteries tends to be most severe in the initial part of the artery, and the

surgeon grafts beyond this region. Graft failures due to obstruction may occur at any time, but most occur early, immediately after surgery.

Balloon Angioplasty

Another highly successful method of widening a narrowed artery eliminates surgically opening the chest and now is preferred to bypass surgery for many patients. In balloon angioplasty, a specially designed balloon catheter is threaded into a leg artery, then moved upward to the narrowed coronary artery under guidance of a TV monitor. Inflation of the balloon ruptures the lining membrane of the narrowed artery, and some of the material in the lining is carried away by the blood, leaving a much wider channel for blood flow.

Angioplasty is simpler and less costly, requires a shorter hospital stay than bypass surgery, and relieves symptoms in many persons. It has been most successful in younger persons with a single blocked artery, although it is used for multiple blockages, too. In about one in four persons, however, the blockage forms again, and a second procedure is required. Angioplasty occasionally triggers a nonfatal heart attack, and emergency bypass surgery is necessary.

Bacterial Endocarditis

Bacterial infection of the valves of the heart or, more rarely, other portions of the endocardium is called bacterial endocarditis. Bacteria usually enter the blood during an illness, such as a sore throat accompanied by fever, or after a dental or surgical procedure. The bacteria normally are destroyed quickly, but if the person has valve disease, the bacteria may set up an infection on the surface of the valve. Untreated bacterial endocarditis almost invariably is fatal. Acute infections generally are caused by a virulent organism and may follow operations, especially those of the urinary tract. Even normal valves then may be involved. There is high fever, and the responsible organism may be grown in a sample taken from the blood. Subacute bacterial endocarditis is less dramatic. The main symptom is mild intermittent fever that responds temporarily to antibiotics. Endocarditis attacks previously damaged valves or congenitally defective valves. Patients who have artificial valves are susceptible, too.

Both acute and subacute endocarditis may cause serious damage to the valve affected, during the infection's active phase or as a result of scarring from the healing process. Most patients respond well to prolonged treatment with antibiotics.

Pericarditis

Infection of the membrane that covers the heart is called pericarditis. Acute cases are marked by fever and usually pain in the middle of the chest or slightly to the left of the middle. Deep breathing accentuates the pain. The infection usually is caused by a virus, although in rare instances bacteria may be responsible. A scratch sound called a pericardial rub is heard in most cases. The electrocardiogram and echocardiogram usually show characteristic abnormalities, and the chest X ray may reveal an enlargement of the shadow of the heart because of excessive fluid formed by the pericardium. Occasionally, the fluid is so excessive that proper filling of the heart chambers is impaired, and the fluid must be removed with a needle or by surgery. Viral pericarditis usually subsides without treatment, but it sometimes recurs. Bacterial pericarditis responds to antibiotics.

The Heart Transplant

The first complete heart transplant was performed in 1966, and the procedure now is done routinely in many hospitals. At first, the transplanted heart was frequently rejected because the body's immune system identified it as foreign and acted to repel it. Since development of the drug cyclosporin, the problem of rejection has been greatly reduced. Many persons have lived 10 years or more with a transplanted heart, and some have undergone more than one transplant.

Heart transplant is most commonly considered when all or a large portion of the heart muscle is diseased, and the disease resists treatment. Age no longer is a barrier, and carefully matched hearts have been successfully transplanted into infants and persons in their sixties. Sometimes, because an impaired heart often compromises lung function, too, a heart and lungs are transplanted simultaneously. Success rates in these combination transplants also are high.

Although a heart transplant sounds heroic, it is not much more difficult for a skilled heart surgeon than replacing two heart valves. Indeed, the major drawback to heart transplant is the shortage of donor hearts. The donor heart must be from a relatively young and healthy person who has died from causes not related to the heart. The heart must be removed quickly and carefully preserved in a chemical solution, then rushed to the waiting recipient. A nationwide network has been established to see that donor hearts are immediately transferred to those needing them. Several states have added donor permission forms to driver's licenses, to allow drivers to contribute their organs in the event of death.

The "artificial heart" has received wide publicity, but early efforts were less than successful. None of the recipients of artificial hearts survived long, for reasons not fully understood. Federally supported research continues, but a fully reliable, portable heart is not considered a possibility in the foreseeable future. A form of artificial heart, the left ventricular assist device (LVAD), sometimes is implanted to keep an ailing heart functioning until a donor heart is available, but its use is limited.

CHAPTER 6

BLOOD VESSEL DISORDERS

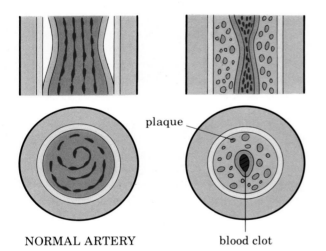

plaque

NORMAL ARTERY

blood clot

AN OBSTRUCTED ARTERY
The cross section at left shows a normal artery, with its central channel large enough for blood to flow through. At right, the artery has been partly obstructed. Deposits of fats, calcium, and smooth muscle cells have built up in the walls, narrowing the channel and providing a site for the formation of a blood clot.

Each thump of the heart pushes blood into a network of pipes called arteries. The blood travels through ever-smaller arteries until it reaches the microscopic capillaries that nourish the tissues. Then, having yielded its oxygen, it returns to the heart through another network of tubes, the veins. The arteries, veins, and heart, along with the lymphatics, are known as the vascular system.

Veins are larger than arteries, with thinner walls. They are equipped with valves to prevent backflow, because the blood in them is moving against the force of gravity. Venous circulation is smooth and even, in contrast to the pulsating movement of arterial circulation. Otherwise, the vessels are similar. They are made up of three layers: the tough outer casing, the fibrous middle layer, and the smooth inner bore. Disease or age can cause change in these layers. The result is vascular disease or disorders of the blood vessels.

OCCLUSIVE ARTERIAL DISEASE

The normal inner channel, or lumen, of an artery is smooth. In occlusive arterial diseases, however, the channel becomes narrowed or blocked and the blood flow is obstructed. The obstruction may occur suddenly (spasm), or gradually.

Arteriosclerosis Obliterans
(hardened and obstructed arteries)

Arteriosclerosis, the most common form of arterial disease, is the condition in which the arteries thicken, harden, and lose their elasticity.

This process usually is accompanied by a condition called atherosclerosis. Deposits of calcium, fats (especially cholesterol), and smooth muscle cells build up in arteries. The deposits, called plaques, provide sites where blood clots may form.

A blocked artery does not always cause destruction of tissue it supplies. A new network of small arteries will develop around the blocked area. This collateral circulation keeps the tissues alive, although it may not supply enough blood during exercise.

The hardening and deterioration of arteriosclerosis can affect any artery. If the arteries that supply the heart are affected, chest pain during exertion (angina pectoris) or a heart attack (myocardial infarction) can occur, as described in Chapter 5, "The Heart and Circulation." An obstruction in the arteries that lead to the brain can cause a stroke. If the blockage occurs in the arteries supplying the legs, walking becomes painful. If the problem isn't treated, gangrene and ultimate amputation result.

Causes. Arteriosclerosis obliterans affects almost all adults in some form, but the location, severity, and rate of development vary greatly. Heredity undoubtedly plays a part. The female hormone estrogen appears to provide protection, so that the disease is rare in women until age 50, when estrogen production declines.

A major factor in atherosclerosis appears to be excessive blood fats (lipids), particularly cholesterol. The increased amount may be related to both heredity and diet. Smoking, high blood pressure, obesity, diabetes, physical inactivity, and emotional stress also are risk factors.

Symptoms. The first symptom of arterial disease is usually a distinctive form of limping known as intermittent claudication. After walking a certain distance, the person develops pain, cramping, or weakness in one or both legs, which disappears within two to five minutes after he stops walking. The symptoms can be felt in the arch of the foot, the calf, thigh, buttock, or arm; they come sooner when walking fast or uphill. Pain at rest indicates a worsening of the condition. Severely painful skin ulcers and gangrene are the final result.

Treatment. The patient who smokes must stop. Nicotine causes contraction of the arteries.

A good exercise program is important. Leg exercises help improve circulation around the blocked artery. The patient should strive to walk at least an hour every day. Jogging, cycling, and swimming are encouraged.

Infections and injuries of the legs and feet should be prevented, because they will heal poorly. Shoes should be soft and comfortable, and fit properly. A lotion containing lanolin should be used regularly. Many amputations can be avoided with proper foot care and avoidance of extremely hot and cold temperatures.

Loss of excess weight also is important. A low-fat diet high in unsaturated fatty acids is advisable.

Angioplasty has revolutionized the surgical treatment of arterial disease, and often is preferred to the measures described above. This technique of reopening blocked arteries is described and illustrated in Chapter 5, "The Heart and Circulation."

Although most commonly directed at coronary arteries, angioplasty actually may be used for virtually any artery. A catheter is inserted into a leg artery and guided by monitor to the point of narrowing. The narrowing then may be reopened by the sudden inflation of a tiny balloon or by clearing away plaque with a laser beam. In the vast majority of cases, the artery remains open.

Drug treatment for arterial disease also is widely prescribed. These medications and their effects also are discussed in Chapter 5.

Buerger's Disease

Buerger's disease (thromboangiitis obliterans) affects the small and medium arteries and the veins in the arms and legs. The disease occurs almost exclusively in smokers.

The pain of Buerger's disease ranges from the lameness of calf muscles when walking to severe, steady pain of ulceration and gangrene. Toes and fingers are most commonly affected. About 40 percent of patients have blood clots in the veins.

ARTERIES AND VEINS

Pulmonary arteries carry blood to the lungs to receive oxygen. Blood then returns to the left side of the heart and is pumped to all parts of the body. The arteries are shown below, in the detailed "road map."

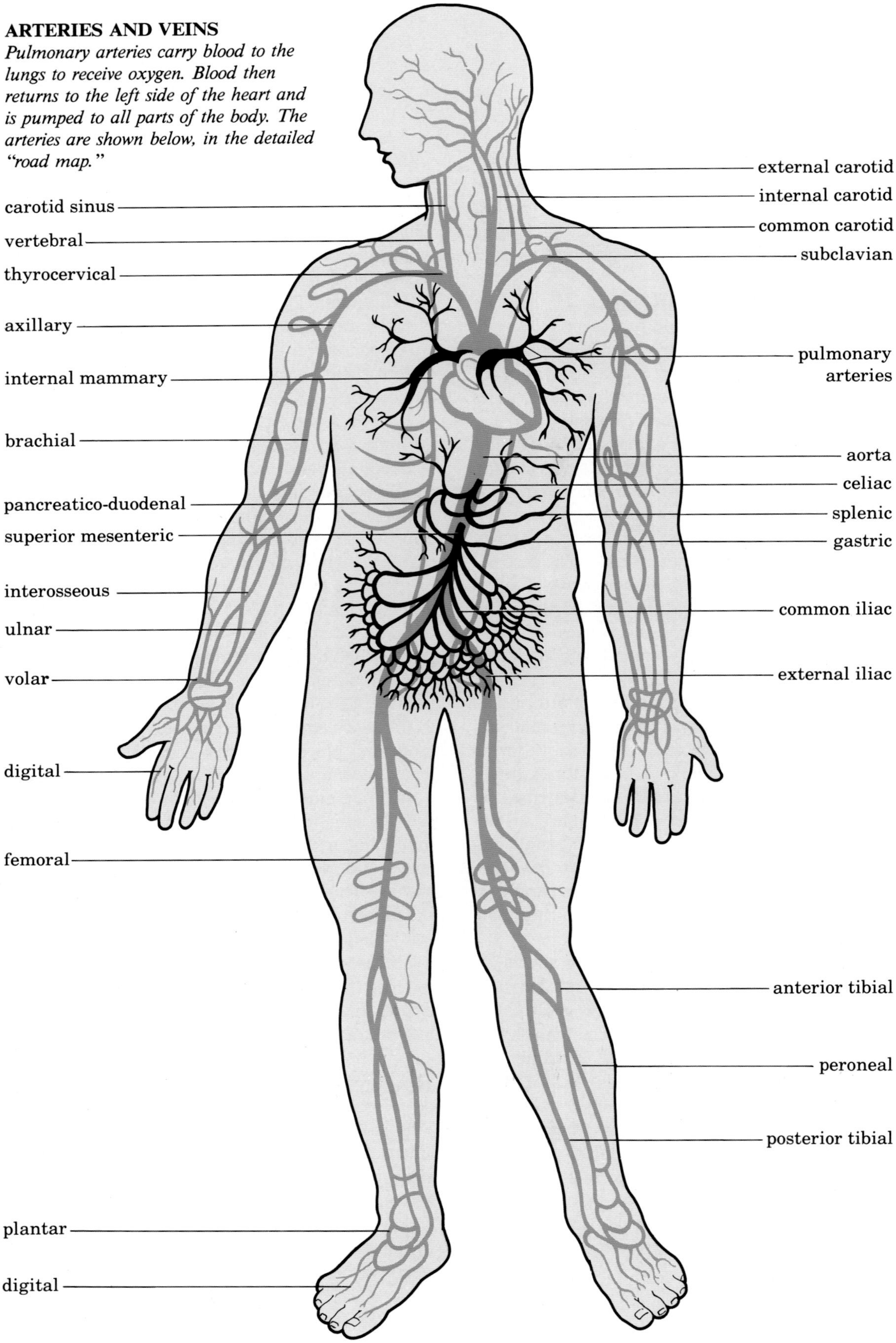

carotid sinus

vertebral

thyrocervical

axillary

internal mammary

brachial

pancreatico-duodenal

superior mesenteric

interosseous

ulnar

volar

digital

femoral

plantar

digital

external carotid

internal carotid

common carotid

subclavian

pulmonary arteries

aorta

celiac

splenic

gastric

common iliac

external iliac

anterior tibial

peroneal

posterior tibial

The body's veins return blood to the heart after oxygen and nutrients have been distributed to the tissues. Smaller vessels feed into ever-larger ones until the blood is collected in the right atrium of the heart. Then it is transported to the lungs, replenished with oxygen, and eventually returned to the tissues.

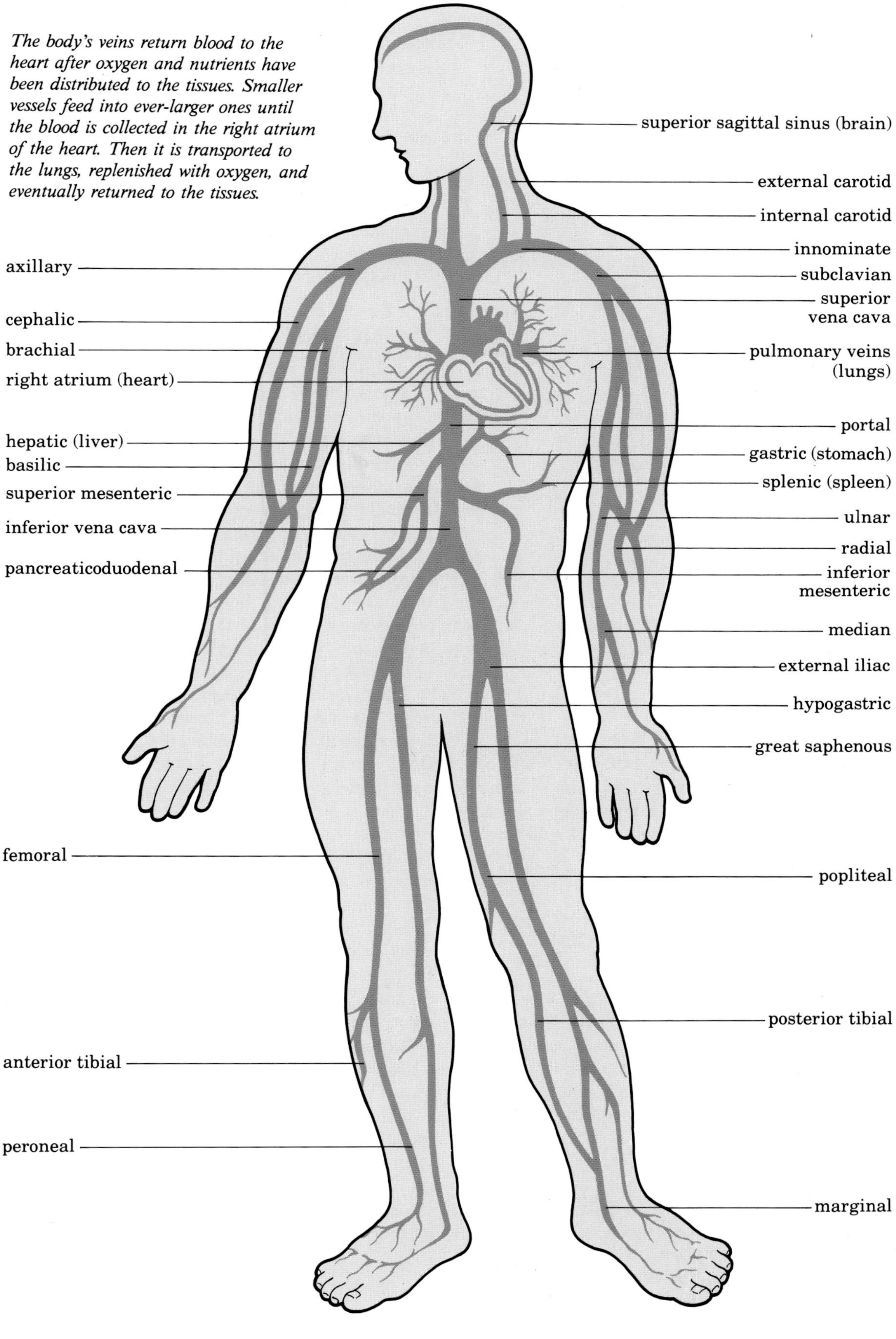

superior sagittal sinus (brain)

external carotid

internal carotid

innominate

subclavian

superior vena cava

axillary

cephalic

brachial

pulmonary veins (lungs)

right atrium (heart)

portal

gastric (stomach)

hepatic (liver)

basilic

splenic (spleen)

superior mesenteric

ulnar

inferior vena cava

radial

inferior mesenteric

pancreaticoduodenal

median

external iliac

hypogastric

great saphenous

femoral

popliteal

anterior tibial

posterior tibial

peroneal

marginal

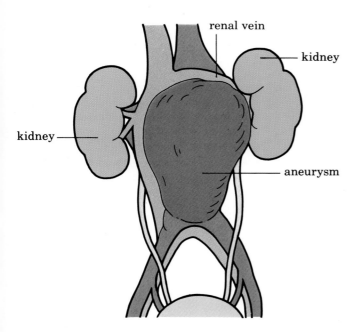

ARTERIAL ANEURYSM
The aorta, the body's main artery, is the most common site for an aneurysm, or ballooning of a narrowed arterial wall. Above, the aorta has ballooned just below the renal arteries supplying blood to the kidneys, displacing kidneys, blood vessels, and ureters. Aneurysms often can be treated surgically.

All patients with Buerger's disease should abstain from tobacco in all forms, including chewing tobacco and snuff. Many patients will then improve markedly. If the patient cannot stop smoking, the disease may progress until amputation becomes necessary.

ARTERIAL ANEURYSMS

An aneurysm is a ballooned, dilated area of an artery. The hardening and loss of elasticity resulting from arteriosclerosis is the major cause. The structural reason is damage to the middle layer of the arterial wall. The artery then begins to balloon out from the pressure of the blood flow.

The aneurysm produces no symptoms until it enlarges and exerts pressure on adjacent organs and tissues. Later symptoms may be caused by thinning of the aneurysm wall and blood leakage.

The most common aneurysms occur in the abdominal aorta, the body's main artery. They usually start just below the renal arteries, which branch off to supply the kidneys. The major symptom is

pain in the upper abdomen or lower back, extending into the groin and the legs. Pain often indicates rapid enlargement or leaking of the aneurysm. If not treated, the aneurysm usually will rupture, causing intense pain and leading to death.

The preferred treatment for aneurysm is to remove the affected portion of the artery surgically and replace it with a synthetic fabric graft. Whether smaller, symptomless aneurysms should be removed depends on the patient's age and general health. Results of surgery for aneurysms are good.

VARICOSE VEINS

More than six million American women suffer from varicose veins, characterized by swollen and bluish "cords in the legs." The condition results from a disorder of the valves in the veins—the irregularly spaced, cuplike structures that open as the blood flows upward to the heart, then close to prevent it from dropping back toward the feet.

There are two sets of leg veins. The superficial veins lie near the skin surface; the deep veins lie far beneath it, next to the arteries and bones. The major connection is in the area behind the knees and in the groin. The systems also connect by a number of communicating veins.

The muscles of the legs help support the deep veins. During walking or moving, contraction of these muscles forces the blood upward. The superficial veins are most likely to become varicose because they have less muscular support.

Causes. Some persons are born with weak veins or valves. In others, disease or injury causes the damage. When the valves can no longer prevent backflow, abnormal pressures dilate the superficial vein system.

Most women and men who suffer from varicose veins have parents or grandparents who have had them. Vein valves also can be affected by obesity, pregnancy, or tumors. Varicose veins develop in elderly people when veins lose elasticity.

Symptoms. A feeling of heaviness in the legs, especially after standing, is a common early symptom. Others include fatigue in the leg muscles, swelling of the ankles, tenderness or soreness, itching around the ankles, and leg cramps at night.

In a woman with an abundant fat pad under the skin, varicose veins may not be visible in the thigh. In the calf and lower leg, however, masses of blue cords may stand out.

Complications. When blood reverses its flow and drops back down the varicose veins, it comes to a standstill in the lower legs, a condition called venous stasis. Swelling around the ankles is an early sign. When the stasis and swelling continue for long periods, a light brown color may develop as a result of tiny hemorrhages. The skin becomes thin and fragile, and a rash may appear. Leg ulcers or sores may follow.

Rupture of a vein can occur when the vein is covered only by a thin layer of skin. The vein may bleed, although bleeding is easily controlled.

Patients with varicose veins face a slightly increased risk of blood clots. These clots usually can be treated at home with rest, elevation of the leg, and a heating pad or warm cloths.

Nonsurgical treatment. Elastic stockings and sometimes elastic bandages are used to counteract the stagnation of blood flow and swelling. For people with mild cases and no complications, light support or panty hose may be sufficient. For more severe cases, a heavier stocking may be necessary. Patients who already have the complications need heavy elastic stockings. A stocking that reaches the knee is usually enough.

Surgical treatment. Enlarged, varicosed superficial veins may be tied off and removed, a process known as stripping. Afterward, the deep veins must carry the blood from the legs to the heart. The operation generally successfully eliminates symptoms. Most vein stripping is done because women do not like the appearance or discomfort of elastic stockings.

THROMBOPHLEBITIS

Thrombophlebitis is an inflammation of a vein associated with a clot. The term is usually shortened to "phlebitis." About 70 percent of cases occur in women.

Superficial phlebitis involves the leg veins just beneath the skin; at times the superficial vein is a varicose vein. It is an annoying condition but not dangerous. Typically, there is a sore, reddened, warm area in the calf or thigh, and a tender cord can be felt. The leg usually is not swollen. Treatment consists of applying warm, moist packs to the inflamed area. Rest with the leg elevated helps to speed healing. The inflammation usually disappears after seven to 10 days.

Deep thrombophlebitis is potentially dangerous. Because the deep veins generally are much larger, the clots are larger. They also are more likely to

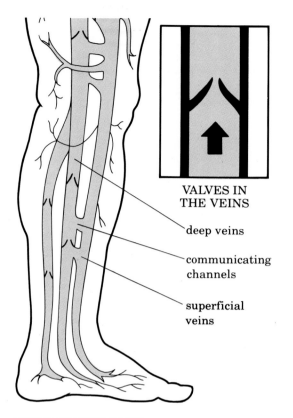

VALVES IN
THE VEINS

deep veins

communicating
channels

superficial
veins

VEINS OF THE LEGS
The main connections between the superficial and deep veins of the legs are behind the knee and in the groin. A series of communication channels also connects them. The inset drawing shows one of the cup-shaped valves that open to allow blood to flow toward the heart, then close again to prevent backflow. Varicose veins develop when the valves are not working properly, permitting stagnation qnd pooling of blood. They are most common in superficial veins, which have less muscular support than deep veins.

break loose and lodge in the lung. This event is called a pulmonary embolism and can cause death.

The signs and symptoms of deep phlebitis can be mild with slight discomfort and minor swelling, or severe with excruciating pain and massive swelling. The diagnosis can be confirmed by X rays.

Once deep phlebitis is diagnosed, hospitalization is necessary. Anticoagulants, or "blood thinners," are given, intravenously at first, and later by mouth. Rest in bed is necessary for a few days. Anticoagulants are continued for three to six months. Elastic stockings may be necessary if swelling of the leg persists.

CHAPTER 7

THE BLOOD

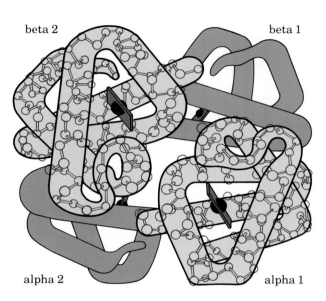

beta 2 beta 1

alpha 2 alpha 1

THE VITAL MOLECULE

The hemoglobin molecule of the blood's red cell is at the heart of life. It carries oxygen to every cell of the body. The molecule consists of four intertwining amino acid chains, which comprise the "globin" part of the molecule. Tucked into the loops of each chain is a small square representing the "heme" portion. An atom of iron is held at the center of each heme. These four atoms capture oxygen molecules in the lungs and transport them to the muscles, brain, and all other organs. The iron atom of the heme gives blood its red color. The hemoglobin molecule vastly multiplies the amount of oxygen that can be dissolved and carried in the blood.

We do not think of blood as an organ, but it is—the only fluid organ in the body. It also is one of the heaviest, second only to the skin. Blood constitutes about 7 percent of body weight, distributed to every nook and cranny of the body. Blood transports fuel, carries away waste, and is vital to all aspects of existence. It is literally "life's blood."

The five quarts of blood in the human body consist of solid particles (the red and white blood cells, as well as substances carried in suspension) and a liquid called plasma. The cells constitute about 40 percent of the five-quart volume, and the plasma constitutes about 60 percent.

The blood system consists of more than the blood itself. Several other organs are part of the system.

THE BLOOD SYSTEM

Bone marrow is the red, pulpy tissue found in the webs of the "flat" bones such as the ribs, pelvis, and spine. Red marrow produces blood cells. Yellow marrow in the cylindrical bones of arms and legs is fat, but it can change to active red marrow when the body needs more than the normal number of blood cells. The fatty marrow is a reserve organ, important because normal blood cells can be produced only in the marrow.

The spleen is an organ about the size and shape of an open hand. It lies in the abdomen, behind the lower ribs on the left side. Most of the aged, worn-out blood cells are destroyed by scavenger cells (phagocytes) in the spleen. The spleen also participates in immune reactions, producing antibodies to attack invading viruses and bacteria, and it manufactures some of the white blood cells, called lymphocytes.

Lymphatic tissue is present as small islands in the spleen. It also is found in dozens of lentil-size lymph nodes in the neck, armpits, groin, chest, and abdomen, and in the tonsils, adenoids, and thymus. If the spleen is removed, these small organs, together with the scavenger cells in the liver, become the destroyers of worn-out blood cells.

Functions of the Blood

The blood is a fluid organ circulating through a system of collapsible tubes. Tough-walled arteries carry blood from the heart at high pressure and thin-walled veins return it. The blood has three functions: transportation, filling the blood vessels, and self-sealing, called hemostasis.

Transportation. The surfaces of the body include the skin, the digestive surfaces of the stomach and intestine, the respiratory surfaces of the lungs, and the excretory surfaces of the kidneys. The circulation of the blood connects them with the inner parts of the body where the vital chemistry is working. The blood carries into the body the substances necessary to life, and it carries out the waste products.

Substances transported by the blood can be divided into three classes: solids, liquids, and gases—food, water, and oxygen. Transport is extremely rapid, with materials moving from the surface to the interior in a matter of seconds.

Filling the blood vessels. When the blood volume is too large, it distends the blood vessels. The heart and lungs cannot operate efficiently. Heart failure can result, and the lungs fill with fluid. On the other hand, too-small blood volume can have the same result.

Hemostasis. When a blood vessel is punctured, it is vital that we not lose this blood and the important substances it carries. Thus, after a few minutes, the rate of blood flow begins to diminish and finally stops. The blood itself forms a plug in the hole. This self-sealing process is brought about by blood cells called platelets, which clump and clot to form a plug.

Components of the Blood

Blood is composed of red cells, white cells, and platelets, together with the fluid plasma in which the cells are suspended and in which many materials are dissolved.

Blood cells are formed when a progenitor cell, or stem cell, divides into two cells. One remains a stem cell that can divide further. The other is a primitive blood cell called a blast. Within four or five days, the blasts mature to form blood cells for delivery to the bloodstream.

Red blood cells. One form of blast, the erythroblast, matures to become an erythrocyte, or red cell. During maturation, these blasts create an enormous amount of the protein hemoglobin, the pigment that gives blood its red color. The function of the complex hemoglobin molecule, illustrated in this chapter, is to carry oxygen from the lungs to all other organs, and the function of the red cell is to carry hemoglobin. The average red cell moves through the heart and bloodstream, transporting hemoglobin, about once a minute. During its four-month life span, a red cell travels almost 100 kilometers (62 miles), continually bumped, crushed, jostled, and squeezed. But when it expires, it is not from injury but from old age.

In its prime, the red cell is equipped with lively chemical machinery to repair its injuries and maintain its vitality. When these chemical reactions run down, it withers. The surface no longer can repel the phagocytes, which ingest all blood cells when their time has come.

Platelets, the smallest blood cells, are disks so tiny that the volume of a pinpoint could contain about 250,000 of them. They are most important in maintaining the walls of the blood vessels. They plug tiny crevices and help to fill holes or wounds. Injury of the blood platelets provokes a chemical reaction that starts the coagulation of blood. Thus, the platelet is the keystone of the blood's hemostatic function.

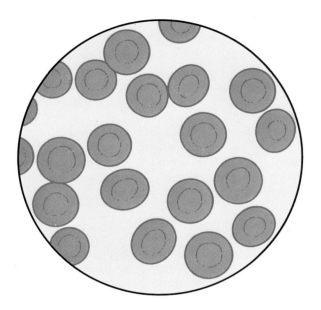

RED BLOOD CELLS

Red blood cells, here magnified 1,000 times, are tiny disks with a slightly concave surface. Their important task is to carry hemoglobin, the protein that transports oxygen from the lungs to all other organs. Hemoglobin gives blood its red color. The red cell prevents the loss of hemoglobin into the urine and tissue. Red cells have a life span of 100 to 120 days.

White blood cells (leukocytes) perform their missions outside the bloodstream. Summoned by a chemical signal, they cling to the vessel wall and escape through cracks between the cells.

There are three basic varieties of leukocytes—granulocytes, monocytes, and lymphocytes—and subcategories of each. They are illustrated in this chapter. All are produced in the marrow from corresponding blasts: myeloblasts for granulocytes, monoblasts for monocytes, and lymphoblasts for lymphocytes. Some lymphocytes also are produced in the lymph nodes and spleen.

Granulocytes, which come in three types, are somewhat larger than red blood cells. All contain chemically active substances concerned with the functions of the cells.

Neutrophilic granulocytes are the most numerous leukocytes. Their function is to prevent or combat infection. They ingest bacteria and kill them. Neutrophils accumulate in areas of infec-

tion, forming a wall to limit spread of infection, and they form pus. Pus, in fact, is a slurry of "used" neutrophils.

Eosinophilic granulocytes increase during allergic reactions, and the blood eosinophil count is high in many parasitic infestations. How the eosinophils function in parasitic disorders, however, is not known.

Basophilic granulocytes contain histamine, which causes an inflammatory reaction. The basophil thus plays some part in inflammation.

Degranulation is the process by which all granulocytes accomplish their function. The granules contained in each granulocyte release their active chemicals and digestive enzymes into the cell itself (that's how the neutrophils destroy ingested bacteria) or into the cell's environment (that may be how basophils contribute to inflammatory reactions). The cell is destroyed in the process.

Monocytes are phagocytes, or scavenger cells. They leave the bloodstream to cruise through the tissue spaces, devouring dead or foreign material, reducing these particles to their component fats, carbohydrates, amino acids, and minerals, and releasing these substances to be reused.

Lymphocytes are the second most common white cells. They are at the center of the body's immune system. From the lymphocytes are derived the antibodies that defend the body against foreign substances.

Blood plasma. Blood cells make up about two-fifths of the blood volume. The fluid portion in which the cells are suspended is the plasma, a pale yellow liquid with the consistency of a thin glue. Dissolved in it are the plasma proteins, various salts, and the fats, carbohydrates, minerals, and vitamins needed to nourish the tissues reached by the circulating blood.

The plasma proteins are incredibly diverse. Albumin is present in the greatest amount. Its prime function is to retain water in the blood, offsetting the blood pressure that tends to squeeze water through the capillary walls into the tissues. When there is too little albumin, the legs become swollen with fluid in the tissue spaces. Albumin's ability to "bind" water develops oncotic pressure.

Albumin is a carrier of various body chemicals such as calcium and the bile pigment produced when hemoglobin is destroyed. It also is a source of nutrient protein for growing cells.

Globulin is the name for all other plasma proteins. Here is a summary of their functions.

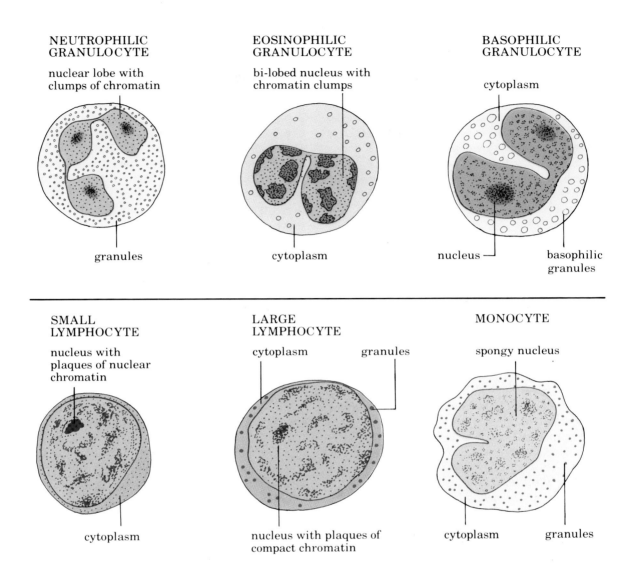

NEUTROPHILIC GRANULOCYTE

nuclear lobe with clumps of chromatin

granules

EOSINOPHILIC GRANULOCYTE

bi-lobed nucleus with chromatin clumps

cytoplasm

BASOPHILIC GRANULOCYTE

cytoplasm

nucleus

basophilic granules

SMALL LYMPHOCYTE

nucleus with plaques of nuclear chromatin

cytoplasm

LARGE LYMPHOCYTE

cytoplasm

granules

nucleus with plaques of compact chromatin

MONOCYTE

spongy nucleus

cytoplasm

granules

WHITE BLOOD CELLS
Six types of leukocytes, or white blood cells, are from top left neutrophilic granulocyte, eosinophilic granulocyte, basophilic granulocyte and from bottom left small lymphocyte, large lymphocyte, and monocyte. All are enlarged about 2,500 times. Neutrophils, the most common, combat infection. Lymphocytes deal with immune reactions. Monocytes are scavengers that remove dead or foreign material from the tissue spaces. The function of eosinophils and basophils is uncertain.

Coagulation system. When blood is damaged, it turns from liquid to a solid clot. A soluble globulin called fibrinogen is altered to become an insoluble fibrin. The feltlike fibrin mesh entraps all of the cellular elements, forming a solid mass.

But clotting does not happen easily or quickly. Reluctance to clot preserves the fluidity of the blood. We are protected from unnecessary clotting by several safeguards, including the smooth surfaces of the blood vessels; a complex chain of reactions, all of which are essential before fibrinogen is converted to fibrin; the blood's continual motion; and anticoagulants in the plasma. When injury is severe enough to override all of these safeguards, the blood does clot, diminishing and stopping blood loss.

Immune system. Like the coagulation system, immune reactions are complex. In the bloodstream, as elsewhere in the body, they center on the relationship between antigen and antibody, which is described in detail in Chapter 23, "Allergy and the Immune System." Various types of blood cells play key roles in the process.

Complement, another complex system of globulins, also helps in the injury and destruction of the antigen targets. It consists of ordinarily inactive enzymes activated by antigen-antibody reactions.

Carrier globulins obtain a substance in one part of the body and deliver it to another. For example, the iron-binding globulin called transferrin picks up two atoms of iron in the spleen after red cells have been destroyed, and delivers the iron to the bone marrow, where hemoglobin in new red cells is formed. Certain hormones are transported by specialized globulins.

Nutrition and Blood

Considerable quantities of "raw materials" are required by the blood. Six grams of protein are needed for just one day's production of hemoglobin, for example. The structure of cell surfaces requires fat. Carbohydrate drives the chemical reactions to fabricate the blood cells. The vitamins are essential "lubricants" or catalysts.

Iron metabolism. Red cells require an enormous investment of iron, more than all the other tissues of the body combined. The body takes good care to prevent loss of this essential element. Unlike other nutrient metals, iron cannot be excreted. Excess iron taken into the body, whether by absorption of food, by medication, or by blood transfusion, must be put into storage. Every cell in the body requires at least a "trace" amount of iron. The iron content of muscle, as myoglobin, is essential for oxygen transport. Iron is in cellular pigments resembling hemoglobin. Some of these pigments move oxygen within the cells, and others store a small amount of oxygen.

A small "obligatory" loss of iron occurs in the constant shedding of cells from the skin and coverings of the other surfaces, but the loss is offset by absorbing one milligram from the 10 to 20 we consume in our daily diet.

Bleeding can deplete the iron supply. To offset the loss, the intestine permits more iron from food to enter, as much as three to six milligrams per day. When iron pills are given, as much as 20 to 30 milligrams can be absorbed.

Vitamins and blood formation. Vitamin B_{12} (cobalamin) and folic acid are needed for blood cells to mature normally in the marrow. Vitamin B_{12} is present in all foods of animal origin. The daily requirement of one microgram is small, but a completely vegetarian diet (containing no milk, eggs, or fish) can, over a long time, cause vitamin B_{12} deficiency. B_{12} cannot be absorbed without the presence of a substance called intrinsic factor (IF), secreted by the stomach. Vitamin B_{12} deficiency thus can occur when a lack of intrinsic factor prevents proper absorption of the vitamin. Fortunately, the concentration of B_{12} in blood can be measured, and supplementary B_{12} given if needed.

Folic acid (foliage = green leaves), another of the B-vitamin family, is abundant in leafy and yellow vegetables. Folic acid, which is adequate in a balanced diet, is essential for rapid proliferation of cells. During periods of extreme proliferation, such as pregnancy, folic-acid supplements often are given.

Blood Tests

The measurement of substances in the blood encompasses more than tests pertaining to hematology. Because the blood transports nutrients, oxygen, hormonal signals, wastes, and the amounts of these substances carried by the blood can be measured to provide clues to the functions and malfunctions of all the body's organs and systems. The methods of blood testing and the information they disclose about many functions of the body is discussed in Chapter 2, "Tests and Procedures."

DISORDERS OF THE BLOOD

The Role of the Marrow

Blood cell production is controlled by feedback systems described on pages 68–69. When more cells are needed, the marrow increases output. The step-up can be evoked by blood loss, excessive blood cell destruction, or an increased requirement, such as during infections.

Normally, part of the marrow consists of fat cells. If increased production is required over a long period, fat storage tissue is converted into functional manufacturing tissue. In certain diseases, fat cells replace functional tissue, resulting in too-little production for normal demand, a condi-

THE LYMPHATIC SYSTEM
The thin lines represent lymph vessels, which collect fluid from the tissues and return it to the blood. Collections of spots in the armpits, groin, spleen, and tonsils are lymph nodes. The nodes are clusters of lymphatic tissue that filter out debris and, when necessary, manufacture antibodies against infection. The arrows show the direction of lymphatic flow.

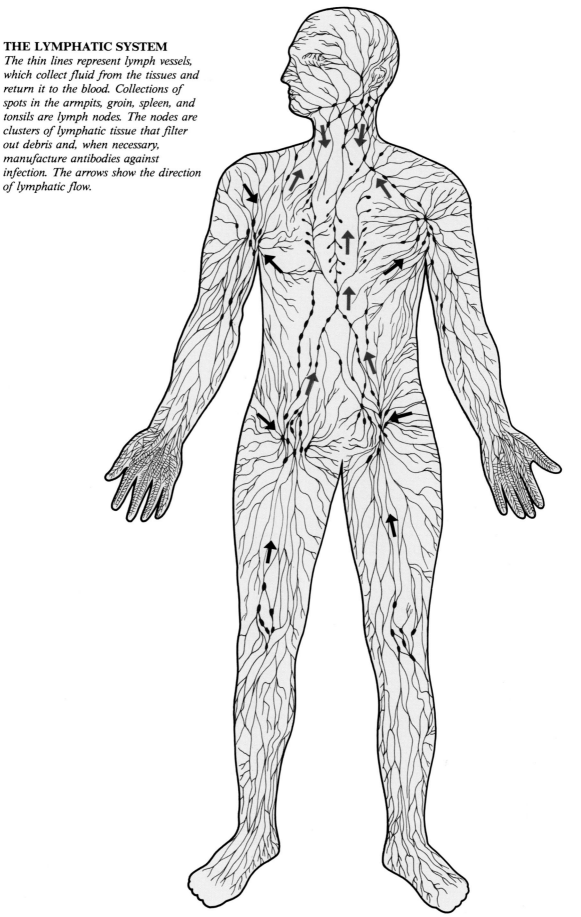

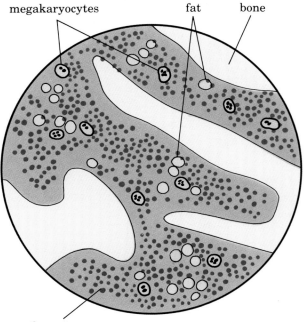

megakaryocytes   fat   bone

erythrocyte

BONE MARROW
The bone marrow in cross section displays the webby structure of the T-bone in a steak. The smooth strips are bone. Between them is the cellular tissue of the marrow where the blood cells are manufactured. Empty circles are fat storage cells. The largest cells in the tissue are megakaryocytes (top left), which produce blood platelets. The smaller circles represent developing red cells (erythrocytes) and white cells.

tion called aplastic anemia. In other diseases, functional tissue is replaced by abnormal cells, scar tissue, or cancer. Sometimes, the marrow cells themselves become abnormal, as in leukemia.

The Role of the Spleen

At the end of their normal life span, most red cells and platelets are devoured by phagocytes, usually in the spleen. But the spleen's scavenging function also can be taken over by other organs with phagocytic cells, as described earlier.

A malfunctioning spleen may increase its phagocytic activity to an abnormal degree, resulting in premature destruction of blood cells. The marrow responds to the best of its ability, but production may be inadequate, and the number of cells in the blood diminishes.

The spleen also is an organ of the immune system. This function can become perverted so that antibodies are produced against *normal* constituents of the blood, especially the blood cells. These autoantibodies attach themselves to blood cells and can cause them to dissolve, or coat them in such a way that the cells are attractive to the body's phagocytes and are eaten.

Hypersplenism is the name given to abnormal activities of the spleen.

Red Blood Cell Disorders

Anemia occurs when the concentration of red cells (and equivalent hemoglobin) is less than normal, usually because production of red cells is insufficient to meet requirements. Insufficiency can result from less-than-normal production or greater-than-normal requirements, or a combination of the two.

The symptoms of anemia are those of insufficient oxygen. The anemic person becomes quickly short of breath or easily fatigued. In general, more severe anemia causes more severe symptoms, but people vary greatly in their ability to tolerate anemia. Young people are more tolerant than older ones. The speed of onset also is a factor. When anemia develops slowly, we adapt to it.

Aregenerative anemia. When the marrow is incapable of producing (or generating) enough red cells for normal replacement, the resulting anemia is called aregenerative. This can result from lowered volume of productive marrow due to aplastic anemia or hypoplastic anemia; a lack of erythropoietin, the chemical secreted by the kidneys that normally stimulates red cell production; insufficient iron in the body; disturbance of hemoglobin synthesis; chronic inflammation; or cancer.

Hemolytic disease occurs when red cells are destroyed prior to their normal life span of 100 to 120 days. When the severity of destruction exceeds the marrow's ability to compensate, the result is hemolytic anemia, or hemolysis.

In most hemolytic diseases, the phagocytes remove and digest abnormal red cells just as they remove normal, aged red cells. This condition is called intracellular hemolysis. In less common forms, the red cells burst in the circulating blood, and their hemoglobin is dissolved in the plasma (intravascular hemolysis); sometimes the plasma turns red and pigment spills into the urine, coloring it red, brown, or black (hemoglobinuria).

When large numbers of red cells are destroyed, large amounts of hemoglobin are broken down, too, yielding great quantities of yellow bile pig-

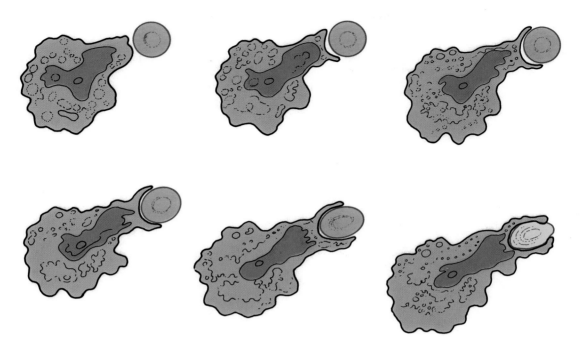

A SCAVENGER CELL
Devouring a worn-out red cell, a phagocyte (scavenger) gradually engulfs its prey. In the final frame, the red cell is pale because it has lost its

hemoglobin. A red blood cell survives about four months before it is devoured. The components of hemoglobin are reclaimed for further use.

ment. Some of the pigment accumulates in the blood, leading to a faint yellow discoloration of the whites of the eyes. This condition is called hemolytic jaundice.

Extrinsic hemolytic anemias result from disturbances of the red cell's environment. Causes include crushing (sometimes temporarily suffered by distance runners, marching soldiers, and even joggers, in the soles of the feet); extensive burns; freezing of tissue (red cells burst on thawing); near-drowning; exposure to certain industrial chemicals; infections, especially the deadly falciparum form of malaria, also known as blackwater fever; immune reactions; and incompatible blood transfusions.

Transfusing blood of an incompatible group into a person causes a reaction between antibodies in the plasma and blood-group antigens on the red cell surface. The red cells often are damaged so severely that they burst. The combination of immune reaction plus hemoglobin destruction can cause serious kidney damage. This is why cross-matching tests are essential before blood transfusions.

Hemolytic disease of the newborn (erythroblastosis), which usually involves the Rh blood-group system, is explained in Chapter 28, "Pregnancy and Childbirth." Tests now are available to detect this destructive disease, allowing for protective injections for the mother, or, sometimes, prenatal transfusions for the fetus.

Autoimmune hemolytic disease develops when the immune system produces antibodies against its own red blood cells. It may develop as a complication of lymphoma, as part of another autoimmune disease such as lupus erythematosus, or as a temporary complication of an infection such as viral pneumonia or mononucleosis. It also occurs independently of associated disease.

Intrinsic red-cell defects primarily are hereditary. They include disorders of the cell membrane, abnormalities of the hemoglobin molecule, and malfunctions of the complex chains of chemical reactions that maintain the fabric of the cell.

Hereditary spherocytosis is transmitted as an "autosomal dominant" disorder of the red-cell membrane. The red cells' normal disc shape thickens, and cells survive an average of only two weeks. Because the marrow can produce seven or eight times the normal number of red cells, the person may show no symptoms except mild jaundice and an enlarged spleen. However, the condition can be severe enough to require transfusions

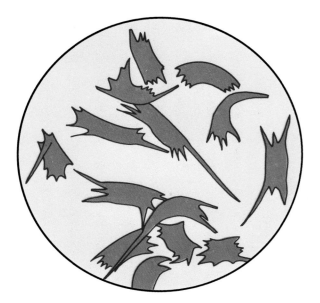

SICKLE CELLS
"Sickle cells" from a person with sickle-cell anemia are illustrated. Normally these red blood cells are concave discs. But when they are stressed by lack of oxygen, lack of water, or fever, the hemoglobin becomes stiff instead of fluid and the cells assume a curved, rigid configuration. When many cells sickle at the same time, "sickle-cell crisis" occurs.

and interfere with growth and development of children. Gallstones develop in most victims. Removal of the spleen cures the disease.

Hemoglobinopathy. Hereditary disorders of the hemoglobin molecule alter some characteristics of the molecule, such as its solubility, its stability, or its affinity for oxygen. There are many forms of hemoglobinopathy, but with a few exceptions, most are rare in the U.S.

Sickle-cell hemoglobin is present in 10 percent of American blacks, occurring in about one in 400 births. With a sickle-cell gene received from one parent, the individual's red cells contain 25 to 35 percent of sickle-cell hemoglobin and 65 to 75 percent normal hemoglobin A. This person is a "healthy carrier" of the sickle-cell gene. When genes come from both parents—a "double dose" of the recessive gene—no hemoglobin A is formed by the victim. When its oxygen has been removed by the body's tissues, the dissolved hemoglobin in the red cells stiffens into needle-shaped crystals, curving the normally pliable disc into an elongated, hard "sickle" shape, as illustrated above. The sickle cells have a life span of about two weeks.

Sickle-cell anemia's major danger is the propensity to crisis. With fever, dehydration, insufficient oxygen, or a disturbance of the body's acid balance, the number of red cells changing shape greatly increases. They become logjammed in small blood vessels, completely blocking flow and preventing oxygen from entering so that more red cells stiffen. The tissues suffer from lack of blood flow, pain develops, and areas of tissue may die.

The sickle-cell crisis is difficult to treat. The patient needs adequate water to prevent or correct dehydration, and often supplementary oxygen. In severe cases, transfusions of normal red blood cells are required.

Homozygous hemoglobin-C disease causes a mild anemia with pallid red cells. Crystals of hemoglobin form in the red cells and are removed by the spleen, thereby reducing the amount of pigment. Two to 3 percent of American blacks are carriers of the trait.

Hemoglobin Yakima and Hemoglobin Chesapeake are hemoglobins that cannot easily release their molecules of oxygen. As a consequence, the feedback system controlling red cell production is stimulated to demand extra red cells. Polycythemia (described below) results.

Thalassemia, or Mediterranean anemia, refers to a group of hereditary disorders of the control of globin synthesis.

When a thalassemia gene is received from only one parent, a mild anemia usually results. Red cells are smaller than normal and contain less hemoglobin. With a double dose, from both parents, the results are devastating. Thalassemia once was thought to be confined to persons of Mediterranean ancestry, and a disproportionate number of cases still are found in this group. However, variants have been found all over the world. Thalassemia now can be detected prenatally by methods of amniocentesis, as described in Chapter 4, "Medical Genetics."

Homozygous thalassemia (Cooley's anemia) is a severe disease marked by overproduction of red cells but inadequate production of hemoglobin. The hemoglobin-deprived red cells have a brief life span. The overactive marrow crowds its cavity, causing the bones of young victims to swell, weaken, and break. Spleens and livers are massively enlarged. Iron storage disease may damage the heart muscle. Continual transfusions are necessary, but transfusions may increase the iron overload and further injure the heart.

Enzyme abnormalities of red cells. Red blood cells depend upon enzymes to break down glucose and release the stored energy. Dozens of enzymes participate. Each is susceptible to genetic mistakes such as those in the hemoglobin molecule.

G6PD deficiency. More than 15 hereditary abnormalities of the enzyme glucose-6-phosphate dehydrogenase have been discovered. The most common occurs in about 10 percent of American black men because the genetic code for the enzyme is carried on the X or sex chromosome.

In the American type of G6PD deficiency disease, G6PD behaves normally in young red cells, but activity gradually diminishes. Nevertheless, enough activity persists to protect the cells against ordinary oxidative stress, the kind involved in normal respiration. Enzyme activity is deficient only with more severe challenges. Some antimalarial and sulfa drugs, or virus infections can provoke an acute hemolytic anemia.

Iron-deficiency anemia, the most common nutritional anemia, rarely results from lack of iron in the diet, except when the iron requirement is temporarily increased during pregnancy or during the rapid growth of early childhood and adolescence. It almost always is evidence that the body is losing blood. It is most common among young women, a consequence of menstrual bleeding. Most women lose only about an ounce or two per menstrual period. Perhaps 5 percent menstruate heavily and require iron tablets or iron supplementation.

When iron-deficiency anemia is found in men or in women after menopause, the source of blood loss must be sought. Possible causes range from nosebleed and hemorrhoids to stomach ulcers and cancer of the colon.

Iron-deficiency anemia is characterized by small red cells deficient in hemoglobin. In severe cases, the skin may be unhealthy, with cracking at the corners of the mouth, thin nails, hair that sheds easily, and itching. A sore and smooth tongue is a common sign.

The sure cure for iron-deficiency anemia is to correct the problem causing the blood loss. When that is not possible, the balance can be restored by taking iron tablets with meals.

Vitamin B₁₂ deficiency. Pernicious anemia most commonly is the result of B_{12} deficiency, occurring primarily among the elderly.

Vitamin B_{12} cannot be absorbed by the intestine unless combined with a substance called intrinsic factor (IF) secreted by the mucous membrane of the stomach. In pernicious anemia, the mucous membrane thins and shrinks, and ceases to secrete IF. The patient becomes anemic because the vitamin is essential for normal blood-cell production. The deprived bone marrow contains large cells (megaloblasts) that produce large, short-lived blood cells. The result is a hemolytic anemia.

B_{12} also is necessary for proper functioning of the nervous system, so the first clue to deficiency may be numbness and tingling of hands or feet, staggering gait, or loss of control of bowel or bladder function.

Injections of B_{12} rapidly correct the anemia, but nerve damage may be irreversible.

Folic acid deficiency. The daily requirement of folic acid needed for proliferation of cells is about 50 micrograms. When diets are low in yellow or leafy vegetables, or vegetables are overcooked, folic acid may be deficient. Pregnant women, persons with hemolytic anemia whose blood-cell production is increased, and victims of sprue, a disease in which the small intestine absorbs food poorly, have an increased need for folic acid. Folic acid tablets rapidly cure the anemia, and in cases of sprue, intestinal absorption improves.

Endocrine-deficiency anemia is a deficiency of hormones associated with inadequate red cell production by the marrow and consequent anemia.

Erythropoietin, a hormone produced in the kidneys, instructs the marrow to produce red cells. Severe disease or removal of the kidneys can reduce or halt the hormone's output and cause anemia. Erythropoietin now is available in medicinal form to correct this.

Removal of the thyroid or spontaneous loss of thyroid activity results in a deficiency of the hormone thyroxine. The accompanying mild-to-moderate anemia can be corrected by proper doses of natural or synthetic thyroid medication.

Pituitary gland destruction by disease or surgery also causes a mild-to-moderate anemia. It seldom is serious enough to be a problem, and can be corrected with a combination of thyroid, adrenal, and testicular hormones.

Aplastic anemia. When the productive cells of the marrow diminish, the marrow cavity cannot reduce its volume to the size of the shrunken tissue. Fatty tissue fills the vacant space. A marrow with a preponderance of fat cells is called aplastic. The decrease in marrow can be severe, with a life-threatening lack of granulocytes and platelets. Aplastic anemia can be caused by injury to the small blood vessels that sustain the productive marrow, by autoimmune injury to the marrow cells, or by a neoplasm of the marrow cells in which the "new cells" are incapable of adequate response to the body's requirement.

Polycythemia. The polycythemias result in excess red cells, the opposite of anemia. They occur when the feedback system governing red-cell production misbehaves.

Reactive polycythemia is triggered when insufficient oxygen is perceived by oxygen sensors monitoring the blood in the kidneys. It develops in persons who live at high altitude, when lung disease interferes with oxygen delivery to the blood, when blood vessels bypass the lungs, when abnormal hemoglobin molecules fail to yield oxygen to kidney sensors, when blood flow to the kidneys is inadequate because of blood vessel narrowing or pressure on the kidneys. Some tumors of the liver, uterus, and ovaries also cause polycythemia.

Reactive polycythemia actually is useful to residents of high-altitude areas and under other conditions of general oxygen deprivation, because the concentration of hemoglobin allows each drop of blood to carry more oxygen.

Polycythemia vera results from an abnormality of the marrow that causes it to produce not only too many red cells but also too many white cells and platelets. It usually is a disease of older persons in whom the thick blood and excess of platelets can lead to clotting, causing strokes and heart attacks. These persons also are prone to ulceration and bleeding of the stomach or intestine.

The victim of polycythemia vera is suffused with blood. The face and palms are red; the eyes are bloodshot. Headache is a common complaint, and so is itching. The disease is easily controlled by suppressing the marrow with drugs or by draining off the excess blood.

White Blood Cell Disorders

As with other blood cell diseases, diseases of white cells can be divided into three types: too many cells, not enough cells, and the wrong kind of cells.

Leukopenia (not enough white cells) or granulocytopenia (not enough granulocytes) may result from inadequate production or from too rapid destruction. The causes are similar to those for inadequate red-cell production. Normally, the marrow produces many more leukocytes than we need. Sometimes the white cell count can be low in a person who is completely healthy. Nevertheless, it is important to investigate the possible causes of leukopenia to be certain that the low count is not caused by some underlying disease.

The dangerous leukopenias are associated with a complete lack of granulocyte production, resulting in a lethal susceptibility to infection. The body cannot form pus, and infections are ineffectually opposed by tissue phagocytes, antibodies, and antibiotics. When the marrow disease is reversible, as it may be after injury by medicines, recovery of granulocyte production usually occurs in time to save the victim's life.

Increased destruction of leukocytes can result from autoimmune diseases in which antibodies are directed against white cells.

Lymphocytopenia. Total absence of antibody-producing lymphocytes results in susceptibility to bacteria. Without antibodies to coat the germs, the granulocytes cannot ingest them.

Leukocytosis, the overproduction of white blood cells, may be neoplastic (leukemia) or the result of disease.

Leukemia. Neoplasms (see above) of the blood-cell-producing tissues comprise a family called leukemias and lymphomas.

The cause or causes of leukemia are not well understood. Atomic radiation and heavy doses of X rays have increased the rate of granulocytic leukemia in exposed persons. Certain chemicals like benzol and certain antibiotics have caused aplastic anemia that in some persons has developed into granulocytic leukemia. Despite many clues and much investigation, there is no indication of a genetic cause for leukemia.

Acute lymphocytic leukemia is a disease of children, uncommon after age 20. The lymphatic tissues, lymph nodes, and spleen enlarge. The marrow is largely replaced by abnormal lymphocytes, and the blood leukocyte count usually is high, with large numbers of abnormal cells. There is anemia, with low platelet counts. Fortunately, prompt and aggressive treatment by chemotherapy and radiation can achieve complete remissions in 90 percent of patients without destroying the marrow and incurring the subsequent risks of hemorrhage and infection. Fifty percent of children adequately treated live five years or more free of disease and are presumed cured.

Acute granulocytic leukemia is a disease of adults. It often is insidious in onset, heralded by symptoms of anemia or unexplained fever. The blood leukocyte count may be high or low, but almost invariably the primitive leukemia cells (blasts) are present. Normal granulocytes are decreased; so is the platelet count. The marrow contains characteristic leukemia cells.

Adult leukemia is much more difficult to treat. The drugs used are harsher and can themselves cause death. Repeated treatments often are required. Remissions usually are partial or brief. For younger patients, the outlook is more encouraging than for older ones.

Chronic lymphocytic leukemia usually is a disease of people over 50. It often is a disease of low aggressiveness with long survival. Median life expectancy is five years, and more than a third of the victims live 10 years. Chronic lymphocytic leukemia manifests itself by the accumulation of lymphocytes in lymph nodes, spleen, marrow, and blood. Later, the problems of anemia and lack of platelets become more insistent, and the normal lymphocytes that can become antibody-producing plasma cells may be suppressed, lowering the defenses against infection. Autoimmune diseases directed against red cells or platelets can cause serious complications. Early in the disease, response to treatment by chemotherapy usually is gratifying. Later, chronic lymphocytic leukemia becomes more and more difficult to treat.

Chronic granulocytic leukemia also is a disease of adults and also is insidious in onset. The patient usually does not feel ill. He may go to his doctor because of a lump in his left abdomen (an enlarged spleen) or because of fatigue, breathlessness, or other symptoms of anemia. In most patients, the leukemia can be controlled with mild chemotherapy, but only about half of the patients live much more than three years after diagnosis. Eventually, the leukemia becomes uncontrollable.

Myeloma also is an older person's disease, originating in the plasma cells of the marrow. It often causes wasting of the bones, with X rays showing a characteristic "moth-eaten" pattern. Bone pain and fractures result. Plasma cells fill the marrow cavity, and the counts of normal blood cells are low. Myeloma cells characteristically do not get into the blood. Myeloma cells pervert the normal production of the plasma protein gamma globulin, producing quantities of abnormal gamma globulin and even fragments of gamma globulin. This abundant protein may clog the kidneys, gradually causing kidney failure. Chemotherapy often can inhibit the abnormal production. Radiation can stop the bone erosion, and can be used for pain or when holes appear in weight-bearing bones.

Macroglobulinemia, like myeloma, causes large amounts of abnormal gamma globulin to appear in the plasma. The protein molecules mass together to form "macroglobulins" that cause the plasma to thicken and interfere with platelet function. The thick plasma distends the small blood vessels, increases the plasma volume, and puts a heavy burden on the heart. Some persons respond to chemotherapy. The thick plasma can be removed mechanically by plasmapheresis, described on page 83.

Lymphoma and Hodgkin's disease. Lymphomas are neoplasms of the lymphocytic tissues, lymph nodes, and spleen; usually there also is some involvement of the liver and marrow.

Hodgkin's disease, which can occur at any age, was once almost invariably fatal, but now is curable in more than half of early cases. It is a disease of the phagocytic cells of the lymph nodes. Usually, at the time of discovery and diagnosis, Hodgkin's disease involves one lymph node or group of nodes, often in the neck. A careful surgical operation called a staging laparotomy, or, sometimes, a CT scan, may be performed to determine the extent of the disease. If it has not affected the nodes in the abdomen, intensive radiation is concentrated on the chest, armpits, and neck. If the abdomen is involved, the radiation may be extended to include nodes there and in the groin. An extended course of chemotherapy also may be prescribed.

Non-Hodgkin lymphomas involve lymphocytes or phagocytes. In undifferentiated lymphoma, the abnormal cell cannot be identified. Non-Hodgkin lymphomas are further subdivided into "follicular" types, in which the neoplastic cells are grouped in small spheres within the lymph nodes, and "diffuse," in which they are not. At the time of discovery and diagnosis, non-Hodgkin lymphoma usually has spread throughout the body. The disease is best treated with chemotherapy. In exceptional cases, radiation also may be used.

The non-Hodgkin lymphomas vary in how quickly they progress and in how they respond to treatment. The outlook in follicular lymphoma generally is better than in diffuse lymphoma.

Platelet Disorders

Platelet disorders are associated, on the one hand, with easy bruising (purpura) and prolonged bleeding or, on the other hand, with clots forming in the bloodstream.

Purpura (the Latin word for purple) describes the presence of darkened blood beneath the skin. The blood spots can be large, as in a black eye, or scattered pinhead- or pinpoint-size spots. Sometimes, there are blood blisters in the mouth, or spots on the whites of the eyes.

Purpura represents superficial bleeding from small vessels. The bleeding itself usually is harmless. Senile purpura, the blotches in the tissue-paper-thin skin on the arms of the elderly, is caused by the skin's fragility. Although senile purpura may be unsightly, it is not harmful. On the other hand, purpura can be a sign of serious disease when, for example, it results in bleeding from a lack of platelets.

Thrombocytopenia (not enough platelets) can result from inadequate production of platelets or their premature destruction. The normal platelet count ranges from about 200,000 to 400,000, many more than necessary. But persons with platelet counts well below 20,000, and with purpura and spontaneous bleeding, are at risk. Fatal hemorrhage in the brain is not uncommon.

Platelet production is impaired in aplastic anemia, in leukemia, or as a reaction to toxic chemicals or medicines. Rapid destruction of platelets may occur in infections when platelets stick on bacteria and the combination is devoured by a phagocyte. Diseases that stimulate the clotting system can rapidly destroy most or all circulating platelets.

The immune thrombocytopenic purpuras result from production of abnormal antibodies directed against the platelets. Sometimes, a medicine is the underlying cause. The antibody is directed against the medicine. The medicine-antibody combination sticks to the platelet and injures it, and the combination is then devoured by a phagocyte. Most such immune reactions are temporary. But these purpuras may become a permanent disease and must be treated with other medicines or by removal of the spleen.

Thrombocytosis (too many platelets) occurs after severe injury, strenuous exercise, surgery, blood loss, or chronic inflammatory disease has stimulated platelet production. The counts return to normal when the stimulus subsides. When platelet production has been temporarily impaired, as by alcohol abuse or vitamin B_{12} deficiency, correction of the impairment causes a temporary "rebound" thrombocytosis.

Thrombocythemia is the exaggerated production of platelets. Thrombocythemia is a common phenomenon in polycythemia vera, chronic granulocytic leukemia, and myelofibrosis. Very high platelet counts are risky. Platelets may clump and block small blood vessels. Clots may form on the clumps and block larger vessels. It often is necessary to reduce the platelet count by inhibiting the marrow with chemotherapy. Sometimes, aspirin may be used to make the platelets less sticky.

Platelet disability. Platelets produced in certain neoplastic disorders may be relatively ineffectual. Overuse of certain medicines, including aspirin, may reduce platelet effectiveness. So may the abnormal plasma proteins in macroglobulinemia. The alteration caused by aspirin is of little consequence in healthy people, but may cause severe deterioration in those with low platelet counts or persons susceptible to bleeding, such as hemophiliacs, described below.

Thromboembolism. Thrombus is a blood clot. Embolus is a piece of clot (or other debris) carried by the bloodstream from the place it formed to another place where it lodges. A thrombus formed in the veins of the leg may be dislodged and move up the vena cava, the body's principal vein, through the right side of the heart to lodge in the lung. One formed in the left heart and dislodged may be carried into an arm or leg artery or the brain. Thrombotic disease is the most common cause of death in older people. Strokes and heart attacks result from thrombosis (see Chapter 5, "The Heart and Circulation," and Chapter 10, "The Lungs").

Abnormalities of Coagulation

With one exception, all of the coagulation proteins are essential to normal clotting of the blood. Depletion of any results in a greater tendency to bleed. These clotting factors usually are lacking from birth because of hereditary diseases, but accidents, poisoning, and acquired diseases also may reduce or eliminate some.

Hemophilia. The classic "bleeder's disease," historically famous for its impact on the crowned families of Europe, actually is found in four hereditary forms. Two forms are transmitted genetically as sex-linked abnormalities, meaning that they are passed from unaffected "carrier" mothers to their sons, as happened with the descendants of Queen Victoria. Another form of hemophilia is not sex-linked but is inherited from two carrier parents. The fourth form, known as Von Willebrandt's disease, comes from one affected parent. The latter two diseases affect men and women equally.

Although hemophilia may be discovered in a child at the time of circumcision, the classic "bleeder" usually does not bleed visibly. Instead, his bleeding is internal, often precipitated by a minor fall, and causes large accumulations of blood in the tissues. Bleeding is particularly common in and around the joints. The pooled blood may force the joints apart, leading to hemophilic crippling.

In times past, the only treatment for hemophiliacs was to replace the lost blood with transfusions of whole blood, a hospital procedure. Now it is possible to separate and freeze-dry the missing factor, and it can be transfused by the patient himself or his family at home. Some patients can learn to anticipate when a bleeding episode is coming on, and to transfuse themselves in advance. Home treatment has enabled many young hemophiliacs to lead nearly normal lives.

Sadly, some young hemophiliacs have been infected with acquired immune deficiency syndrome (AIDS) through transfusions of blood contaminated by the AIDS virus. Since this unfortunate consequence was discovered, donor blood has been rigorously tested at blood banks, minimizing the possibility of AIDS infection.

Acquired coagulation disorders. Vitamin K is required by the liver for the synthesis of four types of coagulation factors. Lack of vitamin K causes hemorrhagic disease of the newborn. Before the nature of the disease became clear, as many as one in 300 newborns died. Now, supplemental vitamin K is given at birth until the vitamin can be absorbed from the diet.

Acquired cases of vitamin K deficiency are related to lack of bile, which is essential for absorption of the vitamin. In obstructive jaundice, a blocked bile duct prevents bile from entering the intestine. Jaundiced patients may develop hemorrhagic disease if the vitamin is not injected. Patients who can eat no food also must be given vitamin K.

Disseminated intravascular coagulation occurs when coagulation factors are activated and used up, platelets are destroyed, and fibrin (clot) is precipitated and then dissolved. The reaction is triggered suddenly, usually by the introduction into the bloodstream of some objectionable material: bacteria, incompatible blood cells, or amniotic fluid from the uterus during delivery of a baby. When the disorder occurs after surgery, severe bleeding may occur that is difficult to control. However, the crisis may pass harmlessly except for a chill, a fever, and a drop in blood pressure.

Acquired anticoagulants. Hemophilic patients with severe deficiency of a particular blood-clotting factor (known as Factor VIII) sometimes produce antibodies against the needed factor, which makes treatment difficult. These antibodies also have occurred in nonhemophiliacs as autoimmune disease. Antibodies against other coagulation factors are less common. Lupus erythematosus is a disease in which acquired anticoagulants often are discovered (see Chapter 17, "Arthritis and Related Diseases").

Dysproteinemia. Marrow neoplasms such as myeloma and macroglobulinemia produce large amounts of abnormal plasma protein. Sometimes, this protein may coat the surface of blood platelets, making the platelets ineffective. A purpuric disorder results.

TREATMENT OF BLOOD DISEASES

Transfusion

The art of transfusing one person's blood into another who needs it is a triumph of 20th-century medicine. A few successful transfusions were given in earlier times, but the catastrophe caused by blood incompatibility far outweighed the successes. Only with Karl Landsteiner's discovery of the ABO blood groups in the 1920s was it possible to match donor and recipient and transfuse blood safely and successfully.

Today, miraculously, we can transfuse not only from one person to another, but time after time, from 100 different donors into a single anemic recipient, thus extending the recipient's life for years. The art of transfusion we now take for granted permits surgery that otherwise would be impossible—open-heart surgery, for example.

Although most transfusions are from donor to recipient, being transfused with one's own blood is a valuable alternative. Autotransfusion eliminates the possibility of incompatibility or contamination of blood sources. Blood may be donated in advance of an anticipated elective operation and stored until needed. Autotransfusion now is available at most hospitals.

BLOOD GROUPS

TYPE	ACCEPTS			
B	B			O
AB	A	B	AB	O
A	A			O
O				O

The success of a blood transfusion depends on a careful matching of blood groups. Within the ABO system, O blood can be transfused into any person; AB will accept blood from any other group. A and B accept only their own, plus O. The most common blood type is O.

Transfusion reactions. Meticulous attention to blood grouping and crossmatching has nearly eliminated the reactions caused by incompatibility. When, by error, incompatible red cells are transfused, they are rapidly destroyed and some of their hemoglobin spills into the urine. The clotting system is activated in the bloodstream and the disseminated intravascular coagulation reaction occurs. The patient's blood pressure falls and acute kidney failure may follow.

Less serious incompatibility reactions bring on fever or hives. These are fairly common and not harmful.

One risk of blood transfusion is the transmission of a virus contained in the donated A or B blood. The hepatitis B virus, once a risk in transfusion, now can be detected in donor blood and no longer is a risk to the recipient. However, another form of hepatitis virus, known as non-A, non-B, cannot be detected, and carries a significant risk of inducing chronic hepatitis. Most infected blood, however, comes from those who sell their blood, usually drug addicts, and more stringent screening procedures have reduced substantially the non-A, non-B threat.

The virus responsible for acquired immune deficiency syndrome (AIDS) also can now be detected with almost 100 percent accuracy, and the risk of contracting the fatal disease by transfusion has been virtually eliminated. Prior to development of the test, however (and before the scope of the disease was recognized), a number of persons contracted AIDS in this manner.

Iron storage disease can occur in people who, over the years, receive many transfusions. Because there is no normal channel for excretion of iron, iron given up by transfused red cells must be stored in the body. In time, the increasing concentration of iron begins to injure tissue where the iron is stored: liver, pancreas, heart, and endocrine glands.

Blood Fractionation

Today, there are relatively few transfusions of whole blood. Instead, each unit of blood is divided into its component parts.

Platelet transfusion has provided an enormous improvement in the practice of transfusion, allowing many patients who otherwise might have died of uncontrollable bleeding to be operated upon safely, and patients with adult acute leukemia to be transfused with fresh platelets. Platelets are creamed off almost every unit of blood collected, then concentrated, and platelets from six to 12 units dispensed in a single transfusion. The procedure raises the recipient's platelet count substantially. After treatment for leukemia, the patients can be kept from bleeding until the marrow resumes platelet production.

White blood cell transfusion. Because white cells in the blood are few and their life span is brief, the number in one unit of blood is negligible. To obtain a useful quantity of white cells, the donor is connected to a machine called a cell separator. Blood from one arm is run through the machine and returned via the other arm after the machine removes the white cells. The white cells then are transfused to the recipient. Platelets can be skimmed off and transfused in the same fashion.

Phlebotomy

When too much blood or too many red cells are present, one unit at a time is removed by opening a vein until the volume is restored to normal. Thereafter, an occasional phlebotomy is required to maintain the normal volume. Phlebotomy also is used to treat hemochromatosis, a disease in which the intestine absorbs more iron than the body requires, because storing excess iron eventually damages the storage organs.

Plasmapheresis

Plasmapheresis is akin to phlebotomy, but only the plasma is retained and the red cells are returned to the donor. Plasmapheresis is helpful when the plasma contains a harmfully high concentration of protein. It also can be used to reduce rapidly a dangerously elevated platelet count. Normal people are plasmapheresed to obtain normal plasma protein components.

Bone Marrow Transplants

Bone marrow transplantation is a radical treatment for some cases of leukemia and aplastic anemia. Preparation is rigorous, involving irradiation of the entire body and chemotherapy to destroy *all* proliferating cells of the blood-forming organs. The danger of overwhelming infection then is great because cellular defenses have been completely destroyed. Young adults are the best candidates for the procedure.

During the procedure, marrow cells from a carefully matched donor, usually a relative, are suspended in plasma and transfused. When all goes well, the graft takes, and then precautionary treatment must begin to prevent the transplanted immune system of the donor from generating lethal antibodies against the patient's tissue, the so-called graft-versus-host disease.

The matching of donor and recipient is more difficult than matching for blood transfusion. In blood transfusion, the red-cell antigens are matched; in transplantation, the white-cell antigens are matched. The human leukocytic antigen (HLA) system is so complex that good matches usually can be found only among brothers and sisters. Identical twins are the perfect match.

Splenectomy

Splenectomy, removal of the spleen, usually is performed because the organ has become so massively enlarged that it limits the patient's mobility, and presses on adjacent organs. More than half of the blood pumped by the heart may be diverted into such a large spleen. It also may be removed because it is destroying so many red cells that it causes anemia or so many platelets that it causes purpura, or because of autoimmune diseases centering in the spleen.

The spleen is not an essential organ. Persons without a spleen live in good health. However, there is a remote risk of severe infection by pneumococcus bacteria, and the risk is higher in children. Persons without spleens are vaccinated against pneumococcus and advised to take antibiotics as soon as an infection begins to develop.

Radiation Therapy

Radiation therapy, the bombardment of malignant cells with high-voltage ionizing irradiation, is used especially to treat the lymphomas. A large proportion of patients with Hodgkin's disease can be cured by radiation. In childhood leukemia, the brain often is a "sanctuary" where leukemia cells can escape from chemotherapy. To cure childhood leukemia, these cells must be destroyed. Radiation to the brain and spine can accomplish this. Radiation therapy and chemotherapy often are used in combination.

Radioactive Isotopes

Radioactive isotopes are used to treat neoplasms that can be induced to combine with a radioactive element. Radiophosphorus, for example, "seeks" the cells of certain leukemias and lymphomas. Radiophosphorus often is successful in controlling chronic leukemia, polycythemia vera, and thrombocythemia.

Hormones

Hormones in natural or synthetic form are used to treat disease in two ways. One is to replace a lack of hormone. For example, anemia caused by deficiency of thyroid hormone is cured when the hormone thyroxine is taken daily in pill form. The second way is to combat directly certain blood diseases. Hormones of the adrenal cortex such as cortisone or prednisone in large doses suppress the immune system, and are used to treat autoimmune diseases. In many children with lymphocytic leukemia, cortisone still is used in combination with chemotherapeutic drugs. Prednisone is a part of the formula for the treatment of other leukemias and other kinds of cancer as well. Testosterone, the male sex hormone, in large doses causes polycythemia in normal people. It is used for anemias that do not respond to other treatments.

CHAPTER 8

HYPERTENSION

Few major causes of death in the Western world can be reasonably and easily treated. The killers of history, such as malnutrition and infectious epidemics, have almost disappeared. Most of the problem diseases of today, such as heart disease and cancer, resist cures. High blood pressure (hypertension) is an exception. It is widespread, and it is a major cause of death and illness, but it *can* be treated.

WHAT IS BLOOD PRESSURE?

"Blood pressure" refers to the force blood exerts against the arterial walls during the action of the heart. Systolic blood pressure is the pressure during the pumping phase. In a blood pressure reading, it is the larger (and the first) of the two numbers. Diastolic blood pressure is the pressure during the resting phase. Diastolic blood pressure is the second number in a blood-pressure reading.

Blood pressure is not strictly a matter of the heart's pumping action. It also is affected by hormones secreted by the kidneys and by the sympathetic nervous system, which controls dilation and constriction of blood vessels.

MEASUREMENT OF

BLOOD PRESSURE

Normally, blood pressure is measured indirectly, using either a mercury or, more commonly, an aneroid (dial) sphygmomanometer. A cuff is placed around the upper arm and inflated until blood flow in the artery is stopped. Air gradually is let out of the cuff. Through a stethoscope placed over the artery at the elbow, the person taking the pressure hears a thumping sound. This sound is the systolic pressure, the peak of pressure produced by the heart's contraction. As the pressure in the cuff is reduced, the noise fades. This represents the diastolic pressure.

Both of these measurements are expressed in terms of how high the pressure will raise the column of mercury in the sphygmomanometer. A "blood pressure reading" of 120 over 80 means that the column stands at 120 millimeters of mercury during the pumping phase, and 80 millimeters during the resting phase. The reading usually is written as 120/80.

Many persons measure their own blood pressure at home, which can be helpful to those under treatment in monitoring the effects of medication.

NORMAL BLOOD PRESSURE

Life expectancy is greatest when the blood pressure lies between 100/60 and 130/80. Above 130/80, life expectancy is progressively shortened as blood pressure is increased.

As a rule, both systolic and diastolic pressure are high at the same time. Occasionally one or the other is elevated alone. All the evidence suggests that either elevation is associated with an increased chance of disease.

There is no sharp line between normal and abnormal blood pressure. The incidence of cardiovascular problems rises steadily as blood pressure readings rise. But the rule does not always hold for individuals. So other risk factors, like smoking and family history, must be considered.

HIGH BLOOD PRESSURE

Symptoms of High Blood Pressure

Hypertension causes diseases with symptoms, but hypertension itself usually has no symptoms. Constant or recurrent headaches can be a symptom of hypertension. A feeling of a "full head" or a little giddiness may be produced by high blood pressure. Because high blood pressure is a risk factor rather than a disease, many persons resist treatment because they feel no symptoms.

The Damage of Hypertension

The relentless pressure of uncontrolled hypertension damages the walls of the arteries, including those of the heart, brain, and kidneys. The risks of heart attack and stroke rise sharply.

Several kinds of arterial damage can occur. The small arterioles may leak or burst in the eye, interfering with vision; in the brain, causing confusion, fits, and coma; or in the kidney, interfering with the kidney's ability to rid the body of wastes.

Hypertension also causes the walls of the arteries to thicken. The process narrows the inner diameter of the artery, so the blood flow meets greater resistance, and pressure must be increased to push the blood through. The narrowing of the arterial channel also slows and reduces the blood supply, which is particularly serious in the kidney.

Uncontrolled high blood pressure over a long period may weaken the arterial walls and cause outpouchings (aneurysms) in the small arteries, especially in the brain. These aneurysms may burst and bleed, leading to a stroke.

The heart itself suffers as well. More heart muscle is developed to keep up with increased work demand. Eventually, the heart muscle becomes less efficient as it is stretched too far.

Hypertension apparently helps to hasten the process called atherosclerosis, in which fatty deposits build up in the arterial walls, further narrowing the channel (see Chapter 6, "Blood Vessel Disorders"). The exact relationship between hypertension and atherosclerosis is not known. Probably, hypertension injures the intima, the inner lining of the arteries, so that plaque builds up inside the vessels.

What Causes High Blood Pressure?

Although we don't know what causes high blood pressure in 95 percent of patients, certain factors correlate with blood pressure.

Family history. High blood pressure tends to run in families. The common environment may be a partial explanation. However, the blood pressures of identical twins are more likely to resemble each other than those of fraternal twins, suggesting that heredity is more important than environment. Also, identical twins who were raised apart tend to have similar blood pressures, despite differences in life-style and diet.

About half of hypertensives appear to be "salt sensitive," meaning that even moderate salt intake may predispose them to increased blood pressure. The sodium portion of the salt molecule helps to regulate blood pressure and excess amounts normally are excreted by the kidney. In salt-sensitive persons, either the kidneys or the nerves controlling them may be laggard in excretion, possibly as a result of an inborn deficiency. Another explanation says that the red blood cells of the salt sensitive handle sodium less effectively than those of normal persons. On the good side, the blood pressure of salt-sensitive persons responds better to salt-restricted diet and diuretic treatment than does that of the salt insensitive.

Obesity. The fatter a person is, the more likely he or she is to have high blood pressure. Males with bulging waistlines appear to be at greater risk.

Sodium and potassium. Although the exact relationship between sodium chloride (table salt) and hypertension is not clear, it appears that tribes that eat little salt and a great deal of potassium (generally found in fresh fruit) have little hypertension. It is true that they also are thin, frequently diseased, and engage in strenuous physical activity to collect food—any or all of which could be a partial explanation. Possibly, potassium may prevent high blood pressure by increasing the excretion of sodium.

Emotions and stress. Acute emotional episodes can affect blood pressure. Anger, excitement, and pain can raise the reading. Depression slowly lowers it. However, almost every attempt to find a clear-cut relationship between emotional makeup and blood pressure has failed. At one point, tranquilizers were prescribed for high blood pressure without obvious benefit. It now appears that if stress does relate to hypertension, it is not simple stress but repressed anger and limited options.

Specific Causes of Hypertension

In a tiny fraction of the people with high blood pressure, a specific cause can be identified. Most of these result from irreversible kidney disease. Others include: oral contraceptives (less common now that low-estrogen birth control pills are used more often); drugs and medicines, including the cold remedies phenylpropanolamine and pseudoephedrine, which constrict the blood vessels, and amphetaminelike medications for losing weight; contraction of the aorta, a disease that narrows the great artery from the heart above the kidney; and adrenal gland tumors, which usually are diagnosed by measuring blood or urine levels of hormones, and usually are treated surgically.

WHO NEEDS TREATMENT

A study by the National Heart, Lung, and Blood Institute has given guidance about when high blood pressure should be treated: anyone 50 years of age or older whose diastolic blood pressure is 90 or higher. Those with readings of 90 to 104 mmHg should be treated if other cardiovascular risk factors, such as smoking, high cholesterol, or family history of heart disease, are present.

PREVENTION

Although there is no clear evidence that hypertension can be prevented by staying thin, keeping one's salt intake lower, and eating a lot of green vegetables, root vegetables, and fruit with high potassium content, it seems reasonable to pursue such a course—especially if one is slightly obese and has a family history of hypertension. In addition, persons at risk for developing hypertension should remember that hypertension interacts with other risk factors. It is more important for these persons not to smoke than for someone who has normal blood pressure.

THERAPY

Diet and Weight Loss

Weight loss often is prescribed for mild hypertension, often in conjunction with drugs. The benefits may not be confined to the obese. We still do not know which persons will respond to weight loss with lowered blood pressure, but it occurs frequently enough that even those who are slightly overweight should try reducing.

Salt Restriction

The average American takes in 10 grams of salt a day, more than twice the amount the body needs. Persons who salt food without tasting it take in even more.

A desirable goal for the hypertensive person is to lower salt intake to four grams or less a day. This can be achieved easily if only fresh foods are used. Halving the salt intake will reduce blood pressure 5 to 7 mmHg in the salt sensitive.

Salt Appetite

One problem in reducing salt intake is that people have a salt appetite. Human beings tend to increase their salt intake if they are salt-deprived. But much of our salt intake is habitual.

A person who reduces salt intake will find that the food tastes insipid at first. Salt reduction should be carried out over several months, accompanied by generous use of spices, lemon juice, and pepper. In addition, some persons will find that salt substitute, which is primarily potassium chloride, will readily replace salt.

Drug Treatment

Diuretics help to get rid of salt. Most patients are started on a "thiazide-type" diuretic, which is the most efficient if they have normal kidneys. Diuretics have some side effects. The drugs rid the body of potassium as well as sodium, so the patient using them must try to increase consumption of citrus fruits, lean meats, and leafy and root vegetables. Diuretics also may increase blood sugar and uric acid, and raise blood cholesterol. There also is an association with heart irregularities.

Drugs that interfere with the sympathetic nervous system. Beta-blocking drugs interfere with the function of the nerves' beta fibers, thus reducing the force and frequency of heart contractions. Reserpine, methyldopa, and guanethidine affect the muscle tone of peripheral blood vessels. Some persons on medications have marked depression, loss of interest in sex, diarrhea, and dizziness on standing.

Vasodilator drugs directly open the small arteries. The most common are hydralazine and minoxidil. Both are effective, but they usually are used when a patient has not responded to the combination of a diuretic and a drug that decreases the action of the sympathetic system.

Other drugs. Normally, the kidney secretes renin, and renin then splits a substance from the blood's plasma proteins, angiotensin I. A "converting" enzyme further changes the substances by removing two amino acids. The result is angiotension II, a very powerful blood-pressure-raising substance. A new class of drugs stops the conversion of angiotensin I to angiotensin II. Many hypertensive patients appear to improve markedly with these medicines.

Discontinuing Treatment

The greatest handicap to blood pressure control is that patients feel well, and therefore do not think they need to continue medication. The patient must remember that a normal blood pressure on medication does not mean that the medicine is no longer needed. It means the medicine is working.

CHAPTER 9

THE SKIN

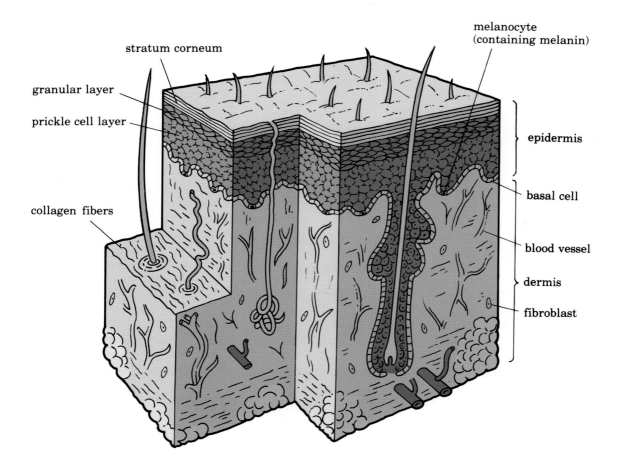

stratum corneum

granular layer

prickle cell layer

collagen fibers

melanocyte
(containing melanin)

epidermis

basal cell

blood vessel

dermis

fibroblast

SKIN LAYERS

A cross section of the skin shows its distinct layers. The thin top layer, or epidermis, is the only visible part. It consists of the stratum corneum, the outermost layer, and the stratum germinativum. New cells originate at the lowest level of the epidermis and gradually rise upward through the prickle cell layer and granular layer to the stratum corneum, where they are sloughed off to be replaced by others

rising from below. The thicker dermis contains primarily fibrous connective tissue known as collagen; it rests on the third layer, the subcutaneous fat. The dermis contains the two types of sweat glands, apocrine and eccrine, which help to regulate body temperature, and the oil or sebaceous glands. The dermis also contains blood and lymphatic vessels, but the epidermis does not.

If you stand naked before a mirror, you can see virtually the entire surface of your skin. From this perspective, the skin seems to be an inactive organ, merely a wrapper to keep the inside in and the outside out. The appearance is deceiving. The layers of the skin are full of activity, performing myriad and subtle functions to shield the body from injury and maintain constant internal conditions.

Although the skin is the boundary where our space ends and the world's begins, it is not impermeable. It blocks entry of infectious organisms and noxious substances, and holds in water and chemicals, but it also allows substances to pass through in both directions, screening them in response to the body's needs. Connective tissue and fatty layers cushion the body against shocks and injuries. The skin's pigment, or coloring matter, protects against the ravages of sunlight. The sun's ultraviolet light stimulates skin to make vitamin D.

The skin plays a key role in regulating body temperature. The thick fatty tissue helps conserve heat. The blood vessels, by constricting and expanding, influence how much heat is lost. When the outside temperature plunges, the vessels narrow, keeping the heat within the body. When the temperature soars, the vessels dilate, allowing heat to pass through the skin. Moisture from the sweat glands also cools the skin through evaporation.

With its vast network of nerves, the skin helps us feel touch, pressure, temperature, pain, and itch. Its perceptive powers are extremely sensitive. The skin conveys messages about the external world and from one person to another. Touching is the essence of human sexual expression.

From a health perspective, perhaps the most important feature of the skin is its sheer visibility. Skin diseases are easily seen and thus can be promptly treated. Potentially serious malignancies can be detected much earlier than in other organs. And the skin is a mirror that reflects changes in other parts of the body. Examining it can provide clues to internal disease.

Visibility, however, is a two-edged sword. Skin diseases are significant not only because they may impair physical health, but also because they are often unattractive in appearance. The psychological consequences of a disfiguring skin disorder can be more devastating than the physical ones.

VARIATIONS IN NORMAL SKIN

Moles

Moles are raised, usually discolored (pigmented) spots on the skin. They may be apparent at birth and commonly enlarge after adolescence. Moles should be removed if they are repeatedly bumped or irritated, if they have any undesirable cosmetic appearance, or if they undergo changes that suggest malignancy.

The chance that a mole will give rise to cancer is small. There are two exceptions. One is that certain rare families have an inherited tendency to develop a form of cancer called melanoma from moles at a relatively young age. The second exception is that large moles present at birth undergo malignant transformation at an unusually high rate. Persons with a family history of melanoma or large congenital moles should be checked regularly by a dermatologist.

Freckles

Freckles are flat brown spots scattered irregularly over skin that has been exposed to sunlight. The pigment-forming cells in freckles are genetically influenced to synthesize melanin (pigment) more actively than normal after ultraviolet light exposure. The area between them does not tan, but remains a sunburned pink. Freckles are harmless, but they are warning signals that the person is likely to sunburn easily.

AGING OF THE SKIN

Aging of the skin usually has mainly cosmetic significance. As we grow older, the epidermis becomes slightly thinner. The rate at which the cells divide and replace themselves becomes slower. The number of pigment-producing cells decreases. The skin tans less readily and is more easily damaged by ultraviolet light.

The collagen also becomes more stable, making the skin of older people more stiff and less pliable. The skin loses elasticity. When stretched, it does not "snap back" as rapidly as in youth.

Blood vessels break more easily and skin bruises are more common. And, in many areas of the body, the fat layer beneath the skin decreases. The body is not as well cushioned against outside injury, nor protected against heat loss.

The changes in the dermis and in the subcutaneous tissue contribute to the furrows, deep wrinkles, and sagging of aging skin.

Another change that comes with age involves the glands of the skin. Both sweat glands and sebaceous (oil) glands decrease in number and activity. Older people are not able to sweat proficiently and thus may not be able to tolerate hot weather well.

Several types of benign skin growths commonly appear with age. Among them are cherry angiomas (small, bright red, dome-shaped proliferations of capillaries) and seborrheic keratoses (superficial, warty growths tan to dark brown in color).

Sun and aging. Wrinkles and the loss of resiliency of the skin are hastened by sun exposure over many years. Although the effects may look the same as those of natural aging, the underlying changes are different. However, damage to the skin from sun can be minimized by the regular use of sunscreens, discussed below.

Although the normal aging process cannot be reversed, it can be slowed by topical application of retinoic acid (Retin-A), a vitamin A derivative also used for acne. Daily administration of Retin-A, a prescription drug, in cream form has been shown to retard fine wrinkling, improve skin color, and plump up skin. The method, which must be continued indefinitely, will not restore already damaged skin, however, and can cause irritation when first begun, so dermatologists recommend it be used with caution.

Sunscreens

Sunscreen lotions protect the skin against ultraviolet radiation, which can cause sunburn, premature aging, and wrinkling. They come in two forms: physical and chemical. Physical sunscreens, such as zinc oxide, shut out all ultraviolet radiation and prevent tanning as well as burning. They usually are reserved for extremely sun-sensitive areas, such as the nose.

Chemical sunscreens, used on larger areas of the body, are rated according to their Sun Protection Factor, or SPF. SPF relates to the amount of time it will take you to get a mild sunburn while using the product. Ratings range from two to 15 or more. This means, for instance, that if your skin burns mildly after 20 minutes' exposure, a product with a rating of six would let you stay in the sun 120 minutes, or two hours, before you burned to the same degree. Those with a rating of 15 prevent virtually all burning, although higher numbers prolong the protection. Persons who burn easily and never tan should use a product with an SPF of eight or higher; dark-skinned persons who rarely tan may use one with an SPF of two or three. Sunscreens should be applied at least a half hour before going into the sun to allow the product to penetrate the skin. It should be applied liberally, and renewed after swimming, drying with a towel, or if you sweat a lot.

SKIN CARE

The first principle of proper skin care is to do no harm. The misguided application of salves or creams, or squeezing and picking at minor pimples or blemishes, can be detrimental. Moisturizers, greasy cleansers, and oil-based cosmetics may precipitate or aggravate acne in some people. Squeezing a pimple can inflame it more and even lead to scarring. Frequent, vigorous scrubbing in an attempt to rid the skin of acne can produce excessive irritation.

Cleansing

In today's society, washing is more a social custom than a practice necessary for healthy skin. Water alone dissolves and removes most dirt. Soap can remove the skin's natural oils, and regular use of standard soaps can cause excessive skin dryness. It may be better advice to use soaps containing oatmeal or lipid-free lotions or superfatted soaps.

A cold, low-humidity environment dries the skin. Water can be replaced in the skin by proper use of lubricating agents. A bath oil, lotion, cream, or ointment, applied immediately after bathing, will form a film that traps the water. Alternatively, a bath oil can be added to the tub water.

Cosmetics for the Face

The multibillion-dollar cosmetics industry reflects the widespread hope that creams, moisturizers, hormones, vitamins, facial masks, and astringents will benefit skin. The truth is that, although many of these cosmetics may temporarily improve the appearance and comfort of the skin, none of them bring about lasting change.

Overnight creams and moisturizers can make dry skin feel smoother by coating the irregular surface of a flaking outer layer. If a moisturizer is applied after washing, water loss will be retarded.

Astringents are intended to close pores. After their use, the skin may tingle and pores may seem less prominent, but only because the astringent has caused mild irritation and swelling of the adjacent skin. No permanent decrease in pore size occurs.

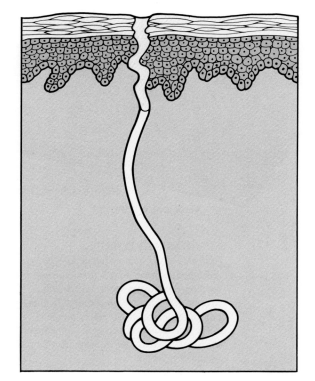

ECCRINE SWEAT GLAND
An eccrine sweat gland's coiled lower portion, which lies in the dermis or subcutaneous (beneath the skin) tissue, secretes fluid. The upper end makes its way through the epidermis in a corkscrew manner to open onto the skin surface. Eccrine glands produce the watery secretion that is important in dissipating excess body heat.

Antiperspirants and Deodorants

Antiperspirants and deodorants affect sweat. An antiperspirant reduces perspiration, usually through the action of an aluminum salt. A deodorant does not affect the sweating process, but reduces or masks odor. Odor occurs when normal skin bacteria decompose the organic contents of the sweat. Most deodorants reduce odor by means of an antibacterial ingredient. A few contain a perfume to mask a disagreeable odor with a more pleasant one. Because the purpose of eccrine sweating is to help maintain normal body temperature, no attempt should be made to control it except in areas where moisture creates special problems, such as on the feet, where it may lead to fungus infection (athlete's foot).

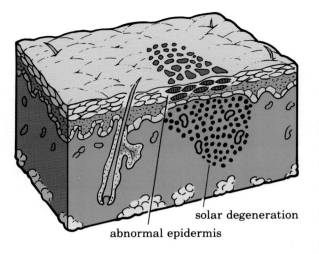

solar degeneration
abnormal epidermis

SUN-DAMAGED SKIN
Skin damaged by sun has a familiar reddened surface, which turns tan as protective melanocytes reach the area. Beneath the surface of chronically sun-damaged skin, protein fibers break down and skin cells assume abnormal shapes. Repeated sun damage can cause permanent harm.

Protection from Sunlight

One of the most important aspects of skin care is to prevent sunburn and avoid chronic overexposure to the sun. Sunburn brings temporary discomfort, and if severe enough to cause peeling, it produces an unattractive mottled appearance. More important, it can damage skin cells. Repeated sunburn eventually causes permanent harm.

A look at chronically sun-exposed skin under the microscope shows striking evidence of damage to the protein fibers in the upper dermis. These changes do not occur in skin that is never exposed to the sun, such as on the buttocks.

The skin's main defense against sun damage is melanin, the pigment that provides color. When sun strikes the skin, it induces the melanocytes to make more pigment. Two or three days later, the melanin becomes visible as a tan. Melanin absorbs and scatters ultraviolet light, allowing less to penetrate to the lower epidermis and dermis.

Fair-skinned people make less melanin than darker-skinned people. Consequently, fair skin is more susceptible to sunburn and the harmful effects of chronic sun exposure.

It is extremely important for people who tan poorly and sunburn easily to protect themselves from ultraviolet light. They should especially avoid midday sun, when the sunburn-inducing rays reach the earth in greatest quantity. Wearing a wide-brimmed hat is helpful but not a complete solution because many harmful rays are reflected from the ground. Sunscreens applied to the skin can partially or totally block the ultraviolet rays.

People who burn upon first exposure to the sun but eventually tan should expose themselves to sun gradually. Starting with a few minutes of exposure will stimulate melanin formation without causing a sunburn. As a protective tan develops, more time may be spent in the sun.

Treatment for Sunburn

The sting of a mild sunburn can be partially relieved by applying cool tap water compresses for 20 minutes several times a day. A bland lubricating cream or ointment applied afterward is soothing, too.

In cases of extreme overexposure, contact a physician immediately. If started early, a three-day course of a corticosteroid taken by mouth can almost completely prevent a potentially severe sunburn. An intense sunburn that has already developed requires continuous cool compresses, topical steroids, and lubricating agents.

DISEASES OF THE SKIN

Acne Vulgaris

Acne affects almost everyone at some time. Outbreaks range from an occasional blackhead or pimple to a festering and scarring process that is long-lasting and emotionally crippling. Although acne flourishes in adolescence and usually diminishes by the late 20s, it can begin late or persist into middle age.

Causes. The acne lesion originates in the sebaceous follicle. Sebum, the oily substance produced in the follicle, empties into the canal through short ducts from the sebaceous gland. The lining of the follicle has an outer layer of horny cells, which are fragile and do not stay together but remain loose within the canal of the follicle. An additional occupant of the canal is a type of bacteria called *Propionibacterium (Corynebacterium) acnes.* The

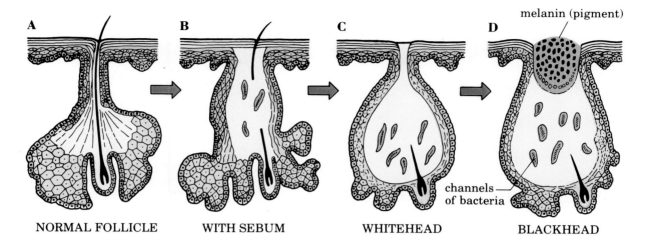

melanin (pigment)

A   B   C   D

channels of bacteria

NORMAL FOLLICLE   WITH SEBUM   WHITEHEAD   BLACKHEAD

THE BEGINNING OF ACNE

These four illustrations show the evolution of a comedo, which is the beginning of acne. A normal sebaceous follicle (left) has large, multiglobulated glands and a tiny hair. In drawing B, its canal is becoming distended, filling with sebum, horny material, and bacteria. The closed comedo, or whitehead, in C has a microscopic pore. In D, expansion of the contents has dilated the opening and produced an open comedo, or blackhead. The dark color comes from melanin, pigment made by cells of the upper portion of the follicle.

white, cheesy material that can be squeezed out of sebaceous follicles is composed of sebum, keratin (sloughed horny material), and bacteria.

Normally, the contents of the follicular canal pass from the follicle and are deposited on the surface. In acne, for unknown reasons, the horny cells form a solid mass that gradually expands to become what is known as a comedo. At first, this cluster, or comedo, is too small to be seen. Later, it enlarges into a visible whitehead, or closed comedo. Still later, the horny material may expand, dilate the opening of the sebaceous follicle, and form an open comedo, or blackhead. The dark color is caused by melanin in the horny cells. Sometimes, a closed comedo may break through the thin walls of the follicular canal and start an inflammation that appears as a pimple.

The usual location of acne on the skin corresponds to the distribution of sebaceous follicles. These are located mainly on the face, chest, upper back, and shoulders.

Acne has no single cause, but several prerequisites can be identified. When a boy or girl reaches puberty, changes occur in the sebaceous glands. The blood level of male hormones (androgens) rises, and the sebaceous glands increase in size and produce more sebum. Except in rare cases, acne is not caused by hormone "imbalance." Normal levels of androgens are enough to play a role in the development of acne in susceptible persons.

Many female patients experience a worsening of acne before a menstrual period. Progesterone, a hormone secreted after ovulation, may in some way influence premenstrual acne, but its exact role is not known.

Bacteria are important in the development of acne. They appear to act indirectly, possibly by altering the sebum or by producing a substance that makes the follicular wall rupture more easily. Certain antibiotics that reduce the acne bacteria also improve the disease.

Cleansing. Persons with acne often feel unclean because of the excessive oiliness of their skin. In fact, compulsive washing can be more harmful than beneficial.

People with acne should wash as often as they feel comfortable, generally once or twice a day. Some soaps made for acne contain abrasive or peeling agents meant to help unseat comedones. Most comedones are not so easily removed, however. Soaps cannot reach down into the follicles where the acne process begins. Abrasive soaps

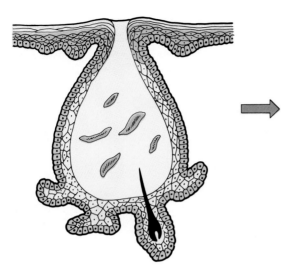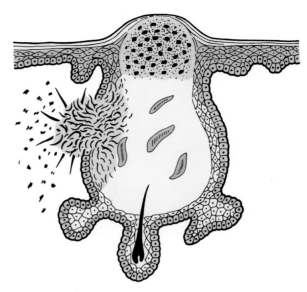

PIMPLE FORMATION
An inflamed pimple occurs when the contents of a whitehead, or closed comedo, rupture through the wall of the hair follicle into the dermis. The result is an inflammatory reaction, seen as a red papule or pustule. If a large portion of the follicle wall is destroyed and swelling isn't great, a nodule or cyst may form.

have an irritant effect. They peel and redden the skin surface by increasing blood flow. Thus, they may speed up the clearing of inflammatory lesions.

Cosmetics. Many women unknowingly precipitate or worsen acne by use of cosmetics. Oily products can make acne worse. The list includes foundation lotions or creams, greasy cleansers, moisturizers, and night creams.

Diet. Although acne patients have been admonished against eating chocolate, potato chips, soft drinks, nuts, and "junk foods," diet has little influence on acne. Some acne patients still feel that certain foods precipitate an outbreak. More likely, the lesion already was being formed, and the suspect food was coincidental. In general, the best advice is to eat a sensible, well-balanced diet.

Treatment. Whether an acne lesion leaves a scar depends on the degree of inflammation. Deep, inflamed cysts are likely to scar. Picking and gouging with the fingernails can worsen scarring.

Treatment decreases both the number of active lesions and the severity of inflammation so that the risk of scarring is reduced. Removing scars after they have formed is not always possible or satisfactory. Preventing scars is preferable.

Therapy for acne falls into two categories: medicines applied to the skin (topical) and medicines taken by mouth (systemic).

Topical medications. Many topical preparations for acne can be bought without a prescription. Most contain sulfur, resorcinol, salicylic acid, or benzoyl peroxide, and act by superficially peeling the skin and enhancing blood flow. Application of carbon dioxide slush and liquid nitrogen works in the same manner.

Two useful topical preparations are retinoic acid (tretinoin) and benzoyl peroxide. Retinoic acid, available only by prescription, is particularly active against blackheads and whiteheads. It helps expel existing comedones and interferes with formation of new ones.

Benzoyl peroxide is marketed under several brand names, some of which require a prescription. Its action is threefold: (1) it expels comedones; (2) it induces peeling and stimulates blood flow; and (3) it suppresses the growth of bacteria.

Several antibiotics also have been incorporated into topical acne medications. These include tetracycline, erythromycin, and clindamycin.

Systemic medications. Severe acne characterized by inflammatory pimples, cysts, and nodules seldom responds satisfactorily to topical medications alone. Antibiotics taken by mouth are then the mainstay of therapy. Improvement is often dramatic, although six weeks or more may pass before results can be noticed. Antibiotics reduce the population of the acne-associated bacteria.

Tetracycline is the antibiotic most physicians choose in treating acne, although several others may be used. The starting dose varies according to the severity of the acne, but continuous low-dose therapy over several years often is necessary.

Long-term use of tetracycline apparently causes few problems. For women, the most common side effect is a yeast infection of the vagina, called monilia or candida vaginitis. The symptoms are vaginal itching and a whitish discharge.

Another vitamin A derivative, isotretinoin (Accutane), has been highly successful in treatment of severe cystic acne, especially in women in their 20s and 30s. However, Accutane has been associated with increased birth defects among offspring of women using it. Despite this record, dermatologists continue to prescribe Accutane as the most effective method of combating the crippling psychological and physical effects of severe disease. They advise women to have a pregnancy test before beginning treatment and to use contraceptive methods during treatment.

Oral contraceptive pills. Some women with severe acne may benefit from estrogen, most easily taken as a birth control pill. Estrogens decrease the size of the sebaceous glands and reduce sebum production. At first, new inflammatory lesions may break out, and improvement may not be apparent for two or more months. The effect may last only a year or so.

Acne temporarily worsens in some women when they discontinue the birth control pill. A woman may even develop acne for the first time. The cause of this "rebound" is unknown.

Ultraviolet light. Many people notice that acne improves in the summer. One reason is that warm sun increases blood flow and inflammatory lesions clear faster. A suntan also partially masks lesions. It is unlikely that ultraviolet rays change the basic process of acne. Probably, benefits come from accelerated clearing of existing acne rather than prevention of new outbreaks.

Cosmetic surgery. The appearance of acne scars sometimes can be improved by surgical removal and replacement with a less noticeable scar. Sometimes a small graft of normal skin is taken from behind the ear, or a depressed scar is made more level by injecting silicone or a substance called fibrin foam. Chemical peeling agents also can help.

Dermabrasion planes the scarred skin with a rapidly rotating brush. Improvement of shallow pitted scars can be achieved in some cases. The procedure usually is restricted to the face.

Rosacea

Acne rosacea, sometimes simply called rosacea, resembles acne vulgaris, but with important differences. Rosacea patients are typically older—usually at least 35. Redness and dilated blood vessels of the nose and central face, rather than pimples, are characteristic. The nose may become enlarged, a condition known as rhinophyma and sometimes called the W. C. Fields nose. Rosacea patients should avoid alcohol, caffeine-containing beverages, and spicy foods, which stimulate the blood vessels to dilate, and cause an exaggerated blushing response, leading to permanent redness. Rosacea usually responds to tetracycline treatment.

Eczema

Eczema is a form of dermatitis, or skin inflammation, in which there is fluid collection or swelling between the cells of the epidermis. It has many causes, comes in many types, and can be acute or chronic. In acute eczema, the skin is red, swollen, and often blistered and weeping. Chronic eczema is characterized by scaly, thickened, red or brownish-red skin. The chief symptom of both is intense itching.

Atopic dermatitis usually runs in families, and may be associated with allergies, hay fever, and asthma. Infantile atopic eczema, often beginning about 3 or 4 months of age, appears on the scalp, cheeks, and neck, with scattered patches elsewhere. By age 2, the rash usually becomes less severe or disappears. It may recur between ages 4 and 10, tending to localize where the skin flexes—the neck, behind the ears, the elbows, or behind the knees. During adolescence and young adulthood, this pattern may become more pronounced.

The skin of a person with atopic dermatitis itches easily, even under normal circumstances. The persistent itching leads to scratching, which causes most of the visible changes in the skin. A person with atopic dermatitis often develops other medical problems. Broken blisters or raw scratches can be invaded by bacteria, causing infection. Patients with cold sores are unusually susceptible to the spread of the virus over their skin, a serious illness requiring hospitalization.

Topical application of corticosteroids is the cornerstone of therapy. The use of moisturizing creams and antihistamine drugs taken by mouth help to alleviate itching.

Contact dermatitis can be irritant or allergic. Irritant contact dermatitis can occur in anyone who is sufficiently exposed to harsh chemicals. It is caused by direct injury of the skin by contact with the irritant. Allergic contact dermatitis, on the other hand, occurs only in those who have developed a specific allergy to the responsible substance.

Cosmetic dermatitis. Often, the person who develops an allergic contact dermatitis from a cosmetic is able to identify the culprit. But a person may use the same product for many years without difficulty, then suddenly become hypersensitive to one of its chemicals. Or, one or more ingredients may have been changed without the user's being aware of it. Hypoallergenic preparations decrease but do not eliminate the possibility of allergy. Tweezers and eyelash curlers, and small sponges used to apply rouge or eye shadow, especially if they contain rubber, may be responsible.

The principal site of reaction to a cosmetic does not always coincide with the place where it is applied. Allergy to nail polish, for instance, often appears mainly on the upper eyelids. This is because the skin around the nails is relatively tough and resistant to contact dermatitis compared to the skin on the eyelids, which often are touched unconsciously.

Perfumes contained in other cosmetics or used alone also are potential offenders. They can cause not only the usual type of allergic contact dermatitis, but also a photo-contact reaction, brought out by exposing the affected area to the sun. The photodermatitis appears as a dark spot with sharply outlined borders corresponding to areas exposed to sunlight.

The first step for persons with cosmetic dermatitis is to eliminate all cosmetics. If the dermatitis subsides promptly, it can be assumed that one of the cosmetics eliminated was responsible. The cosmetics then can be reintroduced one at a time. If a rash recurs, take note of the cosmetic used last. A reaction to that particular cosmetic often can be confirmed by performing what is called a "usage test." Apply the suspect agent to the skin on the inside of the forearm three times a day for two days and observe the area for redness.

Poison ivy dermatitis, the most truculent form of allergic contact dermatitis, is illustrated and discussed in Chapter 23, "Allergy and the Immune System."

Hand eczema. Anyone whose hands are habitually exposed to household or occupational irritants or sensitizers may develop hand eczema. Household users commonly acquire it from soaps, detergents, bleaches, and cleansers. Bartenders, surgeons, dental hygienists, dentists, and kitchen workers similarly are exposed. The problem usually begins with mild dryness, redness, and scaling, and progresses to fissuring and crusting. Sometimes, the fissures become infected.

Protecting the hands from irritating substances is the basic therapeutic approach. Using long-handled brushes for dishwashing helps. Cotton gloves dusted with talcum powder should be worn under rubber gloves to protect against direct contact with rubber, to which some people are allergic. When bathing infants, wear a pair of cotton gloves *over* the rubber gloves as well as under them so that the baby can be handled without danger of slipping. When doing dusty or dirty housework, wear cotton gloves.

Dyshidrotic eczema is characterized by blisters on the palms and soles and between the fingers and toes. The blisters usually spontaneously heal after scales appear in about three weeks. In severe cases painful cracks in the skin occur during this phase. Dyshidrotic eczema tends to be recurrent and chronic. Treatment is similar to that for other types of eczema.

Lichen simplex chronicus. In this disease, the itch comes first, and subsequent scratching produces eczema. Around the ankles, wrists, and back of the neck, chronic scratching thickens and darkens the skin until it assumes a leathery consistency. Repeated scratching also may enlarge the nerves so that the skin itches more easily, and a vicious itch-scratch cycle is set up. Sometimes, the scratching is done unconsciously.

Therapy is aimed at controlling the itch with pills, creams, or ointments, and sometimes local injections of corticosteroids.

Psoriasis

Psoriasis, estimated to strike 1 to 2 percent of Americans, occurs because epidermal cells proliferate too fast and don't have time to reach full maturity. Psoriatic lesions consist of a piling-up of immature cells. The lesions usually are red because the small blood vessels in affected areas are dilated.

The basic cause of abnormal cell proliferation has not been identified. Genetics apparently plays a role.

A small percentage of patients have an associated arthritis (see Chapter 17, "Arthritis and Related Diseases," but the disease only rarely affects general health. To most psoriasis sufferers, the unsightly skin lesions are a greater burden. They appear as thickened red areas covered by white scale. The lesions may itch or develop painful fissures. Diseased skin may be confined to the knees and elbows or may cover the entire body. The scalp often is affected. Fingernail changes range from pitting to thickening and deformity.

Sunlight usually has a beneficial effect on the psoriatic skin. Most patients spontaneously improve in the summer and get worse during the winter. Further evidence of the sun's benefit is that the face usually is mostly clear, even though there may be extensive psoriasis underneath clothing.

Ultraviolet light exposure is the cornerstone of several treatment regimens for psoriasis. If the disease is widespread, therapy often is carried out best in a hospital. In the Goeckerman regimen, coal tar is applied to the affected areas, which then are exposed to artificial ultraviolet light. Patients usually have completely clear skin after three weeks of daily therapy. Once the disease is brought under control, a patient usually is able to manage the disease effectively at home for months.

The Ingram regimen combines application of a preparation called anthralin and ultraviolet light exposure. The Ingram method uses anthralin in a stiff paraffin-containing paste and usually is confined to outpatient centers.

Topical corticosteroid medications are widely used to treat psoriasis. They must be used strictly according to instructions, because they can damage skin if overused or applied to the wrong areas.

Anthralin in cream or ointment form also is available by prescription for home use, and can be effective in improving or clearing psoriasis in some cases. The disadvantage of anthralin is its irritant effect, and it also may temporarily stain the skin.

Psoriasis of the scalp can be discouraging because treatment is time-consuming. It consists of removing the scale by applying preparations called keratolytics (often most effective when used under a plastic shower cap), frequent shampooing, and sometimes the application of corticosteroid lotions. Several types of shampoos are helpful, including those containing tars.

For severe psoriasis, antimetabolite drugs, also used to treat cancer, prevent the excessive prolifer-

ation of the epidermal cells. Unfortunately, their effect is not limited to the skin. They also affect the cells in other organs, such as the bone marrow, liver, and gastrointestinal tract. Antimetabolites must be given in carefully determined doses under close medical supervision.

The PUVA treatment for psoriasis consists of swallowing a drug called psoralen, followed two hours later by exposure to long-wave ultraviolet light (UVA) in a specially designed cabinet. When the psoralen reaches the skin, it becomes activated by the UVA exposure. The process binds the DNA, the large molecule in the nucleus of the cell, and thus inhibits the reproduction of epidermal cells.

Most dermatologists reserve PUVA treatments for patients who have not responded to traditional methods, or for older persons with extensive disease in whom the benefits outweigh the long-term risk of developing skin cancer, which the treatments appear to increase.

Skin Cancer

Skin cancers are the most common malignant tumors. Because they can be readily seen and detected, however, they can be treated promptly.

The two most common types of skin cancer, basal-cell carcinoma and squamous-cell carcinoma, account for 29 of 30 cases of skin cancer, but they usually are discovered while still localized and thus are treated successfully. Malignant melanoma, the least common form, always is potentially fatal unless detected early and treated promptly. In that case, complete cure often is possible.

Chronic sun exposure increases the risk of basal-cell or squamous-cell cancer. Persons most susceptible are those who sunburn easily and tan poorly, such as those of Irish, Scottish, or Welsh background, and persons who work outdoors and receive prolonged sun exposure over many years, such as farmers and sailors.

Sun exposure also plays some role in malignant melanomas. The trend toward more leisure time and travel to sunny vacation spots is believed to explain at least partially melanoma's increase in the United States and northern European countries. Significantly, an increasing number of melanomas now are found on the back and neck in men or on the lower leg and back in women. It probably is no coincidence that these locations have become more exposed to sun as styles have changed.

Relatively few melanomas occur where skin is almost always covered. Still, a small number of melanomas do occur on the buttocks and female breasts, suggesting that factors other than exposure to sunlight play a role.

Basal-cell carcinoma, which accounts for 75 percent of all skin cancers, commonly appears as a small nodule on the skin that eventually ulcerates in the center, intermittently bleeding and forming a crust. Because it usually is painless, the tumor may be neglected for some time. Bleeding and failure of the ulcer to heal usually prompt the person to see a physician.

Although it grows slowly, basal-cell cancer can invade deeply into underlying tissue and bone and be very destructive locally if not treated. Fortunately, it rarely spreads to distant sites.

More than 95 percent of basal-cell lesions can be cured with the first treatment. Surgery, destruction of the tissue by high-frequency electricity, freezing with liquid nitrogen (cryotherapy), removal by laser, and radiation are all effective. A technique called chemosurgery is especially useful for treating tumors that are recurrent, far-advanced, or in locations close to a vital structure such as the eye.

A person who develops one basal-cell carcinoma has an increased risk of developing additional ones. He or she should visit a dermatologist regularly, and always use a sunscreen.

Squamous-cell carcinoma may begin as a small bleeding growth with an irregular surface, but the appearance varies. If treated early, the outlook is good. If left untreated, squamous-cell cancers eventually will spread to the lymph nodes.

Squamous-cell cancer can arise from what appears to be normal skin, but most often occurs in skin chronically damaged by sun. This change is called an actinic keratosis. It usually appears as a faint, red, slightly elevated lesion with a sandpaperlike texture. Actinic keratoses can be quite numerous on the face and backs of the hands and forearms of people who have had prolonged sun exposure, especially those with light complexions who sunburn easily.

Liquid nitrogen may be used to treat actinic keratoses if they are few in number. A medicine containing 5-fluorouracil may be applied when le-

sions are numerous. Retinoic acid (Retin-A) also appears to retard development of keratoses.

Malignant melanomas are classified into three types. Two of the three spread outward on the surface of the skin before invading downward. This characteristic allows diagnosis while the malignancy is still curable by surgical removal. These two types, superficial spreading and lentigo maligna melanomas, together account for about 75 to 80 percent of melanomas. The third type, nodular melanoma, tends to invade downward into the skin at an early stage, so the chance of cure is much lower.

The peak incidence of melanoma is in the late 40s and 50s. Lentigo maligna melanoma tends to affect older people. The most common location for melanoma is the back, except for lentigo maligna melanoma, which most often develops on the face from a large, flat tan spot.

Early, curable superficial spreading melanoma usually begins as a brown spot on the skin. The lesion gradually enlarges and assumes characteristic features: an irregular border, variation in color, and an irregular surface. The colors usually are predominantly brown, but shades of brown and black with areas of red, white, and blue may be present. Frequently, the easiest clue for a patient is the irregular border, which clearly is different from the smooth, regular borders of benign moles.

Large moles present at birth, sometimes referred to as bathing trunk or garment congenital nevi, have about a one in 10 chance of developing melanoma. If possible, these moles should be removed surgically during childhood. If complete removal is impossible, they should be examined for malignant change at least annually.

A definite diagnosis of melanoma is made by examining a biopsy specimen under the microscope. The type of treatment then is determined by how deeply the cancer has invaded the underlying tissue. In the most superficial cases, surgical removal of the melanoma plus a border of normal tissue, sometimes requiring a skin graft, usually is all that is necessary. In more advanced cases, lymph nodes may be removed. Chemotherapy and agents to stimulate the body's immune system are given for deep melanomas or those that have spread elsewhere in the body.

Parasitic Infestation

Pediculosis means an infestation of lice. These parasites feed specifically on human blood. Infestation occurs in three forms, all characterized by severe itching.

Head lice (pediculosis of the scalp) are more common in children than adults. Epidemics among schoolchildren are common. The head louse is transferred from one child to another by shared clothing, combs, and brushes. The lice produce small wheals in the scalp, temporary skin swellings that itch intensely. Scratching often opens the skin and leads to secondary bacterial infection, or impetigo, which in turn causes lymph glands to swell as they mobilize to fight the infection. Examination of the scalp usually fails to reveal adult lice. Instead, numerous tiny white nits or eggs can be seen firmly attached to the hair shafts, especially on the back of the head and above the ears.

Pubic lice (pediculosis pubis) infest the hairs of the pubic region. The pubic louse is short and squat and has clawlike legs; hence, infestation with the pubic louse commonly is referred to as "crabs." Occasionally, the crab louse also infests the eyelashes, beard, or armpits. Both nits and adult lice can be seen, along with small, rust-colored specks representing digested and excreted blood. The pubic louse is transmitted from person to person and on clothing, bedding, and towels.

Body lice (pediculosis corporis) are not common in the United States, but sometimes occur among elderly indigents and vagrants. The body louse lays its eggs in the seams of clothing, and attacks the skin in areas that are in constant contact with underwear, such as the waist, shoulders, and upper back.

Treatment. Gamma benzene hexachloride (Kwell), a prescription drug available as a shampoo, cream, or lotion, kills both lice and nits, but the dead organisms may remain attached to the hairs. They can be loosened by applying a solution of equal parts of white vinegar and water under a towel for an hour, and then removed with a fine-toothed comb. Afterward, all clothing, bedding, towels, and hairbrushes should be laundered.

Scabies is an intensely itchy parasitic infestation caused by a mite. The female mite, barely visible to the human eye, burrows a tunnel in the top layer of the skin and lays eggs. The burrow may resemble a fine, black thread with a minute blister at one end. Most commonly affected are the webs between the fingers, the waistline, underarms, nipples, elbows, buttocks, and penis. The head almost never is involved, except in infants.

Scabies usually is acquired through intimate contact with infested people. In rare instances, the mite that causes scabies in animals (mange) takes up temporary residence on human skin and produces itching.

Once scabies is diagnosed, gamma benzene hexachloride applied from the neck down and left on for 24 hours usually is prescribed. All potentially infested clothing, bedding, and linens should be washed in hot water or dry-cleaned. Itching often lasts for a week or more.

Fungal Infections

A distinct group of fungi called dermatophytes can live in the superficial layer of the epidermis, nails, or hair. Dermatophyte infection is commonly referred to as ringworm because the lesions often assume a ringlike shape.

Warmth and moisture increase the likelihood of fungal infections. They frequently occur between two skin surfaces where moisture can't easily evaporate, such as between the toes or in the creases of the thigh.

Tinea corporis, fungal infection anywhere on the skin except the scalp, may produce no symptoms or may be only mildly itchy. Typically, lesions are round, light red, and scaling, with a well-defined border. The skin may be clear in the center. A few lesions may be treated with an antifungal cream applied daily for several weeks. Widespread cases often require an oral medication, griseofulvin.

Athlete's foot (tinea pedis) is the most common dermatophyte infection. It primarily affects adults, many of whom are so accustomed to the scaling on their soles and the moist skin between their toes that they accept the condition as normal.

Athlete's foot may cause small fissures in the skin that allow bacteria to enter and set up infections. The fungi can spread to other areas, such as the nails, groin, and hands. Once a fungus has infected the toenails, eradication is very difficult.

The first step in treatment is to eliminate moisture from the feet, especially between the toes. Feet should be thoroughly dried after bathing and a powder applied regularly. If possible, open shoes or sandals should be worn to expose bare feet to open air. Topical creams or lotions with antifungal ingredients can be prescribed.

Tinea cruris ("jock itch") infects the inner surface and upper parts of the thighs. It is seen most often in men. Treatment consists of keeping the area dry and frequent application of an antifungal cream or lotion.

Tinea manus, fungal infection of the hands, causes fine scaling with minimal redness on the palms. It almost always is accompanied by athlete's foot. Topical treatment alone may be effective, but griseofulvin sometimes is used.

Onychomycosis means fungal infection of the fingernails or toenails. The nails become thickened, white or yellow, and crumbly.

Topical medication is ineffective. Griseofulvin must be taken for five to six months, and sometimes relapse occurs afterward. Toenails are even more difficult to treat. Medication must be taken for an average of one year, and many cases do not respond even then.

Tinea capitis, fungal infection of the scalp, affects more children than adults. It is contagious and may occur in epidemics. The usual appearance is patchy areas of scaling, broken-off hairs, or even bald patches. Sometimes, a localized painful, boggy, swollen area of inflammation occurs. Tinea capitis now can be cured with griseofulvin.

Yeast Infections

The yeast *Candida albicans* lives normally in the mouth, gastrointestinal tract, and vagina. Under certain circumstances, its normal relationship can be disturbed and it can cause disease. Predisposing factors include pregnancy, antibiotic and birth control medications, diabetes, and chronic debilitating illness. Candidiasis also occurs in AIDS victims and others whose immune systems have been suppressed.

Cutaneous candidiasis appears in several forms. Paronychia is a painful inflammation around the nail involving the cuticle. It is most common in people who frequently immerse their hands in water, such as housewives and dishwashers. Perléche is a moist red area at the corners of the mouth. Since warmth and moisture favor the growth of the yeast organism, a common location for candidiasis is between touching skin surfaces. Monilia intertrigo occurs between the buttocks, in the thigh creases, under female breasts, and under folds of fat. Sometimes the finger webs, especially between the third and fourth fingers, are affected.

Thrush is a yeast infection of the mucous membrane, either the mouth or vagina. Oral thrush is most common in newborns. Vaginal moniliasis may be a complication of pregnancy and medication with oral contraceptives and antibiotics. It can be transmitted to a male sexual partner.

Most forms of candidiasis can be treated with an absorbent powder, after which the affected areas are exposed to air or a fan several times a day. In nail infections, the hands must be protected from water. Medications are available by prescription.

Viral Infections

Warts. Although all warts are caused by the same or at least closely related viruses, warts may vary in appearance. Common warts start as pinhead-size, skin-colored elevations that gradually grow to become larger, raised lesions with a rough surface. They most often are located on the backs of the hands.

Filiform and flat warts are most common on the face. Plantar warts are located on the sole of the foot. Calluses usually form over them, and they may be painful because of pressure against nerves during standing or walking.

Condyloma acuminata (venereal warts) are most commonly found on the penis or around the vaginal and anal areas. They begin as small, isolated bumps but later group together in clusters resembling cauliflower. Venereal warts usually are acquired through sexual contact.

The wart virus is contagious, but whether a person becomes infected depends more on the inborn immune system than on the amount of exposure. Recipients of kidney transplants or cancer patients who must take drugs to suppress the immune system have an increased incidence of warts. Warts may be destroyed without scarring—by freezing the cells with liquid nitrogen, zapping them with electric current, or applying acids.

The treatment for plantar wart "shells out" the wart with minimal injury to the surrounding skin. Venereal warts usually are treated with either liquid nitrogen or a strong chemical. The treatment, incidentally, should include sexual partners.

Molluscum contagiosum consists of one or more firm, dome-shaped bumps that are flesh-colored to pink and have pearly white centers with a tiny depression. The disease is transmitted from person to person by direct contact or spread by the hands from an affected area to another part of the body. Molluscum contagiosum is common in children, usually concentrating on the face, chest, and abdomen.

The lesions usually go away spontaneously, but sometimes last for years. They can be removed by scraping or by applying liquid nitrogen or acids.

Herpes simplex is a virus that causes the common but distressing cold sore. Most people are infected in childhood, but the initial infection usually causes no symptoms. Less often, a child, usually between the ages of 1 and 5, will become ill with fever, enlarged lymph nodes, and painful sores in the mouth. Recovery is usually complete within two weeks.

Once a person has been infected by herpes simplex, the virus goes into a latent phase. Later, the virus becomes reactivated and causes a cold sore on the outside of the lip. In some people, emotional stress, physical illness such as the common cold, sunburn, or menstruation predictably triggers an outbreak. The cold sores tend to occur repeatedly in the same site.

At present, there is no cure for herpes simplex infections, although numerous treatments have been tried. Blisters are thought to heal faster if a local drying agent such as alcohol is applied. Secondary bacterial infection can be prevented by washing the area with an antiseptic solution.

Remember that the blisters of a herpes simplex infection are contagious to others and occasionally may be spread by the hands to other parts of the body, including the eye. Herpes simplex infection should be suspected if the eye becomes pink and painful in the presence of herpes lesions in other areas.

Herpes simplex also can affect the genital area. Small blisters that quickly break are found on the vulva, vagina, and cervix in women and on the penis in men. The first infection is very painful, especially in women, who may experience such discomfort that urination and even walking and sitting are difficult.

Recurrent infections can occur after the primary outbreak subsides. Reexposure to the virus is not necessary. Fortunately, the symptoms from recurrent infection usually are mild. Because the blisters harbor the virus, sexual relations should be avoided until the blisters have healed to prevent spreading.

Genital herpes is a special problem to a pregnant woman. The infant can contract a fatal infection when passing through an infected birth canal. In such cases, cesarean section usually is done.

Treatment with acyclovir, an oral medication, helps to relieve symptoms of acute herpes infections and also may prevent recurrent attacks.

Bacterial Infections

Impetigo is a common, superficial bacterial infection of the skin caused by streptococcal or staphylococcal bacteria. Children often are affected, with small itchy blisters appearing on the face. The blisters easily rupture and leave yellowish-brown crusts on a red oozing base. Sometimes, impetigo occurs on skin where there is a minor cut or abrasion.

Impetigo is contagious, but it responds readily to an antibacterial cleanser and topical or oral antibiotics.

Folliculitis is a mildly painful infection around hair follicles, usually caused by staphylococcus bacteria. Tiny pustules appear at the base of each hair. Common locations are the thighs and buttocks. Friction and exposure to grease or oil can increase susceptibility. Frequent washing with an antibacterial cleanser helps eliminate the infection, but sometimes antibiotics are necessary.

Boils begin around hair follicles but extend outward and downward to form a pocket of pus called an abscess. The cause usually is staphylococcus bacteria. A furuncle is a deep infection of a group of adjacent follicles, often draining at multiple sites.

Boils are painful because of the expanding pus, which becomes visible when it "comes to a head." Small boils can rupture and heal spontaneously. Large boils need medical attention because incision and drainage, and sometimes an antibiotic and pain medication, are required.

Pigmentation Problems

Vitiligo is a loss of skin pigmentation caused by the disappearance of melanocytes. Common sites are the backs of the hands; the face, especially around the mouth and eyes; and the genitalia. The involved areas appear white and are most noticeable in dark-skinned persons.

Absence of melanin leaves the areas unprotected from sunlight, so they sunburn easily. Sunscreens should be used. To improve appearance, temporary stain can be painted on the white areas.

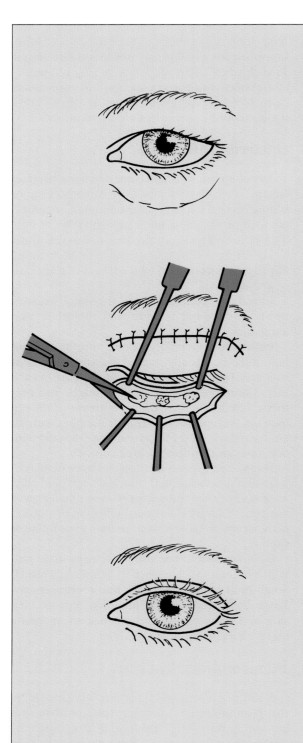

Cosmetic Surgery

Surgical techniques to improve the appearance have become increasingly popular and can now be performed on an outpatient basis. Eyelid surgery (blepharoplasty), illustrated here, removes bags and wrinkles from upper and lower eyelids. An incision is made following the natural creases above the eye. Fat and excess skin are cut away and the incisions are sutured. Face-lifts (rhytidectomy) are done to take up the sagging skin around the jaw and neck. An incision is made along the hairline and around the ear, where it is least visible. The skin is then separated and lifted from the underlying muscles and stretched more tautly toward the hairline. Excess skin is cut away and the skin edges are sewn together.

Improvement in appearance usually lasts three to five years, after which the procedure may have to be repeated. Chemical peel, a form of chemosurgery, removes wrinkles, scars, and blemishes by applying an acid solution to the face that peels away the top layer of skin. The effect is temporary, and may have to be repeated within a few months. Nose surgery (rhinoplasty) reduces the size of a nose or remodels its contours. Incisions are made inside the nostrils. Humps and bulges are sawed off; some cartilage may be removed and the bones broken and reshaped. Liposuction is used to reduce fatty deposits around the hips, buttocks, thighs, and abdomen. An incision is made and a tubular instrument inserted, through which the excess fat is sucked out, and the incisions closed with sutures. Tummy tuck (abdominoplasty) flattens the abdomen by cutting away excess fat and wrinkled skin. Most cosmetic operations are expensive, are not always covered by health insurance, and may require periods of healing ranging from a few days to a month.

Melasma consists of darkened patches on the cheeks and forehead. It occurs mainly in women who take oral contraceptives or who are pregnant, and sometimes is called the "mask of pregnancy."

Treatment must prevent further darkening by sunlight and promote lightening of the darkened areas. A sunscreen that blocks out all light is recommended. Hydroquinone cream will gradually decrease pigmentation, but the dark areas can be more quickly lightened by a prescription preparation containing tretinoin plus a corticosteroid.

Pemphigus and Pemphigoid

These two diseases are characterized by blisters. Pemphigus blisters occur in the epidermis when cells lose their adhesion to one another. Only a thin layer of cells remains to form the roofs of the blisters, so that they easily rupture. Most patients with pemphigus develop blisters in the mouth as well as on the visible skin. The painful blisters may interfere with eating.

Blisters in bullous pemphigoid form lower in the skin, just beneath the junction of the epidermis and the dermis. They are larger than in pemphigus and remain intact longer.

Pemphigus affects mainly middle-aged persons; bullous pemphigoid occurs primarily in the elderly. Treatment includes corticosteroids and antimetabolic drugs.

Common Benign Conditions

Heat rash (miliaria) results when eccrine sweat ducts are blocked so that trapped sweat cannot reach the surface of the skin. Tiny, clear bubblelike blisters are produced. In deeper obstruction, redness surrounds the blisters.

Heat rash breaks out when sweat glands react to a hot environment, fever, or prolonged exertion. Sunburn is another common cause.

Lowering the surrounding temperature is the key to treatment. Once sweating stops, the rash clears spontaneously within a few days.

Pityriasis rosea consists of multiple scaling patches, usually affecting young people during the spring and fall. It is self-limiting, lasting six to eight weeks. Often a "herald patch" precedes the appearance of other smaller lesions. All are pink to salmon-colored, oval, and scaly, and have a crinkly surface, sometimes resembling ringworm. They commonly are located on the back and chest, where their branchlike arrangement resembles a fir tree. The rash usually is not itchy. The cause, though unproven, is thought to be a virus.

Dandruff and seborrheic dermatitis both stem from an increased production of scales on the scalp. Simple dandruff is noninflammatory, but seborrheic dermatitis is characterized by scaling and redness, not only in the scalp, but also in the eyebrows, the creases behind the ears, and on each side of the nose. Red patches also may occur on the chest or in the armpits and groin.

The chronic condition can be controlled but not cured. A special shampoo will slow down the production of scales and wash away those already formed. Tar shampoos are helpful but may stain light-colored hair. If the scalp is very red, a physician may prescribe a steroid solution or spray. Seborrheic dermatitis on the face, chest, and other areas responds readily to topical medications.

Seborrheic keratoses occur most frequently on the face, chest, and back. They are brown or black, have a waxy, slightly elevated surface, and vary in size from a tenth of an inch to three-fourths of an inch in diameter. Seborrheic keratoses need not be treated. If they itch or are of objectionable appearance, they can be removed easily.

Cysts (wens) are cavities in the skin that are filled with the fatty secretion sebum, the protein keratin, and cells. They usually occur on the chest, back, face, and scalp. The two main types, epidermal cysts and pilar (sebaceous) cysts, look alike but display different structures under the microscope. Cysts are painless unless they become infected. They can be removed for cosmetic reasons.

Hives, itchy, well-circumscribed, pink swelling in the skin, usually result from an allergic reaction to a food, drug, or insect bite and are discussed in Chapter 23, "Allergy and the Immune System."

Lichen planus affects the skin with small itchy, angular, purplish bumps. In the mouth, where they can be painful, the lesions appear as a lacelike network of fine white lines. Lichen planus usually lasts several months but can be chronic and persist for years. Treatment is aimed at relief of itching.

Ichthyosis refers to the fishlike scales of dry skin. The most common and least severe type, ichthyosis vulgaris, usually appears in infancy and is inherited from a parent. Some victims also have atopic dermatitis. Tiny bumps tend to develop around the hair follicles on the upper arms and thighs, a condition known as keratosis pilaris. In its mildest form, ichthyosis may be noticed only as dry skin. Emollients such as Eucerin applied after a shower or bath help.

Keloids are thick, rubbery, elevated scars that occur after injury to the skin or surgical incisions. The skin of the chest and back is quite susceptible. Keloids are especially common in blacks. Some-

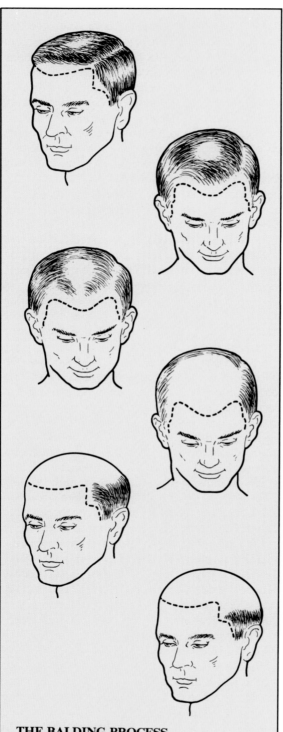

THE BALDING PROCESS
*Common male baldness follows a
pattern. The hair recedes from the
forehead, temple, and crown, as shown,
and the bald areas tend to merge, but a
fringe around the ears and back of the
head usually remains.*

times, keloids can be satisfactorily reduced in size by local injection of corticosteroids.

Erythema multiforme is characterized by distinctive lesions in concentric circles, resembling a target. It usually is found on the hands, feet, forearms, and legs. Although most patients recover completely, in rare instances the problem can be fatal. Certain drugs can cause erythema multiforme, as can herpes (cold sores) and a certain type of pneumonia.

HAIR DISORDERS

Common Baldness
(male pattern baldness)

Male hair loss is part of the normal aging process and occurs in monkeys, apes, and chimpanzees as well as in humans. During balding, the hair follicles become smaller and the hairs they produce change from coarse dark terminal hairs to soft, thin, unpigmented vellus hairs. Hair loss occurs in a characteristic pattern. It tends to affect the parts of the scalp around the temples first, and later involves the crown. Eventually, the two areas may merge.

The scientific term for common baldness is androgenetic alopecia. This term encompasses the two major factors in this type of hair loss—the male hormones or androgens and a hereditary predisposition. The precise relationship between androgens and baldness is being investigated. It is thought that the smaller hair follicles in the frontal scalp metabolize hormones faster than unaffected follicles. But it is not known why androgen causes the hair follicles to shrink in the scalp area yet simultaneously stimulates growth of the beard and axillary and pubic hair. Although we know that genes play a role, the exact inheritance pattern is not clear.

Men vary greatly in how much hair they lose and how quickly. Family history is a useful guide. In general, early, extensive hair loss suggests an unfavorable outlook. On the other hand, thinning of the hair first noticed after age 40 is quite unlikely to evolve rapidly into significant baldness. About 5 percent of white males show the first sign of baldness before age 20. One or 2 percent develop extensive baldness by age 30. By age 60, about 80 percent of men show some evidence of hair loss.

Women also may lose their hair as they get older, but the process begins later and progresses less rapidly. In women, thinning usually occurs all over the head.

For some men with limited amounts of baldness, minoxidil (Rogaine), a medication originally developed for hypertension, in an emollient form will restimulate hair growth. Benefits appear only after twice-daily treatment over several months. New hair growth appears to be confined to those whose hair loss is recent, limited to the crown, and about the size of a silver dollar. Contrary to advertising claims, no magic salve can be rubbed on to cure baldness, and no treatments can start the hair growing again.

Hair transplantation is the favored approach, but it is expensive and time-consuming, and is suitable only for men whose hair is abundant enough to provide a donor site, usually on the back of the scalp, above the neck. Plugs of hair about half the diameter of a pencil are removed, and the resulting holes gradually shrink to form inconspicuous scars. Plugs of the same size are taken from the bald scalp and discarded. The donor plugs then are fitted into the holes in the bald area, where they grow just as they did in the old site. Usually, several hundred plugs must be transplanted to fill in the bald area.

Alopecia Areata

In this condition, which affects both sexes, the hair is lost in a localized spot, most commonly on the scalp, but sometimes in the male beard. The initial bald spot usually is the size of a dime or a quarter.

In most cases, the hair returns spontaneously after several months, but sometimes appears lighter in color than the surrounding hair. In a few people, the bald spot enlarges to include much of the scalp. In rare cases, all of the scalp hair is lost.

Treatment usually is not necessary because spontaneous regrowth occurs. In more extensive and persistent cases, corticosteroid injections temporarily stimulate regrowth, but do not alter the course of the disease. A wiser approach is the purchase of a wig.

Excessive Hair Growth

Excessive hair growth (hirsutism) in women may be caused by an abnormal increase in androgen production from an endocrine disorder or a tumor. It often is accompanied by acne and menstrual irregularities.

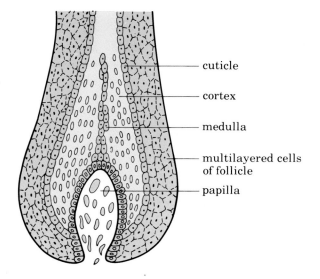

THE HAIR SHAFT
The three components of the hair shaft, from outside in, are the cuticle, cortex, and medulla. Surrounding the hair are several layers of cells in the follicle that take part in the formation of the shaft. The papilla is a protrusion of the dermal skin layer from which the follicle arises.

Some normal women have dark hairs on the face, abdomen, thighs, and around the nipples. This is in part genetically determined. A woman can feel that her hair growth is normal if her mother and sisters have a similar pattern.

To remove unwanted hair, the simplest method is shaving. Chemical hair removers (depilatories) dissolve hair, but may irritate the skin. Tweezing out hairs usually is reserved for the eyebrows. In some salons, waxing is used to remove hairs. Warm wax is applied to the skin and allowed to cool. The wax then is quickly pulled away from the skin, taking with it the hairs in that area. Bleaching is satisfactory for some people, but bleached hair may look unnatural in dark-skinned women.

Electrolysis is the one method of hair removal that can be permanent. A very fine needle is inserted into the hair follicle and an electric current applied. The hair then can be removed easily. The follicles are briefly swollen afterward. Occasionally, tiny, firm red bumps appear, usually lasting several weeks. Because a hair-bearing area always contains some hairs in the resting phase, electrolysis must be done over several months to achieve permanent hair removal.

THE LUNGS

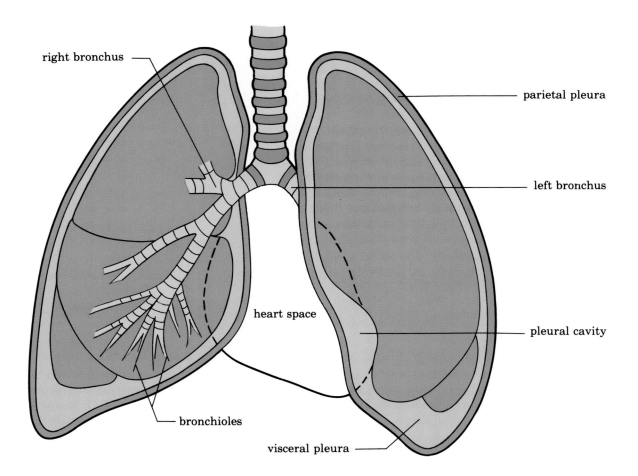

right bronchus

parietal pleura

left bronchus

heart space

pleural cavity

bronchioles

visceral pleura

STRUCTURE OF THE LUNGS

The cone-shaped lungs are located behind the ribs and in front of the heart. They are contained within a glistening membrane, the visceral pleura, another membrane, the parietal pleura is located on the inner surface of the chest. The left lung has two lobes; the right lung, three. Air is brought into the lungs via the bronchial tree, which, treelike, separates into smaller and smaller branches called bronchioles. Alveoli (air sacs) at the terminus of each bronchiole (lower drawing) consist of microscopic air cells where vital oxygen is exchanged for carbon dioxide in the process called respiration.

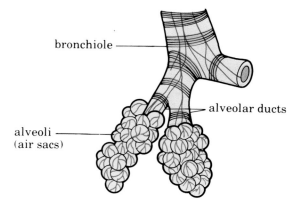

bronchiole

alveolar ducts

alveoli
(air sacs)

The lungs and the heart work closely together to sustain life. All cells of the body need a continuous supply of oxygen to perform the process of combustion known as metabolism, which provides energy. It is the task of the respiratory system to furnish this oxygen and dispose of the waste product, carbon dioxide. Blood pumped by the heart picks up oxygen in the lungs and carries it to the cells, then returns to the lungs with carbon dioxide.

The illustrations in this chapter show the structure of the lungs, identify the parts, and explain their functions. Many methods are used by physicians to assess and examine the lungs, even though they are hidden from direct view. X rays and CT scans, described in Chapter 2, "Tests and Procedures," are the mainstay of these examinations. Some of the other methods are illustrated in this chapter.

Among the most important tests are those of pulmonary functions. These include tests of the arterial blood, to determine how well oxygen is being delivered, and of lung volumes, to determine how efficiently air is being inhaled and exhaled.

The most important measurements of lung volume are tidal volume, vital capacity, residual volume, and total lung capacity.

Tidal volume represents the amount of gas moved during each cycle of inhalation and exhalation while a person is resting. Vital capacity and residual volume are measured by fully expanding the lungs with air and then expelling it as completely as possible. The volume exhaled is the vital capacity; the amount remaining in the lungs is the residual volume. Total lung volume is the sum of the vital capacity and residual volume.

These values are determined by a spirometer, which also can measure the amount of air exhaled in a given period. In the test for forced expiratory volume in one second, the patient fills the lungs and then blows the air out as rapidly as possible. The amount expelled in the first full second is measured and recorded. The amount exhaled at other intervals also can be measured. The time required for total expiration also is a useful measurement. Measurements of forced flow are particularly important in testing for categories of obstructive lung disease.

The flow-volume curve, a less routine test, helps to disclose obstructions of the larynx, trachea, and large airways. The test compares airflow from the mouth with lung volume.

Symptoms of Lung Disease

When the lungs are not functioning properly, the most common symptom is breathlessness, technically known as dyspnea. Dyspnea also may be present in disorders of the heart, blood, muscles, and nervous system.

In the condition known as primary hyperventilation, patients experience breathlessness, yet no underlying lung disease can be detected. They gulp air in deep, rapid breaths until acid and mineral levels in the blood become disturbed and produce numbness and tingling of the lips, muscle spasms, dizziness, and fainting. The so-called hyperventilation syndrome appears to be a psychological problem, and there are indications it runs in families. The best treatment appears to be reassurance and psychiatric counseling.

Coughing is one of the most common human symptoms. Everyone coughs intermittently or chronically. Like breathlessness, a cough is not always an indication of lung disease. It can be triggered by conditions ranging from a bad cold to the aftermath of a hearty bout of laughter.

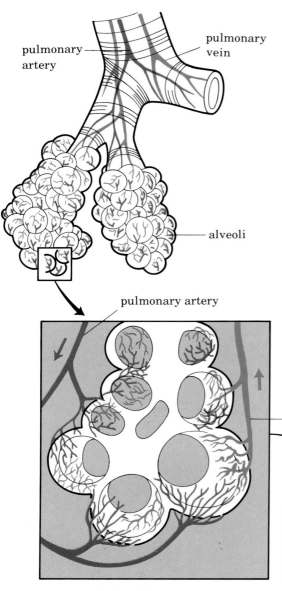

A cough is primarily a defensive weapon against an irritating or infective environment. The throat, trachea, and large airways are studded with nerves sensitive to irritation. When stimulated by infection or an airborne irritant, these nerves send impulses to the cough center of the brain. The message to cough is relayed to the muscles that produce the cough, primarily those of expiration, especially in the abdominal wall. The cough mechanism is a forceful expiration against a closed upper airway. Pressure builds behind the closure, until a sudden release results in a high-velocity expulsion of air, not unlike the controlled explosion that occurs in the barrel of a gun.

Sputum, the mixture of mucus, pus, cellular debris, and other material expelled in clearing the throat, tells much about what is happening in the respiratory system. Its color, consistency, and odor all provide hints about the underlying condition of the lungs. Samples are studied microscopically or cultured in the laboratory in search of disease-causing organisms, or examined for distinctively abnormal cells. Blood in the sputum (hemoptysis) frequently indicates serious lung disease.

Sputum differs from other secretions, such as saliva or postnasal drip. Its occasional presence in a cough is not necessarily a sign of lung disease.

THE GAS EXCHANGE
The heart of respiration is shown in these three drawings. At top, the pulmonary artery brings blood loaded with carbon dioxide from the veins to the alveoli. The pulmonary vein returns it, enriched with oxygen, to the heart. The middle drawing shows the microscopic blood vessels in the thin walls of the air-filled alveoli. At bottom, an air cell shows how oxygen molecules diffuse into the blood and carbon dioxide molecules diffuse out of it.

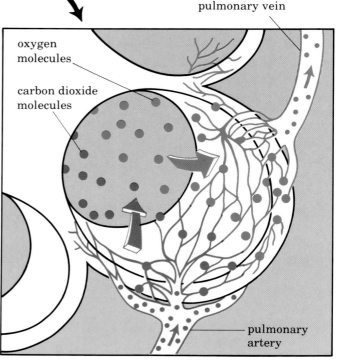

But the chronic presence of cough with sputum *is* a warning of possible lung disorders.

Chest pain is not necessarily an indicator of lung disease. The skin, muscles, and bones of the chest, heart, or esophagus can cause the pain. The parietal pleura, the glistening membrane that lines the chest walls, is highly pain-sensitive, but the visceral pleura, its counterpart membrane that covers the lung and rubs against it during breathing, does not sense pain, nor does the lung itself. (The pleurae and the pleural cavity between them are illustrated on page 106.) Various pulmonary diseases produce pleurisy, a sharp localized chest pain that worsens with coughing, sneezing, or deep breathing. To avert the pain, many persons voluntarily restrict or "splint" their breathing on the affected side.

Respiratory Assistance

When disease-weakened lungs are not strong enough to supply oxygen and eliminate carbon dioxide, and thus not strong enough to sustain life, a machine must help out. There are several types of breathing-assistance equipment.

The essential requirement of breathing assistance is an airtight connection between the trachea and the gas source, which may provide room air, oxygen-enriched air, or pure oxygen. The seal is made by one of two methods. In endotracheal intubation, a flexible tube is inserted into the trachea through the mouth or nose. The inner tip is surrounded by a doughnut-shaped rubber balloon. When inflated, the balloon firmly anchors the tube and seals it into an airtight system. The second method, surgical tracheostomy, consists of inserting a short tube into the trachea through a small slit in the neck. Here, too, an inflated balloon anchors the tube and makes an airtight junction with the trachea.

If breathing support appears to be required for only a short time (as with acute, severe pneumonia), endotracheal intubation is preferred over tracheostomy. On the other hand, endotracheal intubation for more than two weeks might cause pressure damage to the larynx or tracheal wall. Because the tube passes between the vocal cords and makes direct contact with them, voice changes

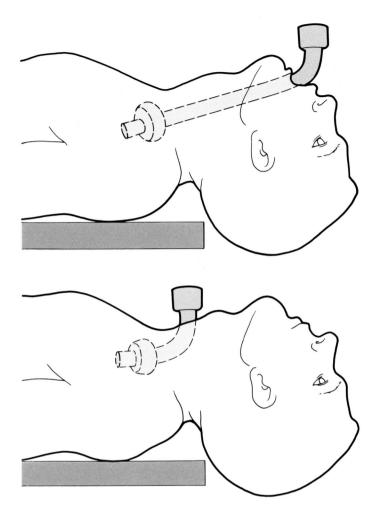

BREATHING ASSISTANCE
When disease-weakened lungs are not strong enough for normal respiration, a machine must help. Two methods of providing an airtight connection to a breathing-assistance device are shown. In endotracheal intubation (top), a clear plastic tube is inserted into the trachea through the mouth or nose. In surgical tracheostomy (bottom), the tube is inserted through a slit in the neck. Endotracheal intubation is preferred for short periods. Tracheostomy is used when aid is needed for a week or more.

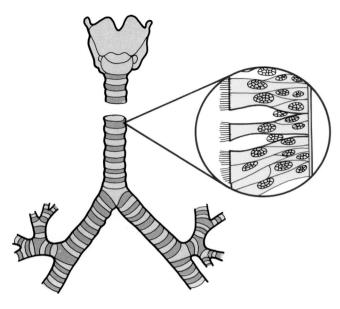

CLEANSING THE LUNGS
Billions of hairlike cilia (see in the close-up) sweep bacteria and other foreign bodies from the respiratory tract by rhythmically beating back and forth, moving like a field of grain in a light breeze. Air passages are lined with cilia, which form a kind of escalator to move material up and out.

can occur. Furthermore, the endotracheal tube makes swallowing difficult. In those cases, tracheostomy is preferred.

Once the tube is in place, it is attached to a ventilator. The machine drives gas into the lungs during inspiration and allows it to escape during expiration. Commonly used ventilator models deliver oxygen-enriched gas, and a triggering device permits the patient to breathe at his or her own tempo. The pace can be regulated for the individual patient.

For the less-ill patient, oxygen can be delivered in concentrations of up to 100 percent by a loose-fitting plastic face mask or double-pronged plastic tubing inserted into the nostrils. A lightweight oxygen container is slung from the shoulder like a purse. The amount of oxygen is tailored to the body's need during exertion.

Despite its central role in pulmonary care, oxygen is not a cure-all. High concentrations given for long periods can damage lung tissue and other body organs. In emphysema or chronic bronchitis patients, oxygen can depress respiration. For this reason, physicians prescribe oxygen with the same care that they prescribe drugs.

A special form of physical therapy also is used to assist breathing. Doctors call it postural drainage with percussion. During infections, the lungs often cannot clear themselves of secretions. The physician may then lower the patient's head, elevate the feet, or tilt the body into various positions with the aid of props and pillows to drain the lungs by force of gravity. These changes of posture are supplemented with percussion, clapping the chest wall by hand or with a mechanical vibrator to loosen the secretions clogging the airways.

Aerosol drugs may be administered directly with a hand-held spray device. These units are particularly important in asthma because the muscle-relaxing medication can be placed where it will do its job with minimal side effects. Pocket-size containers of aerosol antiasthma drugs are available and extremely effective.

DISEASES OF THE LUNGS

Obstructive Lung Diseases

Obstructive lung diseases are characterized by resistance to airflow within the lungs.

Asthma is the most treatable obstructive lung disease. An asthmatic attack usually starts with tightness in the chest and a cough, immediately or soon followed by breathlessness and loud wheezing. The breathing difficulty may become progressively worse. By the time many patients seek medical help, they are in the early stages of suffocation.

Asthma is as frightening as it is mysterious. Attacks may occur without apparent explanation, or they may be provoked by a specific identifiable cause. They may stop spontaneously, or resist the most vigorous therapies. No age group is spared, but asthma counts children among its most frequent victims.

There are two main types of asthma:

Extrinsic asthma is provoked by allergens or irritants—dust or other substances in the air. It often occurs in persons with a specific circulating blood protein called an immunoglobulin, which is structured in such a way that it binds to a foreign protein, the allergen (see Chapter 23, "Allergy and the Immune System"). When a person with the allergy is exposed to a substance he is sensitive to, a reaction occurs on the surfaces of certain cells, which in turn release chemicals, or mediators, into the circulation. The chemicals cause the bronchial muscles to contract and produce the secretions and tissue swelling characteristic of asthma.

Intrinsic asthma appears to occur without an external asthma-provoking irritant. Intrinsic asthma is more common in adults than in children and is more difficult to treat. About 10 percent of its victims have grapelike growths in the nasal lining (called nasal polyps), and attacks may be worsened by use of aspirin and other anti-inflammatory drugs.

The chief difference between an asthma victim and others is that the asthmatic's air passages are unusually sensitive. Many of us have minor breathing difficulty in smoggy air or dusty rooms, but the magnitude of difficulty is small compared to that of persons with asthma.

The view that the asthmatic's air passages are different is supported by the fact that even everyday events lead to attacks. Emotional crises have long been known to induce asthma attacks. It is now known that cold temperature and exercise do, too. Interestingly, certain types of activity are more likely to trigger an attack than others. Running, for example, is more asthma-producing than swimming.

Treatment of asthma has made great strides in recent years. Drugs that relax airways, known as bronchodilators, are the mainstay. They can be administered orally or in aerosol form by the victims themselves in mild or moderate attacks. When the attack is severe, the drugs are given intravenously.

For persons whose attacks are triggered by a known allergen, avoiding exposure to the allergen is obviously desirable. When this is not possible, hyposensitization injections (to pollens, dusts, foods) may be useful, especially in children. These

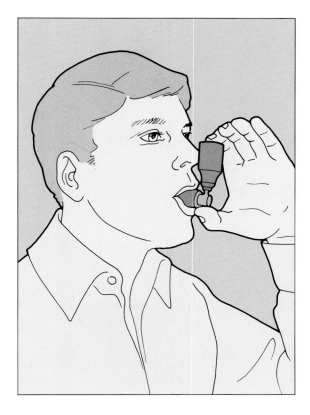

USING AN INHALER
A metered-dose, hand-held aerosol inhaler enables patients to spray drugs directly into the lungs, where they are most needed. The unit shown is synchronized by the patient with the beginning of a deep breath so that the spray is carried to all parts of the lung.

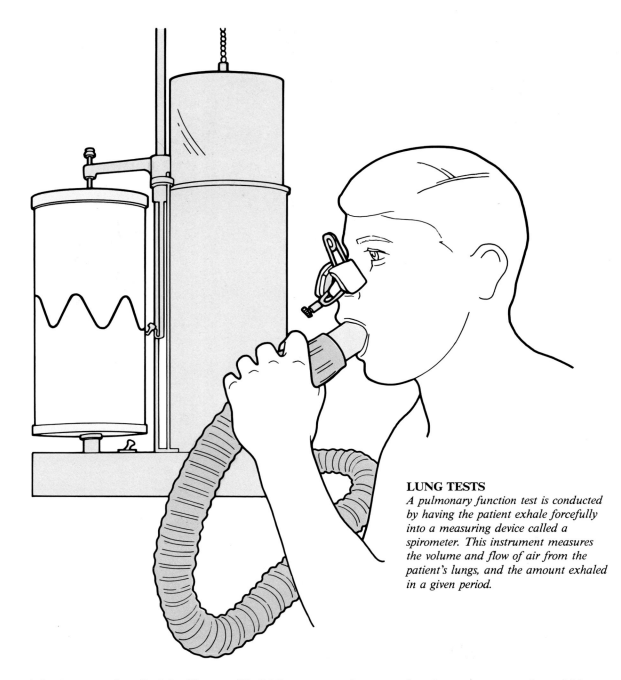

LUNG TESTS
A pulmonary function test is conducted by having the patient exhale forcefully into a measuring device called a spirometer. This instrument measures the volume and flow of air from the patient's lungs, and the amount exhaled in a given period.

injections are described in Chapter 23, "Allergy and the Immune System." Despite asthma's discomfort, the outlook for asthmatics is good, and their expected life span is normal.

Bronchitis, an inflammation of the air passages of the lung, may result from acute infection, chemical irritation, or other causes. The most prevalent type, chronic bronchitis, is said to exist in anyone having a cough and expectoration for at least three months a year for two consecutive years. Many environmental substances cause bronchitis or make it more severe, but cigarette smoking is overwhelmingly the most important.

Like asthma, the underlying problem in bronchitis is obstructed airflow. Unlike asthma, however, the obstruction is caused mainly by greatly increased mucous secretion because of irritation and thickened bronchial wall linings. Unfortunately, these problems are considerably less reversible than asthma's muscle contraction. Bronchitis vic-

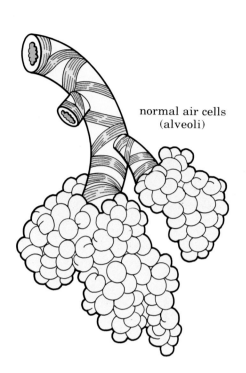

normal air cells
(alveoli)

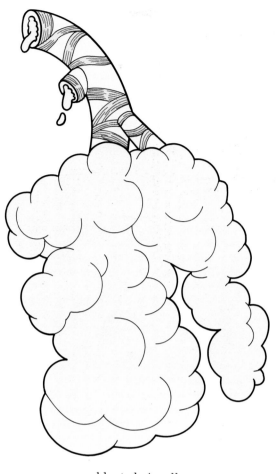

EMPHYSEMA

Overinflation of the air cells is the mark of emphysema, an increasingly common disease, especially among men. The cell walls break down and available surfaces for gas exchange are reduced. The drawing at left shows normal alveoli. At right, mucus and pus obstruct a bronchiole, causing emphysema.

bloated air cells

tims are especially vulnerable to infection, because the overabundant secretions are fertile soil for bacterial growth.

A cough and sputum are the prime symptoms of chronic bronchitis. The cough is most prominent in the early morning. As the disease progresses, shortness of breath appears, first during exertion and later at rest, too. A late and serious complication is heart failure caused by the increased work necessary to pump blood through a severely diseased lung with reduced blood oxygen.

Therapeutically, the greatest benefit occurs if the patient stops smoking. Coughing and sputum production diminish and may cease. Other treatment is directed at preventing infection and providing breathing support.

Emphysema takes its name from the Greek word for "inflation." Like other obstructive lung diseases, it is characterized by enlarged lungs.

The first symptom of emphysema is progressively worsening breathlessness. A cough is typical; wheezing, less so. There is little sputum. At first, the lungs are of normal size, but gradually they enlarge.

The breathing difficulty of emphysema results from lung destruction and scarring, primarily in the branches of the airways that end in the respiratory bronchiole and the alveolar sacs, a single unit that is known as the acinus. Panacinar (throughout the acinus) emphysema affects mainly the alveoli; centrilobular emphysema (involving the central acinus) predominantly destroys the bronchiole itself. Paraseptal emphysema attacks lung tissue at the outer edge of the lung. In all three, destruction is complete, involving both alveolar tissue and blood vessels. The naked eye can detect the grossly empty spaces where tissue has been ravaged.

As with bronchitis, the first step in treatment is to stop smoking. Bronchodilators and antibiotics may make breathing easier. Some doctors prescribe exercise to teach victims to slow the respiratory rate.

One reason that treatment is similar for bronchitis and emphysema is that most patients have a combination of the two. Some doctors make no attempt to differentiate between them, but lump the conditions together as "chronic obstructive lung disease," often shortened to COLD.

Cystic fibrosis is primarily a children's disease, the result of an inborn defect of the glands affecting the respiratory and digestive systems (see Chapter 29, "Taking Care of Your Child"). Its symptoms frequently show up soon after birth. Mucus secreted by the lungs is abnormally thick and sticky, and cannot be cleared. The accumulated secretions are a breeding ground for recurrent bronchial infections. The digestive system is affected, too, because of inadequate secretion of digestive enzymes.

In past years, cystic fibrosis victims frequently died in infancy, weakened by repeated infections or succumbing to respiratory difficulties. Because of improved care, including breathing support, survival is steadily increasing. Research also has identified mild forms of the disease that do not become evident until adulthood.

Cystic fibrosis qualifies as an autosomal recessive disorder, meaning that both parents are carriers of the defective gene but are symptom-free themselves. In affected families, each child has a one-in-four risk of having the disease at birth.

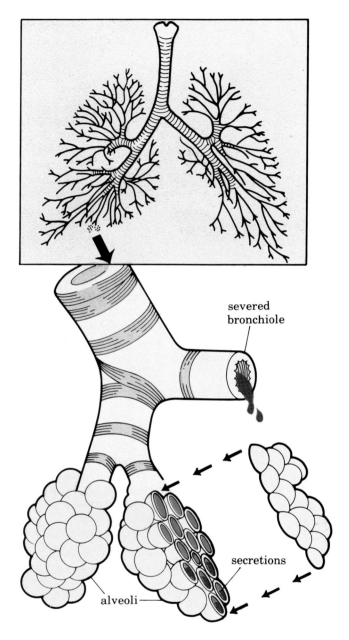

BRONCHITIS

Coughing and spitting are characteristic symptoms of bronchitis. The closeup view of a section of the bronchial tree shows dripping from a cutoff bronchiole. The lower drawing, an exploded view of the alveoli, shows secretions in air cells that normally contain only air.

Bronchiectasis is the localized destruction and deformity of sections of the bronchial tree. The two major symptoms are a cough and heavy sputum production. Severe sufferers may cough 24 hours a day. Paroxysms of coughing may raise ounces of foul-smelling, occasionally blood-streaked mucus and pus.

Treatment aims to reduce the amount of sputum and to remove any that remains. Antibiotics help to cut down infected secretions, and drainage and percussion dislodge the thick sputum. In cases of persistent, serious bleeding, it sometimes is necessary to remove the affected area surgically.

Restrictive Lung Diseases

Unlike obstructive diseases, in which the lungs become enlarged, restrictive diseases reduce lung size. Forced expiratory flow is reduced, too, but in restrictive diseases, the percentage of air forcibly exhaled in one second remains normal—about 80 percent. In obstructive diseases, the one-second exhalation represents a significantly lowered fraction of the lung's total volume.

Pulmonary fibrosis is a general term describing a thickening and deformity of the alveolar walls. It may arise from a virtually endless list of diseases: viral, bacterial, fungal, and parasitic infections, a large number of environmental and occupational pollutants, some forms of chronic heart disease, and several diseases of unknown origin.

Regardless of cause, pulmonary fibrosis produces scar tissue that replaces normally elastic lung tissue. The stiffer lung requires much more energy for expansion. Eventually, lung volumes shrink. The rate of breathing increases, but the amount of air moved in each breathing cycle decreases. Patients in advanced stages of the disease appear to be panting even at rest.

The first signs of fibrosis are shortness of breath, a dry cough, and a peculiar swelling of the tips of fingers and toes around the nail beds, called clubbing. Listening to the lungs, a physician often hears "crackling" sounds, like cellophane being crumpled and uncrumpled. The chest X ray shows undersized lungs marked by small indistinct shadows representing thickened and scarred alveolar walls.

Many cases of fibrosis are of unknown origin. The only widely used medical treatment is the administration of corticosteroids, which are thought to limit scar formation.

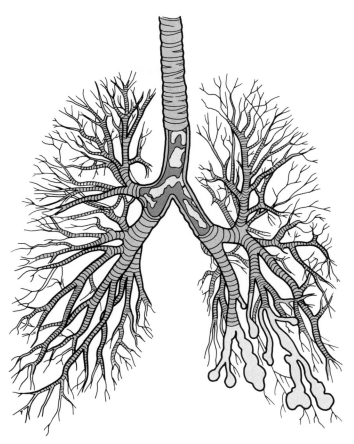

BRONCHIECTASIS
Destruction and deformity of bronchiectasis usually starts after childhood damage from serious pneumonia or other disease. Obstructive foreign bodies and infections that produce abscesses and pus also can be responsible. The dilated, pus-filled outpouchings of the diseased bronchial tree at right contrast sharply with the normal bronchial tree at left. Since development of immunization and antibiotics, bronchiectasis is much less common.

Nerve diseases. Proper breathing requires the muscular power of the chest wall and diaphragm, controlled by healthy nerves and muscles. Many disorders of the nervous system can impair these controls. These include Guillain-Barré syndrome, muscular dystrophy, and spinal cord injury, described in Chapter 11, "The Brain and Nervous System," and poliomyelitis, described in Chapter 32, "Infectious Diseases."

Skeletal deformities of the spine and thorax interfere with breathing because of bony stiffness of the chest wall and limited expansion of the rib cage. The effect is like fitting a tight girdle around a normal chest. The most common of these abnormalities is kyphoscoliosis. Kyphosis is the curvature of the upper spine, commonly called hunchback. Scoliosis, a curvature of the lower spine, is less noticeable unless severe. Usually, the two occur together.

A second type of common chest wall deformity involves the sternum, the shieldlike bone located between the breasts. Sometimes, this bone protrudes abnormally from the chest (pigeon breast) or is deeply indented (funnel chest). Pigeon breast (pectus carinatum) seldom affects normal breathing. Funnel chest (pectus excavatum) is mostly a cosmetic concern, but a severe defect can cause disability if it interferes with action of the heart or if it restricts the volume of air the lungs can handle. These deformities usually are apparent at birth and may run in families.

Infectious Diseases of the Lungs

A huge number of different viruses cause a gamut of respiratory diseases. The common cold is an example. Most upper respiratory viral infections are more nuisance than serious. However, many viruses have the potential to cause serious illness in the lower respiratory tract. Those affecting the upper respiratory tract are covered in Chapter 15, "Ear, Nose, and Throat."

Epiglottitis is an inflammation of the epiglottis, the flaplike structure over the opening of the trachea that prevents food from entering the airways during swallowing. Viral or bacterial infection can cause the epiglottis to swell and obstruct the airway. Tracheostomy may be needed to assure proper breathing until the infection subsides. Swelling of the epiglottis is predominantly a childhood condition, but also occurs in adults.

Laryngitis can be caused by viruses. It is an inflammation of the vocal cords, producing hoarseness or loss of voice.

Tracheobronchitis is a viral infection of the trachea and large airways, often producing a cough and chest pain.

Pneumonia is any infection of the air spaces of the lung, whether viral or bacterial.

Viral pneumonias are caused by many types of viruses, but the most common is the influenza virus. Viral pneumonias differ from those caused by bacteria because they are preceded not only by upper respiratory symptoms but also by symptoms elsewhere. These include stuffy nose, sore throat, watery eyes, headache, muscle aches, fever, and severe fatigue. The lung infection itself is marked by chest pain, shortness of breath, cough, and high fever. Most otherwise healthy patients endure relatively mild illness and recover spontaneously without seeing a physician. As with the common cold, treatment usually consists of bed rest, fluids, and analgesics such as aspirin.

Influenza. Typically, "flu" begins with sudden weakness and fatigue accompanied by sore throat, nasal stuffiness, and headache. Fever, a dry cough, and chest pain follow. Most patients must remain in bed for the duration of illness.

Flu frequently occurs in periodic worldwide epidemics. At about 10-year cycles, the influenza-A virus undergoes spontaneous changes. During any viral infection, the victim develops resistance to the offending virus so that, if exposed again, he or she normally is immune to reinfection. By periodically changing its structure, the influenza organism bypasses the immune defenses of previous victims. In effect, the flu virus is continually in the process of changing to new types capable of reinfecting the same persons. In the close-knit contemporary world, the rejuvenated virus quickly sweeps from one area to another, targeting whole populations immune to its old form, but defenseless against its new one. The epidemic virus is frequently named for the locale where it first was identified. "Hong Kong flu" and "Asian flu" are examples.

Flu does not occur only in periodic epidemics. Each winter there are local outbreaks or isolated cases. But in spite of the virus's periodic changes, effective vaccines against each prevalent strain usually can be developed. Vaccination is especially important for the elderly and chronically ill, in whom influenza produces the severest disease and complications.

Mycoplasmal infections. An organism known as *Mycoplasma pneumoniae,* classified somewhere between viruses and bacteria and sharing properties of both, also infects the respiratory tract. In the lungs it causes a pneumonia resembling viral pneumonia and Legionnaires' disease. This usually mild illness differs from viral infections because it can be treated with antibiotics.

Bacteria cause a variety of respiratory diseases, the most significant of which are pneumonia and lung abscess.

Bacteria reach the lungs by many routes, such as spreading from infection elsewhere in the body, but the most common is simple aspiration.

Once bacteria reach a suitable site in the lungs, they begin to multiply and provoke an inflammatory reaction. The air spaces fill with bacterial products, pus, and inflammatory fluid. The disease may be distributed along airways (bronchopneumonia) or in specific lobes (lobar pneumonia). Under treatment, this material is converted to liquid and expelled from the lungs, usually without damage to underlying tissue. Occasionally, an especially harsh bacterium, such as staphylococcus, can cause permanent damage. Such infections, known as necrotizing pneumonias, produce small areas of destroyed, "liquefied" lung replaced by pus. This is known as a lung abscess. It leaves behind an empty defect or a fibrous scar.

The symptoms of bacterial pneumonia are a sputum-producing cough, fever, chills, and chest pain. The sputum occasionally may be blood streaked. Chest pain indicates that the pneumonia involves the pleural lining. Lung abscesses appear on X rays as round masses containing both fluid (pus) and air. All the pneumonia-causing bacteria are susceptible to antibiotics. Treatment often is supplemented with physical therapy. Patients with other underlying chronic lung disease may suffer temporary respiratory failure. Postural drainage and chest percussion help eliminate the inflammatory material.

A percentage of severe pneumonias claim lives despite antibiotics, so preventive measures are important. A vaccine has been perfected to defend against one bacterium, and is recommended especially for the elderly and chronically ill.

Tuberculosis has been a scourge of mankind since prebiblical days. Today "TB" is far less a threat than in days past, thanks to dramatic advances in treatment and prevention, but it still disables and claims lives. It has made a slight comeback recently in the immunosuppressed systems of AIDS victims.

The offending organism, *Mycobacterium tuberculosis,* is readily recognized under the microscope by its distinct, rod-shaped appearance, clubbed at both ends. It usually is spread by inhalation. Although the lungs are most commonly involved, TB can spread to any organ in the body. The disease can persist for months or years. If undetected, it rapidly can become fatal. It also can smolder for life.

The early stages of TB usually are surprisingly free of symptoms. A cough, weight loss, fever, and night sweats come much later, when the disease has become established. Lung function is not seriously affected during early stages, but progressive destruction ultimately leads to fibrosis and breathing difficulty.

Tuberculosis is diagnosed by finding tuberculosis organisms (tubercle bacilli) in the sputum or other body fluids and tissues. A test to demonstrate past exposure, indicating that walled-off organisms still may be in place, involves injecting a small amount of tuberculin, a purified protein extract of tuberculosis organisms, into the skin of the forearm. A previously infected individual reacts with prominent inflammation at the site of the injection.

A group of antibiotics specifically effective against the tubercle bacillus now can be given by mouth. A patient with moderately advanced disease might be hospitalized for only two to three weeks. With prolonged multiple drug treatment, the cure rate is close to 100 percent.

Legionnaires' disease, named because the first known outbreak struck a convention of American Legionnaires in 1976, results from a previously unknown bacterium now named *Legionella pneumophila.* Since 1976, cases of Legionnaires' disease have been reported all over the world.

Patients are severely ill with a cough, shaking chills, diarrhea, chest pain, and poor appetite. Almost all develop high fever. The X-ray findings mimic a variety of other pneumonias, leading to mistaken diagnosis. Fortunately, this organism

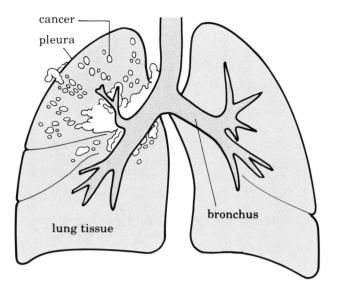

cancer
pleura
lung tissue
bronchus

SPREAD OF LUNG CANCER
The drawing shows a primary cancer of the main bronchus, with infiltration into the lung tissue, extension through the pleura, and invasion of neighboring lymph nodes, which permit the malignancy to spread to other organs of the body. Cancer originating in the stomach, uterus, breast, pancreas, prostate, or thyroid often spreads to the lungs.

can be checked by the antibiotic erythromycin, and most patients recover completely.

The disease appears to be spread by inhaling droplets from contaminated water sources, such as air conditioners and cooling towers. The organism also has been found in natural streams. If the water-borne hypothesis holds, it may be possible to prevent Legionnaires' disease by chemical treatment of potential water sources.

Fungal diseases are organisms slightly more complex than bacteria that live in soil and rarely cause disease. A few types of fungi, however, can trigger diseases that affect the lungs. In the United States, the most common are histoplasmosis, blastomycosis, coccidioidomycosis, and aspergillosis. Each is named for the fungus that causes the disease. Together, they account for about 100,000 illnesses a year.

Most of the fungi, except for Aspergillus, which is distributed worldwide, seem to prefer the soils of certain geographic areas. *Histoplasma* and *Blastomycetes* are found in the Mississippi and Ohio River valleys and in certain mid-Atlantic states. *Coccidioides immitis* is peculiar to the arid regions of California, Arizona, southern Utah, Nevada, New Mexico, and west Texas. Often, fungi are found in the droppings of birds and fowl.

Once they are airborne, the spores enter the body by being inhaled into the lungs. They are quickly spread by the bloodstream to all parts of the body. In acute cases, the symptoms—fever, cough, and chest pain—resemble those of influenza or a bacterial lung infection. More stubborn cases resemble tuberculosis, and in the past were often mistaken for it. There is progressive lung involvement, along with weight loss, fatigue, weakness, fever, and coughing. The rare cases that spread beyond the lungs can cause serious illness and require hospitalization, particularly if the eyes become involved.

No treatment is entirely satisfactory, because the most effective drug has serious side effects. Fortunately, most fungal infections are self-limiting, curing themselves within a few weeks without specific medication.

Pulmonary Embolism

During circulation, solid materials form in the veins and are swept along through the vessels until they reach the lungs (see Chapter 7, "The Blood"). Lodging in the opening of an artery, a particle, or embolus, can completely or partially block the blood flow. A blockage or embolism in the heart's right ventricle can be abruptly fatal.

The most common source of blood clots is the veins in the legs. Often, clots develop there during an illness or injury requiring prolonged bed rest and inactivity. This is the main reason surgical patients are directed to dangle their feet or walk with support as soon as possible after an operation. Clots also occur in otherwise healthy persons during long periods of sitting, such as long automobile trips. (Elderly passengers should stop to exercise

LUNG CANCER DEATH RATES IN THE U.S.

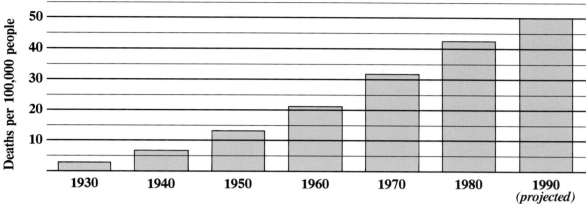

The number of lung cancer deaths per 100,000 Americans has risen sharply since 1930 and shows no sign of abatement (see projected figures for 1990, above). Most lung cancer cases are attributed to cigarette smoking.

every hour or two during a long drive.) With a resumption of activity, the clots may break loose and migrate to the lungs to lodge as emboli.

Clots in the legs, a condition called thrombophlebitis, may have no symptoms or may cause local swelling and pain (see Chapter 6, "Blood Vessel Disorders"). The first warning that they have moved to the lungs may be chest pain, cough, shortness of breath, and blood-spitting. The use of ultrasound and impedance plethysmography now allows leg clots to be detected readily. A lung scan using a radioactive dye helps to reveal lung clots.

Most commonly, leg clots or pulmonary emboli are treated with bed rest and drugs that inhibit blood-clotting, known as anticoagulants. Bed rest appears to reduce the risk of dislodging clots and their subsequent movement to the lungs. Anticoagulants, given by either mouth or injection, prevent enlargement of the clots and can help slightly in dissolving them.

Occasionally, the segment of vein containing the clots may be surgically sealed off from the rest of the circulation. This technique is used for patients who cannot tolerate the usual amounts of blood thinner.

Lung Cancer

The lung cancer death rate for men has increased more than 25 times since 1935. The number of lung cancer cases has more than doubled for both men and women, and now has surpassed breast cancer as the leading form of cancer among women. Five-year survival rates are not improving significantly.

Cigarette smoking is unequivocally identified as the main factor behind the rise of lung cancer. Only 10 percent of all lung cancer patients are nonsmokers. Certain industrial substances such as asbestos, nickel, chromium, arsenic, radon, and halogenated ethers also cause lung cancer, but smoking clearly is the most important risk factor. Not all smokers, however, develop tumors, which means that other factors must contribute.

Typically, lung cancer victims have no complaints while the tumor is small. The luckiest persons are those whose cancers are accidentally discovered when a chest X ray is taken for unrelated reasons. For the less fortunate, the first clue may be weight loss and general fatigue. Still others may bleed from the tumor and expectorate bloody sputum. The first evidence commonly results from spread of the cancer beyond the lungs, such as hoarseness of voice because the nerve to the larynx is involved, or a stroke because of spread to the brain. Chest pain also is a common first clue, usually the result of involvement of the chest wall.

Tumors found in the earliest stages can be removed surgically, often with good results. Lung tumors that have spread require radiotherapy or drug therapy. Radiotherapy involves administering several types of X rays that are more destructive to tumor cells than to normal body cells. Unfortunately, the amount of radiotherapy a patient can tolerate is limited. Drug therapy involves administering certain drugs that are more effective in poisoning tumor cells than healthy cells.

Granulomatous Lung Diseases

The body mobilizes various defenses against infections and other foreign substances. One of them involves lymphocytes, white blood cells that become sensitized to specific chemical substances. When these specialized cells recognize their target chemical in the body, they incite an inflammatory reaction that inactivates the foreign substance, or at least walls it off by surrounding the site of infection with a group of inflammatory cells. The resulting microscopic growth is called a granuloma, and diseases characterized by granuloma formation are called granulomatous diseases.

Sarcoidosis is a generalized granulomatous disease that tends to occur among young adults and is especially prominent among blacks. It typically involves the lungs but can affect any organ.

Seriously affected persons complain of shortness of breath and a dry cough, and may have complaints that stem from other organs. Their chest X rays show numerous granulomata with or without lymph node enlargement. Lung tests disclose reduced lung volumes. Most cases are successfully treated with anti-inflammatory drugs; some patients recover spontaneously.

The cause of sarcoidosis is not known. No infectious agent or other foreign body has been convincingly linked to it. The most popular theory is that this disease represents a disturbance of the body's immune system.

Certain antitumor drugs, combined with steroids, have greatly improved the outlook.

Diseases of the Pleura

The general term for fluid or air accumulation in the pleural cavity is pleural effusion. It comes in several forms and has several causes.

Pneumothorax means the presence of air in the pleural cavity. Often it occurs in paraseptal emphysema, most commonly in the young, and seems unrelated to smoking. Patients lack the usual symptoms of emphysema, but their emphysema-damaged air spaces may spontaneously rupture and leak air into the pleural space.

Hemothorax denotes a blood-filled pleural cavity, usually the result of chest injury or pulmonary embolus. Pus in the pleural space, called empyema, is rare since the advent of effective antibiotic drugs.

Transudative effusions are associated with heart or kidney failure. Exudates contain larger amounts of protein and other large molecules. They usually indicate infection or tumor.

A number of other lung diseases can result in pneumothorax. Injury to the chest wall, such as puncture of the lung by foreign bodies or by fractured ribs, also can precipitate pneumothorax.

The treatment of the pleural disease varies with the cause. Except where large amounts of fluid cause shortness of breath or where tension pneumothorax threatens life, pleural disease generally is not an emergency. When rapid and complete removal of gas or liquid is deemed necessary, a plastic tube is surgically placed into the pleural space, and constant suction is applied. More often, fluid is removed with a small needle.

When effusions recur, an irritative drug may be inserted into the pleural cavity. The resulting inflammation causes the pleural linings to adhere to one another and eventually form scar tissue. This closes the normal pleural space, preventing further accumulation of pleural fluid.

Environmental and Occupational Hazards

Asbestos causes a variety of lung problems. The first to be recognized was restrictive lung disease caused by widespread lung scarring, the result of heavy exposure for many years. Later, it was recognized that such persons are at heightened risk for lung cancer, a risk that is greatly increased if they also are cigarette smokers.

Pleural disease also strikes asbestos workers. This takes the form of calcified scars known as plaques, and occasionally as fluid accumulation in the pleural cavity. Calcification is plainly seen on X ray. The most dreaded of the asbestos-related lung diseases is a malignant pleural growth known as mesothelioma. The treatment of this form of cancer has been unsuccessful.

Silicosis. Silicon is one of the most common elements in the earth's crust. Quartz, sand and sandstones, flint, granite, and other hard stones have high silica content. Silicosis results from repeated exposure to free crystals of silica deposited in the lungs. Persons at high risk for silicosis include sandblasters, hard rock tunnelers, quarry workers, stone cutters, foundry workers, and makers of refractory materials.

The mechanism of lung scarring by silica is better understood than the scarring by asbestos. Silica is a potent killer of lung macrophages, immune-system cells that normally surround and destroy foreign particles, but are not able to do so with a mineral like silica. As repeated generations of macrophages ingest silica particles and are killed by these particles, they release inflammatory chemicals that eventually provoke a scar tissue response.

There are no clear symptoms of early silicosis. The first indication usually is an abnormal chest X ray, with scattered pinpoint punctures throughout the lung. This stage of disease, causing neither symptoms nor functional disability, is called simple silicosis. Fortunately, most patients never proceed beyond this stage. In a few, however, a complication known as conglomeration occurs. The small nodules enlarge and blend into large areas of destruction. Patients become breathless and may approach respiratory failure. In rare instances, the coexistence of tuberculosis may incite the conglomerate phase.

There is no specific therapy for silicosis. Standards for limiting silica particle concentration in the workplace are well established.

Coal miner's lung ("black lung") shares many of the features of silicosis. It is caused by the inhalation of coal dust, which collects in the lung in local formations known as coal macules. A progressive form known as progressive massive fibrosis leads to disability, and sometimes death.

Great progress has been made in establishing safe working levels of coal dust. As in all occupational diseases, prevention is much easier than treatment.

Chemical irritants. A large number of gases used in industrial processes irritate the respiratory system. They include ammonia, hydrogen chloride, chlorine, sulfur dioxide, nitrogen dioxide, and phosgene. The soluble gases, such as chlorine and ammonia, cause upper respiratory irritation

Protecting Your Lungs
- Stop smoking.
- If you have allergic asthma, avoid allergens and irritants.
- If you are over 65 or have a chronic illness, ask your physician about vaccination against pneumonia and influenza.
- If you already have chronic lung disease, notify your physician when fever, increased cough, or increased breathlessness occurs.
- If you have been exposed to tuberculosis, notify your doctor or local public-health agency.

marked by chest pain and a cough. The nonsoluble gases, such as nitrogen dioxide and phosgene, reach the alveoli and small airways, where they cause an outpouring of fluid into the lungs, known as pulmonary edema. Great amounts of alveolar fluid interfere with breathing.

Sometimes, these exposures are treated with supplemental oxygen. Occasionally, steroids are used to treat cases of massive pulmonary edema.

Hypersensitivity lung diseases are caused by an immune reaction directed against certain organic substances inhaled into the lung. In farmer's lung, particles of fungus growing in moldy hay are shaken into the air when the hay is stirred up, then are inhaled deeply into the lung where they are attacked by the body's immune defenses. Fever, chills, and breathlessness follow several hours later. Similar diseases are incited by other fungi, or organic substances such as animal danders or feathers. Only a small percentage of those exposed develop the disease.

CHAPTER 11

THE BRAIN AND NERVOUS SYSTEM

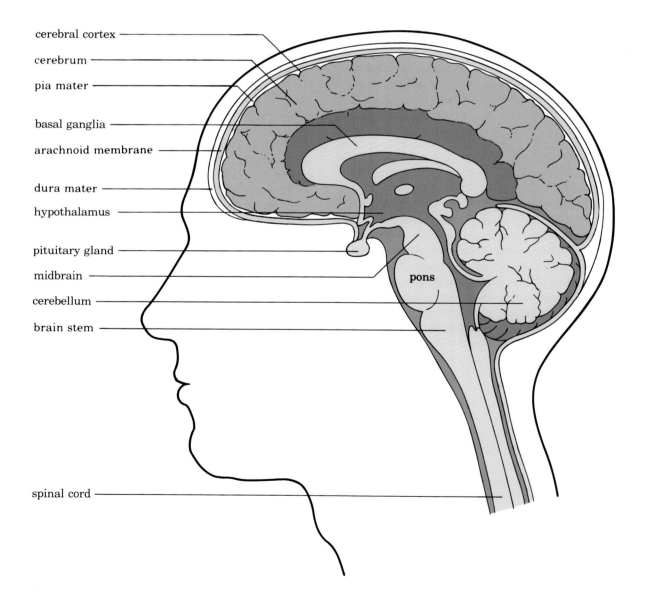

cerebral cortex

cerebrum

pia mater

basal ganglia

arachnoid membrane

dura mater

hypothalamus

pituitary gland

midbrain

cerebellum

brain stem

pons

spinal cord

The basic unit of the nervous system is the neuron or nerve cell. There are at least 40 billion neurons in the human body, 12 billion in the brain alone. Each cell resembles a drop of liquid that has been splashed on a hard surface and sprayed in various directions. The cell body is the central blob. Extending from it are short branched fibers called dendrites. Another long single fiber, called an axon, ends in a brushlike tip. Electrical impulses are carried to the cell body and away from it via these branches.

What we call a "nerve" is a mixed bundle of dendrites and axons. It may have the diameter of a bit of twine, or be as thin as the web of a spider. Each fiber is an extension of a cell body that may lie a great distance away.

PARTS OF THE BRAIN

The human brain is highly specialized, with different parts controlling different functions. The cerebrum, considered the "thinking part," comprises the major portion and occupies most of the skull above the eyes. A fissure divides it into two hemispheres, each with its own functions, and other fissures into lobes. Brain membranes (meninges) cover the cortex, which gathers information and sends messages to and from other parts of the brain. The cerebellum, at the back of the skull, controls balance and muscle coordination. The basal ganglia produce many of the chemicals called neurotransmitters that carry the brain's messages. The brain stem connects the higher brain centers with the spinal cord, enabling the body to carry out the brain's messages. The upper brain stem, or midbrain, regulates many body functions, including sleep and wakefulness. The hypothalamus is situated above the pituitary gland, and through it controls hormone secretion throughout the body.

HOW THE SYSTEM WORKS

Although nerve cells are close to one another, they do not touch. Instead, there is a tiny gap where the axon of one cell approaches the dendrites of another. This gap is called a synapse. A cell may synapse with many other cells. Synapses are the junctions where the neurochemical process that is the basis of all animal behavior takes place.

When a nerve cell body is excited to action, an electrical impulse is triggered that travels along the axon at speeds of up to 270 miles an hour. When the electrical impulse reaches the end of the axon, it causes minute quantities of chemicals called neurotransmitters to be released from tiny globules (packets or vesicles) stored at the end of each axon. These substances cross the synapse and combine with small receptor molecules in the protein membrane of the adjacent cell, initiating a response in the second neuron. Simultaneously, enzymes in the receptor break down the transmitter and inactivate it, so that the sequence can be repeated again within milliseconds. The neuron's response to these events may take one of two forms: (1) The cell membrane may become electrically depolarized, setting off an impulse that is conducted along the length of the cell's dendrites and axons and then transmitted to another cell, or (2) the receptor protein may start a sequence of chemical events that triggers a physiological response, such as the secretion of a hormone or contraction of a muscle. Of course, many thousands of cells acting together bring about the coordinated response.

The chemistry of brain function is one of the most rapidly developing areas of scientific research. At one time, only a few neurotransmitters, such as epinephrine and acetylcholine, were known. More recently, it has been recognized that many neurotransmitters act within the brain, and others are being steadily identified. It also is known that neurotransmissions are closely allied with activities of the endocrine system. Many investigators now believe that many neurological disorders, and even some conditions we classify as psychological problems, are abnormalities of function in the neurotransmitter.

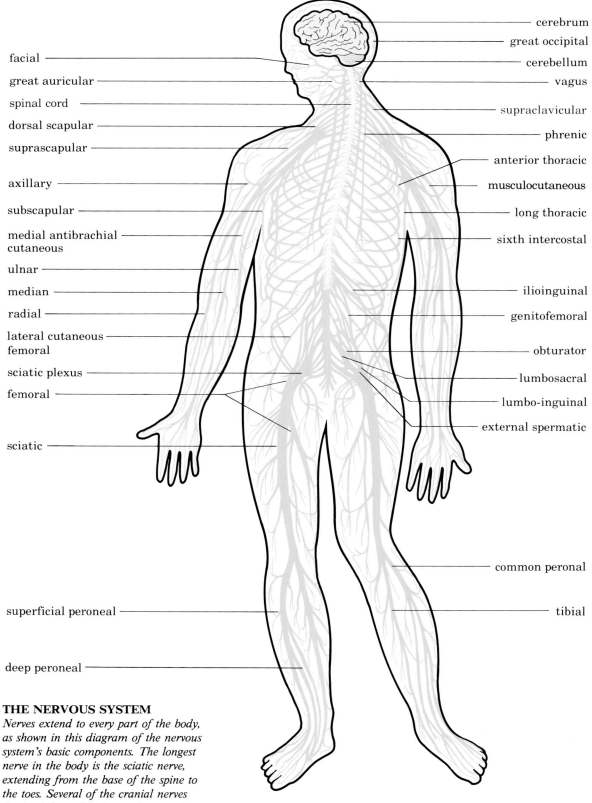

facial

great auricular

spinal cord

dorsal scapular

suprascapular

axillary

subscapular

medial antibrachial
cutaneous

ulnar

median

radial

lateral cutaneous
femoral

sciatic plexus

femoral

sciatic

superficial peroneal

deep peroneal

cerebrum

great occipital

cerebellum

vagus

supraclavicular

phrenic

anterior thoracic

musculocutaneous

long thoracic

sixth intercostal

ilioinguinal

genitofemoral

obturator

lumbosacral

lumbo-inguinal

external spermatic

common peronal

tibial

THE NERVOUS SYSTEM
*Nerves extend to every part of the body,
as shown in this diagram of the nervous
system's basic components. The longest
nerve in the body is the sciatic nerve,
extending from the base of the spine to
the toes. Several of the cranial nerves
(omitted from this diagram) are only a
few inches long.*

THE NERVOUS SYSTEM

Although the nervous system is a unified and coordinated network of interrelated nerve cells, for convenience it usually is classified into three parts. The first is the brain, illustrated on page 122, including the right and left hemispheres of the cerebrum. It also includes the brain stem, which carries messages to and from the cerebral hemispheres, and the cerebellum, which controls balance and coordinates movements. The second part is the spinal cord, which carries messages between the brain and the body. The third part includes the peripheral nerves and muscles.

The hemispheres, cerebellum, and brain stem are contained in the skull, the spinal cord is contained in the vertebrae, and the peripheral nerves run free in soft tissues of the body. The peripheral nerves have two major divisions: the autonomic, with its sympathetic and parasympathetic subdivisions, and the sensorimotor somatic nerves. Each of these major neural structures has many visible divisions and microscopic subdivisions.

Technically, muscles are not part of the nervous system, but because the brain cannot carry out any actions without them, the two usually are considered as a unit.

The Brain

The brain weighs about 3 pounds and is of jelly-like consistency. The brain amounts to only about 2.5 percent of body weight, but it receives 15 percent of the blood supply and 25 percent of the oxygen consumed by the body. The cells in the brain are far more individualized in structure and function than cells in any other part of the body.

Cerebrum. Because of its wrinkled, convoluted appearance, the brain often is likened to a cauliflower set on a stalk. The cerebrum is the flower's bud. It is the major portion of the brain, occupying almost the entire part of the skull above the eyes. The surface is irregular, with furrows (sulci) between mounds (convolutions).

This folded arrangement allows more neurons to be incorporated into the constricted space of the skull than otherwise would be the case. A fissure running from front to back divides the cerebrum into two hemispheres, which are linked by nerve fibers. Other fissures divide each hemisphere into four lobes, and the lobes are further divided into gyri or convolutions. Each area has a specific name and function, and is connected with the other areas by axons and dendrites.

Beneath the meninges, or brain membranes, is the cortex, the outer surface of the hemispheres, composed of nerve cell bodies. Under its gray outer covering is the white matter, which consists of the nerve filaments that carry messages to and from the brain. The cortex interprets information and could be called the brain's thinking part or information processor.

The four lobes of the hemispheres are named frontal, temporal, parietal, and occipital. Each has special functions that in many cases are represented in a similar position in the other hemisphere, but certain activities, including speech, handwriting, and reading, are located on only one side, known as the dominant side. The dominant hemisphere usually is the one opposite the hand used for writing. Because most people are right-handed, the left hemisphere usually is the dominant one.

The back of the brain (the occipital lobe) affects vision. This part of the brain records information that the optical system of the eye has collected and focused on the retina. This screen at the back of the eye is made up of central nervous system cells. Visual information that begins as light is converted here into electrical impulses, which pass from the retina along the optic nerve to the brain. The nerves partially cross each other on the floor of the skull, so that information from the left side of the environment passes across to the right side of the brain, and vice versa. The crossover enables us to obtain a single visual image.

Another function of the cerebrum is the olfactory sense, the sense of smell. The chemicals in the air stimulate tiny receptors in the upper part of the nose ("the small patch") that send their messages through dendrites to the frontal lobe of the brain. Chemicals in liquid are perceived as taste by nerve receptors in the mouth. These messages are correlated with other impulses to give us the impressions we think of as delicious or unappetizing.

Hearing is the translation of air waves by the eardrum into mechanical impulses, which are converted into electrical impulses by the auditory nerve. This nerve carries its impulses into the brain stem and up to the temporal lobes of the brain, where they are recorded and interpreted.

Cerebellum. Helping the body to maintain balance is one task of the cerebellum, which lies at the back of the head, behind the brain stem. Balance requires the integration of several kinds of information that discloses whether the body is in proper alignment with the environment: vision, the vestibular apparatus in the inner ear, and impulses

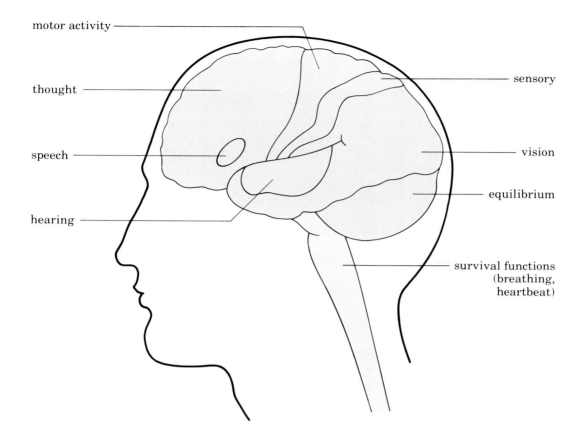

motor activity

thought

speech

hearing

sensory

vision

equilibrium

survival functions
(breathing,
heartbeat)

THE BRAIN CENTERS
Specialized functions have their own distinct areas of control within the brain. The drawing above shows that functions such as speech and

equilibrium are located in different areas. In general, functions on one side are duplicated on the opposite side of the brain.

caused by the effects of gravity. These three sets of data are fitted together in the cerebellum, and outgoing impulses adjust the tension of various muscles to keep the body in balance.

Besides equilibrium, the cerebellum affects muscular coordination and the automatic execution of fine movements.

The basal ganglia are gray concentrations of cell bodies divided into subgroups consisting of the caudate, putamen, lenticular nucleus, and optic thalamus. Each has a special function and receives nerve impulses coming from the lower parts of the nervous system. Each also secretes neurotransmitters. Our conception of the role of the basal ganglia, especially in relation to their secretions, is one of the most rapidly changing in neurobiology.

The brain stem lies almost in the center of the skull, and connects the higher brain centers with the spinal cord. The brain stem is the seat of im-

portant basic and involuntary functions. It is divided into several sections. The hypothalamus (see Chapter 18, "The Hormones and Endocrine Glands") regulates the flow of hormones through the body by its secretions to the pituitary gland, which lies directly beneath it. Growth, puberty, metabolism, and reproduction come under its sway.

In the upper brain stem, or midbrain, just below the basal ganglia, are a series of cell groups prominent in the secretion of neurotransmitters. The most important is the substantia nigra, which secretes dopamine, without which parkinsonism develops. The body of Luys nearby is responsible for control of certain body movements. The midbrain proper contains the reticular activating system, which regulates sleep, wakefulness, and coma. The major nerve controlling eye movement, the third cranial nerve, also is located here.

Below the midbrain is the pons, the Latin word for bridge, so called because it links the upper with the lower brain stem. It contains other nerves controlling eye and facial movements. It also is a major relay station for integration of reflex and voluntary movements with the cerebellum.

The lowest part of the brain stem is the medulla, whose cell groups control many automatic and involuntary functions, such as heartbeat, breathing, intestinal activity, swallowing, and other "vegetative" functions of the body.

Spinal Cord

The nerve tissue of the spinal cord is about the diameter of a clothesline and weighs only 2 ounces. It is enclosed in the bony vertebral column of the back. Except for the 12 pairs of cranial nerves that connect directly with the brain, all the nerves of the body enter or leave the spinal cord through openings in the vertebrae.

A cross section of the spinal cord reveals white tissue on the outside and a gray, H-shaped mass of cells in the center. Sensory impulses of many kinds enter the outside white matter of the spinal cord and travel upward far enough to trigger spinal reflexes at various levels or travel to the brain. Motor impulses travel downward from nerve cells in the brain to reach spinal cells that relay messages to various muscles, organs, glands, and blood vessels.

On each side of the body are 31 spinal nerves distributed evenly in segments down the cord. The "incoming" sensory nerve fibers bring signals from the skin, internal organs, joints, and muscles, and enter the back of the cord and connect with gray matter of the rearward (posterior) horns of the H. In the forward (anterior) horn are the motor nerve cells, which send impulses to the muscles.

Peripheral Nerves

Sensory nerves carry impulses to the central nervous system; motor nerves carry them away from it to bring about action. A sensory nerve warns that a finger is resting on a hot stove, and motor nerves direct muscles to contract and jerk the hand away.

Some nerves are composed entirely of motor or sensory fibers, but other nerves contain both kinds of fibers. Cell bodies of sensory nerves lie just outside the spinal cord, and those of motor nerves lie within it. From these areas, fibers run out to connect with body tissues, muscles, organs, glands, blood vessels, and skin.

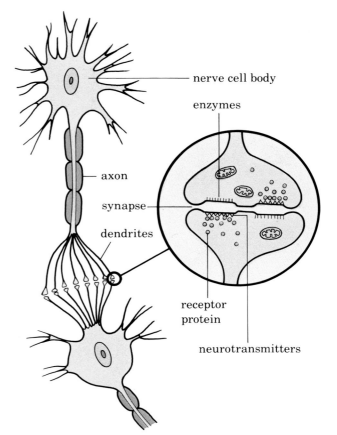

nerve cell body

enzymes

axon

synapse

dendrites

receptor protein

neurotransmitters

THE NERVE CELL
The basic unit of the nervous system is the nerve cell, or neuron, of which we have at least 40 billion. Its main parts are the cell body, where the cell's activity originates, the dendrites, which branch out from the cell body, and the axon, a long single fiber that reaches out toward other nerve cells. Dendrites are excited by impulses from other nerve cells or from external stimuli. Their message is carried to the cell body, which sends its impulse along the axon to another cell. The impulse is transmitted to other cells at a gap called a synapse (enlarged view), where the nerve cells approach each other but do not touch. An individual nerve cell may synapse with many other cells.

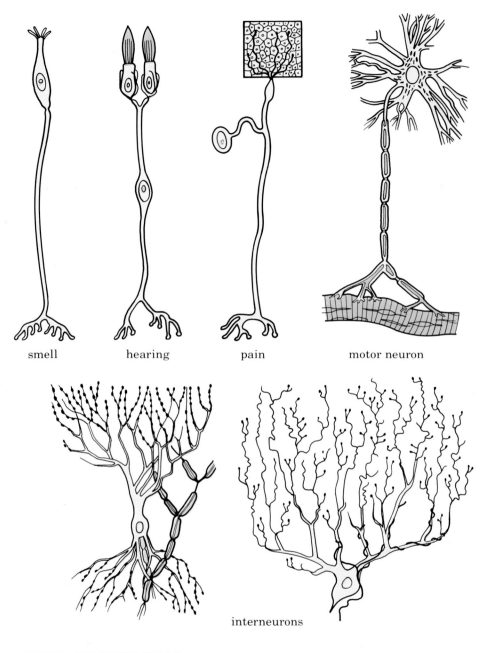

smell   hearing   pain   motor neuron

interneurons

TYPES OF NERVE CELLS

Nerve cells are differentiated according to their function. Sensory neurons have a variety of forms, as shown at top. Each performs a single function. Motor neurons (top right) have only one form. The interneurons in the lower row have a network of axons and dendrites connecting to a single cell body and do not extend beyond the local region. The interneuron at left is from the cerebellar cortex; the one at right is from the cerebral cortex. The structure of nerve cells also varies according to their placement in the body.

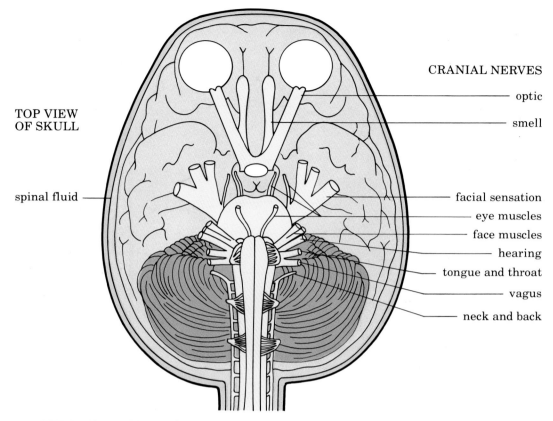

TOP VIEW
OF SKULL

spinal fluid

CRANIAL NERVES

optic

smell

facial sensation

eye muscles

face muscles

hearing

tongue and throat

vagus

neck and back

THE CRANIAL NERVES
Twelve pairs of cranial nerves connect directly from the brain without passing through the spinal cord. They relate primarily to the senses and to facial movements. Three of the pairs control movement of the eyes.

Cranial Nerves

In addition to the spinal nerves, 12 pairs of cranial nerves connect directly with the brain. They are called cranial nerves because they arise from the brain, within the skull.

The Autonomic System

Besides the voluntary motor nerves, which respond to the brain's commands, an involuntary or automatic system of which we are not conscious functions at all times, even while we sleep. This system regulates our bodily environment, maintaining temperature, oxygen supply, nutrients, and blood pressures at proper levels. This system also prepares us for emergencies. It has two complementary parts, the sympathetic and the parasympathetic nervous systems.

Sympathetic nerve trunks lie on each side of the bony spinal column. They connect with spinal nerves, and extend fibers to various organs of the chest and abdomen. Parasympathetic trunk lines originate in the brain and the sacral part of the spinal cord. In general, both divisions reach and control the same organs—lungs, heart, liver, spleen, stomach, pancreas, adrenal glands, kidneys, colon, intestines, sex glands, and bladder—but cause opposite effects.

For example, sympathetic impulses speed the heart and stomach and bowel action. Parasympathetic nerves do just the opposite. One set of impulses causes the muscle coat of blood vessels to constrict; the other causes it to dilate. Interplay between the two systems normally keeps body processes at a steady rate of activity, like stepping on the accelerator to climb a hill and applying the brakes on the downhill side to maintain even speed.

The autonomic system performs another function. For instance, it is more important that the heart pump enough blood into the muscles when we have to run away from danger than for the blood to go to the viscera for peaceful, normal

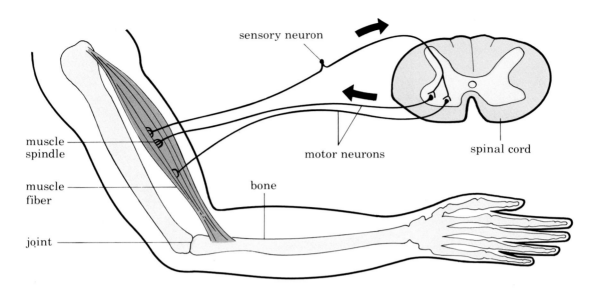

MOTOR-SENSORY NERVES
How a feeling translates into action is shown here. The muscle spindle of the sensory neuron detects a change in posture. The impulse is transmitted to the spinal cord, which sends a message to the nearby anterior horn cells and motor neuron. The message stimulates the muscle fiber to react by contracting, which pulls on the adjacent bone and causes the joint to move.

digestion of food. Autonomic adjustments in such a situation speed the heart and suppress digestion, which can later be resumed comfortably after we have escaped the threat.

It would be a mistake to think of the nervous system as an entirely independent electrical switchboard. The central nervous system and the endocrine (hormone-producing) systems are intimately associated. For instance, when danger threatens, nerves stimulate the adrenal glands to pour epinephrine into the blood and prepare the muscles for action upon order from the brain. But some special nerve cells also secrete neurohormones that in some respects act in a similar fashion. We may think of the nervous system as a rapid-acting electrical system, and hormones as a more deliberate-acting chemical system. The two systems are not independent, but complementary.

SYMPTOMS THAT SUGGEST NERVOUS SYSTEM DISEASE

Headache

Probably the most common complaint on earth is that of headache. Almost two-thirds of all people get headaches at one time or another. About 10 to 20 percent of the population suffer from chronic, recurrent headaches that can be disabling.

The intensity of a headache is not a good clue to the seriousness of its cause. Mild headaches can be early warnings of serious disease, and excruciating ones can have trivial causes.

Doctors classify headaches into several categories. "Disease-related" headaches, about 1 percent of the total, result from some physical ailment, such as inflamed sinuses, tooth infection, head injury, and, rarely, brain tumor. These headaches can be treated only by treating the underlying disease. Tension headaches, the most common type, are said to come from stress and subsequent contraction of the scalp muscles that produces bands of pain around the head. Vascular headaches take their name from the long-held view that the pain results from swelling of the scalp blood vessels. However, muscle contraction usually cannot be detected in tension headaches, and the blood-vessel explanation for head pain has been challenged, so many doctors simply lump all headaches together and treat them on an individual basis. They point out that there is no scientific way to distinguish between headaches, except the patient's own report.

Migraine is a type of recurrent headache that has been known for centuries. Aristotle was an early sufferer. At one time, migraine was believed to be psychological in origin, the mental upset triggering a malfunction of the cranial circulation. Swollen blood vessels presumably pressed on adjacent nerves, producing pain. High-tech methods of visualizing the working of the brain have shown that the disorder stems from a disturbance of the brain's electrochemical system, possibly distantly related to the "nerve storm" of epilepsy.

About 20 percent of adults, predominantly women in the reproductive years, suffer from migraine. So do 5 percent of children. Although people equate "migraine" with "severe," the pain actually comes in many degrees. In some persons, the headache may be triggered by outside stimuli that would not bother others—diet, exertion, bright lights, menstruation. The headache may last for hours or days, and it may recur at long intervals or strike several times a week. Some persons experience nausea, vomiting, diarrhea, and dizziness, giving rise to the popular name, "sick headache." They may be excruciatingly sensitive to light, and forced to take refuge in a dark room.

Classic migraine accounts for 20 percent of all cases but gives the condition its name ("migraine" is derived from the Greek "hemicrania," meaning "half the head"). The patient is forewarned of the attack by an "aura," lasting 10 to 40 minutes, in which he or she "sees" evanescent light flashes like Roman candles, sparkles, or pinwheels. A common aura is "fortification spectra," geometric patterns like the parapets of a fort. Some patients lose vision in one or both eyes and experience tingling in the fingers and tongue, mild confusion, and slurred speech. The aura is followed by a pounding headache that almost always strikes the same side of the head, usually centering over one eye. Some people have an aura but no headache, however.

Common migraine, the form that attacks most persons, involves the entire head. Its victims usually lack the warning aura, but head pain and other symptoms can be equally severe.

Complicated migraine is characterized by paralysis of eye movement, weakness or paralysis of the lips, vertigo, tingling, blindness, and even loss of consciousness. It is very rare, however.

Cluster headache most commonly afflicts men over age 40. It gets its name because attacks occur in clusters, sometimes two to three times in 24 hours for days or weeks. The attack can wake the patient from a sound sleep. Pain usually centers on one eye and has been compared to being stabbed in the eye with a red-hot poker. An individual attack lasts 30 to 90 minutes. Often the affected eye streams and the nose runs or is blocked.

Migraine appears to arise from an upset in the neurotransmitters. The most likely culprit is the neurotransmitter serotonin, which has been shown to rise before a migraine attack. Or the pain may be the result of a disturbance of the brain's own pain-modulating system and the family of neuropeptides called endorphins. Migraine runs in families, and victims may be born with a deficiency of neurotransmitter production.

Treatment of migraine is on two levels. Medication taken after the warning aura may stave off the actual headache. The most commonly used medications are nonsteroidal anti-inflammatory drugs, such as ibuprofen, or the traditional ergotamine tartrate, which has more side effects. Beta blockers, such as propanolol, and calcium-channel blockers, both of which are used in coronary artery disease, also are helpful. Antidepressants have been used, too. Traditional pain remedies, such as aspirin, are a mainstay once the pain strikes. Sometimes they are combined with antiemetics, to prevent nausea. Biofeedback has been used with mixed success.

Cranial arteritis is an inflammation that commonly affects the temporal artery but can affect any scalp artery, or the middle cerebral and ophthalmic artery serving the eye. About one-third of patients may lose vision permanently. The headache may throb at first, but soon becomes severe and burning. The affected arteries are tender and firm, but do not pulsate. Sometimes, weakness, muscle pain, and low-grade fever are present.

Tension headache or muscle-contraction headache usually produces dull and generalized pain. There may be a burning sensation and tenderness of the scalp, which may spread to the neck and shoulders. The headaches may come and go as episodes of stress recur.

Treatment of tension headache usually seeks to uncover underlying conflicts and reduce emotional stress. Mild, nonaddicting analgesics such as aspirin and sedatives are useful. Prolonged tension headache often is associated with depression, so antidepressants may be prescribed, too. Muscle relaxation exercises may help.

Trigeminal neuralgia (tic douloureux) is a particularly severe kind of headache, caused by degeneration of or pressure on the trigeminal nerve radiating from the angle of the jaw. The attack comes as sudden sharp stabbing pains, always on the same side. Sometimes the pain can be relieved with tranquilizers, but surgery may be necessary to relieve the pressure.

Dizziness, Light-Headedness, And Vertigo

Light-headedness and dizziness commonly are lumped together by patients, but are separated by physicians. Light-headedness refers to a subjective feeling of unsteadiness, possibly associated with a sensation that one is about to faint. There may be some blurred vision and ringing in the ears. Dizziness, or vertigo, makes a person unsteady on his feet because of a feeling that he or everything around him is moving. There is no associated clouding of consciousness, but vision may blur if the surroundings seem to be in motion. The reason for distinguishing between the two sensations is that light-headedness usually is caused by reduced blood supply to the brain, while dizziness results from a defect in function of the balancing apparatus that keeps the body in its correct position in space.

Light-headedness. The most common cause of reduced blood supply to the brain is an abnormality in the heart or the blood pressure regulating system (see Chapter 5, "The Heart and Circulation," Chapter 8, "Hypertension," and Chapter 7, "The Blood"). The reduction also may stem from disease of the arteries supplying the brain (see Chapter 6, "Blood Vessel Disorders"). Symptoms of light-headedness also may precede stroke, in which case they usually are accompanied by such symptoms as weakness in one side of the body, loss of vision in one eye, or transient ischemic attacks, which are interruptions of blood supply that can cause lapses of consciousness.

Hyperventilation syndrome also is a frequent cause of light-headedness. A person under stress or anxiety begins to breathe deeply and rapidly, which expels the carbon dioxide in the blood. The blood vessels that supply the brain constrict, lowering the blood supply and inducing a feeling of light-headedness.

Vertigo, the medical term for what is commonly called dizziness, describes the feeling that a person's surroundings are moving—spinning like a top, or pitching and heaving, as if one were standing on a boat tossed about by waves. The cause usually is a malfunction of the balancing apparatus, which includes the labyrinth in the inner ear and its nerves, and the brain stem connecting the cerebellum and cerebrum (see Chapter 15, "Ear, Nose, and Throat").

The diseases that cause this change fall into three major categories: blood vessel diseases, nerve disorders, and diseases of the semicircular apparatus itself. The most common is Ménière's disease or hydrops, described in Chapter 15, "Ear, Nose, and Throat."

An especially severe form of vertigo is one that occurs in some persons whenever they change head position. Even the simple act of lying down, sitting up, or turning the head can induce a violent but short-lived attack. The cause usually is in the inner ear, but may result from a head injury or toxicity to certain drugs.

Pain and Numbness

The skin is full of nerve receptors that sense the environment and send messages to the brain. When this system does not work properly, a person begins to feel pain, numbness, or peculiarities of sensation: a cold object feels painful, for example, or a painful sensation feels hot.

The nerves that leave the skin carry the sensations of pain, temperature, pressure, and vibration together so that any abnormality in the nerve will affect all to a degree. In the spinal cord, the sensations begin to separate, and at the brain stem are "felt" in different locations. An abnormality at the spinal cord or beyond may affect only one sensation, a telltale clue.

The brain also puts these sensations into a meaningful relationship, so that not only are the sensations felt, but the shape of the object and its potential use are recognized by the brain. It is possible, for example, to recognize that something is cold, heavy, and sharp but not to be able to recognize that it is a knife except by looking at it. Certain diseases of the brain destroy the ability to integrate this information or to name the object.

Peripheral neuropathy is the name given to disorders affecting the peripheral nerves. Nerves commonly affected are the radial, ulnar, and median nerves of the arm, and the sciatic nerve in the leg. Herniated discs and tumors of the spinal cord are common nerve root disorders. Neuropathies result from poisoning by alcohol, drugs, or insecticides, and are a common consequence of diabetes.

Sciatica can be caused by compression of the sciatic nerve as it passes through the muscles of the buttock in its long course from the spinal cord to the foot. Sciatica can cause pain down the leg, areas of numbness, loss of reflexes, and sometimes weakness in the foot. Medications, rest, exercises, instruction in proper use of back muscles, and, perhaps, surgery to remove a herniated disc are the best treatments.

Shingles (herpes zoster) is caused by an infection of a nerve cell by a virus related to the chicken pox virus. It causes burning pain and a rash that usually follows the nerve course. Common sites are the trigeminal nerve of the face and nerves of the torso. Steroid medications bring relief. The rash tends to subside and disappear in a few weeks.

Guillain-Barré syndrome (postinfectious polyneuritis) is a disturbance of the nerve roots, sometimes of both arms and legs, along with some of the cranial nerves affecting the face, jaws, tongue, and eyes. Motor as well as sensory nerves are involved, causing weakness, difficulty in breathing, wasting of the muscles, numbness, and loss of reflexes. The disorder may be caused by a postinfectious immune reaction, toxic substances such as insecticides, and serum injections. The patient may need artificial breathing support (see Chapter 10, "The Lungs") because of respiratory paralysis. Symptoms can be relieved by use of steroids.

Compression neuropathy is the direct compression of a nerve as it passes through a narrow canal. In *carpal tunnel syndrome,* the hand is affected, with severe pain in the thumb and fingers, particularly at night. In *crossed-leg palsy,* the nerve to the foot is affected, with tingling, numbness, and temporary loss of power in that leg.

Bell's palsy is compression of the swollen facial nerve as it passes through a bony canal in the skull below the ear on its course to the muscles of the face. Pain below the ear is followed by loss of ability to close the eye or smile on the affected side. The condition is alarming and embarrassing, but normally clears up within several months.

Movement Disorders

Shaking movements, or tremors, have a variety of causes.

Benign essential tremor is the most common form of tremor. Older persons are the usual victims, although it may occur in 40- or 50-year-olds.

Symptoms are a slight shaking of the hands, a sidewise nodding of the head, and/or a tremulous voice. The tremor may be almost imperceptible at first, but usually becomes more and more noticeable. Benign essential tremor is seldom truly disabling, but it may interfere with activities requiring fine movements, such as sewing or writing. The tremor often can be stabilized by drinking alcohol.

Parkinson's disease, or parkinsonism, stems from loss of dopamine-producing cells in the substantia nigra portion of the basal ganglia. It is most common after age 50, although it may occur as early as age 35. The symptoms are shaking (tremor) of the hands, head, and feet, stiffness (rigidity) of the limbs with slowing of movements (particularly walking), and a stooped posture. Except in very advanced cases, the disorder does not affect mental functions or lead to paralysis. The earliest manifestations usually are a slight shaking of the hands during fine movements, but the tremor is clinically different from benign essential tremor. The disorder usually progresses to more widespread symptoms.

The cause of Parkinson's disease is unknown, although an environmental cause is suspected. It is not genetic. Rarely, the symptoms may be caused by damage to the substantia nigra, either by drugs or other chemicals, or by injury.

It sometimes is said that a person with advanced Parkinson's disease is frozen within his own body because the muscles cannot act fast enough to perform the actions necessary for daily living, such as getting out of bed, dressing, eating, sitting down, and standing up. Fortunately, Parkinson's symptoms can be overcome through the use of levodopa, or L-dopa, taken by mouth, to substitute for the missing neurotransmitter dopamine. L-dopa (and a formula called carbidopa), when taken daily in sufficient dosage, can control many of the disabling symptoms. In time, however, L-dopa may lose its punch, and can actually bring on symptoms. Parkinson's also may be treated with Actane, especially in the early stages of the disease. Actane has fewer side effects.

A recent development is adrenal-cell transplant surgery. In this operation, cells from the person's own adrenal medulla, which also produces dopamine, are transplanted to the brain. Early results from this operation are said to have dramatically relieved symptoms in some cases, but long-term results are unclear.

Huntington's disease is hereditary, affecting men and women in their early 40s and 50s. The disease is dominantly transmitted, passed from an affected parent to half of the offspring. Tragically, the child may not know whether he or she carries the disease until symptoms appear in midlife.

The first symptoms usually are an involuntary, barely noticeable movement of fingers, facial muscles, or limbs. As the disorder progresses, these involuntary movements begin to interfere with more skilled movements. Speech is interrupted by sudden facial, tongue, and breathing abnormalities. Mental deterioration occurs in many patients. There may be marked personality change, or sexual and emotional aberrations may develop. Within five to 10 years, the patient is incapacitated. The disorder can be diagnosed by family history or by the characteristic loss of the caudate nucleus. A testing method has been developed, but is not yet in wide use. There is no effective treatment.

Dystonia, also a disorder of the basal ganglia, affects the large muscle groups of the limbs, neck, and body, which contract slowly and cause the patient to be contorted into extremely awkward and sometimes painful positions. Dystonia can result from birth injury, heredity, or unusual reaction to tranquilizers.

Wilson's disease (hepatolenticular degeneration) is a rare but potentially preventable and curable hereditary disorder. The victim is born with an inability to properly use copper obtained in the diet. The metal accumulates in the liver and basal ganglia (see Chapter 22, "The Digestive System"), causing hepatitis or parkinsonlike symptoms. This potentially fatal disease can be cured with a diet low in copper, and medication to remove accumulations of the metal in the body.

Ataxia is the name given to a group of movement disorders whose common characteristic is abnormality of limb placement in response to voluntary movement. The patient is unable to place his or her feet in a desired position rapidly and accurately, and therefore walks with a drunken, rolling gait. In advanced ataxia, the upper limbs also are affected, and the person cannot reach out and touch objects accurately.

The location of this disorder is the cerebellum and its connections. The most common cause is intoxication with alcohol, tranquilizers, street drugs, or toxic substances. In other instances, the disorder is hereditary and develops slowly over many years, often beginning in adolescence. These hereditary ataxias include Charcot-Marie-Tooth disease, with loss of nerves to the limbs, and atrophy of muscles and abnormal sensation; Friedreich's ataxia, affecting the spinal cord; and Marie's cerebellar ataxia, degeneration of the cerebellum. The cause of these genetic disorders is suspected to be enzyme defects in the affected cells, which function normally for years before they begin to die off.

Gilles de la Tourette's syndrome causes an uncontrollable grimacing of the face, coupled with respiratory movements that cause patients to sigh, snort, grunt, and clear their throats. They may even utter obscenities in a loud voice. Treatment with the drug haloperidol may be effective. The cause is not known.

Forgetfulness

Memory is at the heart of human activity, allowing us to learn and then recall the lesson for potential application for years or decades afterward. The neurological basis of memory remains a mystery, however. Loss of memory may arise from many causes, including alcoholism, depression, endocrine disorders (such as reduced thyroid function), or brain injury.

Alzheimer's disease is the name given to a pattern of forgetfulness and disorientation commonly associated with the elderly. Originally the term was applied only to those persons under age 65 who showed evidence of the syndrome; older persons with a similar pattern were said to be suffering from senile dementia. More recently, it has been recognized that the symptoms are the same regardless of age and that they represent a specific disorder, by no means a simple part of aging.

The causes of Alzheimer's disease are not known. Research on deceased victims of the disease has found evidence of distinctive brain changes. Snarls of abnormal nerve fibers have been seen, as have deposits of abnormal protein. The victims usually have lost an abnormal number of brain cells. Although these changes occur to a certain extent in all older people, the amount of change is far greater in Alzheimer's patients.

Several theories have been offered. The most popular theory attributes the symptoms to a deficit

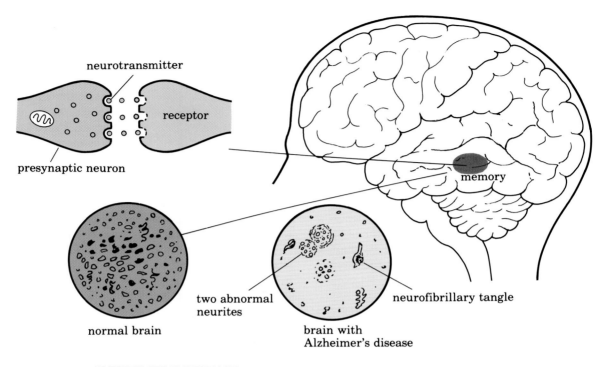

neurotransmitter

receptor

presynaptic neuron

memory

normal brain

two abnormal
neurites

brain with
Alzheimer's disease

neurofibrillary tangle

ALZHEIMER'S DISEASE

The nerve-cell changes of Alzheimer's disease are distinctive, although not fully understood. As shown above, nerve cells in the hippocampal region, which controls memory, are markedly reduced in size and number. Unusual growths called neurofibrillary tangles are found across the surface of the brain. Secretion of certain neurotransmitters is decreased (although some scientists believe that receptors are less able to utilize them). The reason these changes occur—and ways to combat them—is being aggressively studied by scientists worldwide.

of an enzyme needed to manufacture the neurotransmitter acetylcholine, a key chemical in memory formation. Other hypotheses blame the disease on a slow-acting virus or on environmental poisons, particularly aluminum. A genetic component may be involved. Some families have more cases of Alzheimer's than the general population, but the fact that one family member has had the disease does not mean that other members will develop it.

The first indication of Alzheimer's may be loss of memory, particularly for recent events. The indication itself is deceptive, because some memory loss occurs naturally, not only in older people but younger ones as well. Moreover, other conditions, such as depression, drug interaction, or head injury, may cause forgetfulness and confusion. When the person forgets the names and faces of familiar persons, or is unable to remember the beginning of a sentence when it is completed, Alzheimer's may be suspected. Later the person may be confused as to time and place, tend to lose things, and become incontinent. Some persons tend to wander and require continuous surveillance.

Since the cause of Alzheimer's is not known, there is no effective treatment, either to relieve the symptoms or to reverse the process. The only course is good general medical care and tender loving care by the family. Watching the deterioration of a loved one, however, can produce great strain on the relatives, who may be as much in need of sympathy as the patient.

Communication Abnormalities

Aphasia is the name given to the loss of ability to speak or to understand the speech of others. It includes the "deaf and dumb," who have never had normal hearing and as a consequence cannot speak words. Another group, however, has normal hearing but sounds are not properly recorded in the brain because of disease. A third disorder is the loss of the ability to speak even though one hears and comprehends what is said. This type of aphasia is caused by loss of control over the muscles that guide movements of the mouth, lungs, and chest during speech.

Stuttering begins in childhood and sometimes persists throughout life, usually during moments of stress. The cause is unknown, but in some cases it results from mixed dominance, in which the two brain hemispheres compete for control of the neuromuscular apparatus of language.

Dyslexia is a congenital difficulty in learning to read, presumably caused by improper or delayed development of the appropriate brain areas or their interconnections. Dyslexia runs in families, affects males predominantly, and has a tendency to occur in families that have several left-handers. Dyslexics write with letter reversals and at times use mirror writing. It is important to recognize that dyslexic children are not intellectually deficient or recalcitrant. Remedial reading and writing by teaching specialists can produce dramatic improvement.

Sleep and Wakefulness

Sleep is of two types, called REM (for rapid eye movement) and non-REM sleep. They alternate at about 90-minute intervals. In REM sleep, the eyes move beneath the closed eyelids and dreaming takes place. Muscles of the body stiffen and sometimes twitch. The electroencephalogram (EEG) shows a characteristic alteration in rhythm. There are four progressively deeper stages of non-REM sleep, with no eye movement and no dreaming in the usual sense. Each non-REM stage has its characteristic EEG rhythm, too. Disturbances of normal sleep patterns include certain forms of bedwetting (enuresis), sleepwalking (somnambulism), nightmares, and insomnia.

Insomnia is a major complaint of Americans who have been schooled to believe that eight hours of uninterrupted sleep nightly are essential for good health. Studies have shown, however, that there is an enormous range of "normal" requirements for sleep. Some persons are able to function well on frequent short catnaps, while others require a rigid routine of uninterrupted sleep. Because there is no unanimity of opinion among the public or physicians on how much sleep is needed, the tolerable limits of insomnia are unknown, so enormous quantities of sleeping aids and medications are sold annually. Many are harmless, but some create dependency and require increasing use until they are abused.

Some who complain of continuing fatigue have sleep abnormalities that prevent them from achieving stage 3 or stage 4 sleep. Respiratory disorders that obstruct breathing may result in recurrent awakening throughout the night. Snoring can be one clue to this abnormality. Sometimes the breathing obstruction results from obesity. The cure is removal of the obstruction, weight reduction for the obese, and in some cases a tracheostomy to bypass the obstruction of the upper air passages.

Narcolepsy is a disorder in which the person may suddenly drop off to sleep without warning and at inappropriate moments, such as while eating, or at dangerous moments, such as while driving a car. In some cases, this stems from an abnormality in the reticular activating system, the brain's so-called "sleep center." Some persons require brain stimulation through amphetamines. Occasionally, such attacks are accompanied by feelings of body paralysis, weakness, or collapse.

DISORDERS OF THE NERVOUS SYSTEM

Other common neurological disorders include demyelinating diseases, infections, tumors, neuromuscular diseases, and nutritional diseases.

Demyelinating Diseases

Axons and dendrites are enwrapped by cells that contain myelin, a fatty substance essential for normal conduction of electrical impulses. Certain diseases attack myelin and the special cells that produce it, stripping the cells of myelin or causing scarring (plaque). When this happens, the nerve ceases to conduct impulses normally and may even stop conducting completely.

Multiple sclerosis (MS) is the most common of several demyelinating diseases. MS is especially prevalent in the United States, but is not equally distributed within the country, nor around the world. It is concentrated in areas of temperate climate and is rare in the tropics or the Arctic. This suggests to researchers that there may be an environmental or climatic influence.

The disease usually begins during the teens or twenties, and rarely after 35. The onset is sudden and can occur in any part of the central nervous system. It may strike in more than one part, hence the name "multiple." The disease is believed to be autoimmune, a case of the body misidentifying its own tissue as foreign and attacking it. Early symptoms may be subtle and fleeting. Visual abnormality, unsteadiness of gait, tremor, sensory impairment, bladder disturbance, paralysis, and slurring of speech can occur alone or in combination. The plaque of demyelination stops normal nerve function for about two weeks and then begins to heal, resulting in improvement or remission. Healing is seldom complete, however, so full function may not return to the affected areas. Usually the disorder is quiet, without new symptoms, for about two years, whereupon it may recur. With each exacerbation, the patient usually has more loss of neurological function. Some persons, however, never have more than a single attack.

Treatment for MS is nonspecific, because the cause is unknown. Many physicians prescribe corticosteroids to reduce swelling and inflammation during the acute phase. Physical therapy and avoidance of heat are all advocated. Experimental treatments with immunosuppressive drugs and with monoclonal antibodies have shown promise. Although the disease can progress to severe handicap, it is not fatal. About one-third of MS patients are said to hold regular jobs.

Infections

Infections of the nervous system can involve the brain, spinal cord, or nerves, or the roots that emanate from them. Infection of the brain tissue is called encephalitis; infection of the membranes covering the brain and spinal cord (meninges) is called meningitis. Infection or inflammation of the nerve roots is called radiculitis, and infection of the

nerves is neuritis. These diseases, their causes, and their treatment are described in Chapter 32, "Infectious Diseases."

Injury

Injuries to the head and brain most often result from auto accidents or gunshot wounds, and occasionally from falls or sports mishaps. They are most common in the young adult population. Disability and death have been reduced by the mandatory use of seat belts. Helmets for bicyclists and motorcyclists, and safer athletic equipment also have reduced the toll.

Brain injury occurs when the brain impacts against the bony skull, resulting in bruises, lacerations, or bleeding within the brain. Sometimes the injured brain swells with fluid, putting pressure on the cells. There may also be damage if an object penetrates the skull and brain, or from depressed skull fracture, which bruises the brain beneath it.

Mild brain injury that merely stuns or dazes is called a concussion. The person may be confused, dizzy, forgetful of the preceding events, and may vomit. He may briefly lose consciousness. Concussion seldom causes permanent damage, although some patients may experience dizziness, nervousness, restlessness, and headache for weeks or months afterward.

Unconsciousness following a head injury requires prompt medical evaluation. So do persistent vomiting, dilation of one pupil, weakness of the limbs, paralysis, and convulsions following head injury. In fact, it is wise for anyone who has had a head injury, unless it is trivial, to have a neurological examination.

Spinal cord injury usually results from an accident, such as an auto crash, fall, or sports mishap such as a diving or skiing accident. Although seat belts and safer sports equipment have reduced the toll, spinal cord injury remains tragically common.

Damage or severing may occur anywhere in the spinal cord's length, causing impaired function in parts of the body below the point of injury. Numbness or weakness is the initial symptom; there usually is little pain, unless adjacent peripheral nerves have been damaged. Depending on location, lower limbs may be paralyzed because nerve pathways controlling their movement have been cut. Bowel and bladder control also may be impaired. If the injury is higher in the spinal cord, all four limbs may be affected. It is important if an accident victim reports numbness or paralysis not to move him, because further damage may be caused.

Unfortunately, the spinal cord does not naturally heal itself, so disability is permanent, although current research promises eventually to lead to a method of repair. Rehabilitation programs and new emphasis on the rights of the disabled, including wheelchair-accessible buildings and lowered curbs, allow many persons with spinal cord injuries to lead more normal lives than in the past.

Brain Tumor (Neoplasm)

Technically, tumors within the brain, like those that develop elsewhere in the body, fall into two categories, benign and malignant. Because of the confined space within the skull, however, even benign brain tumors can be life-threatening. The intracranial pressure crowds healthy cells and interferes with their normal functions. Tumors can develop deep within the brain, making removal impossible without destruction of other cells. Benign growths are often encapsulated, however. If discovered early in an accessible area, they often can be removed completely. Malignant tumors, on the other hand, often have roots like a plant and removing them completely is difficult. Additionally, the brain is a frequent target for cancer cells spread from a primary tumor elsewhere. Sometimes it is possible to remove the primary tumor but not the satellite growth in the brain.

At first, brain tumor may be difficult to diagnose because symptoms are so vague, or resemble those of other conditions. There may be blindness, paralysis of one side of the body, severe headache, seizures, or loss of consciousness. There may be dimmed vision, reduced hearing, bouts of irritation, or loss of emotion or intellect. Some persons experience strange sensations, such as auditory hallucinations or strange smells. Obviously, none of these clues alone indicates brain tumor, but a pattern, or symptoms that occur "out of the blue," should receive medical attention.

Treatment depends on the location and the type of tumor involved. Surgery is the preferred course for a tumor located near the skull, but sometimes the tumor is so deep in the brain that removal can be accomplished only at the risk of causing further damage or death. In this case, a portion may be removed to relieve intracranial pressure, followed by deep X-ray treatment. Drugs may be used alone or in conjunction with radiotherapy.

Tumors of the central nervous system can originate within the brain or spinal cord from any of the different cell types contained there, or from the meninges that surround the brain (meningiomas).

Neuromuscular Diseases

Weakness is the primary symptom of neuromuscular disorder. The distinction between what would be called "normal" fatigue and weakness indicating disease is often difficult. Many people get tired at the end of the day. But if the person begins to have double vision, difficulty with swallowing, weakness to the point of collapse, and inability to carry out normal activities, particularly if only one part of the body is affected, the symptoms may signal muscle disease. Weakness of the legs often begins with walking difficulties, including frequent stumbling, particularly when climbing stairs or walking over carpets.

Weakness also must be distinguished from fatigue. Fatigue may result from overexertion or exhaustion, or the feeling that one is "out of energy." It usually is felt throughout the body, although it may be confined to muscles that have been overexercised. Weakness, on the other hand, is the loss of ability of a muscle to perform its normal activities when presumably the remaining muscles continue to function normally.

Moreover, weakness may be local or general. Certain diseases result in deficiency of function of specific muscle groups. In myasthenia gravis, the muscles of the face often are the first affected, so that vision, facial movements, swallowing, and perhaps breathing are impaired, but movement of the arms and legs remains strong. In contrast, a disease of skeletal muscle can result in weakness of the limbs, without loss of strength in the muscles of the face and the eyes.

Certain diseases produce characteristic disorders. For example, a person who can stand and walk normally may be unable to arise from a chair. This strongly suggests disease of the muscles that extend around the pelvic girdle, so-called proximal muscle disorder. In another case, a patient may be able to sit and rise normally but repeatedly trips on rugs, steps, or small objects. This would suggest weakness of the dorsiflexors of the foot, and would imply a distal muscle disorder.

Other disorders affect the extraocular muscles that move the eyes. The symptom is double vision, because one eye "lags behind" the other in its movements.

Muscular dystrophy has been identified in several forms, most of which appear to be inherited. Muscles enlarge, then begin to separate, with muscular tissue eventually replaced by fat and connective tissue. The disease is normally characterized by weakness rather than pain, although there may be some pain due to strain on weakened muscles or wrenching of ligaments. The most severe forms are progressive and can require the patient to use a wheelchair. Recent research indicates there are milder forms that go unrecognized and do not lead to disability.

Duchenne muscular dystrophy is a sex-linked disease, transmitted to boys by their unaffected carrier mothers. It strikes early, between the ages of 5 and 15. Muscle wasting is usually confined to the trunk and legs, so that the boy is clumsy, finding it difficult to rise from bed or to stand erect. Facial muscles are rarely involved.

Research has now identified and cloned the defective gene in Duchenne, permitting effective testing for the disease and the hope of eventual gene therapy.

Other dystrophies appear in adolescence or later and may affect either sex. Their course is slower than the Duchenne form. The precise cause of the degenerative changes in the muscle appears to be a defective protein coded by a specific gene. There is no effective treatment.

Cerebral palsy is not a disease, but the name given to a group of conditions affecting muscular control that arise from damage to the developing brain before birth or shortly thereafter. There is no cure, but rehabilitation therapy can help minimize the effects. An important development has been public recognition that intelligence is seldom affected, so that palsy victims are able to hold jobs, attend schools, and lead lives more normal than in the past.

Palsy victims usually are classified into three groups according to the part of the brain that has suffered damage. The distinction is not clear-cut, however, and some persons have mixed symptoms and characteristics. The majority of cerebral palsy victims are spastic. Their tightly contracted muscles make them walk with a lurching gait, fling their arms, toss their heads, and speak in a guttural voice. Damage in this case is to the motor cortex. Most other patients are athetoid, victims of damage to the basal ganglia. They may have constant, uncontrolled motion of the limbs. Less common is the ataxic form, marked by poor balance and frequent falls, and by tremor of the hands and feet.

The symptoms in all varieties range from mild to severe. Some persons are affected in only one limb, or on one side of the body.

The causes of brain damage leading to cerebral palsy are many. It may result from poor nutrition and poor health in the mother, or from her exposure to diseases in early pregnancy. Those that strike during the last months of pregnancy, when the brain and spinal cord are maturing, may be the most dangerous. Birth complications, drugs, infections, and deprivation of oxygen also are causes.

The symptoms usually appear in infancy, when the child is not able to hold the head up, sit erect, crawl, or walk at the expected time. In milder cases, symptoms may not appear for several years. Early rehabilitation therapy is important. Various drugs have been used to relax the contracted muscles, and surgery to sever the nerves that control contracted muscles has sometimes proved successful. The heel tendons also may be lengthened to relax tense calf muscles.

Motor neuron disease or amyotrophic lateral sclerosis (not to be confused with multiple sclerosis) is degeneration of cell bodies of the motor cells of the brain and spinal cord, causing a slowly progressive paralysis and wasting of the muscles used for breathing and swallowing, and of the arms and legs. The hands often show the first signs of wasting and weakness. The legs are affected later. There is no loss of sensation. No specific treatment is available. The cause is unknown.

Myasthenia gravis is a disorder of the synapse between the axon and muscle fibers. The secretion of the neurotransmitter acetylcholine is insufficient to stimulate the muscle fibers to keep contracting. The first few contractions usually are normal, but because the supply of acetylcholine is scant, repeated muscle contractions become weaker and weaker. After a few minutes of rest, the acetylcholine supply builds up again and muscle contraction can be resumed temporarily. This rapid fatigue first involves eye movement, talking, chewing, swallowing, and sometimes breathing and use of the arms or legs. In many cases, the disease can be controlled with steroids, or with medications that inactivate cholinesterase, the chemical that inhibits acetylcholine. Removal of the thymus gland is another remedy. The disease may disappear spontaneously, but some patients need continued medication.

CHAPTER 12

EPILEPSY

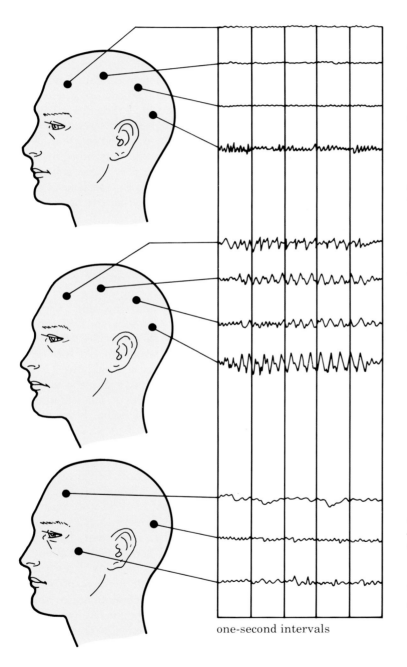

one-second intervals

NORMAL BRAIN WAVES

Epilepsy is a disturbance of the brain's electrical system, which can be depicted by an electroencephalogram (EEG). Electrodes are glued to the scalp to measure electrical voltages, whose pattern then is printed out at one-second intervals, represented by vertical lines. The top drawing shows the EEG of a normal adult. Most normal EEGs show rhythmic waves at a rate of about seven per second. This pattern is called the alpha rhythm.

PETIT MAL SEIZURE

The center drawing shows an EEG during petit mal seizure. A momentary lapse of consciousness occurs with each "spike and wave" discharge. These high-voltage discharges appear suddenly and on both sides of the head.

PARTIAL EPILEPSY

The lower EEG is that of a person with partial epilepsy. Sudden spikes arise from the portion of the brain with a scar or other irritation. If the spikes become continuous, a focal seizure might occur, appearing first at the site of the spike, then spreading to other parts of the brain.

Epilepsy is not a disease but a symptom. It is characterized by recurrent seizures or attacks in which the person experiences a sudden change in sensation or consciousness, or uncontrollable movements or spasms of the muscles. The individual brain cells, which ordinarily function in an orderly, independent fashion, fall into step and begin to beat rapidly and in unison. Because the impulses of the brain are activated by precise and measured amounts of electricity, the condition is one of electrical overload, and the result is overactivity: a seizure.

Characteristically, an epileptic seizure often comes on suddenly and unpredictably, and lasts from a few seconds to 15 or 20 minutes. Between seizures, the person usually is normal. A hard seizure in which there are spasms of the muscles is termed a convulsion.

Depending on the cause, cases of epilepsy fall into two large groups: primary and secondary.

In primary epilepsies, no physical or anatomical abnormality of the brain can be found. The epilepsy results from some constitutional or acquired excitability of the entire brain. Seizures are generalized, involving the whole brain. Although a hereditary factor is suspected, no specific inherited defect appears to be the cause. The first seizure usually occurs between ages 4 and 14. Three out of four cases begin before age 20.

Secondary epilepsies usually result from an injury or an illness that leaves a scar or defect on the surface (cortex) of the brain. The scar irritates the surrounding brain tissues and overexcites them. Seizures originating from such a site or "focus" may start gradually and spread progressively to other parts of the brain. These seizures are spoken of as partial, local, or focal seizures, even though eventually they may involve the whole brain. If there is widespread brain disease or damage, the seizures of secondary epilepsy may originate generalized ones that involve the entire brain. Secondary epilepsies stem from many forms of brain injury, including complications of pregnancy and delivery, meningitis (infections of the membranes around the brain), and accidental head injury.

TYPES OF SEIZURES

Generalized Seizures

The seizures of primary epilepsy usually start without warning.

Tonic-clonic seizures (grand mal) is what most persons mean when they speak of a convulsion or "fit." The person suddenly loses consciousness and the entire body stiffens and becomes rigid. Breath is expelled with a whistling sound or cry, and the victim drops to the ground. Gradually, the rigidity gives way to jerking of the arms, legs, trunk, and head, which lasts five to 10 minutes. When the person regains consciousness, he or she may be lethargic or confused, or may drift off to sleep.

Absence seizures (petit mal) consist of a brief lapse of consciousness, accompanied by loss of awareness and movement. The person develops a blank stare. Eyelids, jaws, and hands may twitch slightly. The person does not fall. As the person regains consciousness, he or she may make a few aimless movements of the hands, but usually recovers rapidly without confusion or loss of memory. The person may continue a conversation as if nothing had happened. Sometimes children who experience petit mal seizures are mistakenly labeled inattentive or daydreamers.

Myoclonic seizures consist of shocklike jerking of the arms and body, so brief that loss of consciousness may not be noticeable. The person may fling objects or drop them without realizing why he or she has done so. In more severe attacks, however, the body suddenly goes limp and the person falls to the floor. Seizures sometimes recur repeatedly over a period of minutes, and occasionally fuse into a generalized attack.

Photosensitive seizures can result in either myoclonic or tonic-clonic (convulsion) symptoms. They occur in a small number of persons who react to a bright light or the rhythmic flashes of a blinking sign or traffic signal.

Partial Seizures

At the beginning of a secondary epilepsy attack, only a part of the brain is affected. The person does not necessarily lose consciousness. A warning or aura may occur, consisting of tingling, numbness, or twitching of the face, hands, or feet, or the appearance of flashing lights or colored balls before the eyes. That may comprise the entire attack, or it may spread to become a generalized tonic-clonic seizure.

Other partial seizures begin with a dreamlike state. The person may pluck at his or her clothes absently or move about in an aimless way. A generalized tonic-clonic seizure may follow, but more commonly the automatic unconscious behavior wears off in five to 10 minutes, leaving the subject confused and disoriented.

DIAGNOSING EPILEPSY

Electroencephalography is a harmless procedure for tracing the rhythm and electrical activity of the brain. Brain electrical activity in most persons follows a regular and predictable pattern, changing in a characteristic way during sleep, upon opening the eyes, or when in deep thought.

An electroencephalogram (EEG) reading that is clearly abnormal is found in about 60 percent of persons with epilepsy, even between attacks, and in almost 100 percent of cases if an attack occurs during the recording. However, such clear-cut abnormalities also are observed in up to 5 percent of the seizure-free population, and in 20 percent of relatives of persons with primary epilepsy.

Computer-assisted tomography, known as the CT scan, is another valuable diagnostic aid (see Chapter 2, "Tests and Procedures"). CT scanners are sophisticated devices that combine X rays and a computer to produce clearer pictures of internal organs than are available from simple X rays. They can record very slight differences in density within the head and can distinguish brain tissue from the water-filled cavities or ventricles within the brain. The picture clearly delineates areas of altered density, such as those produced by scar, tumor, or blood vessel disease. About 50 percent of

the scans taken of persons with epilepsy reveal some anatomical irregularity.

Recently, magnetic resonance imaging (MRI) and video EEG monitoring have been used for epilepsy patients. They are described in Chapter 2, "Tests and Procedures."

TREATMENT

Drugs

Unless an underlying cause can be found and treated, epilepsy cannot be cured. Fortunately, however, the majority of seizures can be controlled by anticonvulsant drugs.

The objective of anticonvulsant drugs is to reduce the sensitivity of the nervous system, and to block brain overactivity that triggers the seizure. It is important to maintain a constant protection level in the bloodstream, so the drugs must be taken on a regular schedule and exactly as prescribed. Withdrawal of the drugs can throw the person into an uncontrollable series of convulsions, called status epilepticus. Changing and discontinuing medication must be carried out over a period of days or weeks to give the body time to adjust.

Most anticonvulsant drugs have some side effects. The most commonly used drugs are:

Barbiturates: phenobarbital (Luminal), primidone (Mysoline), and metharbital (Mebaral). These three medicines are especially useful against generalized convulsions and partial seizures. They do not work well against absence seizures.

Especially at first, phenobarbital can make people sleepy and sluggish. In some children, phenobarbital has the reverse effect. They become cranky and overactive, so other drugs have to be substituted.

Hydantoins: phenytoin (Dilantin), ethotoin (Peganone), and mephenytoin (Mesantoin). They are particularly effective for various generalized convulsions and for partial seizures. Unlike phenobarbital, hydantoins have little sedative effect, but can have serious side effects.

Carbamazepine is the most widely used drug in some forms of childhood and adult epilepsy because it produces neither the sedative effect nor the hyperactive behavior caused by phenobarbital, nor the side effects of phenytoin. Most neurologists consider it first for general and partial seizures.

Valproic acid (Depakene) is especially effective against absence (petit mal) and myoclonic (muscle jerk) seizures, and can prevent grand mal (convulsion) seizures in some patients.

The suximides: ethosuximide (Zarontin), methsuximide (Celontin), and phensuximide (Milontin). Until the introduction of valproic acid, ethosuximide was the best drug for control of absence (petit mal) attacks. The combination of valproic acid and ethosuximide still is used.

The benzodiazepines: clonazepam (Clonopin) and diazepam (Valium). Clonazepam and diazepam, the so-called tranquilizers, are powerful anticonvulsants. Clonazepam is especially effective against absence and myoclonic attacks.

Phenacemide (Phenurone) is a powerful anticonvulsant, especially effective against psychomotor seizures. It has little sedative effect and is well tolerated by most people. But it, too, has serious side effects and is used only in rare instances.

Surgery

Surgery to remove a portion of the brain area may be undertaken if three conditions are met: the seizures cannot be controlled by medication, the point where they originate is in an accessible area, and the removal will not cause intolerable loss of brain function.

In these circumstances, seizure control has been achieved with very low risk in many cases.

Management of a Seizure

A sudden epileptic seizure can be upsetting for an onlooker, but is no cause for alarm. One sensible step is to prevent the subject from injuring himself or herself by clearing the nearby area of sharp objects.

The head should be placed on a soft surface and clothing loosened around the neck. As the person relaxes, after the rigid portion of the attack, the head should be turned to the side to prevent swallowing of saliva. Open the throat to allow passage of air. This can be done by grasping the angle of the jaw on either side just below the ear and pulling gently forward.

In someone not previously known to have epilepsy, it can be important to observe behavior during the convulsion. This information can be helpful to a physician later.

Status epilepticus. If a seizure continues for more than 15 minutes, or if seizures recur so frequently that the subject does not regain consciousness, there is cause for concern. Repeated or continued seizures can develop into a self-perpetuating condition called status epilepticus, in which stopping the seizures becomes increasingly difficult. Emergency medical care is needed.

Managing psychomotor seizures. Persons experiencing psychomotor seizures may fumble with objects, or walk or even run without knowing where or why they are going. Unless life is endangered, however, someone having a psychomotor attack should be left alone until the episode ends.

Febrile convulsions. Some young children suffer generalized tonic-clonic convulsions during an illness associated with high fever (see Chapter 29, "Taking Care of Your Child").

A single febrile convulsion does not indicate that the child will grow up to have adult seizures, although the chances are slightly higher than for children in the general population. Some children who have experienced febrile convulsions may require anticonvulsant medications to protect against further seizures.

HEREDITY AND EPILEPSY

The role of heredity in epilepsy has been greatly overemphasized. Epilepsy is a symptom of an inherited disease in less than 2 percent of all cases. These diseases, however, usually cause physical defects or mental retardation, and epilepsy is a lesser symptom.

If a woman is epileptic, the risk that her child will have epilepsy is greater than the risk to a child of an unaffected mother. The risk also is higher than normal for children born into a family where a brother or sister has epilepsy. When both parents are affected, the chances increase to about 13 percent, which also is the approximate risk when one parent and one child are affected.

It must be emphasized that these figures are averages of large groups of individuals. The risk for any individual or family can be estimated only on the basis of a complete evaluation by a genetic counselor.

CHAPTER 13

STROKE

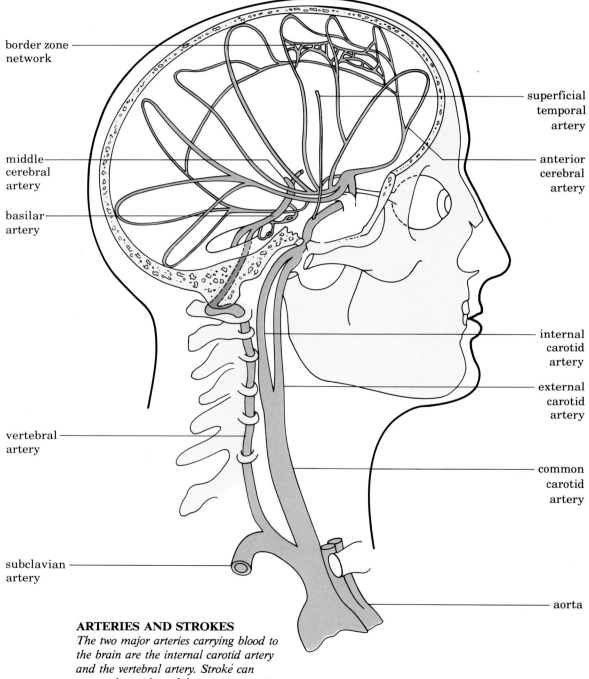

border zone
network

superficial
temporal
artery

middle
cerebral
artery

anterior
cerebral
artery

basilar
artery

internal
carotid
artery

external
carotid
artery

vertebral
artery

common
carotid
artery

subclavian
artery

aorta

ARTERIES AND STROKES

*The two major arteries carrying blood to
the brain are the internal carotid artery
and the vertebral artery. Stroke can
occur when either of these major arteries
is blocked, resulting in damage to areas
beyond the blockage. Afterward, blood
reaches the brain via collateral vessels.*

Stroke (called apoplexy or cerebral vascular accident in old terminology) means a sudden brain disturbance caused by an interruption of the blood supply. It results from disease of the blood vessels supplying the brain. The arteries carrying blood to the brain are most commonly involved, but in rare cases the disease occurs in the veins.

TYPES AND SYMPTOMS OF STROKE

There are three general types of stroke.

Cerebral hemorrhage is caused by rupture of a blood vessel, with bleeding into the brain (intracerebral hemorrhage) or under its covering membranes. Depending on which membranes, this bleeding is called subarachnoid hemorrhage or subdural hematoma.

Cerebral thrombosis stems from obstruction of a cerebral blood vessel when a blood clot forms within its walls. The clot may be caused by abnormal thickening of the blood, damage to the vessel wall from arteriosclerosis, atherosclerosis, inflammation of the arteries, or inflammation of the veins. If the blood supply is stopped completely or is reduced to less than one-fourth its normal level, softening of the brain (cerebral infarction) results, causing permanent brain damage.

Cerebral embolism is obstruction of a cerebral artery by a blood clot or a foreign body that usually has migrated from another part of the body's circulation. Another example is when a clot that has formed on the inside wall of one of the arteries in the neck travels up to the brain and blocks a major artery branch. The clots commonly fragment and lodge in the left middle cerebral artery, which in right-handers supplies the brain areas dealing with speech and the nerve cells controlling movement of the right side of the body.

In stroke victims, interruption of the blood supply causes a corresponding loss of the functions controlled by that part of the brain. This may include loss of speech or slurred speech, confusion, paralysis of one side of the body, paralysis of one side of the face, paralysis of movement of the eyes, unequal pupils, staggering and loss of coordination, loss of sensation to parts of the body, headache, nausea, vomiting, and loss of consciousness.

Severity and Consequences

Besides being classified by cause, strokes also are classified by their severity and consequences.

Transient ischemic attacks (TIAs) are brief episodes of symptoms caused by temporary interruptions of the blood supply to the brain. They last from a few minutes to less than 24 hours, with complete recovery.

Reversible ischemic neurological deficits (RINDs) are small cerebral infarctions, from which there is almost complete recovery within three months.

Recognizing TIAs and RINDs is important because if proper treatment is begun, major strokes can be prevented. At least 11 percent of cerebral thromboses are preceded by warning TIAs, and 41 percent of patients with TIAs will proceed to the permanent damage of cerebral infarction if the condition is not treated properly.

A progressing stroke is caused by infarction of the brain, which usually worsens for five days, and then improves to become a completed or stable stroke, with permanent loss of some central nervous system function. Multiple cerebral infarction can lead to permanent confusion and memory loss. The mortality rate is 30 to 40 percent.

Transient ischemic attacks (TIAs) also may be classified into two major groups according to the part of the brain served by the affected vessels. They are vertebrobasilar arterial insufficiency (VBI) and carotid arterial insufficiency.

Temporary interruption of the blood supply to the brain stem, cerebellum, and occipital lobes (VBI) can cause dizziness, unsteady gait, clumsiness, thick speech, cortical blindness, double vision, and falling spells without loss of consciousness. Temporary interruption of the carotid blood supply can cause weakness of the opposite side of the body, trouble with speech, memory and personality changes, difficulty writing, and loss of sensation on the opposite side of the body.

Apart from TIAs caused by emboli, symptoms also can arise when a carotid artery, middle cerebral artery, or vertebral artery is completely blocked, and the blood supply to the brain's "anemic territory" is supplied by other vessels shunting it around the blockage. When there is a fall in blood pressure or irregular heart action, the collateral circulation may fail and stroke may result.

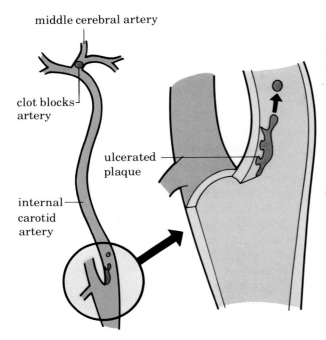

middle cerebral artery

clot blocks artery

ulcerated plaque

internal carotid artery

HOW STROKES OCCUR
Strokes frequently are caused by atherosclerosis of the internal carotid artery of the neck, which supplies blood to the brain, as shown in the left portion of the diagram. Plaque develops on the inner surface of the artery (enlarged view, right), narrowing the channel and roughening the arterial walls. Turbulent blood flow through the narrowed area dislodges the material and carries it to the brain, where it may form a plug in an artery (top left). The result can be a brief interruption in blood supply, called a transient ischemic attack (TIA), or a stroke. The narrowed blood vessel can be reamed out surgically, a procedure called carotid endarterectomy.

INTRACRANIAL BLEEDING

Bleeding within the brain or under its membranes, called intracranial bleeding, is a common form of stroke. Besides cerebral hemorrhage, there are four general types of these hemorrhages.

Cerebral hemorrhage. Patients with cerebral hemorrhage usually have high blood pressure. Onset is characterized by sudden headache, severe loss of brain function, nausea, vomiting, coma, and death within a few days. The death rate for strokes from cerebral hemorrhage is 80 to 90 percent. Fortunately, these strokes are far less common than other types.

Subarachnoid hemorrhage and aneurysm may arise from a congenital defect in the walls of the cerebral arteries. The weak segment stretches and gradually enlarges to cause a ballooning or "blowout" in the wall, called an aneurysm. The thin-walled aneurysm eventually may burst or rupture, bleeding into and through the thin arachnoid membrane that covers the brain. The result is sudden excruciating head pain, stiff neck, nausea, vomiting, and collapse. If the hemorrhage also extends into the brain substance and damages major nerve pathways, it can cause paralysis on one side of the body, dilated pupils, double vision, and paralysis of eye movements, followed by loss of consciousness. The outlook is better if the person remains conscious and if paralysis is minimal. Patients who go into deep coma usually die.

Subdural hemorrhage or hematoma under the outer hard covering (dura) of the brain most commonly arises from head injury, but occasionally from a ruptured aneurysm. The clot must be removed surgically by drilling a hole in the skull or turning a flap of bone to gain access to it (see Chapter 33, "Understanding Your Operation").

Malformed blood vessels. An arteriovenous malformation (AVM) is a tangle of thin-walled vessels, present from birth. These abnormal vessels shunt blood directly from arteries to veins in the cerebral circulation. Because they carry blood under arterial pressure, they are liable to rupture and cause bleeding into the brain.

Other causes. Disorders of the clotting properties of the blood, including hemophilia and sickle-cell anemia, and excessive use of blood-thinning drugs also may trigger intracranial bleeding.

STROKE RISK FACTORS

Stroke can be prevented or lessened by treatment of risk factors that tend to cause arteriosclerosis. These include high blood pressure, diabetes mellitus, elevated fats in the blood, heart disease, obesity, and smoking.

DIAGNOSIS AND PREVENTION

The patient who faces a risk of stroke or who has had TIAs or RINDs should make an early appointment to be examined by a doctor. The examination probably will include a case history, a physical exam, and laboratory tests.

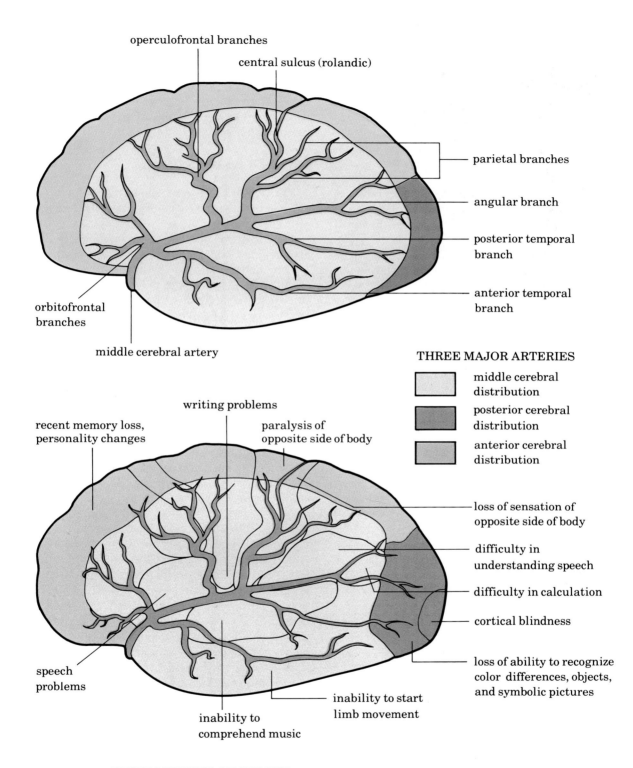

operculofrontal branches

central sulcus (rolandic)

parietal branches

angular branch

posterior temporal branch

anterior temporal branch

orbitofrontal branches

middle cerebral artery

THREE MAJOR ARTERIES

middle cerebral distribution

posterior cerebral distribution

anterior cerebral distribution

recent memory loss, personality changes

writing problems

paralysis of opposite side of body

loss of sensation of opposite side of body

difficulty in understanding speech

difficulty in calculation

cortical blindness

loss of ability to recognize color differences, objects, and symbolic pictures

speech problems

inability to comprehend music

inability to start limb movement

CONSEQUENCES OF STROKE

An interruption of blood supply to the brain can cause a variety of neurological problems, depending on the location of the blockage and the part of the brain supplied by the blocked artery. The top drawing shows the brain's three major cerebral arteries and the portions of the brain supplied by each. The lower diagram shows the location of several brain functions and the neurological problem that results when blood supply is halted to each.

Case history. The person will be asked about stroke and risk factors in blood relatives, because stroke frequently runs in families. The blood pressure will be recorded and blood samples drawn to test for diabetes, high cholesterol, and triglycerides. The heart and major vessels in the neck will be examined for arteriosclerotic plaques.

Physical examination. Neurological tests include evaluation of the state of consciousness, which usually is impaired in severe strokes. Speech, memory, and the patient's orientation to time, place, and person are evaluated. The neck is tested for stiffness, which occurs in subarachnoid hemorrhage.

The ophthalmoscope is used to inspect the optic nerve at the back of the eye. In intracranial hemorrhage or massive infarction, pressure on the nerve or hemorrhages around it may be seen. Paralysis of eye movements, paralysis of one side of the face and body, or loss of sensation may occur.

Laboratory tests. The urine is examined for evidence of kidney disease. Blood samples are tested for the following: red blood cell count, white blood cell count, blood sugar, cholesterol, triglycerides, urea content, and enzymes.

A spinal tap or lumbar puncture may be carried out under local anesthesia by inserting a needle into the lower spine to draw off a small sample of spinal fluid. The sample is examined for fresh blood, found in subarachnoid and brain hemorrhage. The electrocardiogram (ECG) and often the echocardiogram are checked for evidence of cerebral embolism arising from the heart. The electroencephalogram (EEG) may show localized slowing or reduction of brain electrical activity because of stroke damage. A CT scan or MRI helps to locate hemorrhages and infarctions.

TREATMENT

After TIAs or strokes occur, treatment may be surgical or medical.

Surgery

If examination of a patient with carotid transient ischemic attacks discloses large arteriosclerotic or atherosclerotic plaques, some doctors recommend removing them under general anesthesia. This controversial surgery, called a carotid endarterectomy, is accomplished by making an incision in the artery, reaming out the plaque lining and its wall, and sewing the artery together again. A graft of sterile knitted Dacron plastic or vein taken from the leg is then used to restore the artery to its normal width.

Although this operation has been widely performed, several major studies have questioned its value. These studies appear to show that the incidence of stroke after the operation is the same as in persons who have not had the operation.

Medical Management

Medication can prevent the formation of blood clots on the atherosclerotic plaques within the vessel wall.

Many patients with TIAs are treated with one aspirin a day, which inhibits clot formation. Controlled clinical trials have shown that patients receiving aspirin had fewer TIAs and strokes than those who did not receive aspirin. Or, patients may be given anti-blood-clotting drugs of the warfarin (Coumadin) type. These carry a far greater risk of hemorrhage than aspirin, however.

Treatment of subarachnoid hemorrhage begins with complete bed rest. Pain-relieving drugs and sedation usually are required because head pain is severe. Fluids are restricted to minimize brain edema or swelling. Supplementary potassium may be required.

Certain drugs also can enhance clotting of the blood in patients with subarachnoid hemorrhage. The most widely used in the United States is epsilon-amino-caproic acid.

After arteriography has shown the cause of bleeding, intracranial surgery usually is recommended to clip or remove the aneurysm or AVM (see Chapter 33, "Understanding Your Operation") because aneurysm or AVM carries a much greater risk of death or repeated ruptures. Occasionally, if the aneurysm arises directly from the carotid artery, the surgeon may elect to close the carotid artery in the neck gradually in order to reduce blood pressure within the aneurysm.

Treatment of progressive stroke. In general, the recommended treatment of acute, progressive stroke is conservative medical care. Medical treatment is begun with the patient on complete bed rest and lying flat on the back or on the side. The paralyzed limbs are regularly exercised through a full range of motion at least once or twice a day to prevent frozen joints. Blood pressure, pulse rate, and body temperatures are charted daily. Pneumonia and urinary tract infections are common complications that must be watched for. A semi-

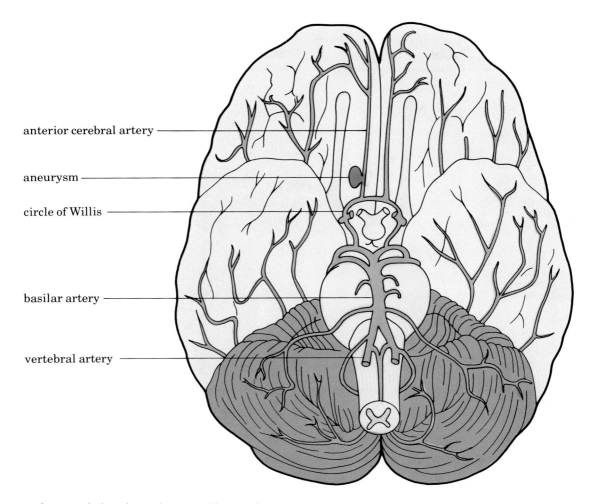

anterior cerebral artery

aneurysm

circle of Willis

basilar artery

vertebral artery

conscious or lethargic patient usually requires a catheter to drain the bladder and must be fed intravenously.

Brain swelling commonly accompanies brain infarction or hemorrhage. No entirely satisfactory treatment has been found, but medication can be given to draw water out of the brain tissue.

After the acute stroke has subsided (usually in four to five days), feeding with a stomach tube may replace intravenous feeding.

Heart Disease and Treatment Of Stroke

More than 20 percent of strokes that do not involve bleeding are caused by emboli from the heart that break off and lodge in the brain. Often the emboli may arise from diseased heart valves, especially the mitral and aortic valves (see Chapter 4, "The Heart and Circulation"). The mitral valve may periodically prolapse (invert like an umbrella blowing out in the wind) and emboli may arise from clots forming on the prolapsed valve.

BRAIN ANEURYSM
A weak-walled, distended area of an artery is called an aneurysm. The balloonlike enlargement is susceptible to rupture and causes hemorrhage under the brain's arachnoid membrane. In this illustration the brain, viewed from below, has an aneurysm of the anterior cerebral artery, a common site. In most cases, an aneurysm can be corrected surgically with a clip so it will not rupture again.

Emboli usually are treated with aspirin or other platelet-inhibiting drugs. Anticoagulant drugs sometimes are used to prevent red clot formation.

If atrial fibrillation is the cause of blood clot emboli, normal rhythm of the heart can be restored with medications. If the blood clots arise from coronary thrombosis or diseased valves, open heart surgery often repairs the problem.

CHAPTER 14

THE EYES

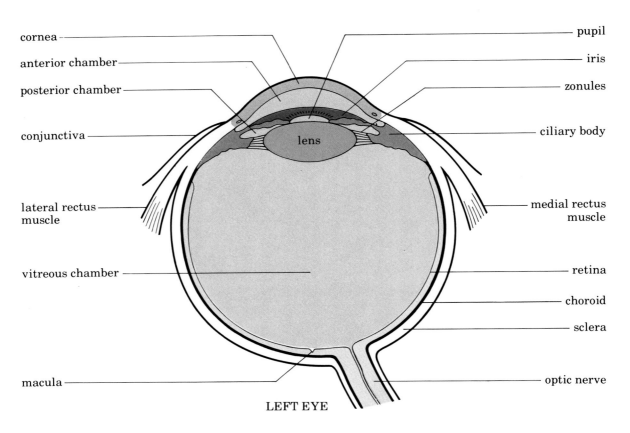

cornea

anterior chamber

posterior chamber

conjunctiva

lateral rectus muscle

vitreous chamber

macula

pupil

iris

zonules

ciliary body

lens

medial rectus muscle

retina

choroid

sclera

optic nerve

LEFT EYE

THE EYE

The eye and some related structures are shown in the cutaway diagram, above. The organ itself rests in a protective socket in the skull called the orbit, and its movement is controlled by three pairs of muscles. The nerve pathways of vision in the brain are shown in the cross section at right. Rays of light falling on the retina excite nerve impulses in the rods and cones of the retina. Nerve impulses follow the pathways of arrows in the optic nerve to the midbrain area and in fibers called optic radiations that make intricate connections in the occipital lobes in the back of the brain.

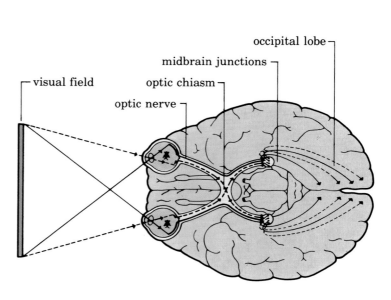

occipital lobe

midbrain junctions

optic chiasm

visual field

optic nerve

How we see is something science is just beginning to understand well. We are learning how light impulses are changed into a visual image in the brain. We know that the eye structures bring the energy into focus on the retina, convert the energy into nerve impulses, and transmit these electric currents over the optic nerve to the back of the brain, then forward to other parts of the brain. It is with the brain, not the eyes, that we "see."

The structures of the eye—those that surround and protect it and enable it to move, as well as those that enable it to collect and transmit visual images—are illustrated on the page opposite.

The process of seeing begins the moment light strikes the outer surface of the eye, because the curved cornea, a convex lens, starts the focusing process by bending light rays inward. The lens does the fine focusing work, becoming thicker to bring objects near us into focus and stretching thinner when we need to focus on objects farther away. Simultaneously but independently, the iris adjusts the size of the pupil and admits as much light as is appropriate for optimal vision. This light-admitting and focusing machinery directs light impulses to the retina's light-sensitive nerve endings, the rods and cones. These cells connect with others, the final connection in the eye becoming the visual fiber layer that coalesces into the optic nerve.

We do not know completely what happens in the visual cortex of the brain to change what was light and now is electrical impulse to the visual imagery we call sight. We do know how the nerve connections are established. The visual image is converted by the optical mechanism to one that initially is upside down. The optic nerve from each eye meets in the optic chiasm where about half of the fibers from one eye cross to the other side, allowing representation from the inner half of each retina to cross to the opposite side of the brain.

CARE OF THE EYES

Eye Examinations

Contrary to common opinion, most people *do not* need an eye examination once a year. No annual checkup prevents ocular disease, although timely visits to an ophthalmologist usually will detect eye problems before they become severe.

A child should be given a routine screening examination at the age of six months and again by the time he or she is 3 or 4 years old. Screening exams are important, because it can be difficult for a parent to recognize that a child has visual problems. Your child's eyes should be tested again around the age of 10 unless school screening tests reveal a special difficulty or specific problems appear earlier.

Because the eyes, like the rest of the body, often have a growth spurt during puberty, teenagers should have their eyes tested every two to four years. Then, unless a person experiences visual symptoms or problems seeing, he or she probably does not need regular biennial eye examinations until about age 40, when most of us develop the need for reading glasses. After the age of 55, we all should seek eye examinations every two to three years unless we experience eye problems. A person will require more frequent visits if he or she has a history of ocular disease, a family history of glaucoma, difficulty seeing, or a general systemic disease such as diabetes, which can result in eye problems.

An initial comprehensive eye examination usually includes the following.

In the first phase, the eye specialist asks your "eye history"—family problems, general medical problems, medications, history of eye problems, eye injuries, glasses. This is highly important in any medical evaluation, for your eyes or for your health in general.

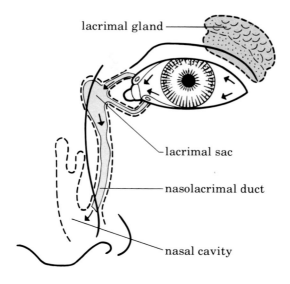

lacrimal gland

lacrimal sac

nasolacrimal duct

nasal cavity

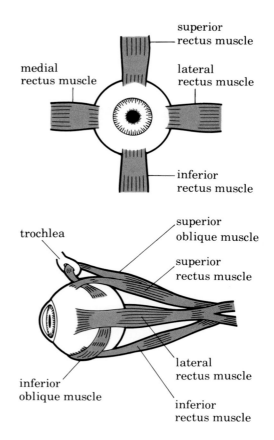

superior rectus muscle

medial rectus muscle

lateral rectus muscle

inferior rectus muscle

trochlea

superior oblique muscle

superior rectus muscle

inferior oblique muscle

lateral rectus muscle

inferior rectus muscle

THE LACRIMAL SYSTEM
Tears produced constantly by the lacrimal and other glands in the upper part of the eye socket flow over the front of the eye to lubricate it. They collect in the lacrimal sac at the inner corner of the eye and drain through the nasolacrimal duct into the nose. That is why the nose runs when a person cries.

HOW THE EYE MOVES
Three pairs of muscles shift the eye vertically, horizontally, and diagonally in a coordinated fashion. The four rectus muscles (top) deal with horizontal and vertical movement. The oblique muscles, shown in the side view bottom, help control up-and-down movement and provide for the diagonal or oblique positions. They also provide the small rotary movement of the eyes. Muscles of the eyes work together to focus on the same object at the same time.

Then, the eye specialist will test your vision with and without glasses, test each eye separately, and test both together. The rest usually is done at a distance of 20 feet or with mirrors to create the effect of a 20-foot examination. It is a distance that, for technical purposes, has been chosen arbitrarily to record visual function. The distance of 20 feet helps define a vision rating. "Normal" vision is 20/20, which means that a person can see at 20 feet what other "normal" people with "normal" vision can see at 20 feet. However, many people see better than 20/20.

The most common method of measuring vision is the familiar Snellen's chart, which tests the ability to distinguish letters of the alphabet in different sizes or numbers or the capital letter E. The chart that uses only the letter E allows testing of preschool children or others who are unable to identify all alphabetical letters or numbers. They can simply indicate which direction the prongs of each "E" face to have their visual acuity measured.

The eye specialist then will look at the external appearance of your eyes, including the eyelids and their linings, the tear ducts, the color and structure of the iris, and the number and location of blood vessels in the white part of the eye. He or she also will check movement.

A refraction, which is testing the eyes for glasses, is done by putting special frames on the nose or by using a Phoroptor. The patient sits in front of this machine, which allows the examiner to test vision with a variety of glass lenses. These determine which modifications will help you see best.

Next, the eye doctor will test for muscle balance to make certain the eyes work together. In this test you look at targets. By covering and uncovering your eyes and using a polarized lens, the doctor determines how well your eyes can fix on the same target and the accuracy of your depth perception.

Next may come a test for clarity of cornea and lens. This test uses a slit lamp, or biomicroscope, that magnifies the front portions of your eye up to 20 times or more. Using the slit lamp, the examiner can observe variations in these structures, which can indicate the presence of eye disorders.

An applanation tonometer attached to the slit lamp allows pressure within the eyes to be measured. Other devices, such as the air puff tonometer or a plunger mechanism called the Schiotz tonometer, are used for screening tests, but the applanation tonometer is the most accurate. Measuring intraocular pressure, a most important test, is relatively simple and painless. It is the most common and reliable means to check for the presence of glaucoma, a leading cause of blindness in the United States and a disease that can be prevented if caught in early stages.

The eye specialist then dilates the pupils by using drops in order to see the back of the eye (the retina). This examination is performed with an instrument called an ophthalmoscope. The examination includes the area of highest resolution directly in the back of the eye, and the retinal periphery, where infections and tumors occur.

At the end of a routine examination, your doctor might prescribe eyeglasses. This usually is done to correct the four most common visual problems: nearsightedness (myopia), farsightedness (hyperopia), astigmatism, and presbyopia.

If you are nearsighted, you probably have an eye somewhat longer than normal from front to back (cornea to retina). You can see to read very well but objects in the distance are blurred without glasses. Nearsightedness is common and readily corrected by wearing glasses or contact lenses.

If you are farsighted, your eyes are shorter than normal. You generally can see things well at a distance and nearby until you approach age 40, when you may need glasses to read.

A third common condition, astigmatism, occurs when the front part of the eye, the cornea, is not perfectly round as a basketball might be, but more curved in one direction than the other as a football might be. The eye bends the light rays as they enter and that distorts the images. To help someone with astigmatism see properly, opticians will grind cylinders into the lenses of glasses according to the prescription written by an ophthalmologist or optometrist. It is not uncommon to be both nearsighted or farsighted and astigmatic.

Contact Lenses

Most people wear spectacles to correct vision problems, but contact lenses have become increasingly popular. The reason for the popularity of contact lenses is not only cosmetic. In cases of profound myopia, contact lenses correct vision better than glasses.

There are two types of contact lenses. Hard contact lenses are made of a hard plastic. Soft contact lenses are made of a slightly different plastic material that has a high water content, which allows them to conform closely to the shape of the eye. Soft contact lenses were developed because some persons found hard lenses irritating. Soft lenses are larger and more malleable than hard lenses. They usually are removed for hygienic purposes nightly, but extended-wear models sometimes are left in place for weeks. Some disposable lenses may be left in the eye for as long as several months, then discarded and replaced.

Regardless of type, it is important to disinfect the lenses regularly. Certain eye infections that develop behind contacts can cause eye damage.

Low vision aids are used by those with substantially lower than normal vision. These are magnifiers or specially constructed high-power lenses and telescopes. They help in cases of macular degeneration in older persons or in pathologic conditions that reduce vision markedly.

Radial Keratotomy

Radial keratotomy, or refractive surgery, is a method of correcting myopia by surgical means. Introduced by Soviet specialists in the early 1970s, the procedure has become popular and has been successful in many cases.

As the illustration on page 155 shows, four to eight radial cuts are made outward from the center of the cornea, near the pupil, almost through the cornea. The pressure of the eye then flattens the cornea, reducing its curvature and changing the focal length. The result is a lessening of myopia. Marked nearsightedness cannot always be corrected by radial keratotomy.

The surgery is carried out on one eye at a time, under local anesthetic. A patch is worn for several days, and the eye remains light-sensitive for a longer period. Although widely performed, keratotomy still is considered controversial. Some doctors object to its use on grounds that myopia can be effectively corrected without surgery, and without the complications associated with surgery.

NEARSIGHTEDNESS

*In myopia (nearsightedness) the image
of an object, unless it is held close to the
eyes, falls in front of the retina instead
of upon it (top drawing), and the object
is seen indistinctly. A concave lens of
proper curvature corrects the condition
by bringing the object into focus on the
retina, as shown in the bottom drawing.*

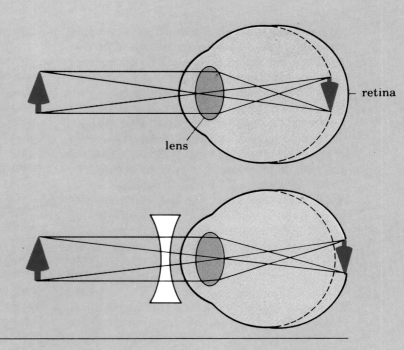

FARSIGHTEDNESS

*In hyperopia (farsightedness) the image
of an object is focused behind the retina
of an eyeball that is too short for the
focusing mechanism (top drawing).
A convex lens brings the light rays
into focus on the retina, ashown at
bottom. Farsighted persons may be able
to see things sharply by thickening the
lens of the eye, a process called
accommodation. However, this involuntary effort involves inner muscles of
the eye and causes eye fatigue if the
hyperopia is of sufficient magnitude.*

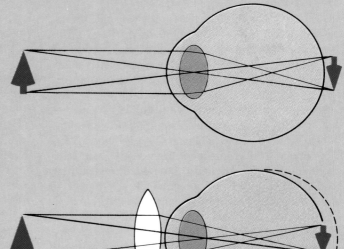

ASTIGMATISM

*Astigmatism is comparable to the
distortion produced by a wavy pane of
glass. The drawing shows light rays 3
and 4 in sharp focus on the retina, with
light rays 1 and 2 focused in front of
the retina. The result is a blurred
image, where the horizontal line is in
focus and the vertical line out of focus.
A cylindrical lens in the proper axis
brings the light rays into even focus and
corrects astigmatism.*

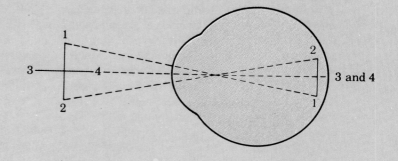

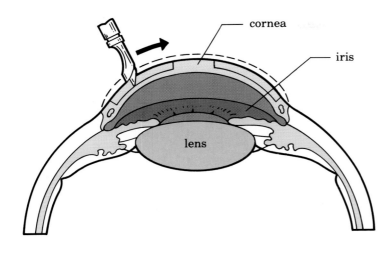

cornea

iris

lens

TREATING NEARSIGHTEDNESS
Radial keratotomy, a relatively new procedure, can correct some forms of myopia by surgical means. As shown, a series of cuts are made partially through the cornea, radiating like spokes of a wheel from the center of the eye. The cuts allow the cornea to flatten from its original curvature, thus shortening the eye's focal length.

HOW THE EYES GROW, DEVELOP, AND AGE

The eyes probably are a baby's most mature organ at birth. They are approximately five-sixths the size of an adult eye and will develop faster than any other part of the body. Although it is impossible to test an infant's vision in the way we test adults, pediatric ophthalmologists using special tests estimate that the normal visual resolution ability of a newborn is somewhere between 20/30 and 20/70.

By the age of three months, a baby can distinguish color, focus on objects near and far away, even put together the sophisticated visual signals that distinguish Mother from any other woman in the room. The child usually develops normal visual acuity between the ages of 3 and 5. By the time he or she reaches school age, a child with normal vision has nearly reached full visual potential.

Like the rest of the body, the eyes change during puberty, reaching maturity before the rest of the body. Just as they experience a spurt in the growth of their bones, many adolescents experience a growth of their eyes as well. The eyes of a young person who previously had no visual problems may grow too large and thus too long—longer, that is, than the lens can accommodate to focus properly. Then, for the first time, a young person needs glasses to correct nearsightedness.

But just as they are one of the first organs to mature, our eyes are one of the first to age. We can measure objectively the effects of aging. As the eyes and their owner grow older, the lens begins to lose its elasticity. Our normal ability to see nearby and distant objects clearly requires that the lens, the focusing mechanism at the front of the eye, make adjustments. These adjustments are made automatically and are a focusing process that many automatic focusing cameras imitate incredibly well. The circular muscle called the ciliary body contracts and relaxes to help the lens change shape. Unfortunately, however, as the protein of the lens progressively hardens, by about age 40, ciliary muscles working through the zonules can no longer compress or stretch the lens enough to change focus from distant to near. The condition progresses throughout life, although the need for progressively stronger bifocals reaches its maximum about age 55.

EYE PROBLEMS DECADE BY DECADE

Because the eyes develop in a chronological fashion, eye problems tend to follow a chronological pattern, too. Occasionally, for instance, a baby is born with cataracts, but cataracts are primarily a problem of later years. Similarly, the need for bifocals usually becomes apparent in middle age. Eye problems usually can be categorized according to the decades in which they commonly occur.

Problems of Childhood

Most babies are born with normal eye function, but it is important for a pediatrician or ophthalmologist to evaluate the infant's eyes at birth. The examination should check the clarity of the cornea, inspect the vascular structure (blood supply) of the optic nerve head, and test for muscular paralysis. The doctor should check for a variety of other problems that are either congenital (present at birth) or inherited (passed down genetically from one or both parents, but not always immediately apparent). These conditions can include cataracts (clouding of the lens), glaucoma (abnormal fluid pressure within the eye), ptosis (droopy eyelid), and strabismus.

Strabismus is by far the most common problem of the early years. It affects 1 to 3 percent of children early in life. In strabismus, the eyes fail to work together to focus on a single object. One eye deviates in or out from the line of focus; the other looks directly at the object. Dissimilar information thus comes from the two eyes. A baby looking out from his or her crib may see parents in one eye and a rattle in the other—a confusing and disturbing message for the brain to sort out.

The brain is an amazingly resilient organ, but when it receives separate and confusing images, it is forced to make a choice. It must decide to see either the parents or the rattle, selecting one and ignoring the other. In time, a "preferred" eye is established because the brain tends to disregard information transmitted by the deviated eye. If the condition is allowed to persist, the visual potential, the brain's ability to process information coming from the "weak" eye, is lost, and that eye may never become a completely functional organ.

Two types of strabismus lead to reduced vision. The more common is esotropia, or crossed eyes. A hereditary factor is involved, but it is not the usual hereditary pattern and therefore not absolutely predictable. Esotropia usually is noticeable to parents during the early months of life.

Exotropia, the outward deviation of one eye, might not be noticed until a child is 6 or 7 years old. Surgery often will be necessary to readjust the eye muscles. Good vision usually is retained in each eye in exotropia.

Ptosis, or droopy eyelid, also causes reduced vision if it droops completely, because the information from one eye is suppressed in the brain and visual potential does not develop.

Years ago, pediatricians believed that a child would "grow out of" strabismus, but this is an erroneous belief. If you seriously believe that your child shows the eye deviation of strabismus, you should have an ophthalmologist's examination promptly. Almost all clinical evidence indicates that the earlier the treatment, the better the chance for normal, binocular vision. Glasses (even bifocals in some cases), surgery, or a combination of surgery and glasses can help align the eyes in the proper direction. Once aligned, the eyes can send similar information to each side of the brain and binocular vision can develop.

Tearing is a common and disturbing disorder in infants, although not generally a sight-threatening problem. Tear ducts drain through a connection into the nose, the nasolacrimal duct, which in an infant is a very small passageway. Not infrequently, the duct does not function properly for weeks or even months after birth, so that the eyes stream steadily. Usually the duct will open spontaneously, but if tearing in one or both eyes persists, an ophthalmologist should be consulted. By a simple and relatively pain-free probe of the duct, he can open the faulty membrane.

Retinoblastoma is a far more serious but relatively uncommon eye disorder of childhood. This malignant eye tumor appears any time from a few months of age to 7 or 8 years. One-third to one-half of cases appear to be inherited. Symptoms often are minimal. A white pupil or a crossed eye are the most noticeable early signs. Generally, children will not complain of pain.

When this disease occurs in only one eye, the afflicted eye usually is removed. If both eyes are attacked, the more seriously affected is removed and its mate is treated by radiation and chemotherapy. If retinoblastoma is caught early, treatment may be successful.

Although most eye problems of childhood are apparent to fathers and mothers, it is important for a child to have an ophthalmological examination before he or she begins school.

The need for visual correction often shows up at this time. It is not always possible for a parent to recognize that a child has seeing problems until schoolwork begins. A school screening examination and an ophthalmologist's exam will disclose nearsightedness, farsightedness, or astigmatism.

Problems of the Teens

Eye injury is the major problem between the ages of 10 and 20. Historically, boys have suffered more eye injuries than girls. However, that may be changing as girls engage in baseball, soccer, and other athletic activities and expose themselves to other accident risks.

The bulk of eye injuries, fortunately, can be treated successfully. Treatments cover a spectrum of medical and surgical techniques. A cut often can be stitched with tiny sutures and the eye covered with a patch until it heals. Antibiotic drops prevent infection and damage. Modern developments in instrumentation save many injured eyes that formerly would have been lost.

In rare cases an eye cannot be saved and must be removed. The procedure sounds horrible, but surgically it is not difficult. A ball of plastic or similar material is implanted in the eye socket and covered with a prosthesis that resembles the eye. The surgeon may affix the plastic globe or ball to the muscles of the eye, or simply place it in the orbit. The plastic eye moves much as the normal eye does, pushed and pulled by the eye muscles and the surrounding tissue. Because a good ocularist usually can duplicate the appearance of a patient's natural eye, the cosmetic outcome generally is excellent, and most people learn to function almost normally with one eye.

"Pink eye" or conjunctivitis (inflammation of the conjunctiva) is a common though minor problem of the teen years (as well as before and after). Pink eye occurs when blood vessels in the eye become congested or engorged, giving the white of the eye a pinkish hue. The condition can result from an injury, or because the eye is rubbed too vigorously, but most commonly the cause is an upper respiratory infection that spreads to the eye. It is most often caused by a virus. Virus pink eye usually resolves itself within several weeks and does not necessarily require medical treatment. On the other hand, bacterial infections usually are accompanied by more puslike discharge and crusting and should be medically treated. They respond rapidly to an antibiotic.

Sties, a frequent and annoying disorder, are localized red spots or swellings that develop near the lid margin of the eye. They are analogous to boils of the skin. Sties are little abscesses of bacteria (usually a staphylococcus infection). They sometimes drain spontaneously, but may require opening by an ophthalmologist.

Chalazion is similar to a sty, but more chronic. It occurs when the glands in the lid margins become plugged but continue to produce their own secretions. Because there is no place for this material to drain, it escapes into the surrounding tissue. The body then sets up a reaction to it. Like sties, chalazion sometimes resolves spontaneously, but may require surgical removal.

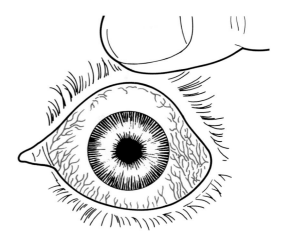

PINK EYE

Conjunctivitis, or pink eye, is a reddening of the outer covering of the sclera. It is most frequently the result of local infection, allergies, irritation, or inflammation within the eye. The condition occurs because blood vessels within this layer of the eye become congested or engorged.

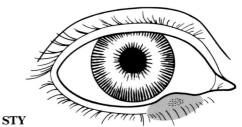

STY

A sty is an infection, usually by staphylococcus organisms, of one of the glands of the eyelid margin. It resembles a boil on the skin. Applications of hot compresses usually bring the sty to a head and pus escapes. If sties occur repeatedly, an antibiotic taken by mouth is advisable.

Problems of the 30s and 40s

The fourth and fifth decades might be described as the Age for Glasses, because by the end of their 40s most people need help in focusing for near vision. The loss of lens elasticity is like gray hair and wrinkles, an unavoidable fact of growing older. Those of us who have difficulty reading the numbers in the telephone directory, or find our arms too short to scan the morning paper, now need glasses. The farsighted lose their previous ability to see objects at a distance. To help focus on

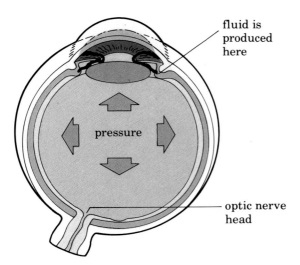

fluid is
produced
here

pressure

optic nerve
head

GLAUCOMA

*A leading cause of blindness, glaucoma
hampers vision because increased
pressure inside the eyeball presses on the
optic nerve. The increase occurs because
too much fluid is produced or because
not enough can leave the eye. Because
of the increased pressure, the most
vulnerable structure suffers first, in this
case the optic nerve head. The disease
must be treated promptly because
damage to the optic nerve cannot be
reversed.*

nearby objects as well as distant ones, some need
bifocals, which are glasses divided into focal
lengths for both close and distant vision. Some are
fortunate and need only minimal correction for
distance or simply require reading glasses that
they can purchase at a drug or department store.

Glaucoma also becomes more common during
the 30s and 40s, although it can occur at any age.
Glaucoma is the result of increased fluid pressure
inside the eye that presses on and damages the
optic nerve, causing a loss of vision. The increased
pressure may be caused by an abnormal production of fluid, by an inability of a normal amount of
fluid to leave the eye (the result of a blocked or
faulty drainage system), or by secondary reactions
to other eye problems or injuries.

Chronic glaucoma, also known as simple or
open-angle glaucoma, is the most common and
vexing form of the disease. Painless and progressive, it can result in blindness if not treated, because of damage to blood vessels supplying the

optic nerve. Many persons notice no symptoms
until some vision has been lost. To treat the condition, the pressure must be reduced.

Usually, the doctor will prescribe a beta-blocking drug in eye drop form. Beta-blockers reduce
the pressure in the eye, although the exact mechanism is uncertain. If this method is not successful,
the beta-blocker may be combined with a drug to
reduce production of acqueous fluid. An older eye
drop, pilocarpine, still is used in some cases. Pills
also may be prescribed.

If drops and pills are unsuccessful, the next step
may be laser trabecular surgery. This office procedure uses a laser beam to burn a series of tiny holes
partially through the eye's trabecular meshwork,
where fluid leaves the eye. The burns seem to
relieve pressure, after which drops may not be
necessary.

In a relatively few cases, trabecular surgery may
be unsuccessful. Then direct surgery may be performed to make a small opening, allowing fluid to
flow directly under the conjunctiva.

Fortunately, chronic glaucoma usually can be
halted if it is detected early. A screening test measures the intraocular pressure in the course of a
regular eye exam. People with a family history of
glaucoma should have the intraocular pressure
and sometimes even their peripheral visual field
measured regularly and routinely. Measuring the
peripheral field (how well we see objects to the side
of the main line of vision) is a critical way to check
the presence of the disorder. If pressure remains
high, the peripheral visual field is affected first.

Closed-angle glaucoma, also known as acute
glaucoma, a less common form, often is an episodic event producing halos in the vision and causing
eye pain. It thus is more readily noticed. It can be
cured with an operation called an iridotomy. The
procedure is performed with a laser, to burn a hole
near the base of the iris. This allows fluid to flow
from where it is produced to where it normally
flows from the eye, and the blockage that impedes
the outward flow of fluid is relieved. If performed
early, the treatment usually is curative.

Secondary glaucoma occurs with inflammations, infections, or injury within the eyeball.
Treatment of the underlying disorder generally
improves the "secondary" glaucoma.

Corneal diseases also appear in the 30s and
40s, although sometimes they do not occur until
the 50s or later. Deteriorating or degenerating corneal tissue is the cause.

Herpes simplex keratitis accounts for a high
percentage of serious corneal scars. The cause is
the same virus that produces cold sores and, like

CORNEAL ULCERS

There are several types of corneal ulcers, but by far the most common is dendritic ulcer, shown in the top drawing. It results from infection by the herpes simplex virus, which also causes cold sores. Corneal transplant, the most successful of transplant operations, is necessary to restore useful vision in severe cases of corneal scarring.

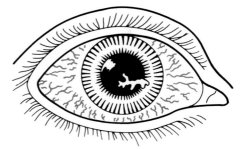

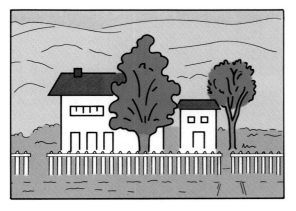

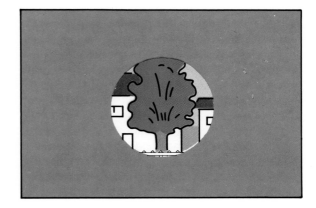

GUN-BARREL VISION

Persons whose vision is impaired by retinitis pigmentosa suffer from a narrowing of the visual field, as if they were looking through a gun barrel. A person with normal vision would perceive the scene on the left. One with retinitis pigmentosa eventually loses

peripheral vision and sees only a small portion of the scene, as shown at right. Similar impairment of the visual field may occur in advanced stages of glaucoma, although in each case it is unlikely that the remaining visual field would be perfectly round.

cold sores, corneal infections tend to recur once the virus has become established. Herpes simplex keratitis is not painful. In fact, the sensation of pain on the normally sensitive cornea is greatly reduced. The infection's particular danger is that it can erode the cornea and produce dense scars that impair vision. Ophthalmologists usually prescribe eye drops, or they may scrape the cornea and patch the eye. Severe corneal disease may require corneal transplant surgery.

In performing a transplant, the surgeon removes part of the diseased cornea and replaces it with a segment of cornea from a donor. The new section then is sutured into place with strands much finer than human hair. Although this procedure is technically difficult, it has become the most successful of all transplant operations. The outcome in most cases is excellent, with sight often restored to near normal.

Retinitis pigmentosa may show itself during the teens, but is more common in the middle years. A layer of the eye, the retinal pigment epithelium containing the rods and cones, begins to degenerate. The process starts at the periphery of the retina and gradually moves toward the macula in the center. People with this condition suffer from marked loss of night vision and narrowing of the visual field, so they sometimes are said to have "gun-barrel vision." Retinitis pigmentosa, like many eye disorders, frequently is hereditary. It is painless and generally progressive, and can result in near blindness, or at least marked narrowing of the visual field. But despite its severity, we know little about how to halt or cure it.

Malignant melanoma, usually thought of as a skin cancer, is the most common cancerous eye tumor in adults. It attacks the pigmented layers of the eye, the choroid and iris. Depending on its location, a melanoma may grow to fairly large size without affecting vision. In some cases the eye is removed, but a long-term study is exploring whether this is the best treatment. The outlook is more favorable than with melanomas of the skin.

Clouding of the vitreous, the semiliquid, gel-like substance in the central of the eye, also can damage vision, especially in later life. The darkening or clouding usually is caused by blood leaking into the eye from hemorrhages on the retina. The hemorrhages result from diseases affecting the blood vessels, such as diabetes, the most common cause, or from a blow or puncture wound to the eye. The blood or tissue blocks vision by preventing light from passing unobstructed to the retina.

A procedure called vitrectomy can be used to clear the patient's vision, if the condition does not spontaneously resolve. Using extremely fine instruments, the ophthalmologist makes an incision through the sclera, the tough outer covering of the eyeball, and removes the vitreous humor from the eye, replacing it with liquid saline solution. Many persons whose vision was severely limited have had significant improvement afterward.

The Later Decades

Cataracts are the most common eye problem that strikes men and women after age 50. They occur when the normally clear lens hardens and becomes opaque with age. The aging lens not only cannot stretch to focus light waves, but blocks light on its way to the retina, obstructing vision.

An estimated nine out of ten 65-year-olds show some sign of cataracts or changes that lead to cataracts, but that does not mean their vision is impaired. A cataract is simply cloudiness of a normally clear lens and if it is in the edge of the lens, no visual loss is apparent. Moreover, a cataract

often develops at such a gradual pace that it does not advance to the point of destroying or impairing eyesight during the person's lifetime. Only when a person is unable to drive, read, or perform the visual tasks necessary in daily life should cataract surgery be considered.

It is important to seek medical help, however, because neglected cataracts remain a leading cause of loss of vision. The early warning signs of the condition are hazy vision or poor night vision. When the cataract victim drives in bright sunlight or at night, the clouded lens will "scatter" light, causing a dazzling effect.

Tremendous advances in cataract surgery have occurred in the past 30 years. More than 98 percent of operations are successful.

To correct cataracts, ophthalmologists in most cases remove the clouded lens and all but its posterior capsule. Either they use an ultrasonic device, which breaks up the lens and capsule and allows it to be removed, or the cortex of the lens and anterior capsule are sucked out by direct aspiration.

Because of smaller incisions, better sutures, higher surgical magnification, and more advanced techniques, cataract surgery usually is performed on an outpatient basis, under local anesthetic. Visual return is rapid and nearly normal in a few days or weeks. In most cases special lenses are necessary for distant vision. Generally, a cataract patient receives a new lens at the time the old one is removed. As the illustration opposite shows, a tiny plastic lens is anchored into the posterior chamber of the eye, using clips that work like a spring to keep the lens in position. Only in a few cases caused by disease or structural defects is it necessary to resort to thick corrective spectacles used by cataract patients in the past.

Retinal disorders are the second most common problem of the later decades. There are three main types: macular degeneration, peripheral retinal degeneration, and retinal detachment.

Macular degeneration is a common disorder after age 70 or 75, but its cause is not fully known. It attacks the macula, the high-resolution or "fine-tuning" center of the retina, which we need for close work such as reading and threading a needle.

Macular degeneration occurs when the blood supply to the macula is reduced, often eventually resulting in hemorrhages, or when other fluid collects in the vicinity of the macula, reducing central visual sharpness. A person with macular degeneration retains vision to the side but has difficulty reading or fine-focusing on any object directly in front of him. Sometimes this reduction is marked, sometimes it is minimal.

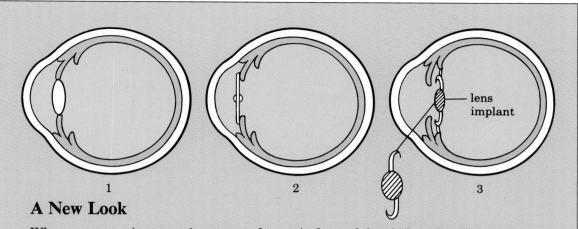

A New Look

When a cataract is removed, a person frequently receives a new artificial lens in the same procedure. Above, drawing No. 1 shows the eye with the lens and cataract removed. Drawing No. 2 shows a new lens implanted in the anterior chamber of the eye, in front of the old lens site. The more common location for the new lens is in the posterior chamber, shown in drawing No. 3. The tiny new lens is positioned and clipped into place with tiny hooks. Improvement of sight is almost immediate.

There are several types of macular degeneration. One is known as age-related macular degeneration. The condition worsens with age, but its cause is not clearly understood. Another form appears to run in families. Certain types of macular degeneration can be treated by coagulating the hemorrhaging vessels with laser burn. The treatment can arrest the progression of the disease but cannot restore lost vision.

A simple home test, the Amsler grid, can be used to detect macular degeneration in its early stages. The grid is illustrated at right.

Age-related macular degeneration is serious, but almost never leads to blindness. Low-vision aids enable many persons to lead normal lives.

Peripheral retinal degeneration is simply the degenerative change or destruction of tissue in the retina's periphery. It sometimes is called "lattice degeneration." There are virtually no visual symptoms because this portion of the eye seldom is used. However, a more serious condition, retinal detachment, can develop from certain peripheral retinal degenerations. Retinal degeneration occurs somewhat more frequently in nearsighted people.

Retinal detachment occurs when a hole in the retina allows liquid vitreous in the center of the eye to seep behind the retina and push it away from its connection to the rest of the eye. The process is much the same as when moisture collects behind wallpaper, producing a fluid bubble. Symptoms include black "floating spots" or a constant dark

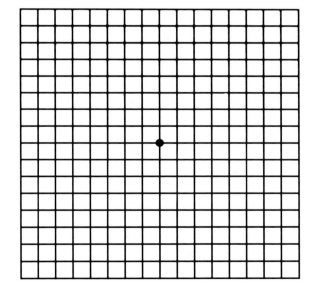

**EYE TEST
FOR OLDER PERSONS**
The Amsler grid provides a simple test for signs of visual change in older persons. Hold the chart at arm's length and focus on the black dot. If the checkerboard lines appear to converge or are wavy, it may indicate age-related macular degeneration, which often can be treated successfully if detected early. Persons over age 55 should test themselves regularly and report any change to an ophthalmologist.

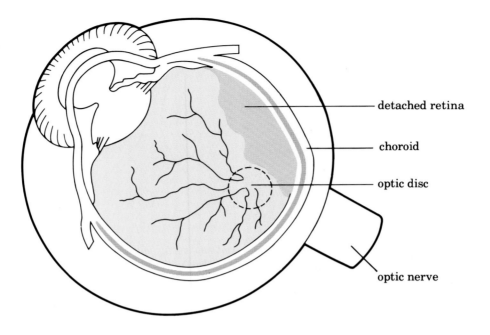

detached retina

choroid

optic disc

optic nerve

DETACHED RETINA
A retinal detachment occurs when the retina separates from the underlying choroid, usually because a hole in the *retina permits fluid to seep under it and lift it. Surgical reattachment is often successful.*

spot in the field of vision. Sometimes the victim feels as if a curtain has been pulled in front of his or her eyes. If the hole is very small and the fluid behind it is minimal, a laser beam may be used to seal off the area. Cryosurgery, or freezing, also may be used. Surgery can freeze or burn the area surrounding the hole so that a scar seals it. A laser beam is one method used for the burning process.

If the hole is large and the amount of fluid is great, an ophthalmologist may place a silicone pillow over the sclera at the site of the hole or an encircling band around the eyeball to force the separated layers together and help seal the hole. If the retinal detachment can be treated before it reaches the macula, there is an excellent chance for good vision. A high percentage of the operations for retinal detachment are successful.

Low-vision aids. Some older people accept the myth that vision naturally dims with age. Others are unduly pessimistic, falsely believing that it is only a matter of time before they become blind. Persons with macular degeneration do *not* go blind. Their ability to read, to recognize friends at a distance, or to perform other tasks that require close visual attention may be impaired, but they retain peripheral vision, which allows them to move around freely. Many still enjoy television.

They can perceive the general movement on the screen but not facial expressions. For these individuals, low-vision aids and appliances can help.

Spectacles with strong magnifying lenses are the best aid for prolonged reading. Other aids are hand-held or stand magnifiers and monocular telescopes small enough to fit into a pocket. There are devices other than nagnifying lenses that are helpful. Examples are colored filters to enhance contrast, large print books and magazines, large print checks and playing cards, large print telephone dials, and special fixtures for appliance dials.

For some people, advice in managing their everyday lives (shopping, cooking, and taking care of themselves and their homes) will be more important than an optical aid. The person who cannot travel safely, efficiently, and alone needs the training offered by schools and agencies for the visually handicapped.

When a person has a corrected visual acuity of 20/200 or less and a visual field of 20 degrees or less, he or she can be classified as "legally blind." That means the person becomes eligible for an extra income tax deduction and can get educational benefits from the state. "Legal blindness" is a legal, not a medical, term. It does not necessarily mean that the person is blind or will go blind.

BLINDNESS

Blindness is confined to no particular age group. Generally, it results from disease or injury, although a small percentage of people are born blind each year.

Research to Prevent Blindness, Inc., a nonprofit foundation dedicated to preventing and curing blindness, estimates that in the United States alone four million new cases of eye disease occur each year and 500,000 are considered "legally blind." According to the National Society to Prevent Blindness, another national nonprofit organization, more than 25 percent of those who lose their sight are blinded by retinal disorders, nearly 14 percent by cataracts, and 12 percent by glaucoma. For more than 11 percent of cases of blindness, the causes are unknown. Most major cities in the United States support a local chapter of the National Society to Prevent Blindness. The Yellow Pages of your telephone directory may list sources of aid under "Blind Institutions." The National Eye Institute, Bethesda, Maryland, is the government's leading research agency in this field.

DIABETES AND EYE COMPLICATIONS

Although not directly a disease of the eyes, diabetes mellitus is a leading cause of serious eye problems. As explained in Chapter 19, "Diabetes Mellitus," long-term diabetes damages nerves and blood vessels throughout the body, including the tiny capillaries in the retina of the eye.

Diabetic retinopathy occurs when diabetes-damaged blood vessels in the retina disintegrate and leak blood, which seeps between the retinal layers and collects there. The pooled blood may detach the retina from the back of the eye, causing blurred vision and even loss of sight.

Background retinopathy is considered an early stage, in which some blood vessels decrease in size and others enlarge, obstructing normal blood flow in the retina. The vessels rupture frequently, and leak blood, which causes the retina to swell. Unless the leaking fluid collects in the macula, however, sight usually is not seriously affected. About 80 percent of cases do not progress beyond the background stage.

Proliferative retinopathy begins with new blood vessel growth on the retina and optic nerve. These fragile vessels may rupture and bleed into the vitreous, causing its clear gellike substance to cloud. Light passing to the retina is blocked and images are distorted. Scar tissue may form on the retina and detach it from the back of the eye, and vessels may even grow into the iris, causing a form of glaucoma. Severe loss of sight and even blindness may result.

Laser surgery, performed in an ophthalmologist's office, successfully seals or coagulates the leaking blood vessels and halts the damage in many cases. The intense heat of the laser beam seals the vessels and forms tiny scars inside the eye, which anchor the retina to the back of the eye. Best results are obtained if diabetic retinopathy is detected early, but even in advanced stages, laser treatment may prevent more severe visual loss. Because of a major study supprted by the National Eye Institute, ophthalmologists may treat diabetic retinopathy with multiple laser burns to the peripheral retina, which seems to prevent progression of the retinopathy to the center of the retina.

In cases where the vitreous has become heavily clouded with blood, the ophthalmologist may perform a vitrectomy, described above, to remove the blood-filled vitreous and replace it with a clear, artificial solution.

A wide spectrum of visual changes, including cataracts, can occur in a person suffering from diabetes over an extended period, and it is important for a diabetic to consult an ophthalmologist if he or she experiences visual changes. Indeed, every diabetic who has had the disease for seven to 10 years should see an ophthalmologist and have regular eye examinations. It also is important to treat the disease itself aggressively. Studies have shown that tight control minimizes the possibility of eye complications.

SYSTEMIC DISEASES THAT AFFECT THE EYE

Other diseases besides diabetes that originate elsewhere in the body can affect the eyes.

Atherosclerosis produces deposits called plaques, which can be found in the larger blood vessels such as the aorta, the body's main artery, or its major branches. Plaques normally do not develop inside the eye because the blood vessels are too small. Frequently, however, small pieces of plaque break off from the walls of the major blood vessels

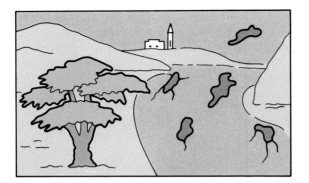 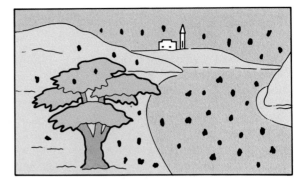

SPOTS BEFORE THE EYES
Transparent "floating" spots across your vision (left drawing), a common occurrence, are normal and should cause no concern. Sudden showers of

black spots that affect your vision, as in the right drawing, may represent a more serious eye problem, and you should see an ophthalmologist immediately.

and lodge in smaller vessels of the eyes. By observing these plaques or recording the history of occasional visual loss, an ophthalmologist often detects symptoms or the evidence of vascular disease.

Arteriosclerosis also can be detected by looking inside the eye. Thickening blood vessel walls or changes that occur when artery and vein cross one another are pieces of evidence that show blood vessels are aging throughout the rest of the body.

Toxoplasmosis, an infection that can be transmitted by the mother to her child before birth, causes a scar on the baby's retina. The child may be born with visual damage, or this scar, containing toxoplasmosis organisms in cyst form, can be reactivated throughout the child's life. Close association with cats seems to be a common, but not the only, cause of this condition.

Histoplasmosis, a fungus disease particularly common in the Midwest, produces a condition in the eyes of younger people that resembles macular degeneration. Treatment is directed at the disease itself. It is difficult to prevent vision loss, however, if the infection centers in the macular area.

Arthritis, particularly the rheumatoid variety and a condition called Sjögren's syndrome, may cause "dry eyes," which are painfully dry and scratchy because the eyes cannot produce enough tears. Juvenile arthritis, particularly that affecting the spine, can inflame the front of the eye and cloud vision. Infrequently it causes loss of an eye due to secondary glaucoma, cataracts, or degeneration of the eye because of the inflammation.

Allergies. As explained in Chapter 23, "Allergy and the Immune System," spring, summer, and fall hay fever sufferers allergic to weeds and pollens often suffer from inflammation of the con-

junctiva as well as irritation of the generalized mucous membrane. Allergies to dust, animals, or cosmetics also produce severe itching, redness, and weeping in the eyes. The proper treatment for these irritations is to alleviate the offending allergen, but short-term symptomatic relief can be obtained with medications applied directly to the eye, such as antihistamines or cortisone. However, cortisone applied topically for prolonged periods can cause glaucoma in susceptible people, and cataracts if used for months.

COMMON SYMPTOMS AND THEIR SIGNIFICANCE

There are many misconceptions about eye problems and treatments. They include:

Spots before the eyes. Small, weblike floating spots almost invariably are caused by the aging process of the vitreous as it changes from a gel into liquid and strandlike components. These strands, which develop patterns like cobwebs or spots, can be annoying but are not serious. They are particularly obvious if an individual looks at a clear wall, moves his eyes, looks at the sky, or "looks for" the spots. In contrast, sudden showers of spots that look like multiple black dots frequently represent a much more serious condition. They result from a break in a small blood vessel and commonly are associated with retinal detachments. If you see hundreds of black spots, you should seek immediate attention from an ophthalmologist.

Headaches. People often blame their headaches on their eyes but rarely are they right. A person who does not have properly prescribed glasses or who is beginning to need glasses often complains of headaches and tired eyes. Once he or she is fitted with the proper prescription, the headaches are alleviated. Headaches in the back of the head generally have nothing to do with the eyes, and usually are stress-related.

Tired eyes. Middle-aged persons who complain that they can read for only a short time won't increase their reading time with eye exercises but can improve it by changing their prescription. In children these complaints may indicate that ability to focus on near objects is inadequate. This so-called "convergence insufficiency"—we all must "converge" in order to read—often can be handled with proper diagnosis and simple exercises. However, "perceptual visual training and eye exercises" generally are of no help and have no documented scientific basis. Dyslexics, persons of normal intelligence who have difficulty reading, should be evaluated for eye problems even though 90 to 95 percent of dyslexia cases have no ocular basis. See Chapter 29, "Taking Care of Your Child," for additional information on dyslexia.

Bulging eyes. Certain people complain that their eyes appear to be bulging. This is most likely a hereditary trait, dependent upon the shape of the orbit which usually is similar to those of one or both parents. However, if you notice that one eye protrudes more than the other or that your eyes are developing a rather marked stare or an upper lid retraction, you should see a doctor. The most frequent cause for this condition is hyperthyroidism (see Chapter 18, "The Hormones and Endocrine Glands").

Eyestrain. Like any other part of the body, eyes will present problems if you overwork them, but these usually are not persistent or severe. If the athlete training for a weight-lifting competition lifts weight for 12 hours a day, it is likely that his body will complain. Similarly, if you read for 12 or more hours a day or watch television for prolonged periods, you may suffer transient headaches, irritations, or discomfort with your eyes. Reading is easiest in proper light, but even reading in dim light will not cause permanent damage.

PREVENTIVE CARE OF THE EYES

An ounce of prevention is worth a pound of cure in eye care. Simple common sense can prevent most eye injuries and problems.

Eye injuries. Individuals pounding metal on metal are asking for trouble. Metal pounded on another metal surface can chip and produce a sliver that can easily penetrate the eye. Goggles may be troublesome, time-consuming, or uncomfortable, but they still are the best way to prevent unnecessary eye injury. If an injury of this nature does occur, immediate treatment is needed.

Trauma. A severe direct blow to the eye sometimes results in a small break of blood vessels inside the eye. The eruption may clear without problems, but it is extremely important that it be examined by an ophthalmologist. The person may require hospitalization and certainly should have pressure inside the eye measured. If the blood does not absorb within a reasonable time, the injury requires ophthalmic treatment.

Red eye. After coughing, choking, or straining in some other manner, you may note a bright red spot in the white part of your eye. Even rubbing your eye can cause this type of bleeding. This subconjunctival hemorrhage is not dangerous, nor is it associated with decreased vision. The blood, contained entirely on the outside surface of the eye, does not penetrate inside and should disappear in seven to 10 days. But if you notice frequent or recurrent red spots occurring spontaneously, you should consult a doctor.

Another type of "red eye" is cosmetic, the result of smog, smoky rooms, dust, allergies, or other irritants. Routinely using eye drops to "get the red out" is unrewarding, except to the manufacturer of the eye drops. The only exception is some cases where prolonged allergenic irritants make drops necessary or helpful on a regular basis.

Chemical burns. Lyes and commercial or home-cleaning ammonias and fertilizers can cause loss of vision or even blindness (see Chapter 35, "Emergency"). Lye burns are many times more dangerous to the eye than acid burns. Acid denatures the protein of the eye immediately but does not continue to cause problems because it neutralizes quickly. Lye will continue to burn for a long time. Individuals working with acid or alkali materials should wear glasses and make extensive efforts to prevent spilling or splashing such material into their eyes. Immediate irrigation and rapid ophthalmic care produce the best outcome if a chemical burn occurs, although severe lye burns carry a high probability for loss of vision or loss of the eye.

CHAPTER 15

EAR, NOSE, AND THROAT

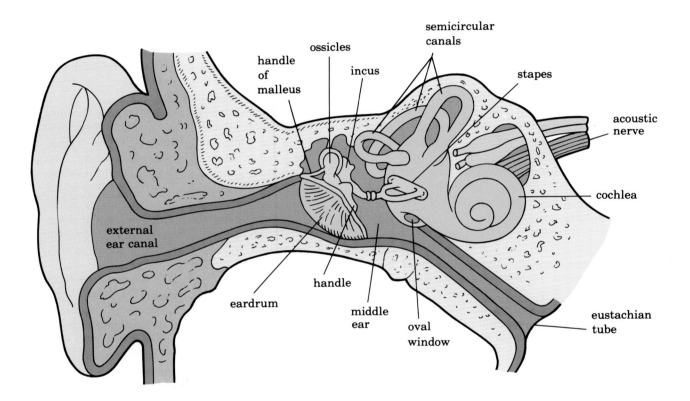

HOW WE HEAR

The structures of the ear enable us to collect sound waves, which are then converted into nerve impulses. Entering the external ear canal at left, the sound waves cause the eardrum to vibrate. The vibrations are transmitted across the middle ear space by three tiny bones called ossicles. The movement of each bone increases the amplification of sound. These movements excite fluids in the inner ear, which excite nerve endings in the acoustic nerve, which in turn carries impulses to the brain for interpretation. The eustachian tube, at lower right, links the throat and middle ear and helps to equalize pressure.

When we speak of something as unnecessary, we sometimes say we "need it like a hole in the head." We have several holes in the head and they are, in fact, quite important to our well-being. The passageways of the ears, nose, and throat, and their internal mechanisms deal with such essential matters as hearing and understanding speech, communicating with others, filtering and warming the air we breathe, balance, smell, tasting and enjoying food, and preparing food for digestion. These passageways enter the head from different directions, but within the bony recesses of the skull they connect, as the illustrations show. As a result, the ears, nose, and throat often are regarded as a unit and thought of as a single medical specialty.

THE EARS

Structure and Function

Sounds are simply air vibrations that have no meaning until they are collected by the external ear, transmitted across the eardrum through the internal parts of the ear, then converted to nerve impulses that travel along the auditory nerve to the brain. The brain unscrambles auditory impulses and interprets what we "hear."

Structurally, the ear is divided into three parts.

The external ear. The pinkish, bendable, question-mark-shaped appendage on each side of the head plays only a minor part in sound reception, although its curving channels do help to funnel sound to less visible parts of the ear. The ear canal, of which we see only the opening and a bit of the tube, also is part of the external ear. It is a passageway about 1¼ inches long, ending at the eardrum, or tympanic membrane.

The middle ear is an air-filled space surrounded by bone and bounded by two membranes, the eardrum on the outer side and a flexible membrane separating it from the inner ear on the inner side. The eustachian tube slants downward from this air space to the back of the throat. Hourglass-shaped, it is about the diameter of a pencil at each end, narrowing at the isthmus in the center to about 1 millimeter. The tube allows air to enter the middle ear space and maintain equal atmospheric pressure on both sides of the eardrum.

The main job of the middle ear is amplification. When a person speaks or a tree falls, sound waves radiate in all directions from the source of the noise. The sound waves travel until they meet resistance. In a listener's ear, that resistance is the eardrum. This tough but delicate membrane is jarred into movement just as any other drumhead vibrates when struck. The vibrations activate the bones of the middle ear, the ossicles, connected in a chain across the middle ear space.

The middle ear bones consist of the malleus (hammer), incus (anvil), and stapes (stirrup). The malleus, the outermost of the trio, is in contact with the eardrum. When sound strikes the eardrum, its vibrations are transmitted to the malleus. These vibrations of the malleus, in turn, stimulate the incus, which passes them along to the stapes, the innermost bone. The amplitude of the vibration increases with each step. The footplate of the stirrup bone is attached to a flexible membrane that covers an opening into the inner ear called the oval window. Moving back and forth like a piston, the stapes sets in motion the fluids of the inner ear. In the short but intricate journey from eardrum to inner ear, the sound wave is amplified as much as 25 times.

The inner ear is the area where the sound vibrations are converted into electrical impulses that eventually reach the brain. When the footplate of the stapes bone moves to and fro in the oval window, it sets off corresponding movements in the fluid of the inner ear.

The rhythmic waves then excite a highly delicate organ that is at the heart of sound reception. Coiled like a snail shell—hence its name, cochlea, from the Latin word for snail—the structure sometimes is described as a spiral piano keyboard.

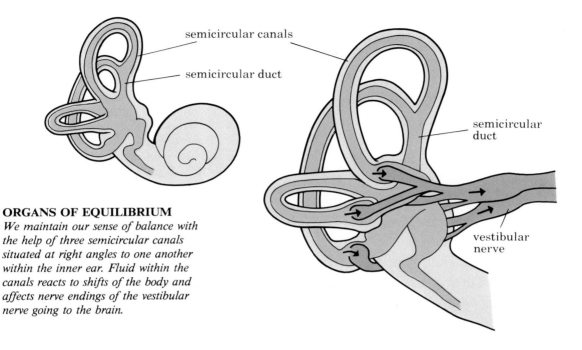

semicircular canals

semicircular duct

semicircular duct

vestibular nerve

ORGANS OF EQUILIBRIUM
We maintain our sense of balance with the help of three semicircular canals situated at right angles to one another within the inner ear. Fluid within the canals reacts to shifts of the body and affects nerve endings of the vestibular nerve going to the brain.

Hair cells at one end of the keyboard respond to sounds at high frequencies, up to 20,000 cycles per second; those at the opposite end respond to low ones, down to 16 cycles per second. The receptors for the bass are at the innermost turn of the spiral. Nerve endings are contained in a complex, slightly elevated structure, the organ of Corti.

As the hair cells of the cochlea are shaken by the oscillations, they initiate an electrical impulse that is transmitted to the nerve fibers, which then merge into the auditory nerve. These impulses are carried into the central auditory pathways of the brain and ultimately to the cerebral cortex, where their pattern is interpreted as a sound.

Balance and Equilibrium

The inner ear also contains two other types of sense organs, which help us to maintain equilibrium. The sense organs of equilibrium, collectively known as the labyrinth, are composed of hair cells and nerve fibers much like those of the organ of hearing. When the hair cells are stimulated by a covering membrane set in motion by movements of another inner-ear fluid, the endolymph, an electrical impulse is transmitted to the vestibular or balance nerve, which connects to the area of the brain that controls the muscles of the eye, trunk, and limbs. When a person moves his or her head, this complex system of canals, sacs, membranes, fluid, and nerves brings about reflex muscle contractions of the eyes and lids that tend to maintain the body in an erect position.

Bone and Air Conduction

Vibrations can reach the hearing nerve directly over the bony structures of the head or by sound waves that strike the eardrum and are transmitted across the middle ear space. The first is called bone conduction; the second, air conduction.

Air conduction predominates in general hearing or listening. Bone conduction is related especially to speaking, and is a kind of feedback control in hearing your own voice.

Air and bone conduction differences are important in tests of hearing. If a person hears air conduction sounds poorly, but bone conduction sounds quite well, the site of hearing trouble is probably in the middle ear. A person who cannot hear bone conduction vibrations probably suffers from nerve deafness as a result of impaired structures in the inner ear.

Impaired Hearing

Relatively few people are totally deaf, but more than 20 million Americans have some degree of hearing loss. Many have a deficiency that stems from growing older. The young ear normally can hear tones in a range of 16 cycles per second up to 20,000 cycles per second. A person older than 60 may not be able to hear sounds above 10,000 cycles per second.

The loss in the high frequency range usually comes on gradually and probably is related to a number of factors: heredity, exposure to noise over many years, or the result of nerve damage caused by such conditions as diabetes, hypothyroidism, or extended use of certain drugs.

Although a slight loss of ability to hear high tones is seldom severely disabling, significant involvement of the entire frequency range will make even ordinary conversation difficult or impossible to understand. The frequency range from 500 to 2,000 cycles per second is crucial for hearing and understanding speech.

Conduction deafness results from a failure of airborne sound waves to be conducted efficiently through the ear canal and tympanic membrane over the middle ear and auditory ossicles to the inner ear. Because of an obstruction along this route, the sound messages never get a chance to stimulate the nerves in the inner ear.

The obstruction that causes conductive hearing loss may occur in the external ear or in the middle ear. The ear canal may be closed by accumulated wax or bony tumors (exostoses) resulting from swimming in cold water. In the middle ear space, fluid accumulation, defects of the eardrum, or fixation of the auditory bones may be the culprit.

Nerve deafness implies damage in the inner ear or its nerve supply. Commonly, the high frequencies are affected more than the middle or lower ranges. Nerve deafness can be sudden or gradual. Besides aging, noise, and drugs, nerve deafness may result from infection of the labyrinth, temporal bone fracture, prenatal infection with rubella (German measles) or other viruses, or meningitis.

Tests of Hearing

The standard unit of loudness of sound is called the decibel. A whisper is rated at 20 decibels; conversation, at 50 to 60 decibels. Train wheels shrieking in a subway is rated 100 decibels; the whine of a jet airplane, 140 decibels.

The easiest and most practical test of hearing is simply to detect whether a person can hear a whisper or normal conversation at a given distance, or to have the person listen to the ticking of a watch. Professional testing may include both speech perception and the perception of tones. In a speech test, the person is tested for ability to understand the complex sound of a word. Tone perception uses a tuning fork with a specific vibrating frequency. The tuning fork is useful in distinguishing conductive deafness from nerve deafness.

A general idea of the type and severity of hearing loss can be obtained with these methods of testing, but more precise evaluation requires an instrument called an audiometer, which emits pure tones that can be graded in decibels. A chart of a person's response to pure tones at different intensities is called an audiogram.

A tympanometer is used to test whether a person (often a child) has fluid in the middle ear or a conductive or perceptive hearing loss. The test shows whether the eardrum and the middle ear ossicles move normally, or whether their movement is limited by accumulated fluid.

The audiometer tests what a person thinks he or she hears. An objective form of testing records electrical waves in the hearing nerve or auditory pathway of the brain in response to a signal, and brain-stem-evoked response audiometry can measure hearing in persons who otherwise are unable to respond, such as infants or stroke victims.

Deaf Infants and Children

Some infants are born deaf or with a serious hearing loss. A warning signal to parents is the failure of a 6-month-old to respond to loud noise. By nine or 10 months, a normal infant can locate a sound quite well and will turn toward it. The deaf infant does not respond.

Another important sign is failure to develop speech by 18 months to 2 years of age. A deaf infant may go through a babbling stage like other babies, but soon gives it up if he or she cannot hear his or her own voice. When a parent notices such signs, the child should be brought to an audiologist or otologist.

Treatment

Hearing aids are the most effective method of combating hearing loss for children and adults. Corrective surgery may be carried out in children after age 10. The hearing aid's main function is to amplify sound. Amplification is useful for nerve deafness or a conduction deafness for which surgery is not advisable. The hearing aid consists of a receiver, an amplifier, and a microphone or stimulator. Today, these components can be compressed into tiny units that are barely visible.

Hearing aids may be classified in three ways.

(1) Power or gain describes the hearing aid's ability to amplify a sound in order to reach the hearing threshold of the impaired ear. Generally, low-gain or low-powered aids are small and can fit in the ear canal or around the ear. Those that require greater power or amplification need a large power source, usually attached around the body.

(2) Monaural or binaural. Monaural aids are fitted in one ear, binaural aids in both. A monaural hearing aid can be quite effective if a person requires amplification in only one ear or, in the case of a bilateral nerve loss, has one ear with better inner ear function. Binaural hearing aids allow the user to locate sound more effectively and increase the sensitivity to hearing by several decibels.

(3) Air-conduction or bone-conduction aids. An air-conduction hearing aid fits into the ear canal and presents the amplified sound to the eardrum. A bone-conduction aid employs a vibrator or stimulator on the bone of the skull, preferably behind the ear on the bulge called the mastoid process. The bone-conducted sound then is perceived directly by the inner ear and hearing nerve. The effectiveness and fidelity of air-conduction aids are superior to bone-conduction aids.

Symptoms of Ear Disease

Vertigo, the feeling of loss of balance, is a prominent symptom of ear disease. It also is discussed in Chapter 11, "The Brain and Nervous System." The victim may feel that his or her surroundings are spinning, or that he or she is falling. The sensation may be accompanied by nausea and vomiting. Vertigo may be sustained, lasting for several days because of a prolonged affliction of the inner ear, such as labyrinthitis, or it may be episodic. Positional vertigo occurs in certain head positions, and usually lasts only seconds.

An early clue is a condition called nystagmus, in which the eyes oscillate because of an imbalance in the eye reflexes. The imbalance is caused by an abnormal train of impulses from the diseased inner ear compared to the normal opposite ear. The standard method of evaluating the ear for a disturbance in the vestibular system is the caloric test, in which cold or warm water is injected into the ear canal. A diminished response in one ear indicates a disturbance in the vestibular system of the inner ear and suggests that more specialized tests are required to determine whether infection, tumor, or other causes are responsible.

Tinnitus, or noise heard in the ear, occurs when some form of inner ear degeneration has occurred. Thumping in the ear may indicate a blood vessel tumor in the middle ear. Any episode of tinnitus should be investigated.

Facial paralysis also may stem from ear problems. The most common form is Bell's palsy, a form of nerve compression described in Chapter 11, "The Brain and Nervous System." Other forms of facial paralysis may signal serious disease in the inner, middle, or outer ear.

Outer Ear Infections

Infection of the external or outer ear is commonly referred to as "swimmer's ear" because of its frequency during the summer months. Essentially, swimmer's ear is an infection of ear canal skin and is more properly termed a dermatitis. It causes a feeling of fullness and extreme discomfort in the ear. Hearing usually is not affected. Pressure on the ear or movement of the jaw joint during speaking or chewing can cause pain. The usual treatment consists of antibiotic ear drops, local heat, and aspirin. The infection usually ends quickly and rarely recurs.

Malignant otitis, a particularly dangerous form of external ear infection, occurs in elderly diabetics. Malignant otitis (also known as necrotizing external otitis) can result in progressive infection into the bone of the skull and its major blood vessels and nervous structures, and can be fatal. External ear infection in an elderly diabetic requires immediate attention.

Infections of the Middle Ear And Mastoid

Serous otitis media, fluid in the middle ear space, is a condition all too familiar to many parents. In its acute form, it can produce excruciating earache in children and cause temporary hearing loss that can become permanent if not treated properly. The fluid accumulation results from dysfunction of the eustachian tube. The condition appears to run in families.

The customary symptoms are poor hearing and recurrent ear infections. Fluid usually can be detected in the middle ear by an examination. Decongestants usually do not help to clear the tube. Treatment is directed at relieving the hearing loss and halting the parade of infections. An incision is made in the eardrum (myringotomy) to drain the fluid behind it, and a tiny ventilating tube is placed in the incision. Healing seals the tube in place and forms a conduit to ventilate the middle ear space. The tubes as a rule are rejected by the eardrum after a few months. If the condition returns, the tubes may have to be replaced. Most cases of serous otitis media will clear spontaneously after a few months, regardless of type of therapy.

Middle ear infections usually follow an upper respiratory infection of the nose and throat. The symptoms are pain around the ear, high fever, and diminished hearing caused by the collection of bacteria and pus. The condition usually clears completely with early antibiotic treatment, but if treatment is delayed or inadequate, the infection may invade the bone around the mastoid cells. The result, acute mastoiditis, causes swelling behind the ear and high fever. Thanks to antibiotics and early treatment, acute mastoiditis is rare today.

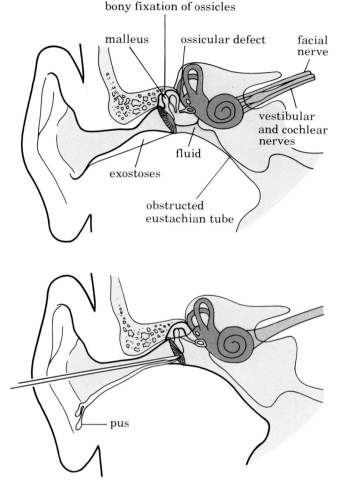

EAR INFECTIONS
Infection can occur in the external or middle ear. Exostoses (top drawing) are a form of bone overgrowth that narrows or obstructs the external ear canal. Middle ear infection is common in children and can have serious consequences if not treated properly. When the eustachian tube is obstructed, fluid accumulates behind the eardrum, preventing the drum from moving normally and providing a site for infection. An untreated infection can cause a bony fixation of the ossicles. To remove fluid, a myringotomy (lower drawing) is performed to make a tiny hole in the eardrum, equalizing pressure and promoting drainage.

REPLACING THE STAPES
Otosclerosis is a mysterious bone overgrowth in the area of the oval window. The growth limits movement of the tiny stapes bone and prevents transmission of sound vibrations to the inner ear. The top drawing shows limitations of the stapes when bone grows over it. The condition can be corrected by surgical techniques in which the stapes bone is removed and replaced with an artificial substitute, often a Teflon piston (lower drawing).

Chronic middle ear and mastoid infection may occur when skin grows into the middle ear and the mastoid through a perforation in the eardrum. The skin then may form a sac or a cyst with a skin lining. The outer layer of cells of the membrane, as they are discarded, accumulate in the sac, liquefy, and produce a foul-smelling ear drainage. This cyst, or cholesteatoma, is able to erode bone. A chronic inflammatory process may be set up, eventually involving such important structures as the labyrinth, facial nerve, and dural covering of the brain. Although local antibiotic therapy can help, the only consistent way to restore the hearing mechanism is surgical removal of all infected tissue and repair of the eardrum and middle ear ossicles. The chances for successful repair of an eardrum are better than 90 percent.

Inner Ear Infection

Infection of the inner ear is called labyrinthitis and may be caused by bacteria or virus. Symptoms of bacterial labyrinthitis are perceptive hearing loss and sustained vertigo. The condition usually results from an extension of infection in the middle ear and mastoid compartment. Total nerve deafness and loss of balance may follow. It is important to prevent the dangerous complication of meningitis infection of the brain membranes, by the proper use of antibiotics and drainage of the inner ear.

Trauma

Temporal bone trauma may result from a head injury that produces a skull fracture. Longitudinal fracture involves the middle ear and the ear canal. The usual symptoms are bleeding from the ear and hearing loss because of blood in the middle ear space. About one in four persons also suffers facial paralysis. Surgery usually is recommended if there is conductive hearing loss.

Transverse fracture of the temporal bone occurs through the inner ear and the internal auditory canal, producing nerve deafness and sustained dizziness. No treatment can preserve inner ear function in this form of fracture. Surgery is reserved for cases in which facial paralysis also has occurred.

Direct damage to the eardrum can be produced by a penetrating injury from a toothpick, hairpin, or cotton-tipped stick inserted into the ear canal and then accidentally pushed toward the eardrum. The usual result is severe pain and bleeding from a laceration of the ear canal skin. If the victim also loses the sense of balance, emergency surgical attention is required.

Acoustic trauma occurs when high-energy sound waves damage the hair cells of the inner ear. The first exposure usually leads to a temporary loss of hearing, which gradually returns over a period of hours. This is referred to as a "temporary threshold shift." Repeated exposure to the same noise level can bring irreversible hearing loss.

Ear-Damaging Drugs

Antibiotics called aminoglycosides can damage the structures and function of the ear. Neomycin, kanamycin, dihydrostreptomycin, and vancomycin primarily damage hearing by attacking the hair cells of the cochlea. The loss worsens with prolonged use of such drugs and is irreversible.

Streptomycin and gentomycin affect balance. The symptoms initially are loss of coordination and balance. If the drug is continued, nerve deafness may occur, too.

Other commonly used drugs with ear-damaging potential are aspirin and quinine. Aspirin is toxic in prolonged high doses, greater than 15 to 20 tablets per day. Quinine produces an irreversible nerve hearing loss that may be transmitted from a pregnant woman to her fetus.

Birth Defects

The most common birth defect is failure of the outer ear to develop (agenesis) or development of a very small outer ear (microtia). These usually are accompanied by a closed or absent external ear canal (atresia). An abnormally small outer ear can be reconstructed by a series of plastic operations. Lack of an external auditory canal when the inner ear is normal causes a conductive hearing loss, which can be treated surgically or by use of a hearing aid. Surgery usually is reserved for cases in which both ears are involved.

Tumors of the Temporal Bone

A frequent malignant tumor occurs primarily in the elderly—skin cancer arising from the lining of the ear canal. The indications are pain and bleeding from the ear canal. Early diagnosis and treatment either by surgery or radiation is essential.

The most common tumor, however, is a benign growth that arises in the middle ear space. The initial symptom of glomus jugular tumor usually is a pulsating ear noise (tinnitus) accompanied by hearing loss. The tumor usually is removed surgically, unless it is so large that an operation might endanger the patient's life. In that case, radiation therapy may be used.

Conditions of Unknown Cause

Otosclerosis is the formation of a bone overgrowth in the region of the oval window that limits movement of the stapes bone (stirrup). Because the bone transmits sound pressure waves across the ear, impairment produces a gradual conductive hearing loss. This hearing loss usually begins in the 20s and 30s, is more common in women than men, and frequently is hereditary. Loss is gradual and progressive. Both ears usually are affected. An operation called a stapedectomy is carried out under local anesthesia through the ear canal. After the tympanic membrane is elevated, the stapes bone is removed and an artificial substitute—a piston or a tiny bit of wire—is inserted into the oval window. The sudden restoration of hearing is dramatic and rewarding. The chances of success are better than 90 percent.

Ménière's disease involves both the hearing and balance organs. In this disorder, a patient has both a hearing loss and episodes of vertigo lasting from one to several hours. The vertigo usually is accompanied by nausea and vomiting. Hearing often is worst during or soon after an attack of dizziness. Ménière's disease usually occurs in only one ear, and has its onset in middle life. Its most dangerous consequence is that the dizzy, spinning feeling may strike without warning.

Although the cause of Ménière's disease is uncertain, it is known that a buildup of fluid occurs in one of the compartments in the inner ear. The membranes then rupture and release a substance that poisons the balancing and hearing nerve fibers. Repeated healing and rupturing of the membranes lead to recurring vertigo and fluctuating hearing loss. No drug has a proven effect on either the hearing loss or the vertigo.

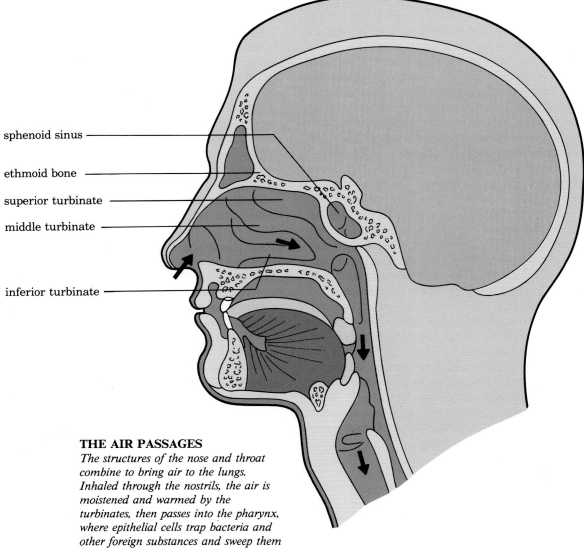

sphenoid sinus

ethmoid bone

superior turbinate

middle turbinate

inferior turbinate

THE AIR PASSAGES
*The structures of the nose and throat
combine to bring air to the lungs.
Inhaled through the nostrils, the air is
moistened and warmed by the
turbinates, then passes into the pharynx,
where epithelial cells trap bacteria and
other foreign substances and sweep them
away to be swallowed harmlessly.
Inhaled air continues through the lower
pharynx to reach the lungs.*

NOSE AND PARANASAL SINUSES

Structurally, the nose is made up of cartilage
and bone—cartilage in the outermost portion and
bone between the eyes, where eyeglasses rest. Both
bones and cartilage come in pairs, one in each side
of the nose. Together they form a skeletal framework that gives support to the external nose.

Internally, the nasal cavity is divided into two
chambers by the septum, a ridge of bone and cartilage that runs down the midline of the nose. Soft
tissue and skin cover the nose, along with facial
muscles that control and change the diameter of
the nostrils.

The respiratory function takes place in the nasal
cavity. It is where the respiratory system begins,
and its job is to prepare inhaled air for entry into
the lungs. The inside of the nose is made up of mucous membrane. As the air passes the nasal membranes, it is moistened by glandular secretions and
warmed by the circulating blood. This air-conditioning system is the reason the lungs are not
chilled even by the coldest air of winter.

The nasal cavity also houses a filtering and
cleansing system. Hairs in the nostrils and finer
ones within the cavity catch particles in the air
before they can reach the lungs, and also remove
bacteria from the inhaled air.

Another vital function of the nose is smell. The smell receptors are located in the top portion of the nasal cavities. In order to be detected, odors must be airborne and soluble enough to be dissolved in the mucous secretions of the nose. Air currents carry volatile odors upward in an arclike fashion before passing into the nasopharynx. We thus may lose the sense of smell because of a simple obstruction in the nose, such as congestion from a cold.

The sense of taste is closely related to smell. The sense organs of taste are located in the tongue. Taste buds are not the minute protuberances or papillae on the surface of the tongue, but are microscopic cellular structures within the tissue of those papillae. There are about 250 taste buds per papilla, but the number gradually diminishes with age to about 90 per papilla. The sense of smell has no way of classifying different types of odors, but taste can be broken down into four sensations: bitter, salt, sweet, and sour. They are distinguished by taste buds in particular surface areas of the tongue.

The central pathways of taste and smell mix, so one is dependent on the other. When an abnormality in taste occurs, smell also is affected, and vice versa. This explains why a cold in the nose interferes with our ability to taste food.

The Paranasal Sinuses

The paranasal sinuses are air spaces that fill the facial bones. They are extensions of the nasal cavities. There are four major pairs of sinuses, with half of each pair on one side of the midline of the face, and half on the other. They open into the nasal cavity by means of tiny openings called ostia. They are called the frontal, ethmoid, sphenoid, and maxillary sinuses.

Disorders of the Nose And Paranasal Sinuses

Injury. Because of its prominence on the face, the nose is particularly subject to injuries. Most involve only the cartilage, but fracture of the nasal bones or dislocation or fracture of the septum calls for the prompt attention of a physician. Failure of these injuries to heal properly can lead both to a misshapen nose and to malfunction of the nasal airway. A broken nose usually is reset by simply elevating the bones into place, but sometimes it is necessary to wire the fractured segments together.

Nosebleed (epistaxis) is the most familiar nasal injury. Bleeding may result from a direct blow to the nose, nose picking, drying of the mucous membrane, or violent sneezing or nose blowing. Most nosebleeds involve damage to the small blood vessels in the lower septum, so bleeding is forward, out of the nostrils. These anterior nosebleeds usually can be controlled by pinching the nostrils together for five to 10 minutes. If bleeding cannot be controlled or if blood flows backward into the throat, packing by an otolaryngologist may be needed to control the flow.

Children often have recurrent minor nosebleeds. These should be brought to the attention of a specialist. In rare cases, repeated nasal bleeding may indicate a tumor.

Infection. The common cold, with its streaming nose, watery eyes, and (often) hacking cough, is the most ubiquitous of ailments. Its technical name (or rather the name for the symptoms it produces) is rhinitis, inflammation of the nasal mucous membrane. If the infection obstructs the sinus openings or spreads into the sinuses, it is called sinusitis.

Acute rhinitis or sinusitis may be caused by a viral infection, a bacterial infection, or both. Besides a running nose, the person may develop a fever. The nasal discharge may be thick and yellow, rather than clear. In sinusitis, there may be pain in the area of the face over the sinuses. Often, the collected fluid or pus and thickened mucous membrane may be seen by X ray.

Rhinitis and sinusitis are treated primarily with antibiotics (mainly to prevent secondary bacterial infection) and decongestants to shrink the mucous membrane and allow better drainage of the sinuses. Viral rhinitis usually is self-limiting.

If a sinus infection is not treated, is treated inadequately, or recurs, changes may occur in the mucous membrane, producing a chronic sinusitis. The result is intermittent pain and headaches over the sinuses, plus a persistent drainage from the nose. Surgery may be necessary to remove the inflamed and infected mucous membrane.

Tumors. Most tumors of the nose are benign. The most common are nasal polyps, which are extensions of the swollen sinus mucous membrane caused by a nasal allergy. Extensive polyps may block the passage between nose and paranasal sinuses and produce a secondary paranasal sinusitis. The polyps must be removed surgically.

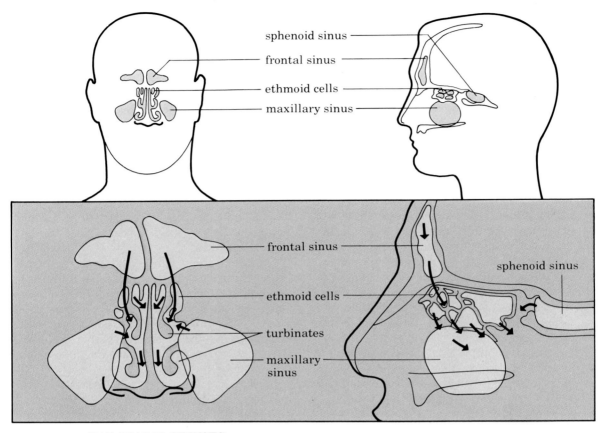

PARANASAL SINUSES
The major sinuses and their locations are: the frontal sinuses above the eyes and behind the root of the nose, the ethmoid sinuses at the root of the nose between the eyes, the sphenoid sinus in the center of the skull, and the maxillary sinuses in the cheekbones. The lower drawing shows the direction of drainage from the sinuses, all of which drain into the nasal cavity.

A second benign tumor of the nose, inverted papilloma, arises from the lining of the nose and ethmoid sinus. This tumor, although benign, should be removed promptly to relieve obstruction and avoid the possibility of malignant change.

Malignant tumors most commonly occur in the maxillary sinus. The first indication usually is a painless enlarging deformity of the bone and obstruction of the tear duct (causing tearing), compression of eye muscles (causing double vision), or compression of nerves (causing numbness). The tumor usually is treated by a combination of radiation therapy and surgery.

PHARYNX AND LARYNX

The throat portion of the ear-nose-throat unit also is known as the pharynx. Usually, the mouth is included in that term, too. The pharynx is a long muscular tube that extends from the back of the nose into the swallowing tube (esophagus). Generally, it is divided into the nasopharynx, oropharynx, and hypopharynx.

The nasopharynx, located above the soft palate and behind the nose, connects the nasal cavity and the oropharynx and plays a key role in the breathing process. The eustachian tubes that ventilate the middle ears connect to the nasopharynx on both sides. A blockage in the nasopharynx may obstruct the airway, eustachian tube, and middle ear.

Adenoid. The most common tissue mass to block the nasopharynx is the adenoid. It is a normal mass of lymphoid tissue, which during childhood infections may greatly enlarge. Snoring is a common result. The obstruction also can cause fluid to collect in the middle ear space, producing a conductive hearing loss. If an enlarged adenoid produces such symptoms or becomes infected, removal (adenoidectomy) becomes necessary.

Angiofibroma is a blood-vessel tumor that occurs only in adolescent boys. Symptoms are difficulty in breathing through the nose, recurrent nosebleeds, and a bulging deformity of the cheek. Although benign, these tumors should be removed because they destroy the surrounding tissue.

The oropharynx forms the rear portion of the oral cavity. It aids in swallowing. The tonsils, masses of lymphoid tissue, occur at the junction of the oropharynx and the oral cavity.

Children's tonsils normally enlarge and become inflamed during periods of infection. The enlargement may partially obstruct the throat and interfere with swallowing or breathing. Sometimes a secondary infection arises in the inflamed tissue, and persists after the original infection has subsided. This condition, called tonsillitis, often includes severe sore throat, high fever, earache, difficulty in swallowing, and swollen lymph nodes in the neck.

Tonsil infections decrease as the child grows older, but tonsillectomy during early childhood remains one of the most common surgical procedures. It usually is not recommended unless the child's health is significantly affected. Most ear, nose, and throat surgeons consider four to five documented cases of bacterial tonsillitis a year for more than three successive years sufficient indication for tonsillectomy (see Chapter 29, "Taking Care of Your Child").

The oral cavity also has roles in chewing and speaking. The tongue and mouth muscles are important for both.

Malignant tumors may occur in the oral cavity, usually on the floor of the mouth or in the tongue. The first indication usually is a sore or irritation, sometimes accompanied by bleeding. A sore area, especially in a person who smokes and drinks heavily, should be examined if the soreness persists for three to four weeks.

The salivary glands provide the saliva in the mouth, which helps break down food and aids digestion. The glands are located primarily in the parotid area near the ear and in the submaxillary area at the angle of the jaw. The most common

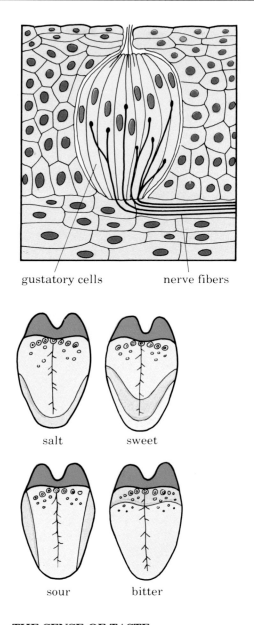

gustatory cells   nerve fibers

salt   sweet

sour   bitter

THE SENSE OF TASTE
A single taste bud is sensitive to only one of the four primary sensations of taste. The taste buds of the tongue are not uniformly distributed. The lower drawing shows the location of buds sensitive to salt, sweet, sour, and bitter tastes. The top drawing, a cross section through a taste bud, depicts how dissolved substances on the surface make contact with spindle-shaped cells, producing impulses that travel over nerve fibers to the brain.

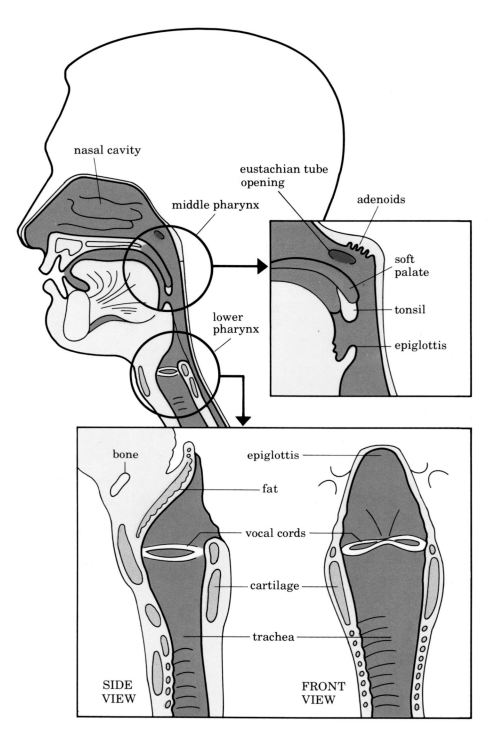

nasal cavity

eustachian tube opening

middle pharynx

adenoids

soft palate

tonsil

epiglottis

lower pharynx

bone

epiglottis

fat

vocal cords

cartilage

trachea

SIDE VIEW

FRONT VIEW

NOSE AND THROAT

Important features of the nose and throat and their interrelationship are shown above. The enlargement at upper right shows the middle pharynx, also known as the tonsillar area. Below, two views of the lower pharynx show how speech and breathing are controlled.

The vocal cords are two muscular bands that contract when we swallow to prevent liquids or solids from entering the lungs. They also rhythmically control the expulsion of air from the lungs into the mouth and throat, where it is formed into words or sounds.

problems are benign tumors, painless masses or lumps in the cheek or in the front of the ear. These usually are removed surgically to prevent malignant change.

The hypopharynx is the lower part of the pharynx and also contains the larynx. Its functions are primarily in swallowing and speaking. Malignant tumors sometimes develop in the swallowing area, or a sac (diverticulum) may collect food. Either can cause difficulty in swallowing. Anyone with a swallowing problem that persists for more than four weeks should see a specialist.

The larynx is the cartilaginous box felt in the front of the neck as the Adam's apple. The vocal cords of the larynx are two muscular bands that contract during swallowing to prevent solids or liquids from entering the lungs. Human vocal cords are trained to control the expulsion of air from the lungs into the mouth and throat. These puffs of air are formed into sounds or words by the tongue, lips, and cheek muscles.

The larynx also has a respiratory role. It separates the vocal cords to allow inhaled air to enter the trachea and lungs. The most common problem with the larynx is infection (laryngitis), causing an inflammation of tissues and spasm of laryngeal muscles. The result is hoarseness and discomfort or pain in the throat. Laryngitis caused by bacteria can be treated with antibiotics, by inhaling steam, or simply by resting the voice.

A special form of laryngitis, laryngotracheitis, occurs in infants and is called croup. It results from a viral infection that causes the cords to swell and narrows the space between them. The condition and its treatment are described in Chapter 29, "Taking Care of Your Child."

Another form of infection in a child's larynx is epiglottitis, an infection of the upper part of the larynx over the vocal cords. Loose membranes in this part of the larynx may swell and completely obstruct the opening. A bacterial infection usually is responsible.

In adults, polyps of the vocal cords, representing accumulations of mucous membrane and fluid-producing hoarseness, may result from prolonged shouting, such as at a football game, talking too much, or inhaling cigarette smoke. These polyps should be removed surgically.

Cancer of the larnyx also is associated with cigarette smoking, particularly if accompanied by heavy drinking. Persistent hoarseness is the primary symptom. Any hoarseness that lasts longer than four weeks should be investigated by a specialist. When the cancer is small and limited to the vocal cords, chances for cure by radiation therapy are more than 90 percent.

If the tumor also involves other regions of the larynx, complete removal of the larynx (total laryngectomy) is necessary. After such an operation, the trachea is brought out to the skin as a permanent opening into the windpipe, and the swallowing tube is sutured closed so that the person may eat normally. The swallowing tube is used to develop a substitute form of speech called esophageal speech. The person is trained to swallow air into the stomach, then belch it up into the mouth to be formed into words by the tongue and mouth muscles. At least two-thirds of those whose larynxes have been removed can learn esophageal speech.

The lymph nodes of the neck are glandular structures that drain the mouth, throat, and larynx and provide a mechanism for the body to limit the spread of infection or tumor from these areas. Enlarged lymph nodes in the neck not associated with infection should be viewed suspiciously as reflecting a primary tumor somewhere in the pharynx, larynx, or nasopharynx. Such a lymph node or lump in the neck, if persistent, should be seen as soon as possible by an otolaryngologist.

CLEFT LIP AND CLEFT PALATE

A cleft in the lip or the palate results from stunted development of the bones and soft tissues of the mouth sometime before birth. The usual cleft is limited to one side of the palate midline and extends into one nostril. In addition to the speech defect that may occur later, feeding difficulties usually occur in infancy because milk backs up into the nose.

Cleft palate usually can be corrected by surgery that brings the tissues together by means of carefully planned incisions and flaps. The surgery usually is performed in infancy.

The results of cleft-palate surgery are so good that there is no excuse for such a defect to go uncorrected. Speech therapy usually is necessary afterward to help the child form sounds.

CHAPTER 16

THE BONES AND MUSCLES

From head to toe, the adult human skeleton consists of 206 bones, as large as the thighbone, and as small as the bones of the ear. With the muscles, tendons, joints, and supporting tissues, they are arranged in an intricate framework that allows the ballerina to glide across the stage, the wide receiver to levitate beyond the pass defender, and the rest of us to walk upstairs or ride a bicycle.

The bones also play an important role in blood-cell formation, and serve as a storehouse for such key minerals as calcium and phosphorus.

Injuries and other disorders of the bones and muscles are among the most common—and nagging—ailments of humankind.

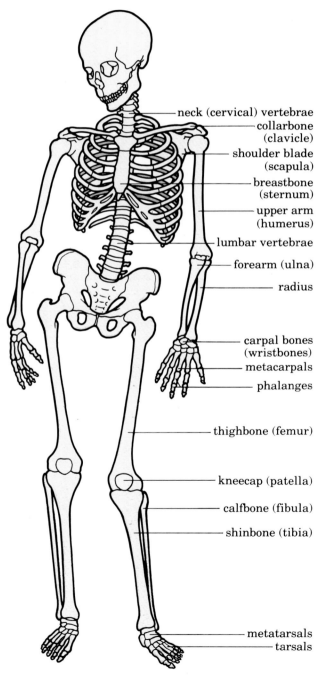

neck (cervical) vertebrae
collarbone (clavicle)
shoulder blade (scapula)
breastbone (sternum)
upper arm (humerus)
lumbar vertebrae
forearm (ulna)
radius
carpal bones (wristbones)
metacarpals
phalanges
thighbone (femur)
kneecap (patella)
calfbone (fibula)
shinbone (tibia)
metatarsals
tarsals

THE HUMAN SKELETON
The major bones of the body, shown here, serve many functions. They not only enable us to move and to maintain posture, but house and protect the vital organs. Names of groups of bones include the spine, pelvic girdle, shoulder girdle, rib cage, and skull. The spine rests on the pelvic girdle and supports the shoulder girdle, rib cage, and skull. Some bones are separate at birth but fuse as we grow older. We thus "lose" about 60 bones as we mature.

MAJOR MUSCLES

The muscles of the human body are almost too numerous to name. Those concerned with movement are illustrated. The topmost layer of muscles is shown on the left side of the figure. Underlying muscles (deep musculature) are named on the right side. Some bones are included as points of reference.

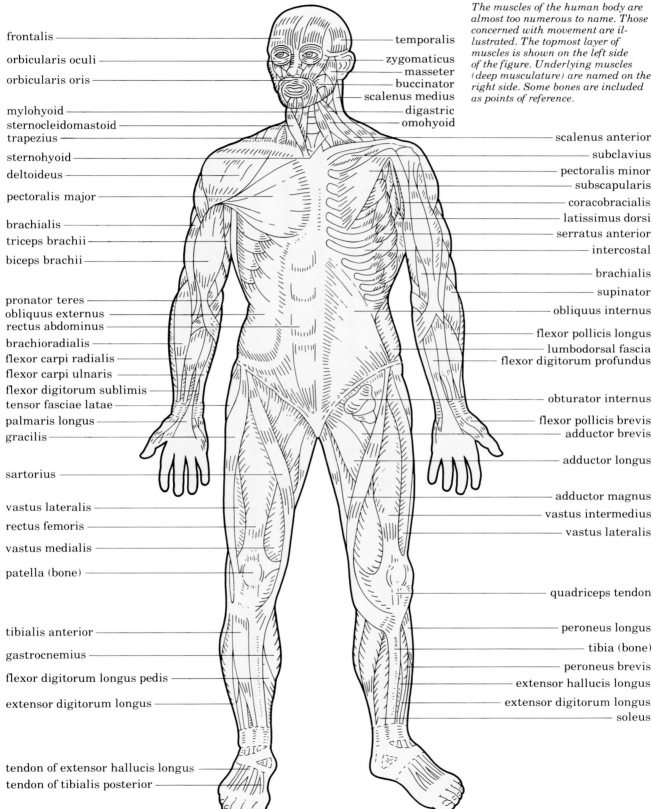

frontalis
orbicularis oculi
orbicularis oris

mylohyoid
sternocleidomastoid
trapezius
sternohyoid
deltoideus
pectoralis major

brachialis
triceps brachii
biceps brachii

pronator teres
obliquus externus
rectus abdominus
brachioradialis
flexor carpi radialis
flexor carpi ulnaris
flexor digitorum sublimis
tensor fasciae latae
palmaris longus
gracilis

sartorius

vastus lateralis
rectus femoris
vastus medialis

patella (bone)

tibialis anterior
gastrocnemius
flexor digitorum longus pedis
extensor digitorum longus

tendon of extensor hallucis longus
tendon of tibialis posterior

temporalis
zygomaticus
masseter
buccinator
scalenus medius
digastric
omohyoid

scalenus anterior
subclavius
pectoralis minor
subscapularis
coracobracialis
latissimus dorsi
serratus anterior
intercostal
brachialis
supinator
obliquus internus
flexor pollicis longus
lumbodorsal fascia
flexor digitorum profundus

obturator internus
flexor pollicis brevis
adductor brevis

adductor longus

adductor magnus
vastus intermedius
vastus lateralis

quadriceps tendon

peroneus longus
tibia (bone)
peroneus brevis
extensor hallucis longus
extensor digitorum longus
soleus

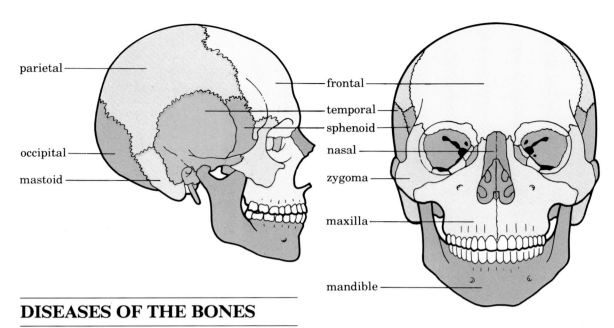

parietal

occipital

mastoid

frontal

temporal

sphenoid

nasal

zygoma

maxilla

mandible

DISEASES OF THE BONES

Osteomyelitis

Osteomyelitis is an infection resulting from the growth of germs within the bone, and is more common in children than in adults. The first symptoms usually are pain and tenderness near a joint. The pain increases rapidly until a child may refuse to move the affected limb. Fever follows; illness is evident. Bone changes may not appear on X ray for eight to 10 days, but the disease usually is diagnosed before that.

Treatment. Antibiotics have revolutionized treatment of what was once a dangerous and crippling disease. Unless treated promptly, however, the infection may become chronic, with local destruction of bone and associated soft tissue abscesses. Unfortunately, extensive infection is difficult to control, and chronic osteomyelitis with draining pus may be present for years.

A complication of acute osteomyelitis is the spread of the infection into one or more joints (septic arthritis). Treatment consists of antibiotics that are administered intravenously. Surgical drainage of the joint also may be necessary.

Another possible complication of osteomyelitis in children is retardation of growth because of damage to the cartilage of long bones.

Osteoporosis

Osteoporosis is a porousness or "thinning" of the bones, with a resulting reduction in bone mass. The apparent cause is a lack or loss of calcium, perhaps because of insufficient production of the

BONES OF THE SKULL
Drawings show front and side views of the bones of the skull. The zigzag lines, called suture lines, are where the bones continue to form after birth to accommodate the growing brain. The bones gradually knit together along these lines to form the brain vault, or cranium. Protection of the brain is the skull's main task.

protein in which the salts are deposited. Although osteoporosis occurs in both sexes, it most commonly strikes women after menopause. More than one woman in four over age 60 is affected.

The most serious consequence of osteoporosis is the fracturing of the thin and fragile bones, especially the vertebrae and hips. More than 200,000 hip fractures a year are attributed to osteoporosis.

Loss of female hormones at menopause is related to osteoporosis in women, but poor nutrition in earlier years and poor assimilation of calcium also may play a part.

Treatment with estrogen is the most effective remedy. Although estrogen replacement therapy has been associated with an increased risk of cancer of the uterus, it now is agreed that a greater risk results from fractures and the lung disease that may develop during a prolonged period of bed rest. An increase in calcium in the diet also is suggested to prevent further loss. In addition, women in their 20s and 30s should consume plenty of calcium or take calcium supplements as a way to bank this mineral for the future.

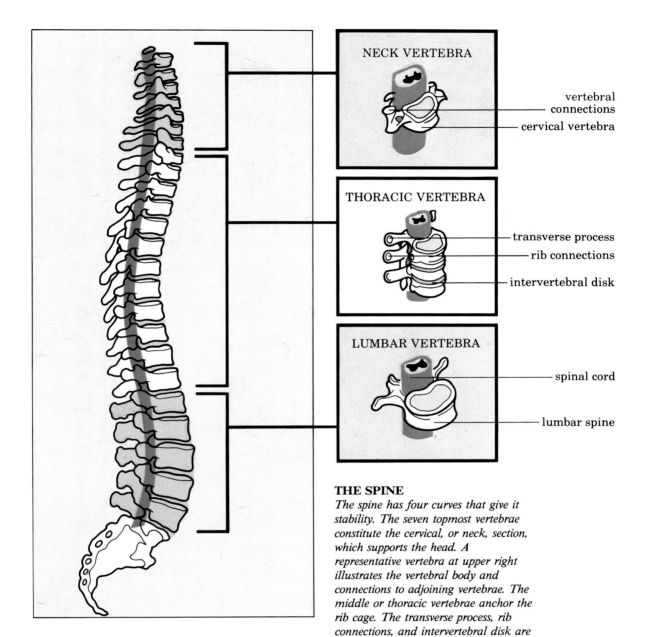

NECK VERTEBRA

vertebral connections

cervical vertebra

THORACIC VERTEBRA

transverse process

rib connections

intervertebral disk

LUMBAR VERTEBRA

spinal cord

lumbar spine

THE SPINE

The spine has four curves that give it stability. The seven topmost vertebrae constitute the cervical, or neck, section, which supports the head. A representative vertebra at upper right illustrates the vertebral body and connections to adjoining vertebrae. The middle or thoracic vertebrae anchor the rib cage. The transverse process, rib connections, and intervertebral disk are shown in the representative section. Heavier vertebrae make up the lumbar spine. They rest on the fixed sacrum, five vertebrae that have fused early in life. The vertebral cross section at lower right shows the placement of protection for the spinal cord.

Paget's Disease
(Osteitis deformans)

Relatively common after age 40, Paget's disease is a chronic process of bone overgrowth, destruction, and new bone formation. Bone becomes deformed and its internal cellular architecture becomes disordered. The patients often have arteriosclerosis and impaired blood supply to the bones. The disease is "spotty," with a predilection for bones of the spine, skull, and lower leg. Spontaneous fractures may occur but heal normally. A hearing aid frequently becomes necessary because of damage to ear bones. The hormone calcitonin may be prescribed to strengthen the bones.

THE SPINE

The erect spine is under stress at all levels, but the greatest stress is between the lowermost lumbar vertebra and the sacrum. A swayback or sag-

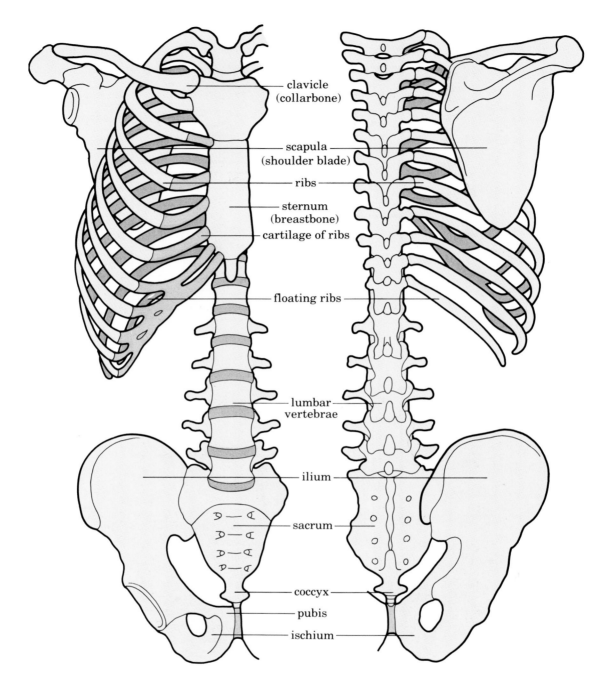

clavicle
(collarbone)

scapula
(shoulder blade)

ribs

sternum
(breastbone)

cartilage of ribs

floating ribs

lumbar
vertebrae

ilium

sacrum

coccyx

pubis

ischium

THE AXIAL SKELETON

The axial skeleton is the body's central framework. The left drawing is the front view; at right, as seen from the rear. Twenty-four vertebrae stacked on top of one another are the main vertical column. The lowest portion, the sacrum, consists of five vertebrae, which fuse into one bone early in life. The clavicle and scapula make up the shoulder girdle. Ribs, sternum, and thoracic vertebrae make up the rib cage; the ilium, pubis, and ischium constitute the pelvic girdle. The junction between the movable lumbar spine and the fixed sacrum is frequently a source of pain.

ging spine is often a source of chronic postural pain because the ligaments are stretched and more weight is borne on the small facet joints than was intended. Decreasing the lumbar curve by strengthening the abdominal muscles usually will correct the painful condition.

Low back pain can be caused by a variety of mechanisms. The most common are acute injury or degeneration of the joints, ligaments, muscles, or intervertebral disks.

Referred pain, which is pain that hurts where it does not originate, can be felt in the back as a result of nerve root irritation. Muscles that are in spasm because of attempts to protect some local injury also can become painful. Sometimes the entire back hurts as the victim hunches and stiffens to guard against painful movement.

Acute back sprain usually is produced by a sudden bending of the spine, as in a fall or a "snatch lifting" motion. The force tears ligaments or compresses disks, producing pain and protective muscle spasms. These injuries usually heal within a few weeks. Some patients must wear a corsetlike support during the healing period.

Chronic back strain, also called postural fatigue, is a condition in which there is no violent, sudden, precipitating incident, but the structures are subjected to prolonged tension greater than they can withstand. Symptoms usually come on gradually. They usually are aggravated if the person is fatigued, but they can be improved by lying down or by physiotherapy.

Treatment is difficult because the main cause of chronic strain is postural fatigue. The outlook is not always good, particularly if it is not possible to change an occupation associated with the fatigue.

Disk trouble. The intervertebral disks are buffers or "shock absorbers" between the bony vertebrae. After age 20, the disks gradually degenerate. Less weight is borne on the pulpy central portion, and added strain is placed on the sensitive outer casing, giving rise to aching pain. The pain usually is confined to the lower back. As degeneration progresses, the pain may be felt in the legs.

Early degeneration of the disk usually does not cause pain, only mild local tenderness, unless strain is added. Treatment should include rest, followed by muscle-strengthening exercises and avoidance of strains.

Ruptured disk or slipped disk. This occurs when the pulpy body at the center of an intervertebral disk ruptures or protrudes through a break in the surrounding casing. When the herniated fragment presses on an adjacent nerve root, severe pain (sciatica) is felt in the buttock, the back of the

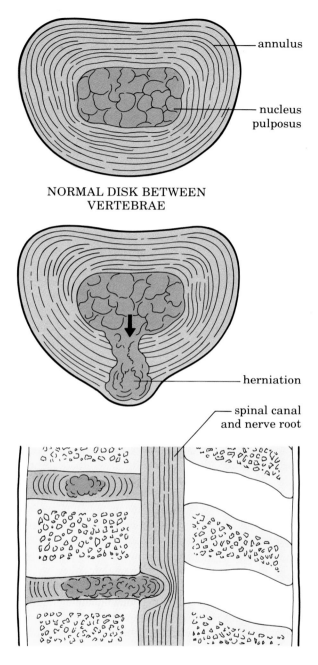

NORMAL DISK BETWEEN VERTEBRAE

annulus

nucleus pulposus

herniation

spinal canal and nerve root

SLIPPED DISK

A "slipped disk" occurs when the intervertebral disk, which acts as a shock absorber between vertebrae, breaks out of its capsule and presses on an adjoining nerve. A cross section of a normal disk viewed from above is shown at top. At center, the casing has ruptured, allowing the nucleus to protrude into a bulge. The side view shows how the bulge impinges on a nearby nerve.

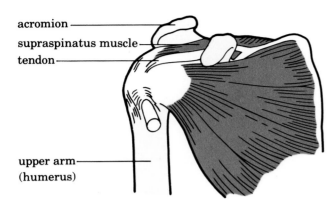

acromion
supraspinatus muscle
tendon

upper arm
(humerus)

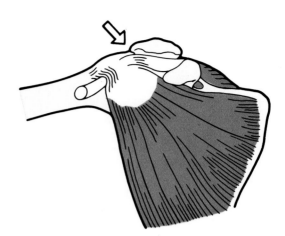

thigh, and even into the foot. Numbness and weakness may follow. The victim often tilts the body to one side (sciatic scoliosis). Pain may be made worse by coughing, straining, sneezing, or making jarring movements.

Treatment usually consists of simple bed rest. Often symptoms will subside, indicating that a herniation did not occur or that the fragment was small and became walled off. If conservative treatment fails, surgery may be necessary to remove the free fragment and the remaining degenerated portion of the disk.

Spondylolisthesis refers to spontaneous forward displacement of a lumbar vertebra caused by a bony defect between the vertebra and the arch enclosing the spinal canal. Spondylolisthesis can exist without backache and often is discovered accidentally during a routine physical examination.

When symptoms occur, they usually appear as a low lumbar backache, with or without accompanying sciatica. Treatment is the same as for disk degeneration. In growing children, the spine may have to be fused to prevent gross deformity.

Scheuermann's disease, sometimes called "adolescent round back," is a common cause of backache among teenagers. For unknown reasons, growth changes give the thoracic vertebrae a wedge-shaped formation that increases the usual thoracic curve. The active stage of the disorder, which lasts from two to five years, may cause pain. In severe cases, bed rest followed by the wearing of a spinal brace, or even a surgical fusion, may be necessary.

Scoliosis, a lateral curvature of the spine, usually appears in childhood. Ribs on one side protrude backward and accentuate the normal curve in the thoracic region. When normal growth ceases, the deformity progresses at a slower rate.

Idiopathic scoliosis is usually recognized before puberty. It occurs predominantly in girls. The

IMPINGEMENT SYNDROME
Impingement syndrome occurs when the arm is raised toward a horizontal position. At left, the arm hangs normally without pain. As the arm is raised, the muscle and tendon are pinched painfully between the upper arm bone and the acromion, or point of the shoulder. The condition often occurs if these tissues are swollen or inflamed. Calcium deposits in the tendons aggravate the problem.

curve is to the right in the chest region and to the left in the lumbar region. Its cause is unknown.

Treatment may consist of bracing, electrical stimulation, and/or surgical fusion. A severe deformity of the chest is to be avoided because it may encroach on the lungs and increase the workload of the heart, even causing eventual heart failure.

Minor deformities can be detected on physical examination. Some schools have screening programs to detect early cases.

Scoliosis sometimes occurs when a person compensates for a sideward tilt of the pelvis produced by a short leg or by an apparent shortening of the leg caused by hip or knee contraction. The scoliosis disappears if the pelvic tilt is corrected.

Torticollis or wry-neck. This deformity of the seven vertebrae of the neck causes a person to carry the head tilted to one side, with the chin thrust forward and pointed toward the opposite side. The muscles on the affected side are contracted. The most common form is found in newborns and is associated with a swelling of the neck muscles. The child's muscles often can be manipulated gently to correct the deformity.

Degenerative arthritis of the spine is discussed in Chapter 17, "Arthritis and Related Diseases."

THE SHOULDER

Impingement syndrome (bursitis). Most shoulder pain is caused by degenerative changes in the small tendons that make up the rotator cuff. The muscles attached to these tendons turn the arm inward and outward and work with the deltoid muscle in raising the arm over the head. Between the rotator cuff and the overlying deltoid muscle is the subdeltoid or subacromial bursa. The two layers of the bursa are lubricated and permit the humerus, or upper arm bone, with its rotator cuff, to glide smoothly beneath the soft deltoid muscle and the acromion, the hard, overhanging projection of the shoulder blade. The deep layer of the bursa becomes locally inflamed when degeneration begins in any of the rotator cuff tendons. As the tendon passes beneath the acromion when the arm is elevated between 60 and 120 degrees, the inflamed bursa is pinched, causing the sharp pain that we know as bursitis. There is usually little or no pain during motion on either side of this middle arc of movement.

Calcium deposits may build up in the degenerating tendons, thereby increasing the inflammation, impingement, and pain. The calcium may liquefy and rupture into the bursal sac. This produces a generalized bursitis and a shoulder immobilized by severe pain.

Treatment may involve exercises and short-wave diathermy, a form of deep-heat treatment. Nonsteroidal anti-inflammatory medications or injections of cortisone derivatives and exercise also are used. A period of rest in a sling may be required as well.

Tendon and muscle tears are common causes of pain around shoulder joints. An incomplete tear of the rotator cuff may result from impingement syndrome. A complete tear greatly hinders ability to raise the arm. Complete tears often are produced by minor accidents, such as falling on an outstretched hand.

The outlook is good if the tear is repaired surgically within a few days of its occurrence. If an operation is delayed, it is unlikely that full shoulder movement will return.

Frozen shoulder is an ill-understood condition. Patients complain of moderate pain and marked limitation of movement. A dull ache comes on gradually in the shoulder and upper arm. Movement is restricted in all directions.

Usually the stiffness gradually disappears, but it may take six months to a year. The pain disappears sooner. Physiotherapy is helpful.

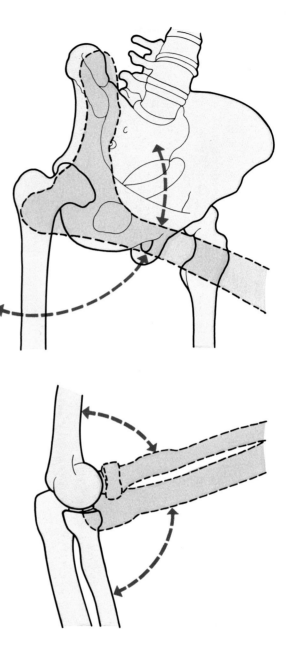

TWO TYPES OF JOINTS
Two types of joints are the ball-and-socket of the hip (top) and the hinge of the elbow. Arrows show the range of motion permitted by each joint. In the ball-and-socket joint, the rounded head of the thighbone, called the femur, fits into a cup-shaped cavity, the acetabulum, in the pelvis. As the femur moves, the head of the thighbone rotates in its socket. The hinge of the elbow permits the forearm to be raised or lowered. It also allows the forearm to be rotated, as in turning the palm up or down.

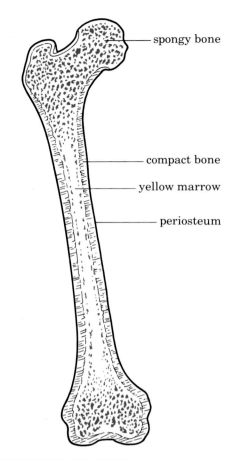

spongy bone

compact bone

yellow marrow

periosteum

THE MAKEUP OF BONE
This cross section of the thighbone shows the components of bone. Spongy bone at either end gives the bone weight-bearing strength. Compact bone is a hard outer tube. The bone shaft contains yellow marrow, a fatty reserve. The periosteum is a tough outer membrane.

Recurrent shoulder dislocation usually occurs when raising or extending the arm without any great violence, even while stretching, swimming, putting on a coat, or brushing the hair. In some persons, dislocations are so frequent that they interfere with daily activities. Often the patient, alone or with the help of another person, is able to relocate the shoulder.

If a primary dislocation is not properly replaced in normal position and immobilized, the risk of recurrent dislocation increases.

Frequent, troublesome dislocations may require an operation to strengthen the joint capsule and slightly limit its range of outward rotation. Many athletes who have suffered repeated shoulder dislocations have been able to continue their careers after a successful repair operation.

The acromioclavicular joint connects the outer end of the collarbone and the acromion process of the shoulder blade. Degenerative changes produce pain. The pain worsens when the joint is used extensively, particularly for overhead work such as painting a ceiling. Bony outgrowth can be felt at the edges of the joint.

Heat, rest, a sling, and aspirin usually are satisfactory. Occasionally, surgery is necessary.

This joint also is prone to persistent dislocation (shoulder separation) brought about by injury. The outer end of the collarbone sticks up beneath the skin. The rest of the shoulder girdle and arm hang lower than the collarbone. Usually little or no treatment is needed, except perhaps a sling.

THE ELBOW

When the arm is held straight by the side, the elbow is bent slightly outward at an angle of about 10 degrees in men and 15 degrees in women. This is known as the "carrying angle."

Cubitus valgus usually occurs because of poor union of a fracture of the lower end of the arm. The deformity is harmless and usually not readily noticeable. Function of the arm is not disturbed, but a possible complication is ulnar nerve neuritis.

The ulnar nerve, which supplies most of the muscles of the hand, passes around the back of the elbow joint and is exposed to direct injury at the point of the elbow known as the "crazy bone." When the carrying angle is greatly increased, the nerve is bent sharply around the angle and repeated injury may damage it, producing numbness, tingling in the hand, and weakness and wasting of small hand muscles. It may be advisable to have the nerve surgically transposed to the front of the elbow.

Cubitus varus, in which the normal carrying angle is reduced, or even reversed, is the opposite deformity. There usually is no disability.

Tennis elbow is a name commonly applied to any disorder causing pain on the outer side of the elbow joint. Only in a few people is it caused by playing tennis. Any activity that requires rotary movements of the forearm and a firm grip of the hand (using a screwdriver, for example) can cause the symptoms. There is pain and tenderness at the rear of the elbow that often radiates down the back of the forearm.

Many mild cases require no treatment. In more severe cases, rest, diathermy, and injection of local anesthetics combined with cortisone derivatives

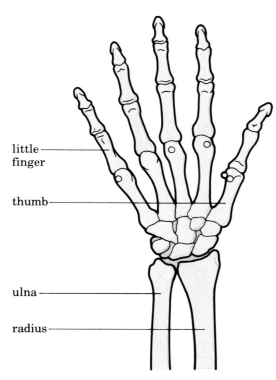

little finger

thumb

ulna

radius

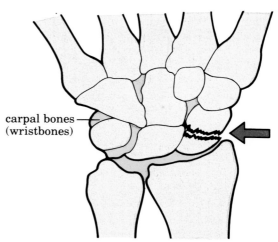

carpal bones (wristbones)

WRIST AND HAND BONES
The bones of the hand and wrist are intricately fitted together to allow fine and delicate movements. The drawing at left shows the relationship between thumb and finger bones and the radius and ulna of the forearm. The closeup drawing shows the eight carpal or wristbones arranged in two rows. The fracture of the navicular bone at the base of the thumb (arrow) is a common injury, often caused by falling on an outstretched hand. A "sprained wrist" is often such a fracture or a dislocation.

are used. Immobilization in a sling or even a plaster cast is often helpful.

The elbow is second only to the knee as a site of osteochondritis dissecans, in which a fragment of cartilage and bone becomes detached. Pain is moderate, and movements usually are somewhat limited. "Locking" of the elbow does not occur until the fragment is completely detached. X rays then may show the bony fragment—a "joint mouse"—lying free within the joint.

Several months of immobilization may be necessary in early cases; once the fragment has separated, it must be removed by incision.

THE WRIST AND HAND

"Sprained wrist" is a common lay diagnosis, but it often is wrong. The true sprained wrist is rare. Symptoms are more frequently caused by a fracture, a dislocation, or arthritis.

Persistent pain in the wrist following an accident is a serious symptom. Fracture of the navicular bone above the thumb is common, and if left untreated, can produce crippling arthritis of the wrist. Falls on the back of the hand can chip small flakes of bone that cause troublesome symptoms for weeks.

If these causes of symptoms can be excluded, true "sprained wrist" can be treated by strapping or temporary immobilization in a plaster cast.

DeQuervain's disease. A common cause of pain in the thumb side of the wrist is a thickening of the sheaths covering two of the tendons that pass to the thumb. The condition is more common among women than men. Symptoms come on gradually. Pain at the base of the thumb radiates to the nail and up into the forearm. Tenderness is present on pressure over the thumb side of the wrist.

Sometimes the condition cures itself if the wrist is immobilized. Cortisone injections into the sheath usually bring prompt relief.

Ganglion of the wrist. A ganglion is a cystic swelling that occurs in association with a joint or tendon sheath. Ganglia occur most commonly as a bulge on the back of the wrist, but also can arise around the knee and ankle.

Usually ganglia produce no symptoms except occasional slight discomfort, and may disappear spontaneously. Aspiration to remove fluid, followed by injection of a cortisone derivative, often will eliminate the cyst.

Carpal tunnel syndrome (median nerve compression). Pressure on the median nerve where it enters the wrist (the carpal tunnel) is a common cause of discomfort of the hand, especially in women over 40. This big nerve passes along the middle of the arm and forearm and enters the hand at the wrist joint, along with all the flexor tendons to the fingers. Thickening of the tendon sheaths and arthritic changes at the wrist tend to reduce the size of the tunnel through which the nerve passes. The nerve is subjected to considerable pressure, with accompanying discomfort.

Symptoms are tingling, vague or sharp pain, and perhaps numbness in the thumb, index finger, and long fingers. The pain is often worst at night. Rest occasionally helps. A cortisone derivative injected into the carpal tunnel often relieves the symptoms. If not, the volar carpal ligament may be partly or completely removed to relieve pressure on the nerve.

Dupuytren's contracture is a thickening of tissue (fascia) of the palm that causes the fingers to be pulled down into the palm. It also can occur in the sole of the foot. It appears to run in families, but the exact cause is unknown. The condition usually starts as a small nodule at the base of the ring finger. As the condition progresses, other nodules appear, and firm bands may spread into the fingers. When the deformity is disabling, it is necessary to sever the constricting band.

Trigger finger results from constriction that prevents free movement of tendons in the sheath of the finger. Despite its name, it can occur in any finger. The tendons develop a "waist" opposite the constriction and tend to swell. The swollen segment often develops into a nodule that has difficulty entering the sheath when the finger is extended. Usually a snap is felt and a click is heard as the finger bends or extends. Cortisone injections can relieve the problem.

Boutonniere deformity, also known as "buttonhole" deformity, results when the central extensor tendon on the base of the middle joint of a finger is cut or ruptured. In the fully developed deformity, the middle joint is bent at a right angle. An immediate operation is needed to reattach the tendon to the bone.

Mallet or baseball finger, in which the tip of the finger bends as much as 45 degrees, is caused by rupture or tearing of the attachment of the extensor tendon. The force to do this is a sudden violent blow on the tip of the finger, as in "miscatching" a baseball. Immobilizing the joint for about six weeks usually realigns the joint.

THE HIP

The hip is a major weight-bearing joint and is subject to many conditions directly connected with the thrust of body weight.

Congenital dislocation. This spontaneous dislocation occurs before or shortly after birth as a result of an abnormality of development, usually a flattening of the acetabulum (the cup-shaped cavity in the pelvis), in which the end (head) of the thighbone rests. Girls are affected at least five times more often than boys. The dislocation occurs more often in one hip than in both.

Warning signs in a newborn are limited outward motion from the hip, particularly when the infant is lying on his or her back with knees bent to 90 degrees, and asymmetrical "folds" of the fat tissue of the leg. The buttock, groin, and thigh folds on the affected side usually are deeper and higher up on the leg than on the opposite side. When the affected hip is moved, a "click" can be heard.

Fortunately, the condition generally is recognized soon after birth.

Treatment. The basic aim is to place the head of the thighbone in the socket and to retain it there until the socket has had time to develop. The most satisfactory method is to stretch tight muscles gradually, then replace the thighbone under general anesthesia, followed by immobilization of the leg and hip joint in a special harness and, later, a plaster cast. After removal of the cast, a bar may be attached to the baby's shoes to hold the legs apart and to limit hip movement. In infants with slight dislocations, splinting may be sufficient.

If the treatment is started within the first six months of life, the results will be excellent in nearly every case.

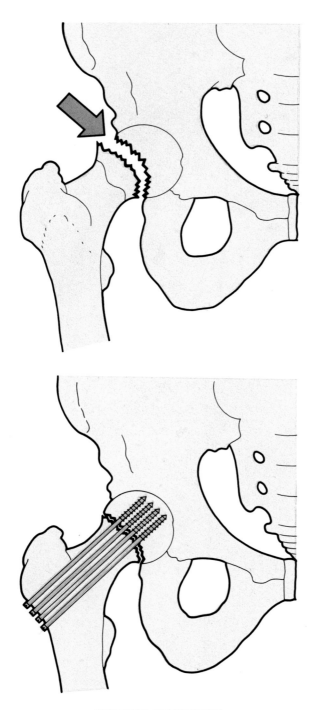

SLIPPED EPIPHYSIS
Slipped epiphysis, which happens in late childhood, is most common at the hip joint, where the rounded head of the thighbone slips from its normal cartilage connection (top drawing), causing an unstable joint, limping, and pain. A cluster of fine-diameter, threaded nails (lower drawing) can hold the slipped parts in position.

Acute suppurative arthritis. Pyogenic (pus-producing) arthritis of the hip in infants and young children usually results from infection elsewhere, such as pneumonia, impetigo, or middle ear infection. The child is obviously sick, has a sudden onset of high fever, holds the hip joint bent, and resists examination.

Fortunately, the infecting organism is sensitive to antibiotics. Sometimes the doctor must surgically drain the hip joint to prevent destruction of bone.

Perthes' disease, a hip disease of children between the ages of 3 and 8, is three times more common among boys than among girls.

The specific cause is not known, but a local reduction of blood supply leads to collapse of the head of the thighbone (femoral head). The condition goes through three stages—onset, activity, and healing—that may cover three years. The onset is marked by pain and a limp. During the active stage, the head of the thighbone softens and deforms. Healing is gradual, but the head may be permanently deformed.

The objective of treatment is to prevent the soft femoral head from being deformed into a grossly distorted shape. Immobilization with braces or in a cast, with the legs held widely apart, seats the ball in the round socket and prevents distortion. Limited weight also is important. Sometimes an operation must be performed to realign the pelvic bone or femur and limit stress on the femoral head.

Slipped femoral epiphysis occurs in late childhood. The rounded top of the thighbone slips from its cartilaginous connection with the rest of the bone and is displaced downward and backward. Usually this is a gradual development, but a fall or injury can cause sudden displacement, with gradually increasing pain in the hip and a limp.

Because the condition worsens until growth has ceased, an operation usually is necessary. If there is minimal slipping, several small screws are inserted across the cartilage plate to prevent further displacement. In extreme cases, it may be necessary to sever and realign the bone.

Degenerative arthritis of the hip and hip replacement. Now the most common and successful form of joint replacement, hip replacement is described in Chapter 17, "Arthritis and Related Diseases."

Knee Injuries

Athlete's knee injuries usually result from a severe impact or twist on a bent, weight-bearing knee. A side tackle on a football player can drive the knee inward and cause strain on the four principal ligaments supporting the joint, as shown in the close-up below. The medial ligament on the inner side of the knee is the one most commonly stretched (strained) or torn, as in the illustration at top. Frequently, the cartilage in the joint (meniscus) also is torn. The tear interferes with joint function, causing swelling and collection of fluid.

Another cause of knee injury in athletes is sudden deceleration with no impact involved. Sometimes, cleats or spikes catching in the turf or other surface cause the abrupt stop. Deceleration injury also occurs in weekend athletes, such as skiers and tennis players, especially if they are poorly conditioned. Older persons sometimes suffer tears when simply squatting or bending. These are due to degeneration of the cartilage.

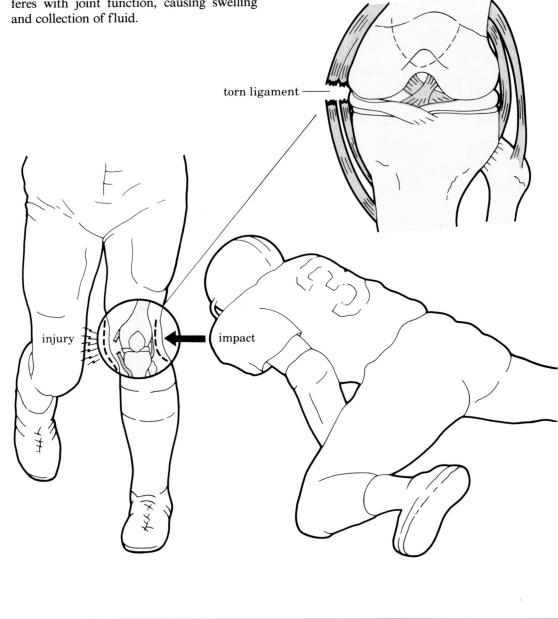

torn ligament

injury

impact

Bursitis of the hip. This bursitis may occur following surgery, but also happens spontaneously in older people, especially those suffering from gout. Pain and tenderness over the point of the hip joint mark the site of the bursa that has become inflamed. When the condition is acute, sufferers find it difficult to lie on the affected side or to walk without a limp.

Heat, rest, and anti-inflammatory medications are used to treat the condition. Injection into the bursa of a local anesthetic combined with a cortisone derivative usually brings pain relief.

THE KNEE

The knee is subject to enormous stresses that must be withstood by four relatively small ligaments: one on each side of and two inside the joint. Those on the sides prevent sideward displacement, and those on the inside prevent backward and forward displacement. Because of the leverage applied through the thigh and leg bones, ligament injuries to the knee are common among athletes.

Patella-femoral syndrome involves the junction of the kneecap and thighbone. The mostly young victims complain of pain under or around the kneecap, catching of the joint, and stiffness. The condition is aggravated by prolonged sitting with the knees bent, stair climbing, deep-knee bending, and climbing hills. The kneecap feels tender, and there is swelling because of fluid in the joint. The cause is not clear.

Treatment consists of exercises to strengthen the quadriceps muscle of the thigh and anti-inflammatory medications. The kneecap is only rarely removed surgically.

Recurrent dislocation of the patella most commonly occurs in teenage girls after injury. The kneecap slips outward, over the edge of the femur. Dislocation can occur spontaneously while walking, running, or turning suddenly. The pain is acute, and the girl is unable to straighten her knee. Another person can easily extend the joint to straighten the knee, and the patella slips back into position.

After the first dislocation, the inner border of the kneecap usually feels tender, indicating the point where the quadriceps tendon has pulled away. The joint is filled with fluid. The torn tendon must be repaired surgically, followed by four to six weeks with the knee immobilized. A vigorous exercise program to restore strength to the quadriceps muscle is necessary afterward.

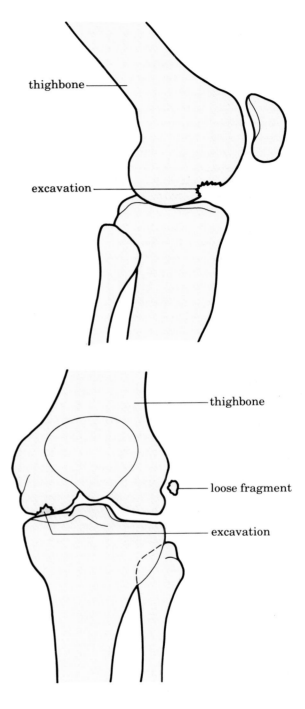

"JOINT MOUSE"
A "joint mouse" is a loose bit of bone and cartilage in the joint cavity, most commonly found in the knee. It may occur because a local reduction of blood supply causes the death of a small area of bone and its overlying cartilage. The dead fragment separates from the rest of the bone and floats in the cavity.

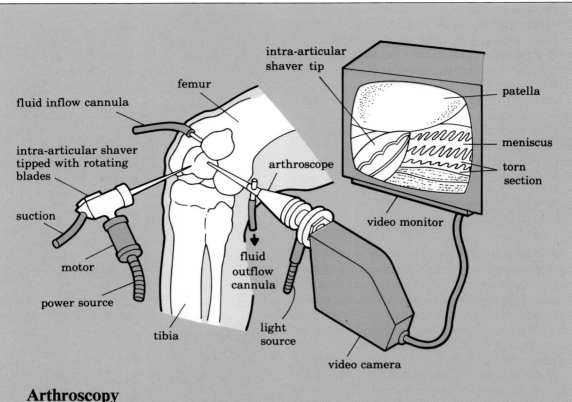

Arthroscopy

Arthroscopy is a method of joint repair that eliminates open surgery. It is called "the quarterback's friend" because it often allows athletes to return to action within a week or 10 days, compared to six weeks' recuperation in the past. The orthopedic surgeon uses a lighted arthroscope to visualize the interior of the joint, and monitors it on a TV screen.

Here, an intra-articular shaver tipped with rotating blades is being used to trim away torn knee cartilage. Arthroscopy also can be used to repair ligament damage or remove "joint mice" and can be used in shoulder, ankle, or wrist repair, as well as for diagnosis. Operations usually are performed under regional anesthesia.

Torn ligaments. The four principal ligaments of the knee joint frequently are strained or torn in sports and accidents. If the ligament is completely torn, the best treatment is early surgical repair. Moderate sprains can be treated by immobilizing the knee in a plaster cylinder or brace. Minor injuries are treated by wrapping the knee and avoiding strains during healing.

All ligament injuries cause wasting of the quadriceps muscle, and intensive exercises are necessary to strengthen the muscle and provide future protection for the joint.

Torn cartilage. An acute tear of one of the knee cartilages is common in young athletes. A tear occurs when a substantial twisting force passes through a bent knee. The initial pain is sharp; it is difficult to straighten the knee. The knee is said to be "locked." Swelling soon follows. Fluid (effusion) can be felt, and the knee is tender over the joint line, usually on the inner side.

Bowlegs represent an outward bending of the knee joint. A mild degree of bowing, followed by a period of straightening and even slight overcorrection that may produce knock-knees, is common in children. No treatment is necessary unless the condition persists.

Knock-knees are produced by inward bending of the knee joint. The condition is common in children between the ages of 3 and 5. A severe knock-knee case that continues to the age of 10 requires surgery.

Osteochondritis dissecans usually occurs in late adolescence. A section of the joint surface of a bone dies, along with its overlying cartilage. Eventually the fragment may separate and form a loose body in the joint. The knee joint is affected most often. Injury is probably a predisposing factor.

Treatment consists of surgical removal of the fragment if it has separated and is loose in the joint. If it has not separated, the fragment often can be encouraged to "grow back" by an operation that drills small holes in the fragment to allow new blood vessels to enter from the depths of the bone. In some cases, the fragment requires a metallic pin to hold it in place.

THE ANKLE

Sprained ankle. The most common disability to affect the ankle joint is the all too familiar "turned ankle" (sprain). A misstep on uneven ground can result in a partial tear on the outer (fibulo-talar) ligament. Small blood vessels are ruptured, causing a large collection of blood to form beneath the skin, followed in 24 hours by swelling in the ankle and foot.

Treatment includes rest with the foot elevated, and an ice pack applied to the ankle. Firm pressure also should be kept on the ankle to minimize swelling. The treatment formula often is abbreviated to I-C-E: ice, compression, elevation. An elastic bandage, adhesive strapping, or a walking plaster cast or splint then may be required to support the ankle, depending on the severity of the sprain. A sprain generally is slow to heal, and pain is out of proportion to the severity of the injury. If the lateral ligaments are torn completely, surgical repair may be necessary.

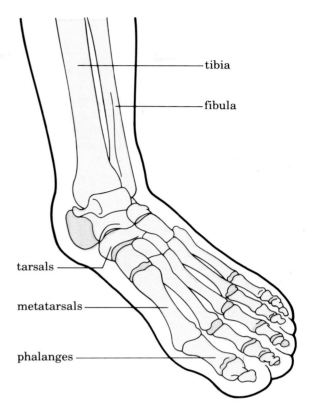

tibia

fibula

tarsals

metatarsals

phalanges

BONES OF THE FOOT
The bones of the foot and their ligaments provide remarkable flexibility and easy, rolling shift of body weight. Despite variations in size and numerous articulations, the bones work smoothly together to support the weight of the body and move it forward. Most people have aching feet at times, but it is not normal for feet to hurt.

Women have more foot problems than men, partly due to the shoes they wear. A bunion, or thickening and swelling of the big toe joint, is common among women. The condition appears to run in families. Bunions often can be corrected surgically.

THE FOOT

Foot strain. The arches and supporting structures in the foot can be affected by acute or chronic strain. Acute strain usually is caused by an isolated incident that grossly overtaxes the foot. Symptoms usually respond to rest. Chronic strain of the foot can be caused by excess weight, excessive fatigue, occupational demands, abnormal gait, and faults or diseases within the foot. Most of the symptoms occur in the midtarsal area.

Treatment requires support for the longitudinal arch sufficiently high to relieve strain on the ligaments of the foot.

Metatarsalgia, pain in the ball of the foot, usually is caused by weakness in the foot muscles. Wearing high-heeled shoes may aggravate the symptoms.

Pain can be relieved by wearing low-heeled shoes with domed supports (metatarsal pads) to distribute the weight over a larger area and relieve the pressure on the metatarsal heads.

Adult Foot Problems

Hallux rigidus (stiff toe) usually is produced by repeated minor injuries or a single major accident that overextends the toe with great force. Degenerative joint disease follows. Relief can be obtained by surgery.

Hammer toe. Hammer toe usually is caused by cramping toes into shoes that are too small. Most often, the clawlike deformity affects the second toe. Symptoms may be alleviated by padding.

SPRAINS, DISLOCATIONS, FRACTURES, AND CONTUSIONS

A well-planned conditioning program does much to prevent injury. In spite of the best-laid plans, however, accidents do happen.

Sprain. A sprain is an injury to a ligament, and a strain is an injury to a muscle or its tendon. All joints in the body are held together by ligaments strong enough to resist normal forces. When violent force is applied, a stretched ligament will tear and a sprain occurs.

Mild sprains do not weaken the joint and usually need only strap support. Severe sprains usually produce a complete tear of a major ligament and are best treated by surgical repair.

Dislocation. A dislocation occurs when the force applied to a joint is greater than that necessary to produce a strain, resulting in displacement of the bone from its normal position in the joint. Dislocations must be reduced (returned to proper position) as soon as possible, and usually an anesthetic is necessary to relax the spasm in surrounding muscles.

Once the bone is returned to its proper position, the torn tissues must be given time to heal before allowing movement in the joint. Three weeks usually is the minimum.

Fracture. A fracture is a break in a bone. When the skin is broken, the fracture is open or compound. When the skin is not broken, the fracture is closed or simple.

A common fracture among older persons is the Colles's fracture of the wrist, caused by a fall on an outstretched hand. The force crushes the radius bone of the forearm just above the wrist, so that the hand can be displaced backward. Because of the crushing, the fracture often heals with a characteristic curve called the "silver fork" deformity.

Among active young adults, ankle fractures are the most common. A spiral break of the fibula, the outer, smaller bone of the leg, often is the result of a twisting fall, as in skiing. A tendon frequently tears loose with the smaller bit of broken bone.

Young children frequently suffer an incomplete or "greenstick" fracture of the long bones, in which the break occurs only on one side, as in a half-broken green branch.

Bone's capacity for repair makes it possible to treat most fractures by manipulations that place the broken ends close enough to each other for good union to occur. Some closed fractures are so grossly unstable that they constantly shift, and need to be immobilized internally by fixing screws or pins.

All types of breaks are treated by the same general principles: (1) reduction of the fracture into a satisfactory position; (2) maintenance of fracture reduction until healing is sufficient to prevent redisplacement; (3) restoration of normal function to muscles, tendons, and joints.

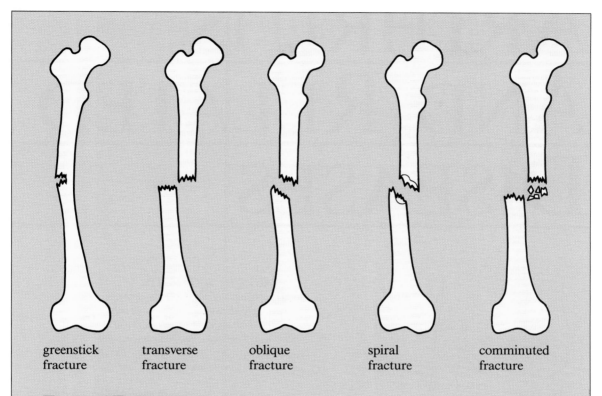

greenstick fracture transverse fracture oblique fracture spiral fracture comminuted fracture

Types of Fractures

Fractures occur in different forms, as the drawing above shows. From left: a greenstick fracture, common in young children, whose flexible bones may break only on one side; a transverse fracture; an oblique fracture; a spiral fracture, a common skier's injury; and a comminuted fracture, in which the bone is crushed into small pieces. A simple or closed fracture does not break the overlying skin. In a compound fracture, jagged ends of the broken bone may protrude. Fractures sometimes are mistaken for sprains; usually only X rays can determine if a bone is broken. Whatever the type of fracture, immobilization in a cast usually is necessary.

Contusion. Often associated with fractures and sprains are contusions of the soft tissues. The usual "black and blue" spots are caused by blows that crush the fatty tissue just beneath the skin, tearing the small blood vessels. These require little or no treatment. A blow with more force can contuse a muscle, causing some tearing of fibers and bleeding within the muscle. This is a far more serious injury in terms of length of disability and pain. Unless the muscle is completely torn apart, however, it will heal together by scar tissue following a period of rest. Complete rupture of a muscle requires surgical repair.

Restoration of function. A vital part of treatment is restoration of function after the fracture has united. When the cast is removed, it is customary to find joint stiffness and muscle atrophy, which is a shrinkage or wasting away of the muscle caused by lack of use. Physiotherapy is of great help in the mobilization of a stiffened limb, but movement and muscle contractions by the patient are the key to success. Most restoration of function occurs during the first three to four months.

CHAPTER 17

ARTHRITIS AND RELATED DISEASES

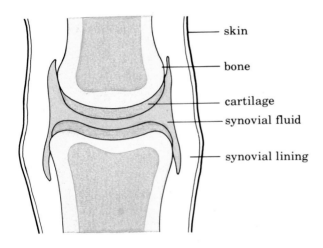

- skin
- bone
- cartilage
- synovial fluid
- synovial lining

STAGES OF ARTHRITIS

The changes of degenerative arthritis begin gradually and may cover many years. The drawing at left shows a normal knee joint (with ligaments not shown for clarity). The synovial lining forms a capsule and secretes fluid for lubrication. Cartilage cushions the end of each bone. In the early stage of arthritis, cartilage softens and cracks, forming an uneven surface and narrowing the joint space. Later, underlying bone attempts to compensate for damage with new growth. Bits of cartilage and bone float in the synovial fluid, interfering with movement. In the advanced stage, cysts develop, joint space is greatly narrowed, and the synovial capsule is distorted by bone spurs.

cartilage degeneration

hardening of bone

cartilage debris

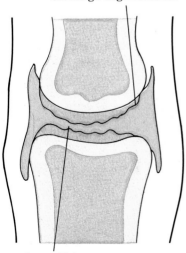

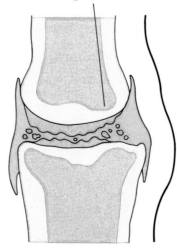

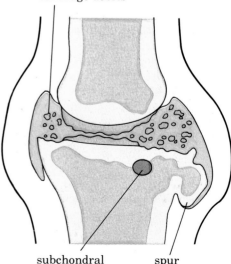

loss of joint space

subchondral bone cyst

spur

There are many types of arthritis. Some are acute; others, chronic. Some are common; others, rare. Some affect a single joint; others, all joints. Arthritis may be associated with generalized illness, but more often it is an entity unto itself. The more than 100 types of rheumatic disease are caused by injuries, infections, metabolic disturbances, or tumors. In many cases, the cause is not known.

The Arthritis Foundation estimates that more than 32 million Americans suffer from one form of arthritis or another. Some types of arthritis are peculiar to certain age groups. For example, rheumatic fever is basically a disease of children. Gonococcal arthritis, a venereal disease, afflicts mostly young people in their teens and twenties. Rheumatoid arthritis most often occurs in young to middle-aged adults, whereas gout occurs in those middle-aged and older. A disorder called polymyalgia rheumatica strikes only the aged. Some forms of rheumatism, such as lupus erythematosus, are more prevalent in women, yet men are more likely to develop a disorder known as ankylosing spondylitis. Men and women are equally prone to most rheumatic diseases. No one is immune from arthritis.

Arthritis is primarily a disease of the joints. A joint is defined as a connection of two movable bones covered by a membrane that secretes joint fluid. The joint itself is covered with ligaments, fascia, tendons, muscles, fat, and skin. The cap of cartilage at the end of each bone provides a relatively low friction surface between the bones. Cartilage is composed of cells that produce a mucuslike substance, and collagen fibers. Both provide considerable strength and elasticity so that the cartilage can act as a shock absorber and combat shearing forces. The joint fluid or synovial fluid is a viscous, light yellow liquid secreted by the membranes that line the joint. It facilitates joint motion, lubricates, and aids in exchange of nutrients the tissues need.

Ligaments are tight bands that link one bone to another across the joint. A ligament's flexibility varies from one joint to another depending upon how much motion that joint is intended to have. Without ligaments, the entire skeleton would collapse. Tendons are tough, spindled ends of muscle composed of densely packed collagen fibers. They, too, attach to bones to impart both stability and motion of the joints. The brain sends messages to the muscles to contract or relax. In response, the joints move.

DIAGNOSIS OF
RHEUMATIC DISEASES

Many rheumatic diseases are readily diagnosed because their symptoms are so characteristic. Symptoms are still the main way to identify rheumatic disorders.

Symptoms and Physical Signs

There are six major categories of symptoms that may occur in rheumatic disorders:

Pain is the major symptom of almost all rheumatic disease. It may arise from the joint or the surrounding structures. It may be mild, severe, constant, or intermittent. Individual response to pain is so variable that no two people react the same way to the same painful stimulus. When a physician evaluates pain for diagnostic purposes, he considers the location, onset, frequency, duration, and severity, among other factors.

Stiffness is the feeling, independent of pain, that the joints are tight and do not move as well as we would like them to. All of us feel stiff for short periods once in a while, especially the morning after a day of vigorous activity. Many rheumatic diseases, notably rheumatoid arthritis, are characterized by prolonged morning stiffness that sometimes lasts several hours.

Weakness and disability accompany some rheumatic conditions, especially when the joints are inflamed or when the illness has been prolonged. In some disorders, local weakness is the predominant symptom. Disability depends on many factors, including the type of arthritis, number of joints involved, severity of the illness, presence of deformities, and quite importantly, motivation. A positively motivated person can minimize disability.

Swelling of the joint may result from fluid within the joint, engorged synovial tissues, bony enlargement, or a combination of these factors. Severe swelling is easy to detect, but mild swelling is less noticeable. Sometimes, the first symptom of a rheumatic disease is swelling of one or more joints, not necessarily accompanied by pain.

Tenderness characterizes most painful joints, but not always. The physician may be able to diagnose a condition by the location of tenderness. For example, patients with subdeltoid bursitis complain of pain in the upper arm, yet the tenderness usually is limited to the outer portion of the shoulder. Heat and redness are additional clues to inflammation. A red-hot, swollen, exquisitely tender big toe is a tip-off to gout.

Deformities, single or multiple, are so characteristic in certain rheumatic diseases that a doctor usually can diagnose the problem solely by examining the deformity. Deformities may be caused by a combination of changes in the joints, muscles, ligaments, tendons, or skin. Deformities do not necessarily imply disability or crippling, but the primary goal of any treatment program is to prevent any deformity from developing.

Special Tests

A physician who suspects arthritis can perform blood, urine, synovial fluid, and X-ray tests. But only in rare instances are any of these tests by themselves critical. Instead, they usually serve only as guides to support the doctor's suspicions.

X rays are important for the full assessment of many types of arthritis because they frequently disclose the destructive process going on within the body, and help to confirm a clinical diagnosis. For example, if a few joints in the hand are inflamed, the physician may not be able to tell whether the patient has rheumatoid arthritis, psoriatic arthritis, infectious arthritis, or gout. The X-ray examination often will easily differentiate among them.

Radioisotopic scanning. The principle of bone and joint scanning is based upon the concentration of previously administered radionucleotide tracers in areas of inflammation and new bone formation. A scan may "light up" an area that the physical X-ray examinations fail to disclose as abnormal.

Electromyography. Skeletal muscles and nerves emit electrical impulses that may be detected just as the impulses emitted from the heart are detected by an electrocardiogram. Electromyographic and nerve conduction studies give vital information about the muscles and nerves. As a result, the disease site can be located precisely.

Arthroscopy, illustrated in Chapter 16, "The Bones and Muscles," is a relatively safe, simple procedure that permits inspection inside the joint, using a large needle, bright light, and magnifying lens. The procedure eliminates the need for major surgery in order to search for tumors, foreign bodies, inflammation, or changes in the joint. Operations also may be performed, but the procedures can be used only in large joints.

Laboratory tests. The red blood cell sedimentation rate is a relatively inexpensive laboratory indicator of inflammation in the body regardless of cause. The test screens out noninflammatory disorders and tells the physician when to investigate further. The test result tends to be normal in noninflammatory rheumatic diseases such as osteoarthritis and fibrositis, but it is higher in rheumatoid arthritis, other connective tissue diseases, infectious arthritis, gout, and polymyalgia rheumatica.

The latex fixation test for rheumatoid factor is a measure of certain protein antibodies in the blood. These so-called rheumatoid factors are higher than normal in 70 to 80 percent of patients

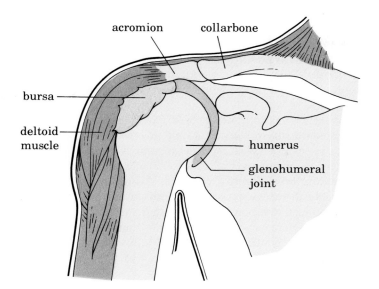

acromion   collarbone

bursa

deltoid
muscle

humerus

glenohumeral
joint

BURSITIS
*Inflammation of a bursa, a lubricating
sac between muscles or between muscle
and bone, can cause excruciating pain.
The most common form occurs in the
shoulder. When the arm is moved, the
swollen bursa may become pinched
between the upper arm bone (humerus)
and the point of the shoulder
(acromion). Sometimes the shoulder is
tender, swollen, and red.*

with rheumatoid arthritis. Factors also may be found in certain other rheumatic and nonrheumatic diseases, so their value in diagnosis is limited. The higher the level of rheumatoid factor, however, the more likely the diagnosis of rheumatoid arthritis.

The antinuclear antibody and LE cell phenomenon (LE prep) help make a more precise and earlier diagnosis of systemic lupus erythematosus and other connective tissue diseases. The test consists of labeling known cellular (nuclear) antigens with a fluorescent material. If antibodies to any of the antigens are present in a blood sample, patterns can be seen with a fluorescent microscope.

Synovial fluid analysis. Normal synovial fluid, the lubricating substance of the joint, consists of extremely large, heavy molecules and is highly viscous. When the joint is diseased, the fluid may

increase in quantity, become inflamed, and contain abnormal elements such as white cells, crystals, sands of collagen, and bacteria. Analysis of the fluid may help to identify the condition.

Biopsy. The removal of a bit of tissue for examination usually implies a search for malignancy. But in rheumatic diseases, biopsy of the joints, muscles, skin, blood vessels, and other structures is done to allow precise assessment of these tissues.

Other tests. Other routine laboratory tests, including complete blood counts, analyses of the urine, and liver and kidney function tests, may be required to check for manifestations of disease outside the joints and to monitor the effects of drugs.

RHEUMATIC DISEASES

Nonarticular Rheumatism

Not all rheumatic diseases affect the joints directly. Nonarticular rheumatism encompasses rheumatic conditions of tissues around the joint—muscles, ligaments, tendons, fascia, bursa—rather than inside the joint. It also includes certain conditions in which pain is felt in joints far from the immediate cause.

Bursitis is an inflammation of a small lubricating sac, or bursa, located between a muscle and bone. Bursae, located throughout the body, reduce friction. One or multiple bursae may become inflamed, a condition called bursitis. Subdeltoid or shoulder bursitis is the best known, but any bursa can be affected. Symptoms include pain while lying on or moving the involved joint. Joint motion often is limited. Sometimes the bursal area is swollen, red, and tender.

Tendinitis is the inflammation of one or more tendons. It often is precipitated by injury. Persons in certain occupations are more likely to develop shoulder bursitis or tendinitis as a result of overuse or misuse of the joint. Symptoms of tendinitis are identical to those of bursitis.

Ligament problems result from strain or a tear. Ligaments also may become painful and tender as a result of chronic irritation. Tennis elbow (epicondylitis), described in Chapter 16, "The Bones and Muscles," is an example.

Bursitis, tendinitis, and tennis elbow are treated with anti-inflammatory drugs, cortisone injections, exercises, protective devices, and surgery in rare cases.

Nerve entrapments occur when nerves become compressed by distortions or inflammations.

Thoracic outlet syndrome occurs when poor posture, local injury, or congenital abnormalities narrow the upper rib cage opening where the nerves and major blood vessels pass from the chest cavity into the arm. The result is arm pain, numbness, and occasionally swelling, especially when sleeping, reaching, or carrying.

Carpal tunnel syndrome is described in Chapter 16, "The Bones and Muscles."

Fibromyositis, also known as fibrositis, is not a disease in the usual sense of the word because neither pathologic nor physiologic changes have been clearly demonstrated. However, the pattern of symptoms and, in many instances, the response to therapy is so characteristic that it is recognized as a disease. Patients with fibromyositis complain of pain in several areas arising from muscles and ligaments and tendons around the joints. The neck, shoulder, back, elbows, and outside of the thighs are common sites. On examination, the doctor finds tender areas that show no swelling, heat, or redness. These often are referred to as "trigger points" because pressure on one may cause pain in other places.

Patients sometimes are found to be under emotional or physical stress or may be depressed. Some experts believe that emotional tension is converted to painful muscle spasms. Treatment varies but generally consists of heat or ice applications, muscle relaxing and analgesic drugs, and injections of a combination of a local anesthetic and cortisone.

Osteoarthritis

Osteoarthritis sometimes is referred to as wear-and-tear arthritis or degenerative arthritis. Most experts agree that the breakdown process begins in cartilage or in bone under the cartilage. In otherwise healthy people, cartilage gradually deteriorates over many years, but in osteoarthritis, the process seems to be accelerated. Sometimes, a single traumatic event appears to be responsible; sometimes, multiple minor injuries appear to be. It should come as no surprise that former professional football players fall victim to osteoarthritis more often than people who have led more sedentary lives.

Some persons appear to be predisposed to develop osteoarthritis in many relatively inactive joints. Doctors suspect, based on experimental evidence, that increased amounts of certain enzymes cause a premature breakdown of cartilage. Also, certain metabolic diseases are associated with osteoarthritis (it is more common in people with diabetes, for example). Heredity plays a role in some cases; osteoarthritis confined to the small joints of the hands tends to run in families.

Osteoarthritis is the most common type of arthritis. Almost everyone over age 70 has osteoarthritis of the neck, although some are not bothered by it. Because deterioration is gradual, most cases of osteoarthritis are not diagnosed before age 40. Both sexes are affected. Women may notice that it appears abruptly after menopause.

Early symptoms are dull pain and stiffness in a few joints. At first, discomfort is most noticeable in mornings, but soon the patient may become aware of aches that come and go during the day. Mild activity or limbering up may lessen the symptoms, but extensive activity tends to worsen them.

As the disease becomes more advanced, pain is persistent and certain activities become laborious, even impossible. The physician's first examination may show little more than tenderness and mild swelling, or there may be bony protuberances (spurs), growths that interfere with joint motion. Redness and warmth are unusual, and rarely is joint motion severely painful until later in the course of the disease.

In advanced cases, the joint may actually crunch when moved, a phenomenon called crepitus. Range of motion is limited. Still later, certain joints may become loose or deformed. The hands may take on a snakelike appearance because of deviations in the small joints. If your fingers are knobby or bumpy, you may have early osteoarthritis. The base of the thumb is a common site, and may cause severe pain and disability.

When osteoarthritis strikes the neck, the disk spaces between the vertebrae almost always are compressed because of degeneration (cervical spondylosis). The process is not always painful, even when advanced. Patients may complain of pain in the back of the neck that shoots to the head or top of the shoulders. Bony spurs may compress nerve roots as they leave the spinal canal, causing pain that radiates into the hand and even muscle weakness in the arms.

Few people escape back pain during a lifetime. In the older age group, osteoarthritis seems the most common cause. The hips cannot be straightened, and the knees are bowed. Osteoarthritis of the ankle usually is a consequence of previous injury.

Osteoarthritis is painful and may limit function, but fortunately it rarely confines the sufferer to a wheelchair or bed.

There are several variations of osteoarthritis. Primary generalized osteoarthritis is a slowly progressive form characterized by involvement of more than one joint, especially in the hands. Modest inflammatory changes take place in the joints. In certain neurologic conditions, such as those caused by diabetes, the sensation of pain is diminished so that some joints cannot receive the body's message to ease up on an overstressed joint. The excess wear and tear causes a destructive "neuropathic arthritis." In avascular necrosis, blood supply to the joint is diminished. Bony tissue dies, and the ease of joint motion is altered. Secondary osteoarthritis sets in.

The method used to manage osteoarthritis depends on the number of joints involved, the degree of disability, and the person's tolerance for pain. A program of joint conservation—instructing the patient how to use the affected joints with minimum strain—helps prevent deformity. Certain occupations, for example, call for continued use of the hands and persistent stress. Protecting the joints with proper splints enables the joints' continued use and impedes the osteoarthritic process. With arthritis of the lower extremities, prolonged weight-bearing and continued stair climbing should be avoided. Canes, crutches, and walkers help remove weight from the joints.

Most rheumatologists have found aspirin and nonsteroid anti-inflammatory drugs beneficial for pain even though inflammation may not be apparent. Injections of cortisone into a few affected joints can alleviate pain, stiffness, and, to an extent, disability.

Surgery is helpful when there is intractable pain and need for improved function of the joint. Operative procedures include débridement (removal of destroyed tissues), arthroplasty (joint reconstruction), and joint replacement, described below. Osteotomy is an operation in which a wedge of bone is removed for better joint realignment.

Rheumatoid Arthritis

Rheumatoid arthritis is a chronic inflammatory condition not only of the joints, but of some internal organs as well. It strikes most commonly between ages 20 and 45. It is characterized by persistent pain, progressive deformity, and at its worst, profound disability. Rheumatoid arthritis usually starts insidiously. In early stages, the hands, feet, and other joints ache and are stiff. The patient has difficulty with fine finger movements such as buttoning. He or she is clumsy and tends to walk stiff-legged because full weight-bearing causes pain in the hips, knees, and toes. He or she has morning stiffness that lasts several hours. The joints gradually swell and become difficult to move. Forming a fist, for example, becomes nearly impossible. At first, symptoms may be intermittent, but gradually they become persistent and involve almost all the joints in the body. Most patients are so tired that even a minimal chore is exhausting.

The inflammatory process eventually invades cartilage and the surrounding structures. The joint capsule, tendons, and ligaments may become contracted or overstretched, and joint deformities may result. Nodules may develop beneath the surface of the skin in areas of friction. The heart, lungs, spleen, eye, and blood vessels may become in-

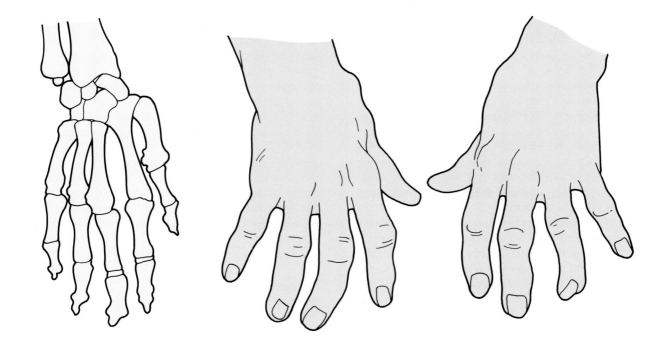

ARTHRITIS OF THE HAND
Small joints of the fingers are a common site of arthritis. Degenerative changes in the joint, joint space narrowing, and spur formation give the fingers a snakelike configuration and a *square appearance at the base of the thumb. The changes are seen on X rays. Arthritis confined to the finger joints appears to run in families.*

volved. Sjögren's syndrome is a complication that causes malfunction and dryness of the lubricating glands of the mouth, eyes, respiratory tract, vagina, and rectum (see Chapter 14, "The Eyes").

The inflammatory change and deformities of advanced rheumatoid arthritis are so characteristic that diagnosis is not difficult. Until significant changes are seen, however, diagnosis may be difficult. Rheumatoid factor (see above) is found in the serum of most patients, sometimes in concentrated amounts. X rays may show loss of bone density, cysts or erosions, and even complete destruction of the joint.

The cause of rheumatoid arthritis, despite thousands of experimental investigations, is not known.

The most prevalent theory is that a virus, small bacterium, or other microorganism is harbored in the joint. Local tissues form antibodies against the foreign invader, but in the process of interacting with the microorganisms, the antibodies become altered and are no longer recognized by the body itself. The body forms new antibodies to fight the altered old ones (rheumatoid factor). This immune reaction triggers a flood of inflammatory substances that increase the surrounding circulation with swelling, heat, and sometimes redness. Somehow, the process becomes self-perpetuating.

Management of rheumatoid arthritis is complex, but drugs play a major role. Analgesics, nonsteroidal anti-inflammatory drugs, systemic cortisone, cortisone injections into the joints, and a group of drugs called remittive agents, including gold salts, penicillamine, and antimalarial drugs, used singly or in combination, are helpful for most patients. The remittive group is most likely to sustain improvement but must be administered for months or even years, and this group has more side effects.

But drugs used without other supporting methods are likely to fail. Physical and occupational therapies play valuable roles. Heat, cold, exercises, splints, braces, and supportive devices not only prevent and correct deformity, but relieve pain. Most patients fail to realize that a single warm towel over an inflamed joint usually will provide as much relief as a potent analgesic.

Almost all patients with rheumatoid arthritis can benefit from some form of physical or occupational therapy. One of the most important phases of the management of rheumatoid arthritis is joint conservation, because it minimizes stress and prevents further damage.

Thirty years ago, joint surgery in rheumatoid arthritis was virtually unheard of. Today, inflamed joint linings are successfully removed to alleviate pain and impede destructive changes. Joints can be realigned. Numerous surgical restorative procedures are available for most joints, including partial or total replacement. Older patients with rheumatoid arthritis often are concerned about whether they can tolerate the surgery. Generally, age is no barrier.

Juvenile Rheumatoid Arthritis

Three forms of juvenile rheumatoid arthritis are recognized. About 50 percent of patients with juvenile rheumatoid arthritis have what is termed the polyarticular form, which means more than one joint is affected. These children tend to have less morning stiffness and greater involvement of the neck, sacroiliac, and temporomandibular jaw joints. They also have more flexion contractures, in which the joints tense and contract and fail to maintain normal alignment. The jaw may be recessed (micrognathia), and the child may stop growing before reaching normal height. There is a greater tendency for fever and a transient, orange-tinted rash on the torso. Nodules under the skin are rare.

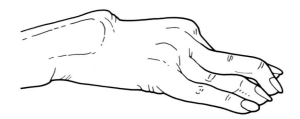

HAND DEFORMITIES
Deformity of the hand joints is common in advanced rheumatoid arthritis. The "swan-neck deformity" is named for its S-shaped curvature of the fingers. Such deformities can make simple acts such as writing or buttoning difficult.

A second type, pauciarticular rheumatoid arthritis, involves fewer joints and affects about one-third of child victims. Knees, ankles, hips, elbows, and wrists are most commonly involved. Fortunately, this type tends to disappear by the teens, although some cases go on to the polyarticular phase. While the joint manifestations of pauciarticular arthritis are more benign than other types, inflammation of the anterior chamber of the eye (iritis) can lead to blindness.

A few children have the acute systemic form of juvenile rheumatoid arthritis called Still's disease. They may become suddenly and seriously ill with high temperatures, a generalized rash, lymph node enlargement, and even involvement of the heart, lungs, and spleen. The joints may appear not to be involved, in which case diagnosis often is difficult.

Rheumatoid arthritis in children is managed as in adults, but with great emphasis on educational programs, physical therapy, recreational programs, and emotional support. Drugs and surgery are used to a lesser degree. Aspirin is a mainstay. Cortisone helps to reduce inflammation but has numerous side effects, including stunted growth.

The treatment goals in children are to reduce pain, prevent deformity, maintain function, and prevent blindness by periodic eye examinations.

Ankylosing Spondylitis

Ankylosing spondylitis, an inflammation of the spinal and sacroiliac joints, strikes mainly young and middle-aged men. Initial symptoms are low back pain on either or both sides. Stiffness is profound, particularly in the morning. Gradually, pain ascends along the spine. The neck tightens, until after several years, it may be difficult or impossible to turn the head. In advanced cases, the spine becomes rigidly straight, so the victim cannot bend or sit.

Almost all persons with ankylosing spondylitis have HLA (human leukocytic antigen) B27, a specific type of genetic marker detected on white blood cells (see Chapter 7, "The Blood"). HLA B27 may be likened to the blood types A, B, or O, but only 4 to 8 percent of the population bear this genetic marker, thus simplifying diagnosis.

Management programs for ankylosing spondylitis emphasize physical therapy to maintain good posture and drugs to reduce inflammation. Aspirin and other nonsteroid anti-inflammatory drugs play a valuable role. Surgery is restricted to realigning badly deformed spines.

Psoriatic Arthritis And Reiter's Syndrome

Most patients are surprised to learn that psoriasis, a chronic scaling disease of the skin (see Chapter 9, "The Skin"), is associated with arthritis. In some cases, arthritis symptoms precede the skin rash. Young and middle-aged adults are the most frequent sufferers. In this condition, which closely resembles rheumatoid arthritis, several joints become acutely or chronically inflamed with pain, redness, heat, and swelling. Involvement in the hand joints and diffuse swelling of the fingers or toes (sausage digit) are striking. It is not clear how psoriasis relates to arthritis.

Reiter's syndrome is a peculiar combination of arthritis, conjunctivitis (pink eye), urethritis (redness and discharge at the opening of the penis), balanitis (inflammation of the penis), keratoderma blennorrhagica (rash on the palms and soles with nail changes), and painless mouth ulcers.

In both psoriatic arthritis and Reiter's syndrome, anti-inflammatory drugs and local injections of cortisone relieve pain and disability. The course of both diseases is unpredictable. Attacks are briefer and lead to less damage than in rheumatoid arthritis.

Gout and Pseudogout

Gout has been known as the "rich man's disease" and "the disease of kings" because it notoriously affects high-livers and overindulgers of wine and food. Anyone may develop gout, however. Middle-aged and older men are most prone; women almost never have gout before menopause.

Gout usually appears suddenly. One or two joints, often adjoining each other, become inflamed. The typical patient reports going to bed feeling well but awakening during the night with excruciating pain, usually in the big toe. Untreated, the attacks usually subside in a few days, but may recur periodically.

Gout strikes people who have excessive amounts of uric acid in the body. Crystals of the acid collect in the connective tissues, notably the joints. Over the years, the crystals coalesce to form larger collections, known as tophi. These are often visible as nodules just below the surface of the skin, particularly in the elbows and hands.

Most attacks of gout occur without explanation, but some are precipitated by stress, injury, increased alcohol intake, and dietary excesses, hence the presumed association with high living.

Treatment of gout is designed to reduce acute inflammation and prevent recurrences. With potent anti-inflammatory drugs or colchicine, an old drug produced from the roots of the meadow saffron, a properly treated attack will subside in 24 to 48 hours. Colchicine also may be prescribed daily for several years to prevent further attacks. Probenecid (Benemid) and sulfinpyrazone (Anturane) reduce blood uric acid by promoting excretion through the kidneys. Allopurinol (Zyloprim) is another effective drug that controls uric acid by preventing its formation. Large crystal deposits may be removed surgically.

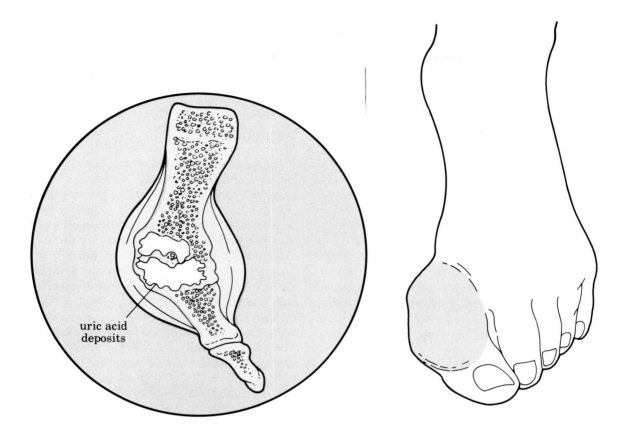

A GOUT ATTACK
An acute attack of gout usually strikes the joint of the big toe, causing swelling and extreme pain. It occurs when crystals of uric acid (urate) are deposited in the joint (enlarged drawing). Gout frequently appears suddenly, often striking while the person is asleep. Pain and swelling may subside within a few days without treatment, but may recur later.

Pseudogout gets its name from its resemblance to gout. But instead of the uric acid crystals, the culprit is a calcium pyrophosphate particle. As in gout, one or several joints are acutely inflamed, but there are no tophi. Treatment includes nonsteroidal anti-inflammatory drugs and aspiration of joint fluid.

Systemic Lupus Erythematosus (SLE)

SLE is prototypical of connective tissue disease, a group of disorders caused by nonspecific, noninfectious inflammation of the supporting systems of the body and internal organs (see also Chapter 9, "The Skin"). The diseases apparently stem from autoimmunity, the phenomenon by which the body forms antibodies against some of its own tissues. The process may strike the joints, skin, blood vessels, nervous system, muscles, kidneys, or lining of the heart, lungs, and other internal organs. Tissue destruction can result.

Full-blown SLE most often strikes women, mostly young to middle-aged; it is rare after menopause. SLE causes fever, arthritis, mouth ulcers, loss of hair, kidney disease, pleurisy, pericarditis (inflammation of the heart lining), seizures, and other nervous system problems. A sun-sensitive rash may appear over any part of the body, but a butterfly-shaped blush over the nose and cheeks most commonly characterizes the disease. All organs may suddenly be affected simultaneously, or they may be affected in turn. The extent of illness in SLE varies. Some patients are desperately ill; others have recurrent, mild episodes for years.

Cortisone derivatives are the mainstay of therapy. Sometimes, high doses by mouth or injection are needed. Other drugs that suppress the immune system also may be tried. Plasmapheresis, a method of removing blood and treating red cells (see Chapter 7, "The Blood"), is used in severe cases.

Systemic Sclerosis
(Scleroderma)

Systemic sclerosis is an uncommon connective tissue disease in which the skin is the major target. It results from excessive deposits of collagen, the main structural protein of the body. Initially, the skin over the extremities becomes swollen and then taut, giving a "hidebound" appearance. Skin may turn color and be punctuated by small ulcers at the fingertips. As the skin tightens, joints contract in flexion, particularly the elbows and fingers. The mouth opening narrows, the nose beaks, and breathing may be restricted because drum-tight skin over the chest limits expansion. Internal organs may be affected, notably the esophagus, lower gastrointestinal tract, kidneys, lungs, and heart. Swallowing may become difficult, and diarrhea may ensue. If the kidneys or lungs are attacked, the disease is fatal.

To a degree, the flexion contractures can be prevented by physical and occupational therapies. Swallowing difficulty can be eased by medication, but the skin cannot be predictably softened. The internal organs, in particular, fail to respond to treatment.

Vasculitis

Vasculitis is characterized by inflammation and blockage of arteries and their branches. There are many different types, each having its own complex of symptoms. The best known is polyarteritis nodosa, in which the blocked vessels prevent blood from flowing to vital organs, damaging them.

A peculiar type of vasculitis is referred to as giant-cell arteritis or temporal arteritis. It involves the blood vessels of the head, almost always in the elderly. On one side of the head, headaches, visual disturbance, and pain on chewing may develop, depending upon which blood vessels are inflamed. Much less frequently, strokes may occur. Temporal arteritis sometimes is associated with polymyalgia rheumatica, a type of rheumatism that affects the elderly and is easily confused with rheumatoid arthritis. In this disorder, the entire body aches, especially the neck, shoulders, back, thighs, and groin. Stiffness may be profound, particularly in the morning. Patients are apt to feel depressed or fatigued, and may appear to be chronically ill. Cortisone derivatives are an effective treatment for temporal arteritis and polymyalgia rheumatica.

Polymyositis

In polymyositis, the muscles become inflamed, causing weakness and a limited degree of pain. Sometimes disability is so profound that the patient finds it difficult to rise from a chair, put on a coat, or lift. Polymyositis may be accompanied by a prominent rash on the face, chest, extremities, and knuckles (dermatomyositis). Diagnosis is made by finding elevated enzymes from muscle in the blood, by special tests to measure muscle activity (electromyogram), and by muscle biopsy. Treatment with high doses of cortisone usually is effective.

MANAGEMENT OF ARTHRITIS AND RELATED DISEASES

Dramatic cures are not likely in arthritis and similar diseases, but as a result of a comprehensive approach to most arthritis patients, marked improvements in pain relief and lessened disability can be achieved.

Drugs

There are many different types of drugs for arthritis, each used in a different way.

Anti-inflammatory drugs. Aspirin and related compounds have been in widespread use to reduce inflammation since the beginning of the century. Most people are familiar with aspirin as a pain killer and headache remedy, but for reasons that are not understood, it also reduces inflammation significantly. Inexpensive and available in many forms, aspirin is the standard against which other nonsteroid anti-inflammatory drugs are measured.

To be most effective, aspirin must be given in proper doses. For the average person, this means 10 to 14 five-grain tablets daily. Most patients can tolerate even higher doses. It is important to take the medication with food to prevent gastrointestinal irritation. Other side effects of aspirin include ringing of the ears, temporary deafness, and small amounts of bleeding through the gastrointestinal tract. In more serious cases, there may be gastric and small bowel ulcers, abdominal cramps, and more extensive hemorrhage. True aspirin allergy, resulting in a rash and wheezing, is rare.

In 1952, phenylbutazone and subsequently a closely related compound, oxyphenbutazone, were introduced as potent anti-inflammatory drugs (grouped with aspirin in the "nonsteroid" category to distinguish them from the steroid cortisone and its derivatives). Several nonsteroid anti-inflammatory drugs have since been approved by the U.S. Food and Drug Administration. These include ibuprofen (Motrin), naproxen (Naprosyn), indomethacin (Indocin), sulindac (Clinoril), and pirox-

icam (Feldene). These drugs do not contain aspirin, but have about the same effectiveness. Side effects vary. Each can cause gastrointestinal upset, but less often than aspirin. Ringing in the ears, deafness, and metabolic disturbances do not develop as with aspirin. However, skin rash and fluid retention are not uncommon. These drugs must be administered cautiously to persons with high blood pressure and congestive heart failure. Usually, a doctor will try them sequentially to identify the most helpful in an individual case.

Unquestionably, the most potent anti-inflammatory agent is cortisone, classed as a steroid hormone, and its derivatives. Synthetic cortisone, or prednisone, can effectively reduce joint inflammation, and inflammation of the internal organs can be brought under control with the administration of relatively large doses.

The response of a sick person to cortisone and its derivatives may be dramatic. Some patients are symptom-free only two days after being extremely sick with a life-threatening illness. But high doses bring numerous side effects. Indeed, all patients who take enough cortisone in large enough doses will suffer some unwanted reaction.

Injection therapy. Cortisone derivatives can be injected safely into joints, bursae, tendon sheaths, and other areas to reduce inflammation. Cortisone administered this way does not enter the general circulation and thus is less likely to cause the multiple toxic effects that occur when it is given by other routes.

Remittive agents. Gold salts, penicillamine, and antimalarial drugs are classed as remittive agents because they are capable of bringing about a complete or partial remission, in which all symptoms and signs of arthritis have disappeared.

Gold salts. Gold has been used for more than 50 years to treat rheumatoid arthritis, although the way it works is not understood. It usually has been reserved for severe cases, but there is a trend toward using it earlier in the disease. Gold is effective; more than half the patients experience good to excellent results. It usually takes at least six weeks to see benefits.

Gold is injected into the muscle weekly at first, but gradually the frequency is reduced to monthly maintenance doses. Recently, an oral form of gold

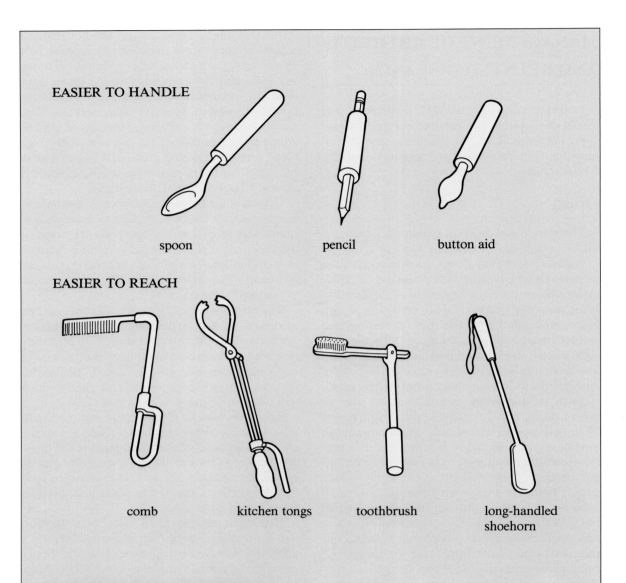

EASIER TO HANDLE

spoon   pencil   button aid

EASIER TO REACH

comb   kitchen tongs   toothbrush   long-handled
shoehorn

Rehabilitation and Self-Help

Keeping the patient independent is an important part of arthritis therapy. Self-help devices like those illustrated here relieve pain and reduce stress loads on stiffened or painful arthritic joints. Many of them may be purchased commercially or may be fashioned at home, or by a physician or physical therapist. Clothing can be altered to make dressing, buttoning, and lacing shoes easier.

Joint conservation methods also may be learned and may be helpful to arthritics. A simple example teaches patients to carry with two extended hands rather than stressing a painful wrist joint by carrying with the handle in one hand. Many books are available on self-help techniques from libraries and arthritis support organizations.

has been introduced and is more effective for some people. Although gold causes side effects, primarily in the skin, kidneys, and blood, these reactions have been exaggerated. Almost everyone can tolerate gold, and if problems develop, the drug can be discontinued temporarily.

Antimalarial compounds like chloroquine and hydroxychloroquine accidentally were found to be helpful in treatment of rheumatoid arthritis as well as malaria. The drugs are administered by mouth once or twice daily and, like gold, take more than six weeks to produce a response. Adverse reactions include nausea and damage to the cornea and retina of the eye. That damage can diminish vision if the drugs are taken in high doses for many years. Therefore, periodic eye exams are necessary.

Penicillamine, used in rheumatoid arthritis, is chemically related to penicillin but is not an antibiotic. It is administered orally in increasing doses until a satisfactory response is achieved. Complete remission with loss of joint inflammation has been seen in many cases. Penicillamine usually is reserved for patients with severe rheumatoid arthritis who fail to respond to other forms of therapy.

Cytotoxic agents, including methotrexate, cyclophosphamine, and azathioprine, sometimes are used. Originally designed for cancer treatment, these agents have proven helpful in some cases of rheumatoid arthritis, lupus, vasculitis, and polymyositis, where they can be lifesaving and sometimes achieve total control. Although dosages are much smaller than in cancer treatment, these drugs retain the potential for serious side effects.

Physical and Occupational Therapy

Physical and occupational therapy programs are exceedingly important in the management of almost all types of arthritis.

Rest. Rest may be interpreted in different ways. Complete confinement to bed is not necessary or desirable. Prolonged bed rest deconditions the body and can cause significant shrinkage and weakening of the muscles. However, both physical and emotional stress often aggravate the arthritic process, so arthritics should not push themselves to the point of fatigue.

Resting the involved joints also is important in order to relieve pain, to prevent deformity caused by overstretched ligaments or tendons, and to allow inflammation to subside. The arms and legs can be rested by use of pillows, splints, casts, and

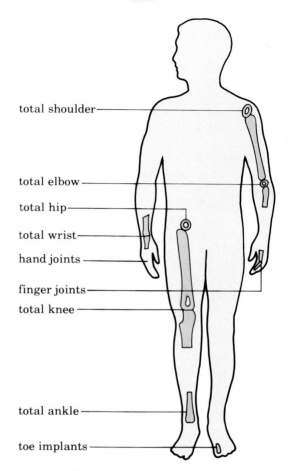

total shoulder

total elbow

total hip

total wrist

hand joints

finger joints

total knee

total ankle

toe implants

REPLACEABLE JOINTS
Artificial joints often can restore motion and eliminate pain and stiffness for many arthritics. The diagram above shows which joints can be replaced. Artificial hip, knee, and finger joints are most successful. Others are still in the developmental stage.

braces. A simple, inexpensive canvas splint for the wrist is desirable for maintaining normal use and alleviating pain.

Exercise. Daily exercise of both arthritic and nonarthritic joints is important in order to maintain functional range of motion, to prevent further deforming changes, and to strengthen weakened muscles. Exercise can prevent pain by gently stretching contracted tendons or by eliminating small degrees of instability. Exercise can be prescribed even if the person is confined to bed. A therapist's help is needed for a few exercises, but most exercises can be performed by the patient independently.

Heat and cold. Heat or cold can help the arthritic joints and the surrounding muscles. Cold appears to be preferred by most patients to relieve pain of injuries, and heat is preferred for more chronic, persistent types of arthritis. A towel must be placed between the hot pack and the skin in all cases to avoid severe burns. There is no support for the colloquialism "the hotter the better." The proper temperature is the one that feels comfortable and relieves pain.

Massage and manipulation. When combined with manipulation of the joints, massage may reduce muscle spasms and improve range of motion. Traction also is used to stretch contracted or improperly aligned joints. In the case of cervical or lumbar disk disease, intermittent traction appears to reduce pain and muscle spasm.

Assistive and self-help devices. Canes, crutches, wheelchairs, braces, and certain shoes are examples of assistive devices that aid movement by relieving pain and reducing stress loads. These devices require instruction by trained personnel.

When, despite all therapeutic attempts, no way can be found to improve function of individual joints so that a person can operate independently, self-help devices may be useful.

Joint conservation. With or without self-help devices, patients can be instructed in the proper use of their joints in daily living. For example, it's often easier for a person with arthritic hands to hold a pot between two extended palms rather than stressing the wrist by holding it by the handle with one hand. Similar physical and occupational therapy can be self-taught or taught by the physician or physician's assistant. More sophisticated therapy programs are best administered by occupational or physical therapists.

Arthritis Surgery

Total joint replacement surpasses the advantages of medication in cases of advanced disease. Relief from pain and significant gains in range of motion can be obtained in all patients. Complications of surgery are not common.

Artificial joints of the hands are made of a silicone rubber compound, Silastic, that is extremely flexible but durable. The larger hip joint usually consists of three components: a high-density polyethylene or plastic cup that serves as the socket of the hip, a smooth stainless steel ball that serves as the head of the thighbone, and a methyl methacrylate cement that holds the two in place. Similar combinations of plastic and stainless steel are found in knee replacements. Total joint replacements have become so successful that other forms of joint surgery, including arthroplasty (remodeling of the joint) and synovectomy (removal of the inflamed joint lining), have become much less common. Other surgical procedures include tendon transplants; osteotomy, in which a wedge of bone is removed so that the limb may be straightened; and joint fusion, which sacrifices joint mobility to provide stability and relieve pain. In addition, impinged nerves may be released by cutting surrounding soft tissues. In some instances, arthritis surgery can be preventive, such as removing a jagged end of a wrist bone that could injure the hand tendons.

Hospitalization

Most patients with arthritis-related diseases do well while living at home. However, hospitalization may be needed for those who fail to respond to outpatient treatment. This is particularly true in patients who require certain treatments not available outside the hospital. Hospitalization may make it easier to provide medication and physical therapy, and is required for most types of surgery. The hospital provides a setting in which the patient can be treated not only by the attending physician but by the orthopedic surgeon, physiatrists (specialists in physical medicine), psychiatrists, psychologists, social workers, vocational rehabilitation counselors, occupational and physical therapists, and arthritis rehabilitation nurses.

Weather, Spas, Acupuncture, and Diet

Weather. It is not an old wives' tale that patients with arthritis become achy before a storm. Controlled scientific studies have proven that most patients worsen within a few hours after the start of a drop in barometric pressure and a rise in humidity. Indeed, some patients claim to be greatly improved in the southwestern part of the United States, where the climate is dry and the atmospheric pressure is stable. Patients who are contemplating a move solely for relief should be warned that changes in job, removal from precipitating stresses, relaxation, and different patterns of exercise also might be responsible for improvement. The decision to move to a different climate must be based on medical, psychological, and economic factors.

Spas throughout the world, particularly in Europe, promise relief and even cures for arthritis. These warm baths, most of them alkaline, frequently do make the patient feel better, at least temporarily. But cures are not to be had for most types of arthritis as a result of spa therapy. Although some spas have been operating for centuries, the effects of mineralized water still are not proven.

Acupuncture has been used effectively in certain types of musculoskeletal conditions, but in the systemic forms of arthritis with multiple joint involvement, results have been disappointing. In the few investigative studies completed, objective signs of inflammation have not been altered by use of acupuncture.

Special diets for rheumatoid and other types of arthritis sometimes are recommended in publications. Under certain circumstances, a low purine diet may help patients with gout. A weight-reduction diet may ease the pressure on the joints in an obese person. Otherwise, the role of diet in causing or relieving arthritic symptoms is not clear.

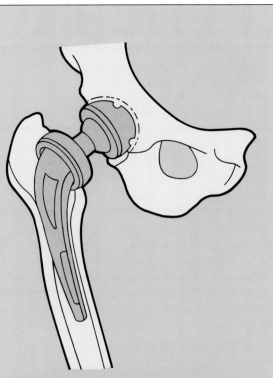

Total Hip Replacement

Replacement of the hip joint has become one of the most commonly performed, and successful, orthopedic procedures. The hip socket is replaced by a polyethylene or plastic cup cemented into place; a stainless steel ball is then fitted into the head of the thighbone, and moves smoothly in the new socket. The person usually can walk with crutches within a few days and without crutches in a few weeks. Near-normal movement is restored in more than 90 percent of cases. In many persons, both hips may be replaced. With time, further degeneration may cause the joint to loosen, but a second replacement then may be performed.

CHAPTER 18

THE HORMONES AND ENDOCRINE GLANDS

Hormones (the word comes from a Greek word meaning to excite or stimulate) are chemicals secreted into the bloodstream by special cells. Carried by the blood, hormones reach other cells in the body and stimulate these cells. The exact number of hormones produced and secreted within the human body is not known, and perhaps never will be. (There may be as many as 100.) Altogether, the hormones make up one of the major control systems for regulating the body's activities.

Most hormones are secreted by special tissues that do little or nothing else. These are the endocrine glands, the glands of internal secretion. In some cases, a hormone comes from a specialized cell that is not a gland, but part of another organ. There are hormone-producing cells in the stomach, intestinal walls, kidneys, heart, skin, even the brain.

Although we often refer to this control system for regulating body activity and metabolism as the "endocrine system," the functions and activities of the system are not limited to the endocrine glands. The functional unit of the endocrine system is the hormone, not the gland.

Deficiencies of hormone production or secretion can have widespread effects throughout the body.

THE ENDOCRINE GLANDS
The endocrine glands distributed throughout the body produce most hormones, but others are made in the brain, stomach and intestine, and perhaps elsewhere. Hormones act on parts of the body far from the site of production, and also interact with each other. Most hormones are present in only very small amounts, and only recently have some of them been identified. Male and female endocrine systems are the same except for the gonads, or sex glands.

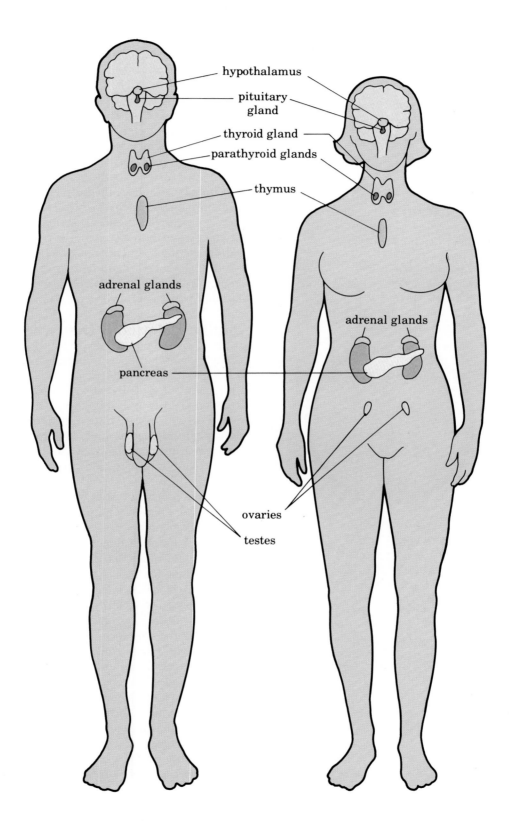

hypothalamus

pituitary gland

thyroid gland

parathyroid glands

thymus

adrenal glands

adrenal glands

pancreas

ovaries

testes

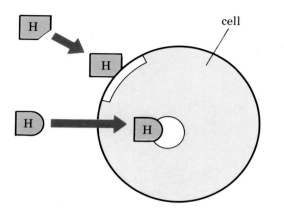

A HORMONE IN ACTION

In order to act, a hormone (labeled H in the drawing above) must attach to a specific receptor on the cell surface or inside the cell. Like a key and lock, only certain hormones fit certain receptors, allowing them to act on the cell body.

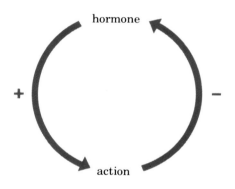

THE FEEDBACK SYSTEM

Secretion of a hormone stimulates a cell's action, indicated by the plus symbol in the drawing. When action reaches a certain level, secretion is shut off by the action itself, indicated by the minus symbol. The system is called negative feedback and helps the body to maintain homeostasis, its state of normal balance.

The Hypothalamus and Pituitary

The pituitary gland, in the center of the skull, underneath the brain, used to be called the body's master gland, the maestro that directed all the other endocrine glands. It is now known that the pituitary is under the direction of the hypothalamus, a portion of the brain directly above it. The hypothalamic-pituitary relationship guides many of the body's functions, including reproduction, metabolism, and even reaction to stress. Hormones cued by the hypothalamus and secreted by the pituitary stimulate other glands to secrete their own hormones, which "switch on" these functions. An intricate feedback system notifies the pituitary when the action has been completed, and the stimulating hormones are switched off again.

The hypothalamus and pituitary are illustrated on page 217, and a listing and explanation of pituitary hormones appears on page 218.

Pituitary Hormone Deficiency

If a pituitary hormone is not being produced, or is being secreted in insufficient amounts to carry out its function, or if secretion is so great that the target organ is overstimulated, characteristic symptoms will be seen. If thyroid-stimulating hormone is missing, for example, the thyroid will be underactive or hypothyroid. Symptoms include fatigue, lethargy, puffiness, and, occasionally, weight gain.

The two principal causes of pituitary hormone deficiency are pituitary tumors and hypothalamic disease. Sometimes the hypothalamic disease stems from a kind of tumor known as craniopharyngioma, but other times its cause is unknown. Careful testing for each of the pituitary hormones will define which ones are missing so the treatment can be designed specifically for that patient.

A child who lacks growth hormone can be given injections of the substance and will grow to a fairly normal height. Human growth hormone is expensive and is now made entirely in the laboratory using techniques of recombinant DNA. Whether this expensive hormone will work in other types of short children needs further study.

Replacing the other missing pituitary hormones is less difficult because a different hormone usually can be substituted. For example, thyroid hormone will compensate for the lack of thyroid-stimulating

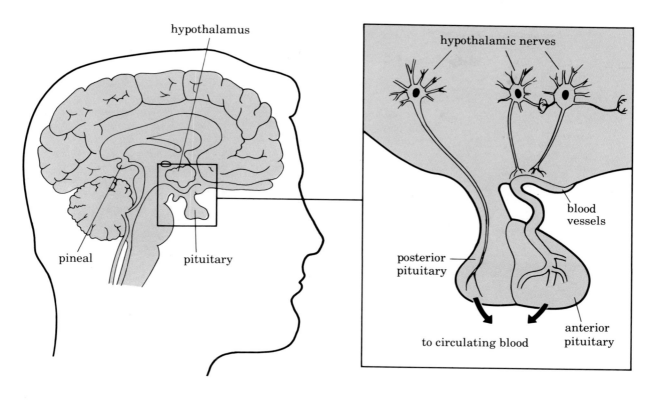

THE HYPOTHALAMUS AND PITUITARY

The hypothalamus in the brain connects to and controls the pituitary gland. Hypothalamic nerves run into the posterior pituitary and secrete posterior pituitary hormones directly into the blood. Other portions of the hypothalamus secrete hormones into blood vessels that carry them into the anterior pituitary and stimulate secretions of hormones directly from there into the circulating blood. Still other hypothalamic nerves appear to act in other parts of the brain. The pineal gland's function is not clear. In other animals, it is influenced by light and plays a role in reproduction.

hormone (TSH). For a deficiency of follicle-stimulating hormone (FSH) or luteinizing hormone (LH), testosterone usually is the treatment in men and estrogen in women.

Correcting pituitary hormonal deficiency does nothing for the disease that caused it. Since the cause is often a tumor in the pituitary, the usual approach is either surgery or radiation. In the past, pituitary surgery was difficult and somewhat hazardous, because the gland lies deep within the skull. In recent years, a surgical technique called transsphenoidal hypophysectomy, which enables the surgeon to go back under the nose to the pituitary, has made the operation much safer.

Excessive Pituitary Hormones

Too much pituitary hormone production usually is limited to only a single pituitary hormone and almost always is caused by a pituitary tumor.

Excessive growth hormone secretion causes acromegaly in a fully grown person or giantism in a person who has not yet reached adulthood. Acromegaly literally means an increase in the size of the hands and feet, but there also is enlargement of the nose, jaw, tissues over the eyes, and many of the internal organs, such as the liver and heart. The facial features become coarse with thickened skin and the tongue enlarges. Acromegaly usually is slowly progressive and is hard to detect in its early stages. Family and friends may not even

Gland	Hormone
Hypothalamus and brain	Thyrotropin-releasing hormone (TRH) LH-releasing hormone (LRH) Growth hormone-releasing factor (GHRF) ACTH-releasing factor (CRF) Prolactin-releasing factor (PRF) Somatostatin Neurotensin Substance P Endorphins/enkephalins Catecholamines: norepinephrine, epinephrine, dopamine
Pineal	Melatonin
Anterior pituitary	Thyrotropin (TSH) Follicle-stimulating hormone (FSH) Luteinizing hormone (LH) Corticotropin (ACTH) Growth hormone (GH) Prolactin (PRL)
Posterior pituitary	Vasopressin (ADH) Oxytocin
Thyroid	Thyroxine (T_4) Triiodothyronine (T_3) Calcitonin
Parathyroid	Parathyroid hormone (PTH)
Adrenal cortex	Hydrocortisone (cortisol) Aldosterone
Adrenal medulla	Epinephrine Norepinephrine
Ovary	Estradiol Progesterone Relaxin Inhibin
Testis	Testosterone Inhibin
Placenta	Estradiol Progesterone Chorionic gonadotropin Placental lactogen
Pancreatic islet	Insulin Glucagon Somatostatin
Kidney	Renin (leads to angiotensin II) Erythrogenin (leads to erythropoietin) Activated vitamin D (from skin)
Thymus	Thymosin Thymopoietin

THE PRINCIPAL HORMONES AND GLANDS

Each hormone has a distinctive role (or roles) to play in the body. Those secreted by the hypothalamus influence the anterior and posterior pituitary, which in turn secretes hormones that "switch on" the other glands. Thyroid hormones regulate metabolism. Parathyroids influence calcium in the blood. Placental hormones are present only in pregnancy. Although most of the pancreas produces digestive juices, specialized cells in the islets of Langerhans make hormones, including insulin, which help to regulate sugar in the blood.

notice the changes because they occur so gradually. Looking at old photographs may suddenly disclose what has happened over the years.

Giantism is acromegaly that begins before the bones have stopped growing. The ultimate height can reach 8 to 9 feet. Note, however, that the overwhelming majority of basketball players and other tall persons are naturally tall, the product of genes and nutrition, not disease.

Both acromegaly and giantism decrease life expectancy and should be treated. Because the cause is almost always a pituitary tumor, the treatment is radiation, surgery, or a combination of the two. With treatment, many of the changes in the soft tissues will return toward normal. Changes in bones such as the jaw, however, are permanent.

Sometimes a child, usually a girl, grows far sooner and more rapidly than her peers. Her parents become worried and remain so even though growth hormone measurements are normal. The problem is cultural, not physical. In our society, it is easy to be a tall man but difficult to be a tall woman, and very difficult to be a 10-year-old who towers over her classmates.

The ultimate height of a rapidly growing girl can be limited, although most physicians would advise against it. The easiest method is to induce early puberty by giving the girl estrogens. By giving estrogen well before puberty occurs, one can stop bone growth at a younger age.

Excessive prolactin secretion can cause galactorrhea, which is secretion of breast milk anytime except after giving birth. The condition is more common in women, but occurs in men, too. Men may have no accompanying symptoms except impotence. Women often have disrupted menstrual periods or the periods may stop entirely. Here, too, the cause usually is a pituitary tumor. The usual treatment is surgical removal of the tumor.

Excessive ACTH secretion causes a similarly excessive secretion of hydrocortisone from the adrenal cortex and leads to Cushing's disease.

THE THYROID GLAND

The thyroid gland is in the front of the neck and weighs about an ounce. It has two lobes, lying on each side of the midline and joined just below the larynx. If the neck muscles are thin, you can see the thyroid gland move upward during swallowing. An enlarged thyroid or a lump on the gland thus can be felt or seen on examination.

The thyroid takes iodine from the blood and makes it into the two thyroid hormones, thyroxine (T_4) and triiodothyronine (T_3), which it then secretes on signal from the pituitary hormone thyrotropin, or TSH.

The thyroid hormones together act to maintain the metabolism of the entire body. They enhance oxygen consumption, speed up chemical reactions, and help the brain develop and function properly. They help determine whether we are hungry or full, energetic or tired, nervous or calm. With too little thyroid hormone, we become mentally sluggish and physically lethargic. With too much, we become jumpy, irritable, and ravenous.

Thyroid secretion is an excellent example of how hormones are controlled by negative feedback. Secretion of the thyroid hormones depends on the secretion of thyrotropin (TSH), which in turn is controlled by TRH, the thyrotropin-releasing hormone from the hypothalamus. When T_4 and T_3 reach the proper levels, negative feedback inhibits further secretion of thyrotropin. An interruption anywhere in the chain can disturb normal thyroid function. Thyroid hormone deficiency, or hypothyroidism, occurs if either TRH or TSH is missing, or if the thyroid itself is defective, which is by far the most common cause. An overactive thyroid (hyperthyroidism) produces too much thyroid secretion and is almost always caused by a thyroid problem.

For the elderly, the consequences of poor thyroid function are less clear-cut. Mild hypothyroidism occurs in 4 to 7 percent of persons over age 60, especially in women. But the symptoms are nonspecific and resemble those occurring in many older persons, such as tiredness or changes in memory.

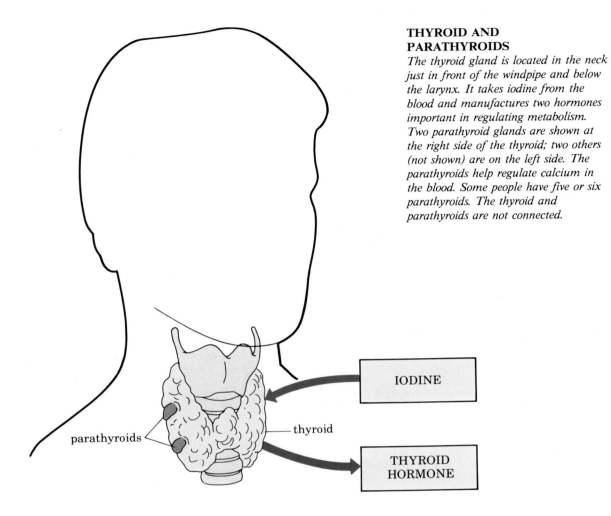

IODINE

THYROID
HORMONE

parathyroids

thyroid

Most hypothyroidism is caused by damage to the thyroid gland itself, and is called primary hypothyroidism. In the newborn, the likely cause is abnormal development of the thyroid. In adults, it usually is caused by either chronic inflammatory destruction of the gland or by previous treatment of hyperthyroidism, which has tilted the balance from too much hormone to too little.

Primary hypothyroidism caused by chronic inflammation of the thyroid usually occurs because of a faulty immune system. The body mistakenly attacks its own thyroid. This immunologic defect often runs in families. The defect also may be part of a pattern in which other glands, especially the adrenals and parathyroid, are affected.

The treatment of hypothyroidism is to replace or supplement the missing hormone. Most patients take daily tablets of synthetic thyroxine (T_4), but the proper interval and amount of thyroxine is not the same for everyone. The correct amount is the dose that brings the thyrotropin down into the normal range.

Because a sluggish thyroid is blamed for "that tired feeling" and a general lack of energy, many people take thyroid hormones as a kind of nonspecific tonic. Taking thyroid hormones as a pep pill is a definite mistake. No one should take thyroid hormones without a well-defined diagnosis of thyroid insufficiency.

Hyperthyroidism

Almost everyone has known someone with an overactive thyroid. The hyperthyroid person is jumpy and irritable, sweats a lot, often loses weight, and may have protruding eyes. Most have a large thyroid or goiter (goiter simply means a large thyroid). Most cases of hyperthyroidism are caused by Graves' disease, which, like many cases of primary hypothyroidism, results from a faulty immune system. In this case, the thyroid is over-stimulated. In fact, it is not unusual for both hyperthyroidism and hypothyroidism caused by immune defects to occur in the same family.

In some people, the disease spontaneously reverses itself. But the usual hyperthyroid person with Graves' disease requires active treatment. Possible treatments include antithyroid drugs to block the synthesis of thyroid hormone, radioactive iodine, or surgery. The latter two destroy most but not all of the thyroid gland. Because radioactive iodine and surgery frequently lead to the opposite extreme, hypothyroidism, several years later, they generally are not used in younger persons. An antithyroid drug controls hyperthyroidism in all cases if the dose is large enough, but the hyperthyroidism may return when the drug is stopped. Careful follow-up is necessary for life.

Subacute Thyroiditis

Sometimes a person will get a "sore throat" that lasts for several weeks or even longer. The problem may actually be an inflamed thyroid. The thyroid is tender, the overlying skin is often red and warm, and there may be a fever. When this happens suddenly, it is called acute thyroiditis. More often, the condition develops over several days or weeks and is called subacute thyroiditis. Large amounts of thyroid hormone may be released into the bloodstream, causing a temporary form of hyperthyroidism. Once the inflammation subsides, the hyperthyroidism disappears.

If the thyroiditis is mild, simple measures such as aspirin may quell the symptoms. If it is more severe, treatment may include thyroid hormone, which appears to suppress the gland's activity, or anti-inflammatory drugs.

Goiter, Thyroid Nodules, And Thyroid Cancer

Goiter means an enlarged thyroid and is not a specific disease. Sometimes the enlargement feels bumpy, so it is called a nodular goiter. Nodular thyroids are fairly common in the United States, affecting 4 percent of the population. Most of these people are euthyroid, meaning they have normal hormone levels. In the past, iodine deficiency was probably the cause of many euthyroid goiters, but today's American diet contains sufficient iodine.

Diffuse or nodular goiter can be left untreated if it does not seem to be growing and if the person's hormone levels are normal. More often, the patient is treated with modest doses of thyroid hormone on the assumption that a slight degree of thyroid deficiency exists. Treating nodular goiter with thyroid hormone may make the nodule shrink or disappear.

Thyroid cancer can be a major concern when there is a thyroid nodule. If several nodules can be felt, the likelihood of cancer is quite small, so concern centers on people who appear to have only a single nodule. In reality, even these usually have several nodules, which are found only after removing the thyroid surgically. The evidence indicates that 5 to 10 percent of these nodules contain tissue that looks like cancer (carcinoma). The overall mortality from thyroid carcinoma is quite low, however. What is carcinoma under the microscope often is not biologically malignant. Some of the nodules containing carcinoma even shrink or disappear after treatment with thyroid hormone.

Findings that increase the suspicion of biologically malignant carcinoma in a thyroid nodule are: a nodule that is extremely hard to the touch, does not move on swallowing, is associated with hoarseness, or gets larger rather than smaller after taking thyroid hormone. Another important clue is radiation treatment to the head, neck, or upper chest years before. The previous radiation increases the chance that a thyroid nodule contains cancer. Sometimes a radioactive scan or "picture" shows little or no radioactivity in the nodule. When it is "cold," the likelihood of carcinoma is higher.

Thyroid carcinoma also is slow growing, usually allowing ample time for the patient and doctor to assess the effect of giving thyroid hormone. T_4 may be given by mouth for several months to a year, while the nodule or lump is being observed. If the nodule shrinks, no further treatment is necessary and the patient can continue to take T_4. If the nodule continues to grow, however, surgery may be performed.

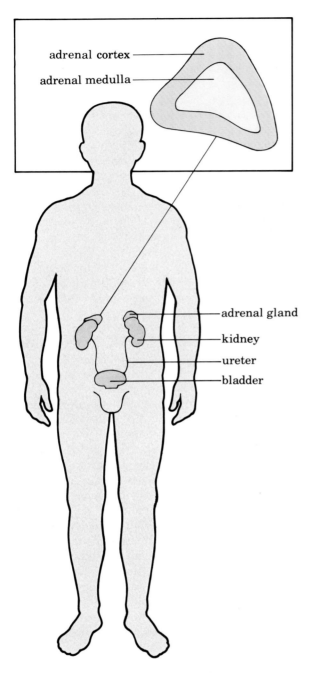

ADRENAL GLANDS
The adrenal glands are located atop the kidneys but have no direct connection to them. The cortex, or outer part, makes the two steroid hormones hydrocortisone and aldosterone, which influence many body functions, including sugar metabolism, heart contractions, and blood pressure. The medulla, or inner part, is an entirely separate gland and makes epinephrine (adrenalin), and norepinephrine.

THE ADRENAL GLAND

There are two adrenal glands, one on top of each kidney. Each adrenal gland is in fact two separate glands. The outer portion, the adrenal cortex, makes two principal hormones, hydrocortisone (also known as cortisol) and aldosterone. It also secretes small amounts of male and female hormones (androgens and estrogens). The inner portion of the gland, the adrenal medulla, makes its own two hormones, norepinephrine (noradrenalin) and epinephrine (adrenalin).

The functions of the adrenal hormones are described in the chart at left.

Adrenal Insufficiency

Lack of adrenal cortical hormones can be caused by direct damage to the adrenal cortex (primary adrenal insufficiency or Addison's disease) or to a deficiency of ACTH from the pituitary (secondary adrenal insufficiency).

Severe Addison's disease causes weakness, lethargy, lack of energy, mental depression, lightheadedness, and an inability to think clearly. The skin darkens, and is sometimes mottled, with black freckles and milky patches. There may be both loss of salt into the urine, causing the person to eat extra salt, and a tendency toward low blood sugar (hypoglycemia). Sometimes, the symptoms are catastrophic, including shock and complete cardiovascular collapse. This is known as acute adrenal insufficiency.

Treatment of adrenal insufficiency is now fairly straightforward. When cortisol is deficient, the treatment is to give supplemental cortisol (hydrocortisone) or cortisone. When aldosterone is lacking, a synthetic mineralocorticoid, called 9-alpha-fluorohydrocortisone (Florinef), is used instead. Many patients with primary adrenal insufficiency must take both cortisol and Florinef. Still, the usual daily medication alone is not complete treatment because any severe stress increases the body's need and can cause acute adrenal insufficiency. The person must be careful to carry an extra supply of cortisone or hydrocortisone and take it in the event of injury. He or she also should be equipped with a bracelet, necklace, or wallet card informing others of the condition.

Excessive Adrenal Function

When there is an overactive adrenal cortex, the extra hormone is either cortisol or aldosterone, but not both.

Cushing's syndrome is caused by too much cortisol. The person is obese, sometimes only in the body without fat arms or legs, usually has a red face and thin skin, and may have high blood pressure. The thin skin stretches easily, which leads to stretch marks (striae). Women may have extra hair on the face or chest, and the menstrual cycle may be disrupted or stop. There can be metabolic effects such as a higher blood sugar, thin bones that can lead to fractures, and poor protein synthesis, which can cause weakness and poor healing.

A common cause of Cushing's syndrome is simply taking too much glucocorticoid prescribed for other diseases, such as asthma and arthritis.

Spontaneous Cushing's syndrome is usually caused by a small pituitary tumor secreting too much ACTH. Sometimes the extra ACTH does not come from the pituitary but from a malignant tumor elsewhere in the body, such as a lung cancer (ectopic ACTH secretion). Less often, Cushing's syndrome is caused by an adrenal tumor secreting too much cortisol. Yet another cause is excessive drinking.

Treatment of spontaneous Cushing's syndrome is basically surgical. A pituitary tumor usually can be removed by transsphenoidal hypophysectomy, the procedure described earlier. An alternative treatment is to remove both adrenal glands. Sometimes conditions are not right for surgery, so radiation or drugs are used instead. When Cushing's syndrome arises as a side effect of glucosteroids for asthma or arthritis, medication must be adjusted or stopped. When the disorder is induced by alcohol, the solution is to stop drinking.

The Adrenal Medulla and Disease

Destruction of the adrenal medulla rarely causes deficiency of epinephrine or norepinephrine, the "fight or flight" hormones, because the sympathetic nerves throughout the body make up for the shortage. Sometimes, however, a large part of the sympathetic nervous system, including the adrenal medulla, is damaged. This can lead to low

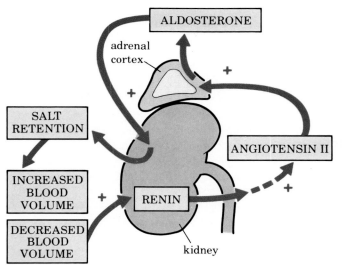

HORMONES AND BLOOD VOLUME
When the blood volume falls because of dehydration, lack of salt, or massive bleeding, a complex process takes place. The kidney (center) senses the loss and secretes into the blood a hormonelike substance called renin. Renin causes the formation of angiotensin, which in turn stimulates the adrenal cortex to secrete aldosterone. The circuit is complete when aldosterone acts on the kidney to prevent it from excreting salt in the urine, thereby helping it to retain salt in the body. The blood volume increases and tends to return to normal because most of the blood is simply a weak solution of salt water.

blood pressure, with light-headedness and fainting, and a tendency toward low blood sugar. Treatment is difficult, mainly involving drugs similar to norepinephrine but longer lasting. Treatment also can include medication to retain salt, which increases the blood volume, making fainting less likely to occur.

Excessive secretion of epinephrine and norepinephrine is almost always caused by a pheochromocytoma, a tumor in one or both adrenals. This tumor may cause high blood pressure, headache, palpitations, and sweating. Occasionally the tumor is found outside the glands.

Nonfunctioning Adrenal Tumors

An occasional adrenal tumor has no effect on hormone production. Because there are no hormonal effects, the tumor may grow quite large before it is finally detected by sheer size or perhaps by the pressure it exerts on the kidney. Surgery is the treatment, but if the tumor is malignant, drugs also may be used. Recently, many nonfunctioning adrenal tumors have been disclosed by routine computerized tomography (CT scans) of the abdomen. Most are harmless, but those larger than 2 inches in diameter usually are observed closely.

CALCIUM, BONES, AND HORMONES

Calcium is important for every tissue in the body. The amount of calcium in the blood stays within a narrow range. Whenever there is too much (hypercalcemia) or too little (hypocalcemia), tissue function deteriorates and characteristic symptoms occur.

Calcium salts also are the primary component of bone and are mainly responsible for its strength. Blood and bone calcium are closely interrelated. Bone contains more than 2 pounds of calcium and

acts as a storage site to be drawn upon whenever the blood calcium falls too low. The other primary source of calcium for the blood is the diet. Most comes from milk or milk products.

If the blood calcium is to stay constant, there must be careful regulation of absorption of dietary calcium, or resorption of bone, and of urinary losses. The hormones that regulate calcium are parathyroid hormone (PTH), calcitonin, and vitamin D. Vitamin D, although called a vitamin, is actually a hormone made by the skin under the influence of sunlight. In fact, even though vitamin D is now added to milk by law, most of the vitamin D in the blood is made by the skin.

Parathyroid hormone is secreted by the parathyroid glands, so called because each pair is located near the lobes of the thyroid gland. Parathyroid hormone causes the blood calcium to rise by stimulating bone cells to break down bone mineral and by stimulating the kidney to resorb calcium that otherwise might be excreted in the urine. Parathyroid hormone secretion is controlled by the level of blood calcium in a simple negative feedback fashion. When calcium goes up, secretion goes down.

Vitamin D released from the skin into the blood becomes potent only after passing through the liver and the kidneys. It stimulates calcium absorption from the intestine and also acts on bone to enhance both the formation and resorption of bone calcium.

Calcitonin lowers the blood calcium. It comes from parafollicular cells in the thyroid gland.

Hypocalcemia, a severely low level of blood calcium, causes irritability, muddled thinking, spastic muscle contractions, and even seizures. The condition often results from a deficiency of parathyroid hormone (hypoparathyroidism). The defect may be present from birth or may be caused by immune destruction of the parathyroid glands (as happens with the thyroid or the adrenals), or may result from previous neck surgery that has damaged the parathyroids. The ideal treatment would be to substitute parathyroid hormone, but it is not available. So doctors use large doses of vitamin D, or perhaps the more potent "1,25-D" form, and give extra calcium by mouth.

Vitamin D deficiency produces a modest degree of low blood calcium levels, but the main effect is on the bones. When the deficiency occurs in children because of a poor diet and little exposure to the sun, the disease is called rickets. The

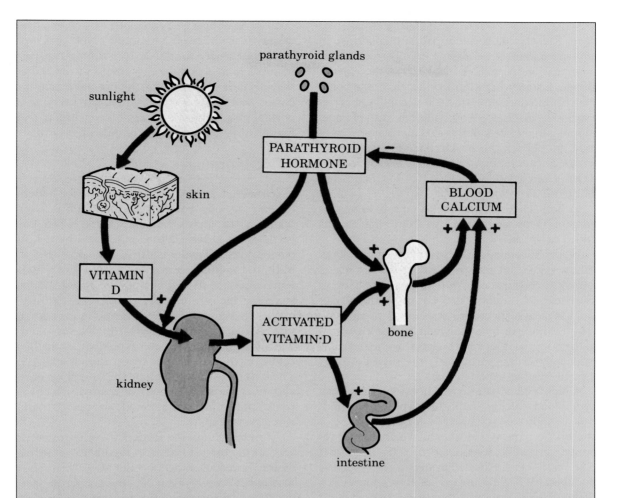

Regulating Calcium

The right amount of calcium in the blood is needed for most bodily processes as well as to build strong bones. Hormones, sunlight, the skin, the bones, and calcium in the diet all interact to maintain calcium levels.

Sunlight acting on the skin produces vitamin D, which is converted into its active form in the kidney under the influence of parathyroid hormone. The activated vitamin helps absorb calcium from the food we eat after it reaches the intestine, and helps deposit calcium in the bones. Along with para-

thyroid hormone, the activated vitamin D helps reclaim calcium from the bones and kidneys when it is needed. The negative feedback of blood calcium on the secretion of parathyroid hormone is an important part of the process.

Loss of calcium from the bones causes a disorder called osteoporosis, which is common among postmenopausal women and the cause of many fractures and joint replacements. Women are advised to eat plenty of calcium-rich foods throughout life.

growing bones become structurally weak and bend. Rickets is now rare in Western countries. In adults, vitamin D deficiency may be more common than suspected, particularly in the elderly. Besides a somewhat low blood calcium, the bones may be thin and somewhat soft, a condition called osteomalacia. Osteoporosis, another form of bone-thinning due to calcium loss, is increasingly common in older women. Decline in secretion of female hormones plays a key role. Osteoporosis is described in detail in Chapter 16, "The Bones and Muscles."

In both children and adults, the treatment is vitamin D by mouth and calcium supplements added to the diet.

Hypercalcemia, excessive calcium in the blood, causes vague and nonspecific complaints such as lethargy, constipation, "not feeling well," or, if severe enough, coma. Usually, excessive blood calcium is caused by excessive secretion of parathyroid hormone or by a malignant tumor elsewhere in the body, such as a lung cancer. Sometimes it is caused by drugs, particularly the thiazide drugs used in treating hypertension.

A high level of parathyroid hormone along with high blood calcium indicates hyperparathyroidism. Usually this is caused by a benign tumor of one of the parathyroid glands, which can be removed surgically. Sometimes the offending gland is an "extra" gland located in an odd place, such as the chest. When the degree of hypercalcemia is slight, phosphate salts by mouth can be used without surgery.

When a malignant tumor causes the high blood calcium, treatment is aimed at the tumor.

THE HORMONES
AND REPRODUCTION

An individual need not reproduce, but the species must or it perishes. In fact, a person who lacks the hormones needed for reproduction lives a fairly normal life in most ways.

For successful reproduction, there must be a precise sequence of events leading to the birth of a child (see Chapter 28, "Pregnancy and Child-birth"). At almost every step of the way, one hormone or another is important. Not only are hormones needed for the development of the spermatozoa in men and the eggs (ova) in women, but they also are necessary for the normal sexual behavior that leads to fertilization, for carrying a normal pregnancy to a successful conclusion, and for ensuring the production of milk after birth.

Male Hormones

In males, testosterone is responsible for masculinizing the body, both when a male fetus is developing in the uterus and at puberty, when boy becomes man. Testosterone is secreted by the interstitial cells (Leydig cells) of the testes. Before birth, testosterone secreted by the testes of a male fetus causes the development of the male genitalia, including the scrotum and penis. Fetal testosterone also acts on the brain to "prime" it for normal male sexual behavior after birth. During childhood, testosterone secretion actually is lower than before birth, but it rises again during puberty. Then, it causes hair growth on the face, pubic area, and other parts of the body, increased size of the penis, a major increase in muscle size and strength, and a growth spurt.

At puberty, too, the rising level of testosterone acts on the brain to develop the libido, or sexual desire. Testosterone acts on the testes themselves to stimulate development of active and fertile spermatozoa. Testosterone also develops the prostate gland and seminal vesicles that contribute fluid to the semen (see Chapter 25, "The Male Reproductive System").

The actions of testosterone are sometimes due to the hormone itself, as in muscle. But in other tissues, such as the prostate gland, the testosterone is converted to dihydrotestosterone, an active product of testosterone. A testosteronelike steroid that has more action on muscle than on the penis or hair growth is called an anabolic steroid. Anabolic

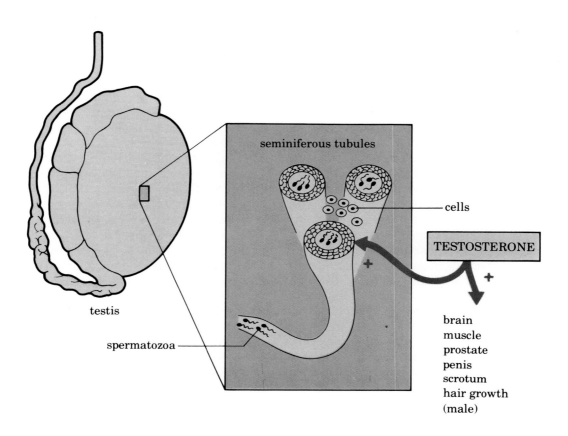

seminiferous tubules

cells

TESTOSTERONE

+

+

testis

brain
muscle
prostate
penis
scrotum
hair growth
(male)

spermatozoa

THE MALE HORMONES

The testis, located in the scrotum, is the male gonad, or sex gland. It makes sperm and the male hormone testosterone. Testosterone helps in sperm manufacture. In the blood, testosterone causes the bodily changes we associate with being male, including face and body hair, increased muscle, and male sexual behavior. Sperm and testosterone production are influenced by two hormones secreted by the pituitary gland, which in turn is controlled by the hypothalamus.

steroids are sometimes used by athletes to increase muscle strength, but evidence of their success is weak, and prolonged use may lead to infertility.

Besides secreting testosterone, the testes make new spermatozoa. Both FSH and LH from the pituitary and testosterone from the Leydig cells contribute. Sperm formation occurs in the seminiferous tubules that make up the bulk of the testes. Inside each tubule are cells that develop into the spermatozoa. Next to them are supporting cells called Sertoli cells. FSH acts on the Sertoli cells, and LH stimulates testosterone secretion from the nearby Leydig cells.

Female Hormones

The female hypothalamic and pituitary hormones are the same as the male hormones, and the general pattern of reproductive hormones is similar. LRH from the hypothalamus increases the pituitary secretion of FSH and LH hormones, which in turn stimulate the ovaries. The important difference is that the ovaries secrete different steroid hormones, estradiol and progesterone, and do so cyclically, at intervals about four weeks apart. Although the male secretion of luteinizing hormone and testosterone and the production of spermatozoa are reasonably constant, in women, the egg and the ovarian hormones are released in a monthly pattern that causes menstrual bleeding.

Estradiol brings about breast development, maturation of the genitalia, and redistribution of fat that occurs in adult women. It also develops the libido (sexual desire), another example of a hormone acting on the brain. The adrenal androgens may be responsible for the growth of hair in the pubic area and armpits. Girls also have a growth spurt at puberty, although it usually is not as great as in boys. Growth is due mostly to estradiol.

After puberty, the menstrual cycle often is irregular, but eventually settles into a regular pattern. After each menstrual bleeding, FSH and LH act together to stimulate growth of a single ovarian follicle, a group of cells surrounding the egg. The follicle grows during the first half of the menstrual cycle, called the follicular phase, and secretes increasing amounts of estradiol. Estradiol helps stimulate growth of the endometrium, the lining of the uterine cavity, to receive a fertilized egg.

About midway through the menstrual cycle, the higher level of estradiol triggers a burst of LH and FSH secretion from the pituitary, a positive feedback effect. The sudden high level of LH causes the enlarged follicle to erupt, releasing the egg, which begins its travels down the fallopian tube (oviduct) toward possible fertilization. The follicle collapses, then rapidly changes into a denser, solid structure called the corpus luteum ("yellow body"), which lasts until the next menstrual bleeding. The second half of the menstrual cycle is thus called the luteal phase. The corpus luteum continues to secrete estradiol and also progesterone.

The combination of estradiol and progesterone from the corpus luteum makes the endometrium develop into a suitable place for the implantation of a fertilized egg. If fertilization occurs (in the fallopian tube), the egg begins to divide and forms a small cell mass called the blastocyst. It takes about one week for the blastocyst to travel down the fallopian tube into the uterus. By then, the endometrium is properly developed to receive it. The blastocyst implants into the endometrium and begins to develop into the placenta and the fetus.

If no fertilization takes place, the corpus luteum begins to fail. It makes less and less estradiol and progesterone. Without them, the developed endometrium deteriorates and is carried away in the menstrual flow about two weeks after ovulation. The reason pregnancy stops menstrual bleeding is that part of the implanted blastocyst begins to form the placenta and makes hormones that keep the corpus luteum alive. In a sense, menstrual bleeding is a failed pregnancy.

During pregnancy, the placenta secretes several hormones of its own. Human chorionic gonadotropin (HCG) acts exactly like LH. Its main function seems to be the maintenance of the corpus luteum for a few weeks. (Its presence is the basis for pregnancy tests.) After a while, the placenta also makes estradiol and progesterone, and the hormonal output of the corpus luteum is no longer needed. HCG also stimulates testosterone secretion by the testes of a male fetus. The large amounts of progesterone and estradiol contribute to the growth of the uterus and to the breast development needed for lactation after the child is born. Progesterone also keeps down uterine contractions and prevents premature birth.

We do not know why pregnancy ends and birth occurs when it does, but it may be because of a fall in progesterone and a rise in estradiol. Estradiol tends to increase uterine contractions. Apparently, the combination of more estradiol, lowered progesterone, and secretion of oxytocin from the posterior pituitary causes progressive contractions that eventually bring on birth.

Lactation, or milk secretion, begins shortly after delivery. During pregnancy, the breasts develop in preparation for lactation largely because of placental estradiol and progesterone, and because of increased secretion of prolactin (PRL) from the mother's pituitary. Lactation usually does not occur during pregnancy because estradiol and progesterone, while they develop the breasts, block lactation itself. After birth, placental estradiol and progesterone disappear, relieving the blockage.

The high prolactin persists because it comes from the mother's pituitary. The breasts then engorge and milk secretion begins. When the infant suckles at the breast, oxytocin secretion from the posterior pituitary is stimulated; oxytocin causes the small milk glands in the breast to contract and the milk squirts out. Suckling also tends to maintain prolactin secretion. Thus, both prolactin and oxytocin are important hormones for effective nursing. If the mother does not nurse the child or if the child stops nursing later, milk secretion stops, too, in part because prolactin and oxytocin secretion cease when there is no suckling.

While the mother is nursing, ovulation usually does not occur. But this is at best an unreliable contraceptive because the inhibition of ovulation is not always complete. Why nursing inhibits ovulation is not clear, but the high prolactin probably interferes with secretion of FSH and LH. When nursing stops, FSH and LH secretion resume in a few months, and the pituitary-ovarian-uterine cycle begins anew.

Disorders of Reproductive Hormones

Disorders of reproductive hormones rarely cause death, but the psychological and emotional effects can be devastating. Disturbances of sexual function and inability to have children are not matters most men and women take lightly. Neither are such problems as excessive body hair or menstrual difficulties, including absence of menses. Hormonal defects are not always the cause of these disorders, but generally a careful study of the appropriate hormones in the man or woman is still needed before a hormone defect can be ruled out.

In men, common problems include impotence (inability to get and maintain erection for successful sexual intercourse), decreased libido (lack of interest in sexual activity), and infertility (inability to father children despite apparently normal sexual function). Impotence, loss of libido, and infertility are described in Chapter 25, "The Male Reproductive System."

Gynecomastia, which means female-like breasts, commonly occurs in boys at puberty. It is of no concern then, because it usually goes away. But gynecomastia at other times of life may indicate excessive production of an estrogen as a result of a tumor of the testes, or in rare cases the result of a tumor of the adrenal or some other organ.

Rarely, a boy may start to masculinize and begin the changes of puberty several years early. This is called sexual precocity, and means he is producing too much testosterone, at least for his age. Sometimes caused by a tumor, sometimes by a metabolic defect in the adrenal cortex, sexual precocity also may reflect early maturation of the whole hypothalamic-pituitary mechanism for puberty. It is important to identify the cause, because if the condition is untreated, bone growth will stop too soon and the boy will become a short man.

Amenorrhea, the absence of menstrual flow, occurs when the ovary does not secrete estrogen so that the endometrium does not develop. Amenorrhea and other disruptions of the menstrual cycle are described in Chapter 26, "The Female Reproductive System." Infertility, the inability to conceive, also is discussed in that chapter.

Hirsutism. Some women have too much facial or body hair, or at least they think they do. Often, the "extra" hair is normal, particularly if it is light in amount and limited to the upper lip, face, and chest, and if other women in the family show a similar pattern. If the hair growth seems greater in amount or extent or if it has recently increased, there may be an endocrine cause, especially if accompanied by infertility, irregular periods, or even amenorrhea. A possible explanation may be a tumor in the ovaries or adrenals. More often, there seems to be a functional defect. In the ovaries, defective function can lead to large, cystic ovaries that make abnormal amounts of testosterone. The condition is called the polycystic ovary or Stein-Leventhal syndrome. Measurement of blood testosterone may not be much above normal, and often it is not easy to tell if the excess is coming from the ovaries or the adrenals. If there are clear-cut polycystic ovaries, medical or surgical treatment to cause ovulation will certainly help. If not, oral contraceptives or adrenal corticoids may suppress testosterone secretion enough so that the hirsutism improves. Only occasionally, however, does the excess hair disappear altogether.

DIABETES MELLITUS

The major characteristic of diabetes is the body's inability to regulate the level of "sugar," or glucose, in the blood.

There are two basic types of the disease. Type I diabetes, also known as juvenile diabetes, ketosis-prone diabetes, or insulin-dependent diabetes, affects only 15 percent of diabetics. They usually develop it as children or young adults and usually are thin. These persons have a total or almost total lack of the hormone insulin, which is necessary to maintain normal sugar levels in the blood. They usually need daily injections of insulin to prevent a dangerous condition called ketosis, in which glucose and acids in the body reach harmful levels.

Type II diabetes, also called mature-onset or adult-onset diabetes, ketosis-resistant diabetes, or non-insulin-dependent diabetes, usually develops after age 40, and victims usually are overweight. These persons continue to make insulin, but not enough to keep their blood glucose level normal all the time. Although, like insulin-dependent diabetics, they are at risk of developing long-term complications, they usually have enough insulin of their own to avoid ketosis.

PHYSIOLOGY OF DIABETES

Diabetes centers on a malfunction of the pancreas, a large organ lying behind the stomach (top drawing). The pancreas contains small islands of tissue known as islets of Langerhans (center drawing). The islets are made up of four types of cells (bottom drawing). Beta cells, the most numerous, are the body's only source of insulin, a hormone that regulates glucose in the blood. Alpha cells produce another hormone, glucagon, also involved in glucose regulation. The role of the somatostatin and polypeptide cells is uncertain.

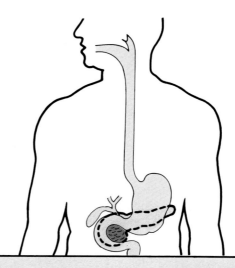

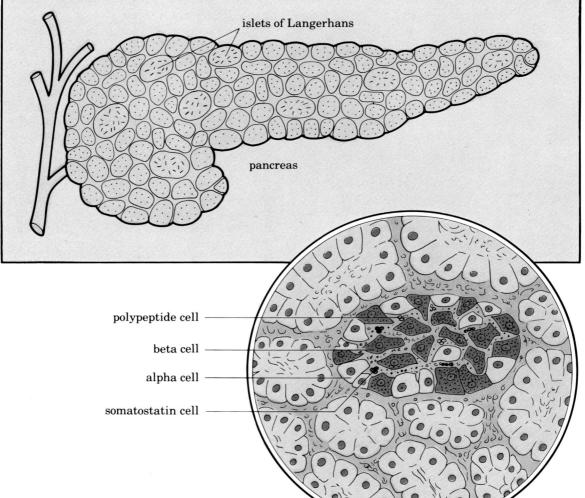

islets of Langerhans

pancreas

polypeptide cell

beta cell

alpha cell

somatostatin cell

How does a person know whether he or she has diabetes? When should a physician suspect the disease? In an adult with Type II diabetes, the onset may be gradual and very subtle, with almost no noticeable change in habits or apparent health. In a child, the disease often begins dramatically.

Type I diabetes sometimes appears during a period of stress such as illness, but in most cases, no precipitating condition can be identified. The disease usually starts in childhood, including the teens, or less commonly during young adulthood. It can be heralded by fatigue and weakness. The young victim may urinate frequently and be compelled to get up during the night to do so. Thirst may be constant, accompanied by increased appetite. But despite "eating like a horse," the new diabetic loses weight. He or she may notice muscle cramps or blurred vision, and may suffer from lingering infections or slow-healing wounds.

Type II diabetes has the symptoms of frequent urination, excessive thirst, and increased appetite, but they are less common than in juvenile diabetes. Instead, the mature-onset diabetic may suffer urinary or skin infections, especially yeast infections in the vagina (causing itching and a whitish discharge) or red, itchy irritation in the groins, armpits, and under the breasts. Sometimes small, raised reddish-yellow spots appear on the skin because of increased fat in the blood. Some persons develop numbness and burning or tingling of the hands, feet, or legs. A few suffer blurry vision or frequently have their eyeglass prescription changed. And, like juvenile diabetics, many adult-onset diabetics feel tired and run-down.

These symptoms, especially in combination, should lead one to consult a doctor. Diabetes is common, easy to test for, and easy to treat. Prompt treatment may minimize complications and reduce risk of associated diseases of the eye, kidney, and nervous system.

Gestational diabetes affects about 2 to 3 percent of pregnant women, who previously have not been diabetic. The disease disappears after childbirth, but 40 to 60 percent of those affected will become diabetic in later life. Gestational diabetes shows no symptoms, and the mother's health is not endangered. However, there is a greatly increased risk of stillbirth, birth defects, or large birthweight babies. All pregnant women should have a diabetes screening test at 22 to 24 weeks of pregnancy. Gestational diabetes normally can be controlled with diet, but insulin injections sometimes are necessary. A woman who develops diabetes in one pregnancy will be affected in future pregnancies.

CAUSES OF DIABETES

Although the causes of diabetes still are not understood, much has been learned in recent years about who is at highest risk. Both juvenile and mature-onset diabetes tend to run in families, and the two types behave as if they were separate diseases, seldom occurring in the same family.

But heredity is not the only factor, and diabetes is not passed from parent to child in an easily predictable way. A person's environment and life-style interact with heredity to determine whether a person will become diabetic.

In mature-onset diabetes, being overweight is the major risk factor. The exact role of obesity is unclear, but it may be that larger fat cells or larger numbers of fat cells demand more insulin than the body can produce (relative insulin deficiency) or that the fat cells do not take up and utilize insulin properly (insulin resistance). Whatever the reason, losing weight and increasing exercise definitely improve Type II diabetes.

Obesity is a problem that fat parents tend to pass on to their children, probably through both genes and life-style, so they also pass on their increased risk of diabetes. The increasing incidence of diabetes in the United States may be explained by the American tendency to overeat (40 percent of the population is obese). The connection between diabetes and obesity has been studied among Yemenite Jews, who formerly lived in the desert, usually were thin, and had a low incidence of diabetes. As they moved to the city, the frequency of obesity increased and so did diabetes.

In juvenile diabetes, heredity plays a more evident role. For instance, the children of two juvenile diabetic parents have about a 30 percent chance of becoming diabetic. In research on cells and organ transplants, scientists have studied many protein antigens, or "markers," that occur on all human cells. Each of us has our own set of antigens. Researchers have found two particular antigens that occur frequently in juvenile diabetics,

COMPARING THE TYPES OF DIABETES

	Juvenile	Adult
Other names	Insulin-dependent Ketosis-prone	Insulin-independent Ketosis-resistant
Percentage of all diabetics	15%	85%
Age of onset	Usually before 25	Over 40
Body type	Thin	Overweight
Insulin	Absolute deficiency	Relative deficiency
Onset	Very rapid	Gradual

making them wonder whether the "genes" for diabetes are passed on in association with the genes for those particular markers.

Viruses also have been implicated in diabetes. As early as 1864, a Norwegian scientist noticed that diabetes increased after a mumps epidemic. Since then, about 20 viruses or virus particles have been connected with diabetes, so it seems likely that no single virus sets off the disease. Diabetes occurs in children more often at ages when they are likely to be exposed to certain virus strains for the first time. Some researchers have suggested that the body, in fighting off a virus infection by making protein antibodies and special cells to attack the invading virus, inadvertently makes antibodies that attack some of the protein markers on its own cells. This backfiring of the normal immune mechanism has been shown to occur in other diseases, described in Chapter 23, "Allergy and the Immune System." Another possible mechanism is that an altered protein is produced by the insulin-manufacturing beta cells in the pancreas, or an altered cell surface occurs that is perceived by the body as foreign. Thus, a person with the cell markers associated with diabetes develops the disease because antibodies produced to fight off a routine virus infection attack not only the virus, but the person's own beta cells.

Other factors can set off diabetes or aggravate it. As people grow older, their diet may change and they may get less exercise, altering the glucose-insulin balance. Certain drugs may elevate blood glucose levels, including those used to treat high blood pressure. Apparently birth control pills sometimes interfere with insulin. Thyroid hormones and cortisone may raise the blood glucose through complicated actions on the metabolism.

DIAGNOSING DIABETES

Besides the common symptoms, other factors may influence a doctor to test a patient for diabetes: a family history of the disease, an early heart attack, an unusually high blood sugar level during a hospital stay, a tendency for a woman to have unusually large babies, or a propensity to develop skin sores that heal slowly. Tests are available, and the American Diabetes Association (ADA) has established criteria for diagnosis of the disease.

The initial screening test measures the fasting blood sugar level. This test determines the amount of glucose in a small sample of blood obtained first thing in the morning, when the patient has eaten nothing since the night before. If glucose levels are normal, it indicates that the person is making enough insulin to keep glucose within the proper range. If glucose is higher than normal, it may mean that the body is not producing enough insulin, and that storage fuels are breaking down and raising the blood sugar in response. A fasting blood sugar level greater than 140 milligrams of glucose per deciliter of blood, obtained on two separate occasions, is considered by the ADA as evidence of diabetes.

If the fasting blood sugar is normal, or the test is inconclusive, a glucose-tolerance test is recommended. The person is given 75 grams of glucose by mouth; two hours afterward, blood sugar is measured. The glucose puts stress on the beta cells by creating a demand for insulin, and their ability to produce insulin is measured by whether the blood glucose level has returned to normal two hours after eating. A two-hour blood glucose 20 percent above normal levels is considered an indication of diabetes. Most doctors repeat these tests when they obtain a high reading, however, and also take into account that blood sugar levels normally are slightly higher in older people.

Testing the urine for glucose is another way to look for diabetes, and is important for insulin-taking diabetics to do at home. It is of little value, however, in diagnosing the disease, because glucose levels in the blood may rise to two or three times normal before the kidneys begin to spill glucose into the urine. Part of the job of the normal kidney is to conserve glucose, not excrete it, and a diabetic's blood glucose may rise dangerously high before this conservation mechanism is overwhelmed and the urine test becomes positive.

COMPLICATIONS OF DIABETES

The long-term effects of diabetes are serious and involve every organ of the body. Compared to the normal population, diabetics are 25 times more prone to blindness, 17 times more prone to kidney disease, five times more prone to gangrene, and twice as prone to heart disease. Although heart disease is the leading cause of death among diabetics as a whole, juvenile diabetics are particularly vulnerable to kidney failure. In fact, half of juvenile diabetics die of kidney failure by the time they have been diabetic for 25 years.

Given these figures, it is understandable that research efforts to find the causes of diabetes' complications and to understand their relation to high blood sugar have been intense. There is mounting evidence that controlling blood sugar helps prevent damage to the eyes, kidneys, and nerves. Normal blood glucose levels also improve the function of blood cells and the body's metabolism. But doctors are less optimistic that control of blood sugar lowers the diabetic's high risk of heart disease and damage to large blood vessels.

The disease does damage in a number of ways. In the eye, abnormal shifts of water and chemicals can impair vision by causing swelling of the lens (which may improve when blood glucose is brought back to normal). The patient may experience blurry vision. If the blood sugar level is elevated for a prolonged time, cataracts may develop and eventually require surgery. Glaucoma is common, and can impair vision if not treated.

The most dangerous visual complication is diabetic proliferative retinopathy, the process of damage and abnormal growth of small blood vessels in the retina of the eye. Less than 5 percent of diabetics become blind, but that is enough to make diabetes a leading cause of blindness. Early retinopathy can be helped by blood glucose control, but more advanced retinopathy may require laser treatment, as explained in Chapter 14, "The Eyes." This seals off the leaking blood vessels and often improves vision, avoiding blindness or hemorrhage and detachment of the retina.

Like the eyes, the nerves of diabetics can malfunction because of chemical abnormalities associated with high glucose levels or because of damage to the tiny supporting blood vessels. The results include tingling or burning of the skin, weakness, dizziness, diarrhea, bladder problems, and impotence. Nerve damage can decrease pain sensation in the hands and feet, which is dangerous for diabetics because foot injuries may occur without the person sensing normal pain.

Kidney failure is a particularly severe consequence of juvenile diabetes, but mature-onset diabetics also are vulnerable. Diabetic kidney damage appears to be related to both impaired blood supply and abnormal glucose levels, and can make the diabetic's kidneys more vulnerable to infection and to destruction by high blood pressure.

Diabetics run a higher risk of heart disease, and have heart attacks at younger ages and with fewer warning signs. After age 40, blood vessels supplying the limbs and skin are affected. In addition, the function of white blood cells diminishes and the combination makes diabetics prone to infection and slow wound-healing. Blood supply to the feet can become so poor that the tissues break down, and an apparently minor cut can fail to heal, become infected, and even lead to gangrene and amputation. For this reason, diabetics are instructed in foot care and warned against going barefoot and against wearing tight shoes and stockings.

Even though control of blood sugar clearly does not *cure* diabetes, it improves so many aspects of the disease that doctors agree every effort should be made to bring high glucose levels down to normal and keep them there.

TREATMENT OF DIABETES

In mature-onset diabetes, treatment concentrates on increasing the natural supply of insulin and its effectiveness in the body. A reducing diet apparently makes the diabetic more sensitive to his own insulin and increases the amount available.

Diet is based on five factors: total calories, percentage and type of carbohydrates, percentage and type of fats, meal spacing, and adjustments for exercise or complicating disorders.

For most patients who are taking insulin, the total calorie intake should be between 1,400 and 2,700 a day, with the exact amount depending on daily activity and desired weight of the patient. (Growing, active young people need more calories.) The usual distribution is 160 to 230 grams of carbohydrates, 65 to 125 grams of protein, and 40 to 60 grams of fat. Fats usually are kept low in proportion to protein in the diabetic's diet. It is important that meals be eaten regularly and on time.

For the diabetic who is not insulin-dependent, three divided meals of approximately equal calories are recommended. The calorie total is normally kept low.

The optimum diet usually is worked out by a doctor and a dietitian. It may have a high fiber content, which has been found to be beneficial in diabetes. Regular exercise is encouraged because it helps the patient lose weight and because it lowers blood glucose. When a patient is very obese or has great difficulty losing weight, doctors may employ a diet high in protein and low in carbohydrates. The diabetic diet centers on well-balanced meals that are tailored to individual needs, likes, dislikes, and life-style.

Often, diet and exercise are adequate treatment for mature-onset diabetes. If blood glucose levels remain too high, most doctors consider insulin injections the best measure. Sometimes, a doctor may prescribe an oral hypoglycemic agent, a pill to lower blood glucose levels.

There are two classes of oral medications. Oral hypoglycemics work by increasing insulin manufacture and release by the beta cells and by affecting glucose metabolism elsewhere, thus lowering blood sugar. The long-term success rate of newer hypoglycemics in keeping glucose levels normal is estimated at 50 percent. Approximately 5 to 10 percent of mature-onset diabetics do not respond

Low Blood Sugar (Hypoglycemia)

The problem of low blood sugar is the opposite of diabetes. Hypoglycemia refers to all the symptoms that occur in a diabetic during an insulin reaction: nervousness, sweating, trembling, drowsiness, and others. Low blood sugar in normal people can indeed produce these symptoms, and recent publicity has touted hypoglycemia as the long-overlooked explanation for the vague feelings of malaise most people experience at times. In reality, the symptoms of hypoglycemia do occur repeatedly in certain people when their blood sugar falls too low, but the disease is not common. Patients with reactive functional hypoglycemia develop a low blood glucose level two to four hours after eating because of an overactive insulin release, primarily in response to carbohydrates. If the symptoms and the low blood sugar level can be demonstrated by an oral glucose tolerance test, in which the patient's blood glucose is measured repeatedly up to five hours after a glucose meal, then the patient may show improvement by turning to a low-carbohydrate, high-protein diet.

Although persons with reactive hypoglycemia do not appear to have an increased risk of diabetes, similar symptoms and low blood sugar may occur three to five hours after eating in a few patients with early diabetes. Rarer causes of hypoglycemia, such as excess insulin release after stomach surgery or excess insulin caused by a pancreatic islet tumor, require more specialized tests and treatment.

WARNING SIGNS OF INSULIN REACTIONS

Pallor	Nervousness	Tingling around the mouth
Headache	Perspiration	Inability to concentrate
Dizziness	Blurred vision	Drowsiness or fatigue
Confusion	Irritability	

At the first sign of any of the above warning signs, give sugar immediately in one of the following forms:

- Sugar—5 small cubes, 2 packets, or 2 teaspoons
- Fruit juice—½ to ⅔ cup
- Carbonated beverage—6 ounces (not diet or sugarless soda pop)
- Candy—Three candy mints or ⅓ candy bar

to oral hypoglycemics; with others, the medication gradually loses its ability to control blood sugar. The percentage of such failures is estimated at another 5 to 10 percent, but sometimes failures are not due to medication but because the person gained weight.

A controversial research project, the University Group Diabetes Project (UGDP), questioned whether those using oral hypoglycemics had higher death rates, especially from heart disease, than other diabetics. Other studies have failed to substantiate the finding, and doctors point out that only one type of oral agent was implicated. A minority of doctors still oppose oral hypoglycemics, but others contend that the pills play an important role in diabetes treatment. The pills occasionally lower blood glucose too far, causing lethargy, nervousness, confusion, and other side effects, so they are not for everyone.

For the juvenile diabetic, diet and exercise also are essential, but the approach is different. Because juvenile diabetics so often are children, they must eat frequently in order to grow. And because they take insulin daily, diet must be carefully regulated to correspond with the insulin dose, keep the blood glucose level as constant as possible, and avoid an insulin reaction from a blood sugar level that is too low. Calorie requirements change as children gain height and weight, and food intake must be spaced throughout the day to avoid rapid zigzags in glucose levels. Juvenile diabetics also must learn to increase food intake on days when they exercise

vigorously, because exercise lowers glucose levels and decreases insulin requirements. Although juvenile diabetic diets usually limit sugar consumption, diabetics always must keep sugar available—candy, juice, soft drinks—to eat in case of an insulin reaction.

Injectable insulin is one of the landmark success stories in medical research. In 1922, two Canadians, Dr. Frederick G. Banting and Charles H. Best, a young student, succeeded in extracting from the islet cells of the pancreas a hormone with which they could control blood sugar levels in laboratory animals. The hormone was insulin. Shortly afterward they treated their first diabetic patient, and the results were dramatic. Although injectable insulin was not then and is not now a cure for diabetes, it quickly revolutionized treatment and kept alive millions of diabetics who otherwise would have died.

Today, injectable human insulin is manufactured primarily by techniques of genetic engineering, eliminating some of the reactive problems of insulin from pork and beef pancreases used in the past. Insulin comes in several preparations, with different durations of effect. The most commonly used types are regular insulin, whose peak activity comes two to four hours after injection, and NPH and long-acting Ultralente insulin, whose duration is 24 hours. Many diabetics take only a single injection of long-acting insulin in the morning.

Others take a mixture of intermediate and regular insulin, or more than one injection per day. The amount of the dose is determined by a doctor, who first prescribes a low dose and then tests the diabetic's blood and urine, slowly increasing the daily dose until blood glucose levels are nearly normal. The diabetic learns how to give himself or herself injections and how to decide whether to raise or lower the dose slightly depending on the presence of glucose in the urine.

Even young children can administer insulin to themselves. Injection is performed under the skin, the site rotated among such areas as thigh, abdomen, hip, and arms.

Although insulin treatment becomes more complicated during pregnancy, illness, or surgery, most insulin-dependent diabetics can become expert at treating their own illness.

A number of self-administered tests now are available to help diabetics. Glucose monitoring techniques are now widely used. A blood sample is obtained by pricking the finger with a small sterile needle, and a drop of blood is placed on a strip impregnated with a chemical reagent. After about a minute, the excess blood is washed off the strip and the color change that occurs can be compared to an established scale to determine glucose content. By taking several samples during the day, a diabetic can continuously monitor blood glucose.

Other tests measure urine sugar levels by dipping a chemically treated strip into a morning urine sample. The tests vary in expense, accuracy, and difficulty of administration. The exact test used by the patient should be determined by both the patient and the physician.

Insulin Reactions

The diabetic, and the diabetic's friends and family should know the symptoms of and treatment for an insulin reaction, which occurs when the body has an excess of the hormone compared to the amount of glucose. Most reactions can be readily checked with a quick-acting sugar (two teaspoons of sugar, a half-cup of fruit juice, six ounces of a regular [nondietetic] soft drink, two candy mints). Symptoms include hunger, nervousness and irritability, trembling, pallor, perspiration, headache, blurry vision, confusion or abnormal behavior, crying, drowsiness, and abdominal pain. Symptoms of low insulin and a very high blood sugar level (ketosis)—a particular danger in juvenile diabetics—also include hunger, weakness, dizziness, confusion, headache, abdominal pain, and passing out. A positive urine test for glucose can help distinguish between the two, but when symptoms occur, it is always best for the diabetic to take sugar at once and call the doctor or go to the emergency room, because both conditions are dangerous.

Special Problems Of the Diabetic

Besides the daily control of blood sugar, the treatment of diabetes demands that a doctor or nurse provide regular counseling and support. The diabetic must assume responsibility for control of the disease. The diabetic must consider what to eat, what to do, and how to care for the body more carefully than most people. A youthful diabetic may rebel against limits on diet or alcohol intake. In the middle years, the diabetic must work harder than other adults to reduce the risk factors for heart disease, such as smoking, high blood pressure, and high cholesterol consumption. Parents of diabetic children learn to live with the frightening risks of ketosis, insulin reactions, and decreased life expectancy, and children of diabetic parents might have to live with a parent's blindness, heart problems, or kidney failure.

General Hygiene

A special consideration for diabetics is general hygiene. Proper care of teeth and gums is strongly recommended. There is ample evidence that diabetics have an increased incidence of both gum and tooth problems, apparently because of the elevated levels of blood sugar. Some of these problems can be prevented by frequent brushing and flossing to prevent plaque formation. A diabetic's skin may be dry and itchy, and may require the use of lanolin creams after a bath or shower to trap water in the skin and prevent cracking. A diabetic should examine his or her feet daily, checking for infection, bruises, cuts, and blisters. Shoes that fit properly are imperative, and new shoes should be broken in slowly. The diabetic should always wear shoes or slippers and never walk barefoot.

CHAPTER 20

TEETH AND ORAL HEALTH

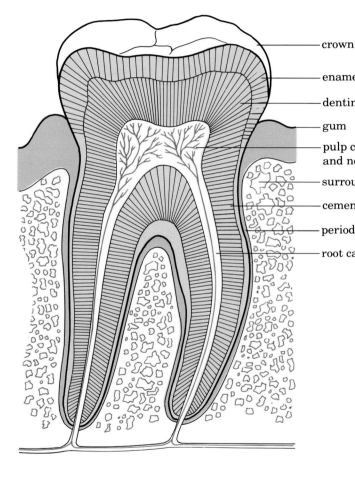

crown

enamel

dentin

gum

pulp contains blood vessels
and nerve fibers

surrounding bone of jaw

cementum

periodontal membrane

root canal

STRUCTURE OF A TOOTH

Each tooth, as shown here in a cross section, consists of a crown and a root. The crown is the visible part above the gum line. The root usually is two to three times as long, fitting into a bony socket in the jaw. Dental enamel coats the crown; bonelike cementum, the root. Dentin comprises most of the tooth and provides elasticity. The dental pulp contains small blood vessels and nerve fibers and provides moisture to the dentin. Blood flow in the pulp can be altered by very hot or cold foods or by infection accompanying tooth decay. Vessels then enlarge and press on nearby nerves, causing the pain of toothache.

Preparation of food for digestion is the primary function of teeth. The 32 teeth of the adult human are designed to bite, tear, and grind food into a semiliquid that can pass down the gullet and into the digestive system. A full complement of healthy teeth permits a wide selection of food and encourages a well-balanced diet. A poor set of teeth or less than a full set of teeth may limit a person to foods that need little or no chewing, provide limited nutrition, and constitute a monotonous diet.

Personal appearance relies on healthy teeth and gums. Many persons become socially withdrawn because of poorly arranged, unsightly, or diseased teeth. Inflamed and swollen gums not only are unattractive, but can cause bad breath. The appearance of the lower half of the face is determined to a large extent by the teeth. The receding jaw and the protruding jaw are two dental abnormalities involving improper "meshing" or contact of upper and lower teeth. Teeth that are missing, drifted, or improperly positioned also may distort the shape of the lips, mouth, and cheeks.

Good speech also depends on good teeth. Many sounds are formed by the position of the tongue or lips against the teeth. People who lack upper front teeth may have difficulty speaking distinctly. Misaligned teeth, overbite, and other irregularities can contribute to problems of articulation and communication.

ORAL DISEASES, ACCIDENTS, AND ABNORMALITIES

Tooth Decay *(dental caries)*

Thanks to fluoridated water and other advances, tooth decay is far less common than in the past. Still, a person who has never had a single dental cavity is rare indeed. The problem is most prevalent during childhood and adolescence, and it begins early. Even 2-year-olds may show evidence of decay. Adults develop fewer cavities only because most of the vulnerable teeth have been attacked and repaired during childhood.

Tooth decay occurs in areas of the mouth where bacteria and food debris accumulate and remain undisturbed. The bacteria react with the carbohydrates of the foods to produce an acid that dissolves tooth enamel. There are three types of decay, categorized by location:

•Pit and fissure decay develops on the biting and chewing surfaces of the rear teeth.
•Smooth-surface decay occurs in areas between teeth, where they adjoin.
•Root-surface decay attacks the lower portion of the tooth crown, where the gum tissue has receded (usually in later life).

Many elements appear to interact in order for decay to develop. They include the tooth and mouth structure itself, inherited resistance or susceptibility, contour of the teeth, composition and arrangement of the teeth, character and amount of saliva, and the presence or absence of tooth-strengthening fluorides in the drinking water from birth. Variations in diet and the presence or absence of certain strains of bacteria also play a part.

Decay usually starts with a single microscopic spot, then gradually widens and deepens until a noticeable and sometimes painful cavity is seen. Once decay has occurred, the destroyed part of the tooth must be treated and restored. This involves removing the decay completely to stop the process from advancing, then shaping the cavity to receive a filling. The purpose of the filling is to restore the original shape and contour of the natural tooth so it can maintain its function. Filling materials traditionally have been made of silver and gold for strength when used in back teeth; tooth-colored materials of porcelain and plastic are used in the front teeth to look natural. Stronger tooth-colored materials now are used in back teeth, too.

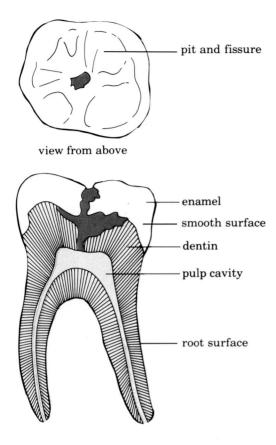

view from above

pit and fissure

enamel

smooth surface

dentin

pulp cavity

root surface

THE DECAY PROCESS
The process of tooth decay, shown from the top and in a cross section, usually begins with acid action that dissolves the enamel of a tooth. At this stage, a dentist can remove the decayed part, fill the cavity, and stop the progress of decay. If decay reaches the dentin and invades the pulp cavity, it may be too late to save the tooth.

Prevention and Control Of Tooth Decay

Because four elements must be present to promote decay, the destructive process can be broken by intervening in several ways:

Diet. Too much sugar is detrimental to health for several reasons. Most important from a dental point of view is that the sucrose of refined sugar provides a special attraction for bacteria.

Sucrose turns up in some surprising foods, including such unlikely candidates as catsup and mayonnaise, "unsweetened" cereals, and white bread. The largest source of concentrated sugar is in candy, pastries, jams, and soft drinks. Children in particular eat these sweets several times a day. Their teeth are repeatedly exposed to substances that can be the basis for harmful acid formation.

Bacteria. Tooth decay cannot occur without bacteria. Research shows that animals without decay develop cavities when inoculated with certain bacteria obtained from animals with decayed teeth. Yet some of the inoculated animals do not develop decay, presumably because some immunological mechanism prevents the bacteria from growing. So it appears to be with humans. Researchers have strong suspicions about which strains of bacteria cause decay, but investigation has not yet identified them positively.

Toothbrushing. To remove the bacteria and the sugars on which they feed as quickly as possible, the best course of action is brushing. Acid begins to form minutes after sugar has entered the secluded areas of the mouth, and formation reaches its peak 15 to 30 minutes later. Thus, teeth should be brushed immediately after eating for greatest effectiveness. Brushing first thing in the morning or before going to bed makes the teeth look better, stimulates the gum tissue, and may make the mouth feel fresher, but it is not much help in controlling tooth decay.

Fluoride. Fluoride (a chemical compound of the element fluorine and some other element, usually a metal) occurs naturally in some water supplies, and has been found to be extremely beneficial in reducing tooth decay. Up to 65 percent fewer cavities have been found among residents of areas with fluoridated water supplies. Those who benefit most are children conceived, born, and raised in areas of waterborne fluoride.

How fluorides work. Chemically, fluoride has a strong propensity to react with calcium, a major building block of teeth. The combination forms a new substance in the tooth that is less soluble in the acids associated with tooth decay. Moreover, fluoride in the tooth substance and in saliva has a bacteria-killing effect. A child who drinks fluoridated water from birth develops strong teeth, and the protective fluorides present in the body fluids during the prenatal period of tooth formation are built into the tooth substances.

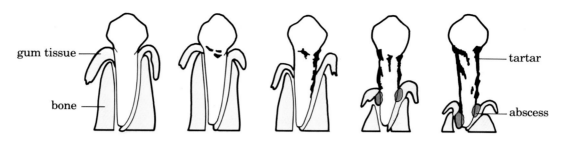

gum tissue

bone

tartar

abscess

PERIODONTAL DISEASE
The stages of periodontal disease are shown above. Hard deposits of tartar, shown in color, irritate the gums and underlying bone. Pockets of infection form between gum tissue and tooth surface. As they become wider and deeper, gums and adjacent bone recede and an abscess forms. The tooth becomes increasingly wobbly in its socket and in the final stage is lost from lack of support. Tartar cannot be removed by ordinary toothbrushing. Removal requires a dentist or dental hygienist with special equipment.

Topical fluorides. Fluorides also can provide a significant amount of protection when applied periodically to the surfaces of the teeth. When fluoride is painted on the surface enamel of the tooth, the tooth takes it up and becomes more resistant to acid. Residents of areas without fluoridated water can have fluoride solutions applied to their teeth by a dentist, usually in the forms of a gellike substance, a liquid, or a mouth rinse.

Another method of receiving fluorides is by mouthwash. Mouthwash containing fluoride is an effective means of combating decay if it is used daily as prescribed. The least effective means of receiving fluoride is by daily use of a fluoridated dentifrice.

Sealants. The biting surfaces of the back teeth usually are the first to decay. A plastic coating, or sealant, can be applied to the fissures and grooves of these teeth to protect against decay. The material is applied by trained dental personnel, requires no drilling, and is painless. The coating provides strong protection for the biting surfaces, but should be used with fluoride therapy for other areas of the teeth.

Periodontal Disease

Periodontal disease is an inflammation that results in destruction of the tissues supporting the teeth. It is a major dental problem and is the primary cause of tooth extraction in persons 35 years of age or older. Many victims are unaware of the problem because it usually develops painlessly and progresses slowly.

Gingivitis. The simplest and most common form of periodontal disease is an inflammation of the gums known as gingivitis. It begins with a slight swelling along the gum margin of one or more teeth. Gum tissue may have a slightly reddish tinge. As the condition grows worse, the puffiness and color change become more pronounced, the "collar" of gum tissue loses its tight adaptation to the tooth surface, and the tissue bleeds on slight pressure. Usually there is no pain, and often the person is not aware of anything unusual.

Periodontitis. If inflammation of the gums is not treated, the gum tissue gradually may separate from the tooth and a pocket may form between the soft gum tissue and the hard tooth surface. Bacteria, saliva, and food debris begin to collect in the pockets. The adjacent bone is destroyed, more attaching tissue is lost, and the pocket deepens and widens. Eventually, the tooth loosens and begins to move during chewing. By the time a tooth becomes noticeably loose or begins to shift so a gap develops, considerable damage already has been done. Many people do not become aware of periodontal problems until this stage.

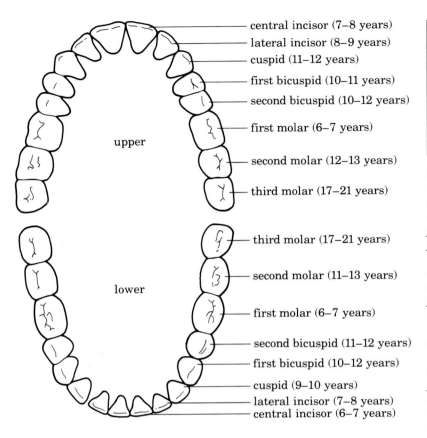

central incisor (7–8 years)
lateral incisor (8–9 years)
cuspid (11–12 years)
first bicuspid (10–11 years)
second bicuspid (10–12 years)
first molar (6–7 years)
second molar (12–13 years)
third molar (17–21 years)

upper

third molar (17–21 years)
second molar (11–13 years)
first molar (6–7 years)
second bicuspid (11–12 years)
first bicuspid (10–12 years)
cuspid (9–10 years)
lateral incisor (7–8 years)
central incisor (6–7 years)

lower

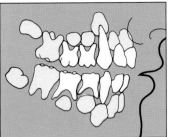

SUCCESSION OF TEETH
The primary and permanent teeth are shown in these drawings. In the side view above, primary teeth are in white, their permanent successors in blue. Primary teeth begin arriving at about six months and continue to appear through the first two years. As permanent teeth grow, they gradually exert pressure on the roots of the primaries until they are finally pushed forward. The view at left shows the final arrangement of the 32 permanent teeth, which begin to appear about age 6 and continue until the "wisdom teeth" arrive at age 17 to 21.

Treatment. Unless periodontal disease is treated early, the task becomes more difficult because the destroyed tissue cannot be replaced.

Calculus removal. In most people, there is a tendency for calcium and other mineral salts contained in saliva to combine with bacteria, food particles, and salivary sediment. This debris is called plaque. In its soft form, it can promote tooth decay. It also can harden into a substance called dental calculus or tartar.

Plaque attaches itself to the teeth in areas along the gum line and between the teeth. Good brushing and other means of tooth cleaning can remove most of the deposits while they are soft. If they are left undisturbed for 24 hours or more, they may solidify.

These solidified mineral deposits irritate the gums and underlying bone. They intensify the destructive process in gum and bone tissues and act as a center for further collection of debris.

The hard and soft accumulations must be removed by a dentist or a dental hygienist, who uses small instruments to scrape off the hard coating and polishing devices to clean and brush surfaces.

Gum surgery. If tooth cleaning does not prevent or cure periodontal disease, it may be necessary to remove the gum tissue that has been separated from the tooth to eliminate areas of stagnation and irritation. Gum surgery produces greater areas of tooth surface to be kept clean, but also makes these surfaces more accessible.

Prevention of periodontal disease includes frequent and thorough scaling of the teeth above and below the gum line, followed by regular brushing. Both must be carried out faithfully.

Tumors

It has been estimated that 2 to 5 percent of all cancers occur in or around the mouth. The cure rate is poor because cancer around the mouth usually invades rapidly and spreads deeply.

Malignancies in the mouth begin painlessly and seldom interfere with oral functions at first. The victim may be unaware of the cancer for some time. The need for early recognition of growths or nonhealing sores in the mouth is an important reason for regular dental examinations.

Irritation appears to be associated with cancer development. That is why rough edges on teeth or fillings should be smoothed as soon as possible. Bridges or dentures that are loose or do not fit properly should be adjusted promptly. Repeatedly assaulting the mouth with extremely hot drinks or highly spiced foods can be hazardous. Oral cancer also is more prevalent among those who smoke or chew tobacco, or consume alcohol.

A condition called leukoplakia may appear as a leathery white patch or patches anywhere on the mucous membrane lining the mouth or covering the tongue. The surface may be smooth and thin, raised and thick, roughened and fissured, or ulcerated. Leukoplakia results from irritation and may become malignant if not treated.

Benign growths, called polyps and papillomas, also can be found in the mouth. These outgrowths of soft tissue often are subjected to irritation during chewing or toothbrushing. Although these tumors are not malignant, they can become so and should be monitored or removed.

Tooth Loss

If a tooth or several teeth are lost, there is a tendency for the neighboring teeth to shift toward the empty space created by the loss. These teeth then may be in such a position that they are less able to tolerate the stress of chewing. Such tooth "migration" also may open spaces between the remaining teeth. This is why it usually is important to insert a bridge to substitute for the missing tooth or teeth as soon as possible.

The rough edges of cavities along the gum line cause irritation that can lead to the destruction of deeper tissues. The edges of poorly fitting crowns or fillings can have the same effect. These defects should be corrected promptly.

Tooth Implants

Tooth implants are a method of attaching false teeth directly to bone instead of relying on natural teeth for support. In most cases, implants substitute for bridgework or partial dentures in filling gaps between teeth, but some types allow the entire lower jaw to be implanted.

In the most common implant, an oral surgeon drills a hole into the upper or lower bone, then inserts a stem of composite material into the hole.

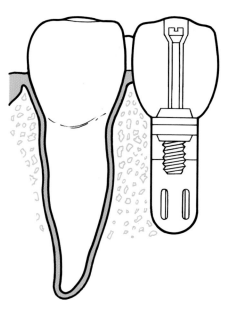

TOOTH IMPLANT
A tooth implant anchors a false tooth directly into the bone. A hole is drilled into the bone, and a stem of composite material is inserted. The bone then grows back and holds the stem securely. The tooth then is screwed into the stem. In the drawing above, the implanted tooth also is supported by the natural tooth adjoining it. Most implants replace molars as shown here, but front teeth also may be implanted.

Within a few months, bone grows back to grip the stem securely. The false tooth then is screwed into the stem. Although most single implants are to replace molars, front teeth also may be implanted.

Other types of implants use a metal frame anchored to the bone in the back and front of the mouth, or to soft tissue covering the bone. Teeth then are attached to the frame. This implant method is most commonly used when all the lower teeth are missing.

Implants are said to be more stable than bridgework or dentures, but some dentists question their long-term durability. Some persons prefer implants because they eliminate shaving down and crowning of healthy teeth, and because they are more attractive cosmetically.

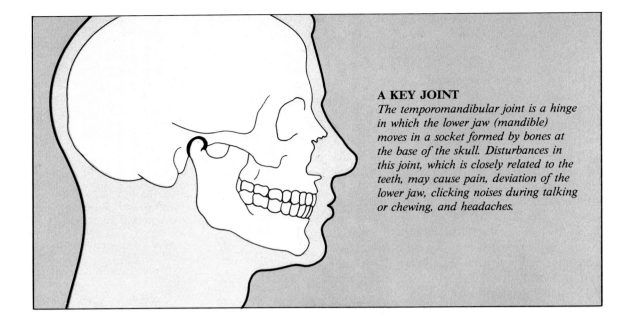

A KEY JOINT
The temporomandibular joint is a hinge in which the lower jaw (mandible) moves in a socket formed by bones at the base of the skull. Disturbances in this joint, which is closely related to the teeth, may cause pain, deviation of the lower jaw, clicking noises during talking or chewing, and headaches.

Temporomandibular Joint Disturbances

The lower and upper jaws are connected on each side by temporomandibular joints. They are in front of the external opening of the ears and consist of an extension upward of the lower jaw (mandible), which has a rounded end fitting into a socket in the base of the skull. The bony parts are held together by ligaments and muscles. The arrangement of the temporomandibular joints is responsible for the variety of movements that the lower jaw can make, including chewing, swallowing, and talking.

The symptoms of temporomandibular joint disturbances include a clicking noise upon opening the mouth or while chewing, an inability to open the mouth fully, a deviation of the lower jaw to one side upon opening the mouth, pain when opening the mouth, soreness in the side of the face, pain in the region of one or both joints when chewing, and recurrent headaches in some instances. The lower jaw may be susceptible to recurrent dislocation of the joints when the mouth is opened wide, because of a weakness in the joint structure.

Dental conditions that may contribute to or cause these disturbances are malocclusion of the teeth or uneven bite. Other causes are: overclosure of the bite, overopening of the bite, poorly fitting dental restorations, and habits such as grinding or clenching the teeth.

Treatment may involve grinding the teeth to adjust an uneven bite, replacement of improper restorations, special appliances to correct habits, corrections of malocclusion, use of physical therapy such as massage and special exercises, and in some severe cases, a complete reconstruction.

Occlusion and Malocclusion

Occlusion refers to the way the upper and lower teeth mesh when the jaws close. A few teeth may strike each other early and thus be subjected to excessive pressure. Or teeth may be positioned so that the force of tooth contact is not directed vertically toward the end of the root, but instead tends to wedge the teeth sideways.

A dentist may adjust the occlusion by carefully grinding certain tooth surfaces. The dentist may even make changes in the alignment of the teeth, or construct a splint to hold two or more adjacent teeth together, providing them with mutual support against the biting strains. Splints usually are used only when teeth already have become loose. They help preserve some teeth for further service.

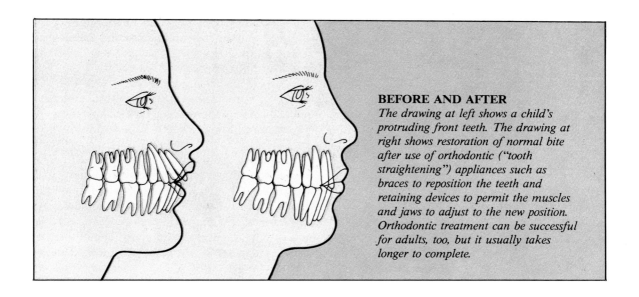

BEFORE AND AFTER
The drawing at left shows a child's protruding front teeth. The drawing at right shows restoration of normal bite after use of orthodontic ("tooth straightening") appliances such as braces to reposition the teeth and retaining devices to permit the muscles and jaws to adjust to the new position. Orthodontic treatment can be successful for adults, too, but it usually takes longer to complete.

Straightening teeth. Heredity is one of the most important factors producing the crowding or spacing of teeth and the way in which the upper and lower teeth mesh when the jaws are closed. Other factors may be the early loss of the primary teeth, dietary and growth disorders, and undesirable habits such as prolonged thumb-sucking.

Poorly positioned teeth can interfere with the proper chewing of foods, impair appearance, and lead to psychological problems. They also are more vulnerable to decay or periodontal disease. Usually, the irregularities are not outgrown but can be corrected.

A number of devices have been developed for applying gentle pressure to move the teeth. They usually include bands around the teeth with wires attached, and are used with other means to reposition the teeth and to influence the growth and contour of the jaws. The treatment also may require removal of several teeth so that sufficient space exists for the teeth to come into proper alignment. The proper time for starting treatment, the time required, and the type of treatment depend on the extent of the malocclusion.

Thumb-sucking. Infants are born with a natural instinct to suck. Thumbs and fingers are readily available to satisfy this need. Thumb-sucking produces no lasting effect on the arrangement of the permanent teeth and the development of the jaws unless the habit continues after age 4. Even then,

potential damage depends on the frequency and intensity of the habit. Persistent thumb-sucking over a period of years, however, may result in unsightly spacing and protrusion of the child's upper front teeth.

Tongue-thrusting may occur when a child has enlarged tonsils and adenoids or has a mouth too small to accommodate the tongue. Other children develop a habit of biting the lips or thrusting the tongue between the teeth during times of tension. Although these habits usually do not noticeably irritate the tongue or lips, sufficient pressure can be exerted over a period of time to alter the position of the teeth and cause jaw malformation.

Space maintenance. Early loss of baby teeth can result in a lack of space that will prevent the permanent tooth from coming into the mouth properly. When a baby tooth is lost early, there is a tendency for the surrounding teeth to attempt to fill the void. It may be necessary for a dentist to insert an appliance to maintain the empty space.

Accidents. A significant number of teeth are lost due to accidents and injuries, but recent advances in safety and prevention, plus government regulation, have helped reduce those losses. Automobile seat belt systems and padded automobile interiors have helped lower the number of facial injuries. The regulations in contact sports for protective equipment have significantly reduced other forms of injury.

It is important to know that a tooth that has been completely "knocked out" can be replanted

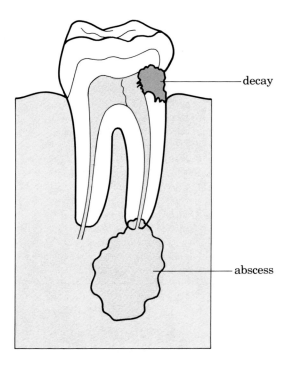

decay

abscess

ROOT ABSCESS
An abscess at the root of a tooth may result from infection caused by deep decay, as shown above, or from irritation or a hard bump. If the pulp is dead as a result, no pain will be felt and the abscess may be discovered on routine X-ray examination. To prevent damage to surrounding bone, the tooth must be extracted or treated by endodontics, in which the pulp is removed and the root canal is filled and capped.

by a dentist if treatment begins within an hour or two after the accident. Success is largely dependent upon how quickly treatment can take place.

TOOTH LOSS
AND REPLACEMENT

An X-ray examination may reveal an abscessed tooth, frequently to the amazement of the patient. This pocket of infection beneath the tooth represents the loss or destruction of tissue. It may have occurred because the pulp or "nerve" within the tooth has died from an irritation, from infection caused by deep decay, or from a hard bump on the tooth that the individual may not remember. Death of the pulp can occur painlessly, or it can cause excruciating pain. As a result of the dead and usually infected pulp tissue within the root canal, the bone around the end of the root may dissolve. This area appears as a dark shadow in the X-ray picture. Affected teeth require treatment or extraction.

Generally, pulp irritation causes pain. This means some form of treatment is required. Years ago, it usually meant extraction of the tooth, but today many teeth can be saved. The pulp is removed while the patient is under local anesthesia, followed by the preparation and filling of the root canal. The cause of the irritated pulp and subsequent toothache most often is a deep cavity.

Sometimes, particularly in children, before the root has fully developed, it is possible to clean out the decayed material and cover the pulp area with a medicated cement. This procedure is known as pulp capping. In other circumstances, the portion of the pulp near the cavity may be removed and the medicated cement carefully placed over the amputated pulp stump. This treatment is known as pulpotomy or pulp amputation. These techniques may keep the pulp alive until the root is fully formed, allowing the conventional root filling to be done later. In some cases, capped pulps remain alive and require no further treatment.

Saving a "Dying" Tooth

Pulp irritation may be so severe that the pulp tissue dies or will die if left in the tooth. If the tooth is to be saved, the pulp tissue must be removed and the canal prepared medically and sealed.

When the pulp has been dead for some time and has not been removed, changes take place in the bone around the root. When a considerable amount of bone has been destroyed, and the end of the root also shows signs of shrinkage and roughening, an operation known as periapical surgery (root resection, root amputation, or apicoectomy) may be performed to save the tooth.

This operation requires the exposure of the root end by making an opening through the overlying gum and bone. The small mass of inflamed tissue is scraped out of the bony cavity at the root end, the root end is sealed, and the window in the gum is closed with sutures. Periapical surgery usually is done on the easily accessible and single-rooted front teeth.

Fractured Teeth

When a tooth is broken off, its dental pulp chamber often is exposed. If enough of the tooth remains to permit the missing crown portion to be replaced with an artificial substitute, the pulp must be removed and the root canal filled. If the pulp is not exposed, a protective cement may be applied to the fractured dentin surface.

Tooth Extraction

Although it is possible today to keep teeth for a lifetime, there are instances in which extraction becomes necessary. Decay may destroy so much tooth structure that restoration becomes impossible. Gum disease, if allowed to advance, also can destroy so much bone and supporting structure that the tooth becomes too loose to be maintained.

Thanks to pain medication and advances in equipment, extraction methods are much improved. Following extraction of a tooth, the wound in the jaw usually heals in a few days without complications.

Care after extraction. Swelling often develops in the face after an extraction. The reaction usually is not serious and can be minimized or prevented by the application of an ice bag or a moist, cold cloth. It should be kept in place for 15 minutes each hour and repeated for several hours.

The mouth should not be rinsed until the day after the extraction. This allows the blood clot to remain undisturbed. After the first day, the mouth can be rinsed gently with warm salt water, made by dissolving one-half teaspoon of salt in eight ounces of warm water. Routine but careful brushing of the remaining teeth should be resumed the day after the extraction to keep the mouth clean and lessen the possibility of infection.

Bleeding usually stops shortly after tooth removal. Some oozing or actual bleeding may continue for several hours or even persist into the next day. Continued bleeding may be controlled by gently using a clean piece of gauze to wipe away the blood that has collected in the area of the wound, then folding clean gauze into a pad of proper size so that when placed over the wound, the teeth can be tightly closed and firm pressure made by pressing the gauze with the teeth against

When Toothache Strikes

Unfortunately, many toothaches seem to strike when a dentist is not available, usually at night. Here are emergency steps to be taken until a dentist can be consulted:

Gently rinse the mouth and affected area with warm water. Remove any debris or food from the tooth cavity and mouth. A small wad of cotton can be used to fill the cavity and protect it from the air and fluids in the mouth. If available, a few drops of oil of cloves can be placed on the ball of cotton. Under no circumstances should any medication or drug such as aspirin be placed in the mouth, on the tooth, or near the affected area. Aspirin can damage tissue and cause a serious "aspirin burn" if left in contact with the gums.

If swelling is present, a cold compress should be placed on the cheek in the area of the swelling for 15 minutes and then removed for 15 minutes. This can be done for several hours to control the swelling. If pain persists, aspirin can be taken.

Even if pain subsides, a dentist should be consulted promptly. Dental problems never heal by themselves.

the bleeding area. The pressure should be maintained for a half hour, and repeated, if necessary. If bleeding persists or occurs in considerable amount, the dentist should be consulted.

Continue eating after tooth extraction. Choose soft foods to avoid disturbing the blood clot. Soft boiled eggs, soups, custards, and ground meat are recommended. Solid foods can be added to the diet as soon as they can be chewed comfortably and without dislodging the clot.

Most extraction wounds heal without complications. If considerable swelling, continued bleeding, or severe or prolonged pain should develop, the dentist should be consulted.

Dry Socket

Dry socket is a complication that sometimes develops following the extraction of a tooth. As the name implies, the blood clot that normally forms in the socket shortly after tooth removal fails to develop or is lost. This leaves the bony wall of the socket bare and unprotected, exposing the bone to bacteria, saliva, and food debris. The lining of the socket contains many sensory nerve endings and when these are open to such an irritating environment, severe pain can develop.

A sedative medication may be prescribed to reduce the pain of dry socket. The area must be kept as clean as possible, and an anesthetic dressing placed in the open socket until nature develops a protective covering for the exposed bone. Healing usually is delayed, and several days pass before the pain disappears.

Crown and Bridge

In some instances, it is necessary to restore or cover the entire crown of a tooth. This usually is done if the tooth has been broken because of decay or injury. The crown is reduced and smoothed with a dental drill, then a cover or crown is made from a model of the patient's tooth. The materials usually are gold with plastic or porcelain similar in color to natural teeth. A crown can be made to look very much like the missing tooth.

When missing teeth are to be replaced, it is possible to fix the new (replacement) teeth permanently by means of a bridge. Teeth adjacent to the space are prepared for crowns, and the entire unit is soldered together and permanently cemented into the mouth. These replacements usually are very durable.

Tooth Bonding

Tooth bonding is a method of covering stains, building up chipped or cracked teeth, or rebuilding old, eroded teeth to make them look better. It sometimes is used instead of crowns because it is not necessary to plane and shave the natural tooth.

A composite resin is painted, or bonded, onto the front surface of the tooth. The coating is hardened under a special light, then it is shaped and polished.

The bonded surface gives a more gleaming smile, but the tooth eventually may yellow or chip after biting on hard foods, so periodic touch-ups may be required.

Partial Denture

This is a removable appliance that replaces one or more missing natural teeth. The "partial plate" is held in the mouth by clasps that grip the adjacent natural teeth. "Partials" must be cleaned after each meal, because food particles can be trapped under them and cause harm to the natural teeth. The partial denture should not be left out of the mouth because the natural teeth may shift position, making the denture fit poorly or not at all.

Complete Dentures

A full set of "false teeth," upper and lower, is necessary much less frequently than in past years. False teeth are considered a last resort, and are seldom prescribed for young people, as they previously were.

Today's dentures are far superior to those of years ago. Materials have been developed that make dentures more lifelike and durable, and less bulky and porous. Modern techniques have improved their fit and function. Individuals can be less concerned with the cosmetic aspects of dentures because they look more natural and are more likely to mesh properly for eating and speaking than in the past. Dentures should be checked and the mouth periodically examined by the dentist to eliminate soreness or tender areas, to assure that the dentures fit properly, and to see that supporting tissue is healthy.

Oral Health During Pregnancy

A misconception still persists that a developing fetus can withdraw calcium from the mother's teeth and thus cause cavities. The old wives' tale, "For every child, a tooth," has not been proven in scientific study. The fetus does require calcium, but the fetal supply does not come from the dental enamel of the mother. If the mother's diet does not provide an adequate supply, the fetus can "steal" calcium from the mother's bones. However, calcium cannot be withdrawn from tooth enamel into the bloodstream and circulated to another tissue, to an organ, or to a growing fetus. It is fixed and can be removed only by external action, such as acid forming on the tooth surface (as in dental caries) or by cutting with dental instruments.

If a woman seems to have more tooth decay during pregnancy, the cause is more likely to be relaxation of oral hygiene or an increase in between-meal snacks. If she has had bouts of nausea and acid regurgitation, the natural acid-neutralizing agents in the mouth may be depleted or less able to combat the acids formed by fermenting food. That is why the pregnant woman should practice meticulous oral hygiene.

Oral Health Products

The American Dental Association, although not a governmental agency, traditionally has evaluated dental products. Those proven to be both safe and effective carry the association's approval.

Toothpaste (dentifrice), the toothbrush, and dental floss remove plaque. Although plaque should be removed at least once a day, the dentist may recommend brushing more frequently for certain oral health conditions.

To remove stains and plaque, the toothpaste must have some degree of abrasiveness, but toothpaste containing too many abrasive elements can affect restoration (fillings) and injure surrounding gum tissue.

Toothpastes containing fluoride provide the greatest benefits. Fluoride dentifrices and a fluoridated water supply can help reduce decay.

Desensitizing toothpastes often are used for teeth that have become sensitive due to erosion of the enamel or exposure of tooth areas below the gum line.

Toothbrushes come in two types, manual and electric. Neither has been proven more effective than the other. The choice depends on individual preference, although some children find a powered toothbrush more interesting and therefore use it more consistently and thoroughly. When considering a manual toothbrush, be sure that the brush head can reach all areas of the mouth. Many persons prefer a soft-bristled brush.

Dental floss. Two types of dental floss can be purchased, waxed and unwaxed. Although unwaxed dental floss may be more acceptable for plaque removal, waxed floss may be easier to use, especially if the teeth are close together. Floss daily, following the procedure recommended by the dentist. Removal of plaque by flossing can be important in maintaining good oral hygiene.

Oral irrigating devices. These devices spray water onto gums and teeth to remove loose food particles and debris. They should not be used *instead* of a toothbrush or dental floss. They can be used as an additional aid in maintaining cleanliness, especially by persons wearing dentures or orthodontic bands.

Mouthwash. Although mouthwash may make your mouth feel or taste better, mouthwash without fluoride has not been proven beneficial in removing plaque and cannot prevent tooth decay or periodontal disease. Mouthwashes that do not contain fluoride should be considered primarily cosmetic and should not be substituted for the toothbrush, toothpaste, and dental floss.

Halitosis. Halitosis is a condition in which a chemical compound or series of compounds produced within the body result in an unpleasant odor on the breath. The condition can be caused by decaying material deep within the tooth or surrounding tissue. Decayed teeth also can cause bad breath, as can periodontal disease and gum infection. Infections in the nasal cavity, sinuses, or upper respiratory tract, a deviated septum, or infected tonsils and adenoids are other causes.

Breath odors may originate in the intestines rather than the mouth or respiratory tract. Garlic or onion odors return to the mouth after being absorbed in the bloodstream, then are exhaled through the lungs.

During sleep, the normal flow of saliva is reduced, so the cleansing action that functions when we are awake and when we chew food is not present. This condition is aggravated by food particles left in the mouth overnight, which are quickly acted upon by bacteria and cause strong odors.

Good oral hygiene is the best way to prevent halitosis. This includes flossing, brushing (even gentle brushing of the tongue), and regular cleaning by a dentist once or twice a year.

CHAPTER 21

NUTRITION

The study of food and its utilization by the body is a relatively new science, but its importance in human health is increasingly recognized. Although humans have long understood that good food is essential for strong bodies, many details of that relationship are only now becoming clear.

Food, as a walk through the supermarket shows us, comes in an astounding variety of "packages." The orange "package" that is the pumpkin bears little resemblance to the yellow banana, yet both are foods. Nor would anyone be likely to confuse grain with a grape. Despite this amazing and colorful array of packages, all foods have one characteristic in common: They are composed of chemical compounds. The early task of nutrition scientists was to classify this great variety of foods according to a meaningful system. Thus, foods are classified according to the substances they contain in the greatest amount—carbohydrates, fats, or proteins.

The chemical compounds that make up the foods are termed nutrients, so called because they provide the nourishment the body needs for normal growth, development, and activity.

THE BASIC 5 FOOD GROUPS FOR ENSURING ADEQUATE DIETS

Milk Group
(two or more cups daily)

Children	3 to 4 cups	Pregnant women	4 or more cups
Teenagers	4 or more cups	Nursing mothers	6 or more cups
Adults	2 or more cups		

Milk alternates that have equivalent calcium content:
Cheddar-type cheese: 1-inch cube = ½ cup milk
Cream cheese: 2 tablespoons = 1 tablespoon milk
Cottage cheese: ½ cup = ⅓ cup milk
Ice cream: ½ cup = ⅓ cup milk
Ice milk: ½ cup = ⅓ cup milk

Meat Group
(two or more servings daily)

Beef, veal, pork, lamb, poultry, fish, shellfish, and organ meats (liver, kidney, heart)

Meat substitutes:
Dry beans, dry peas, lentils, eggs, and peanut butter

A serving consists of:
2 to 3 ounces (no bone) of cooked meat, poultry, or fish; 2 eggs;
1 cup cooked beans, dry peas, or lentils; 4 tablespoons peanut butter

Vegetable-Fruit Group
(four or more servings daily)

A good source of vitamin A should be eaten at least every other day. Sources include broccoli, carrots, sweet potatoes, winter squash, pumpkin, and dark green leaves. Good fruit sources of vitamin A include apricots and cantaloupe.

A good source of vitamin C should be eaten daily. Sources include citrus fruits and juices, melons, fresh berries, broccoli, brussels sprouts, leafy greens, potatoes cooked in jackets, cabbage, cauliflower, spinach, peppers, tomatoes, and tomato juice.

A serving consists of:
½ cup of fruits or vegetables; ½ grapefruit or cantaloupe; 1 medium apple, banana, orange, or potato

Bread-Cereal Group
(four or more servings daily)

All whole grain, enriched, or restored breads and cereals. Ready-to-eat or cooked cereals Cornmeal, crackers, flour, macaroni, spaghetti, noodles, rice, rolled oats, baked goods made with whole grain or enriched flour

A serving consists of:
1 slice of bread; 1 ounce of ready-to-eat cereal; ½ to ¾ cup of cooked cereal, macaroni, noodles, rice, or spaghetti

Fats, Sweets, and Alcohol

Foods that provide low levels of nutrition compared with the number of calories are classified in a fifth group, the fats, sweets, and alcohol group. They include butter, margarine, mayonnaise, salad dressings, candy, sugar, jams and jellies, soft drinks, alcoholic beverages, and unenriched breads and pastries. A minimum number of servings is not suggested because these foods are "extras," providing mainly calories.

CARBOHYDRATES

Simple Sugars (monosaccharides)	Glucose: corn syrup, grape sugar, honey, vegetables Fructose: vegetables, honey, fruits Galactose: produced from lactose in digestive process
Double Sugars (disaccharides)	Sucrose (glucose + fructose): maple, cane, beet, and sorghum sugars; fruits and vegetables Lactose (galactose + glucose): milk Maltose (glucose + glucose): grain sprouts and grain products such as beer
Chains of Simple Sugars (polysaccharides)	Starch: legumes, grains, vegetables Glycogen: stored in liver and muscle for energy Cellulose: found in plants (a fibrous, undigestible structural material) Pectins: ripe fruits (seen commonly as the gel in fruit jellies)

Carbohydrates, our chief form of energy, come in simple, double, and chain forms. Starch is a chain of simple sugars. Carbohydrates are derived primarily from plants, and are a common food source.

Energy: The Chain of Life

The sun is a source of virtually unlimited energy. In the chain of life, all living things depend on it, because without sunlight, plants could not grow, and plants provide the basic food source for all animals, including man.

In a complex chemical process, plants take carbon and oxygen (carbon dioxide) from the air and combine it with nitrogen from the soil and hydrogen from water. These elements are acted upon by the plant enzymes. Then, in the phenomenon called photosynthesis, the radiant energy of the sun acts on chlorophyll cells that contain these elements.

In that reaction, the inorganic compounds hydrogen, nitrogen, and carbon dioxide are converted to organic compounds in the form of sugar and related substances. Photosynthesis creates the primary food of the biological world, glucose (sugar). All other energy-containing molecules, such as starches, fats, and proteins, are derived from glucose directly or indirectly. Glucose also is a basic building block of cellulose, a main component of the walls of plant cells and the wood of trees.

Man needs only three things to survive: food, water, and oxygen. In photosynthesis, two of the three are produced, because not only does photosynthesis manufacture food, it also gives off oxygen as a by-product. Without this simple yet mysterious process, man could not survive.

Energy: How It's Measured

In nutrition, the energy needed for all life processes, such as digestion, the heartbeat, and maintenance of body temperature, is measured in calories. Not all human beings have the same calorie requirements for normal growth, development, and health maintenance, however. The number of calories (or the amount of energy) needed varies with age, height, weight, and recreational or work activities. Although total calorie needs differ from individual to individual, every diet must contain a variety of foods.

CARBOHYDRATES: THE FIRST LINK IN THE FOOD CHAIN

Carbohydrate food substances are derived mainly from plants, and therefore are among the most common food sources. They are composed largely of sugars and starches. Carbohydrates in the form of simple sugar called glucose can be found in such foods as corn syrup, vegetables, grape sugar, and honey. Fructose, another simple sugar, can be found in fruits, vegetables, and honey. Simple sugars are called monosaccharides.

Polysaccharides are chains of simple sugars. Pectin, for example, is the gel formed from ripe fruit in combination with water. Starch, a simple-sugar chain contained in such foods as grains, vegetables, and legumes (peas, peanuts, beans, and alfalfa), is an excellent source of carbohydrates.

Carbohydrates are our chief form of energy. Compared to foods high in protein, carbohydrate foods such as fruits, vegetables, and cereal grains are readily available and affordable. Complex starchy carbohydrates, often containing fiber or bran, require more time to digest, which allows for greater absorption of the nutrients.

Energy from carbohydrates. The process of extracting energy from carbohydrates begins as soon as food is placed in the mouth. Here, starches and other polysaccharides are chewed and mixed with saliva, which contains a powerful enzyme that breaks them down. The breakdown continues in the stomach and small intestine. All carbohydrate foods are broken down into glucose, and the glucose molecules are absorbed into the bloodstream through the intestinal wall. The glucose is then transported to the liver, where some of it is converted to glycogen. This complex carbohydrate is the body's form of readily available stored energy. When the body is saturated with glycogen, the remaining glucose is converted into fat and stored for future energy needs.

FATS: FRIEND OR FOE?

Fats have some properties that other foods do not. No other food substances can provide an essential nutrient called polyunsaturated linoleic acid. The body can synthesize other fatty acids from foods, but only in the presence of polyunsaturated linoleic acid.

Fats also are the most concentrated form of food energy, containing more than twice as many calories as carbohydrates or protein.

Fats from foods also carry the important fat-soluble vitamins A, D, E, and K.

Fats appear in butter, margarine, cream, salad dressings, cooking oils, lard, bacon and other meats, fish, and poultry. Fats also are present in natural foods such as nuts, avocados, and chocolate, and they are found in dairy products of all kinds. Salad oils and cooking oils are 100 percent fat; butter and margarine are about 80 percent fat.

Cholesterol is a naturally occurring material that the body produces. It also is found in various foods of animal origin. Cholesterol is necessary for the proper function of the brain and nervous system, and is found in almost all cell tissues. Cholesterol also plays a role in the digestion of fats and is needed in the synthesis of certain hormones.

The body produces about two grams of cholesterol each day. This amount should serve the body's daily needs. Therefore, eating foods high in cholesterol can raise the level of cholesterol in the blood. Eggs, dairy products, and meats are the primary sources of dietary cholesterol. Much of the cholesterol obtained in the diet, however, is simply excreted.

Americans appear to have higher levels of cholesterol than certain other populations. Why this is so is not known precisely, although our high fat diet generally is blamed. Most researchers, including governmental authorities, assert that high cholesterol figures prominently in heart disease, because excessive cholesterol accumulates in narrowed arteries, allowing clots to lodge and trigger a heart attack. A minority of researchers contend that cholesterol's role has been overstated. Most doctors recommend keeping cholesterol levels down to a moderate range, below 200 milligrams per deciliter (200 mg/dl). Most American males have readings above that level. Methods of lowering cholesterol are discussed in Chapter 5, "The Heart and Circulation."

A SAMPLE LISTING OF PROTEIN SOURCES

	Energy				Nutrients				
	Calories	Percentage of Calories from Protein	Percentage of Calories from Carbohydrates	Percentage of Calories from Fats	Protein gm	Thiamine (B_1) mg	Riboflavin (B_2) mg	Niacin (B_3) mg	Iron mg
Frankfurter 2 oz (57 gm)	172	17	2	81	7.0	0.09	0.11	1.4	0.9
Ham, baked 3 oz (85 gm)	179	61	0	39	25.7	0.56	0.26	4.9	3.2
Meat loaf 3 oz (85 gm)	230	28	23	48	15.3	0.27	0.24	3.4	2.4
Tuna 3 oz (85 gm)	168	62	0	38	24.5	0.04	0.10	10.1	1.6
Egg, fried, large (50 gm)	108	28	0.7	71	6.9	0.05	0.15	0.1	1.2
Egg, hard-cooked, large (50 gm)	82	35	2	64	6.5	0.05	0.14	0.1	1.2
Peanut butter 2 tbsp (32 gm)	186	17	12	71	8.9	0.04	0.04	5.0	0.5
Peanuts, salted ¼ cup (36 gm)	211	15	13	71	9.4	0.12	0.05	6.2	0.8
Peas, blackeye ½ cup (124 gm)	94	23	74	4	6.3	0.20	0.05	0.5	1.6
Corn 5″ ear (125 gm)	114	9	82	10	4.1	0.15	0.13	1.8	0.8

PROTEIN: LINKING THE FOOD CHAIN

Proteins are large molecules constructed of hundreds, even thousands, of smaller molecules. These smaller molecules are called amino acids. Nutrition scientists have identified 22 amino acids. Nine of them are categorized as "essential" amino acids because they must be furnished by the diet. From these 22 substances, the body synthesizes the hundreds of proteins that it requires for its highly specialized functions.

Although protein is vital for growth, maintenance, and repair of bodily tissue, it has other equally important functions. Proteins are present in the structure of enzymes, and thus help break down other foods for digestion. Many hormones that regulate our metabolic processes are proteins. And nucleoproteins are carriers of our genetic potential, or inherited characteristics, in the living cell. Our muscles are made up of proteins that need continual repair and replenishment.

Protein Sources

Protein is found in ample supply in a variety of foods, both plant and animal. Meats and fish are excellent sources, as are eggs, milk, and cheese. Vegetable sources include beans, such as navy beans, soybeans, and kidney beans; a variety of lentils and peas; grain cereals, including rye, oats, wheat, millet, and corn; and nuts such as peanuts and cashews.

Most adult Americans consume more than 40 to 60 grams of protein per day, the level recommended by the Food and Nutrition Board of the National Research Council. For those who prefer a meatless diet, however, it is more difficult to select foods that give the proper balance of amino acids.

Vegetables do not offer complete protein—protein in which all nine essential amino acids are present—with a few notable exceptions, such as soybeans. Therefore, combinations of vegetables must be eaten to achieve the proper balance.

VITAMINS

	Vitamin	Why it's needed	Symptoms of deficiency	Sources
FAT SOLUBLE	**A**	Needed for growth of bones and teeth; for healthy skin and mucous membranes; for normal vision (it is part of visual pigments of the retina).	Night blindness; rough skin and mucous membranes; no bone growth; cracked, decayed teeth; drying of eyes.	Liver, eggs, cheese, butter, fortified margarine, milk; yellow, orange, and dark green vegetables (carrots, broccoli, squash, spinach).
	D	Essential for normal bone growth and maintenance of strong bones.	Rickets (in children), retarded growth, bowed legs, malformed teeth, protruding abdomen. Osteomalacia (in adults).	Milk, egg yolk, liver, tuna, salmon. Made on skin in sunlight.
	E	Necessary for normal red blood cells, muscles, and tissues; prevents oxidation of vitamin A and fats.	Breakdown of red blood cells. Symptoms in animals but not in man.	Vegetable oils, margarine, whole grain cereal and bread, wheat germ, liver, dried beans, green leafy vegetables.
	K	Essential for normal blood clotting.	Hemorrhage (especially in newborns).	Green leafy vegetables and milk, vegetables in cabbage family.
WATER SOLUBLE	**Thiamine (B$_1$)**	Needed to release energy from carbohydrates and for synthesis of nerve-regulating substance.	Beriberi; mental confusion, muscular weakness; swelling of heart; leg cramps.	Pork (especially ham), liver, oysters, whole grain and enriched cereals, pasta, and bread.
	Riboflavin (B$_2$)	Needed for release of energy to cells from carbohydrates, proteins, and fats; maintenance of mucous membranes.	Skin disorders, especially around nose and lips; cracks at mouth corners, eyes very sensitive to light.	Liver, milk, meat, dark green vegetables, whole grain and enriched cereals, pasta, and bread, mushrooms.
	Niacin (B$_3$)	Works with thiamine and riboflavin in energy-producing reactions in cells.	Pellagra skin disorders, especially parts exposed to sun, smooth tongue; diarrhea; mental confusion; irritability.	Liver, poultry, meat, tuna, whole grain and enriched cereals, pasta, and bread, nuts, dried beans and peas. Made in body from amino acid tryptophan.
	Pyridoxine (B$_6$)	Participates in absorption and metabolism of proteins; use of fats; formation of red blood cells.	Skin disorders; cracks at mouth corners; smooth tongue; convulsions; dizziness; nausea; anemia; kidney stones.	Whole grain (but not enriched) cereals and bread, liver, avocados, spinach, green beans, bananas.
	Cobalamin (B$_{12}$)	Necessary for building of genetic material, formation of red blood cells, functioning of nervous system.	Pernicious anemia, anemia; degeneration of peripheral nerves.	Liver, kidneys, meat, fish, eggs, milk, oysters.
	Folic acid (Folacin)	Helps form body proteins and genetic material; formation of hemoglobin.	Anemia with large red blood cells; smooth tongue; diarrhea.	Liver, kidneys, dark green leafy vegetables, wheat germ, brewer's yeast.
	Pantothenic acid	Needed for metabolism of carbohydrates, proteins, and fats; formation of hormones and nerve-regulating substances.	Not known except experimentally in man; vomiting; abdominal pain; fatigue; sleep problems.	Liver, kidneys, whole grain bread and cereal, nuts, eggs, dark green vegetables, yeast.
	Biotin	Formation of fatty acids, release of energy from carbohydrates.	Not known except experimentally in man; fatigue, depression, nausea, pains, loss of appetite.	Egg yolk, liver, kidneys, dark green vegetables, green beans. Made in intestinal tract.
	C (Ascorbic acid)	Helps the maintenance of bones, teeth, blood vessels, formation of collagen, which supports structure; anti oxidant.	Scurvy, gums bleed, muscles degenerate, wounds don't heal; skin rough, brown and dry; teeth loosen.	Many fruits and vegetables, including citrus, tomato, strawberries, melon, green pepper, potato.

Three of the amino acids have been called "limiting amino acids." If a person consumes 100 percent of the daily requirement of six amino acids, yet consumes only 30 percent of the daily requirement of any of the limiting amino acids, the value of the consumed amino acids is only 30 percent.

Thus, in a meatless diet, one vegetable must provide the amino acids that the others lack. However, a glass of milk with each meal will supply any amino acid missing from the vegetables.

VITAMINS: AGENTS
OF CHANGE

Traditionally, vitamins have been defined as organic substances required by the body in small amounts for the processes of life. Generally, these substances must be derived from the foods we eat, because the body cannot produce its own vitamins. (Vitamin D may be regarded as an exception because this "sunshine vitamin" is produced in the skin in combination with the ultraviolet rays of the sun.) Thirteen vitamins have been identified.

Vitamins act as catalysts, or agents of change, causing chemical reactions among the other nutrients to assure the smooth operation of bodily functions. (The chart in this chapter lists the vitamins, their functions, and symptoms of deficiency.)

Most nutrition scientists agree that the role of vitamins is preventive. That is, if vitamins are consumed in the amounts recommended, one will not be susceptible to any of the deficiency diseases. It has yet to be demonstrated that any vitamin *cures* any disease (other than the deficiency diseases).

The U.S. Recommended Daily Allowances for vitamins, set by the Food and Drug Administration, are determined by the amount needed each day to maintain health in healthy people. A safety margin is built in to allow for individual differences in diet and metabolism.

Vitamin Supplements:
Not Without Risk

Millions of Americans supplement their diets with multivitamins. This practice, although generally harmless, may be unnecessary and a needless expense. The average American can receive all the vitamins he or she needs from a varied diet.

The true risk of supplementing the diet with large amounts of vitamins lies in the different ways vitamins are metabolized. Vitamins A, D, K, and E are fat soluble. The fat-soluble vitamins, if not used up in life-process functions, are stored in the body, mainly in the liver.

The remaining nine vitamins are water soluble. Once the body absorbs the necessary amount of vitamin C, for example, the body will excrete the excess. There is little danger of "overdosing" on water-soluble vitamins.

It also would be difficult to consume overdoses of fat-soluble vitamins that naturally occur in food. Yet, there are those who feel that if a small amount of a vitamin is good for you, large amounts are even better. This kind of thinking can lead to serious consequences in the case of vitamins A and D. Vitamins do indeed work wonders by acting on the other nutrients and guaranteeing the smooth operation of the life processes, but they are by no means "wonder drugs" and should not be regarded as such.

MINERALS AND WATER

Another class of nutrients is inorganic in composition and vital for a normal, healthy life.

Like vitamins, minerals are required in minute amounts and are found in a variety of food sources. Unlike vitamins, which do not become a part of the bodily composition but fulfill their function by causing change, minerals do become part of our body structure. Our skeletons and teeth are made largely of calcium. Iron is a chief component of red blood cells. Magnesium and phosphorus are found in our bone structure.

Iron-deficiency anemia is the most common of the deficiency problems. It occurs primarily in women of childbearing age who lose iron during the menstrual cycle, and pregnant women or nursing mothers whose needs for increased iron are not met even with a special diet.

Water. The human body is 50 to 70 percent water. This calorie-free fluid makes possible all of life's processes. It transports blood, passes nutrients through membranes, and is the vehicle by which bodily wastes are excreted.

MINERALS

Mineral	Functions	Symptoms of Deficiency	Food Sources
Calcium	Necessary for hard bones and teeth; muscle contraction, especially normal heart rhythm; transmission of nerve impulses; proper blood clotting; and to activate a number of enzymes.	In children: stunted growth, retarded bone mineralization; poor bones and teeth, skeletal malformation (rickets). In adults: osteoporosis (brittle, porous bones resulting from demineralization).	Milk and hard cheeses, dark green leafy vegetables, small fish eaten with bones, soft cheeses, dried beans and peas, broccoli, artichokes, sesame seeds.
Phosphorus	Necessary (with calcium) to form and strengthen bones, as part of the nucleic acids, and for metabolism of fats and carbohydrates.	Deficiency is seldom seen in humans eating a normal diet. Weakness, bone pain, loss of minerals, especially calcium, from bones, poor growth.	Organ meats, meats, fish, poultry, eggs, milk and cheese, nuts, beans, and peas, whole grains.
Magnesium	Activates enzymes in carbohydrate metabolism and release of energy. Helps regulate body temperature, nerve and muscle contraction, and protein synthesis.	Deficiency is seen only in alcoholism or in people on a diet limited to a few highly processed foods. Weakness, tremors, dizziness, spasms and convulsions, delirium, and depression.	Whole grains, nuts, beans, green leafy vegetables. Processing may result in high losses of magnesium.
Sulfur	Part of proteins, especially in hair, nails, and cartilage; part of the B vitamins thiamine and biotin; takes part in detoxification reactions.	Deficiency not found. A diet adequate in protein (several amino acids contain sulfur) will provide sulfur.	Eggs, meat, milk and cheese, nuts, legumes.
Sodium	Is the major component of fluid outside cells. It regulates water balance, muscle contractions, and nerve irritability.	Deficiency is rare. Nausea, diarrhea, abdominal and muscle cramps. Excess: probably a factor in inducing high blood pressure; certainly a low-sodium diet is essential to reduce blood pressure.	Salt, salted foods, monosodium glutamate, soy sauce, baking powder, cheese, milk, shellfish, meat, fish, poultry, eggs.
Potassium	Major constituent of fluid inside cells. With sodium, needed to regulate water balance, nerve irritability, muscle contraction, and heart rhythm. Necessary for protein synthesis and glucose formation.	Muscle weakness, nausea, depletion of glycogen, rapid heartbeat, heart failure. Excess: not known.	Widely distributed in foods. Fruits, like dates, bananas, oranges, cantaloupe, tomatoes, vegetables, especially dark green leafy vegetables, liver, meat, fish, poultry, milk.
Chlorine	Part of the fluid outside the cells. Takes part in the formation of gastric juice, absorption of vitamin B_{12} and iron. In stomach, suppresses growth of microorganisms in foods.	Vomiting, diarrhea.	One-half of table salt (with sodium).

SAMPLE MEAL PATTERN

Breakfast:	1 serving of fruits and vegetables rich in vitamin C
	1 serving of grain products
	1 serving of milk and milk products
Morning snack:	Optional
Lunch:	2 servings of grain products
	1 serving of protein foods
	1 serving of other fruits and vegetables
	1 serving of milk and milk products
Afternoon snack:	1 serving of protein foods
	½ serving of milk and milk products
Dinner:	2 servings of protein foods
	2 servings of leafy green vegetables
	1 serving of milk and milk products
Evening snack:	½ serving of milk and milk products

This is a sample meal pattern for the pregnant woman or the woman who is breast-feeding. For a guide to the serving sizes, refer to the basic food groups chart on page 442. Because pregnant women are synthesizing new tissue at a faster rate than any other time in their lives, each day they require about 30 grams more protein than the healthy nonpregnant woman. That is roughly the amount of protein in a quart of milk. A nonpregnant woman using this meal pattern could leave out one serving of protein food and one serving of milk or milk products.

Individuals have been known to survive for weeks with no appreciable intake of food. However, losing one-fifth of the body's water without replacing it can be fatal.

Our bodies require at least 1½ quarts of water per day. Most of the water comes from foods with a high water content, such as soup, milk, or other beverages.

NUTRITION'S ROLE IN THE LIFE CYCLE

Because life is a continuum from generation to generation, a convenient starting place for a discussion of nutrition in the life cycle is pregnancy.

Maternal Nutrition

The pregnant woman and her developing fetus or the lactating mother requires a nutritionally sound diet, plus additional amounts of certain nutrient-rich foods.

Studies of large numbers of women in various parts of the world have shown that a woman's weight before pregnancy and her gain during pregnancy are the predominant influence on the weight of the baby at birth. We now know that birth weight is the best indicator of the degree to which the newborn has achieved its growth potential.

Any pregnant woman with an inadequate weight gain (less than two pounds per month), or a weight loss, or a woman who gains excessively (more than two pounds a week), or a woman who plans to breast-feed her baby—all face exceptional nutritional risk during pregnancy.

Diet in pregnancy. A healthy average weight gain during the course of pregnancy is 24 to 30 pounds. Furthermore, the pattern of weight gain should be relatively smooth. The exact number of calories needed will vary. However, every mother-to-be requires more calories than she did before pregnancy.

Pregnant women synthesize complex new tissues at a rate greater than at any other time in their lives. To meet these needs, it is recommended that they consume an additional 30 grams of protein a day, the amount of protein in a quart of milk. The expectant mother also requires increased iron—iron tablets are recommended because it is extremely difficult to consume enough iron in the normal diet—and perhaps folic acid. Sodium (salt) is important for the healthy pregnant woman, too.

Teenage pregnancy. Pregnant teenagers have the most critical nutritional problems. Adolescence, especially in girls, is a time of profound growth and developmental changes. Nutritional

TRACE MINERALS (those needed in minute amounts)

Mineral	Functions	Symptoms of Deficiency	Food Sources
Iron	Transports and transfers oxygen in blood and tissues. Part of hemoglobin in blood, myoglobin in muscles, protoplasm of cells, cell nuclei, and many enzymes in tissues.	Faulty digestion, changes in body levels of enzymes containing iron, cell damage, low iron stores, microcytic anemia (red cells smaller, level of hemoglobin in them is lower).	Liver, eggs, lean meats, dried beans and peas, nuts, dried fruits, whole grains, and green leafy vegetables.
Iodine	Vital constituent of the thyroid hormones thyroxine and triiodothyronine, which regulate basal metabolism and influence growth, mental development, and deposition of protein and fat in the body.	Goiter, and, if the mother has a severe iodine deficiency in the first three months of pregnancy or before conception, cretinism in infants.	Iodized salt is the sure source, plus seafood, vegetables grown near the sea where soil is rich in iodine, and butter, milk, cheese, and eggs if the animal's ration has been rich in iodine.
Manganese	Part of many enzymes. Necessary to synthesize complex carbohydrates, fat, and cholesterol, to use glucose and fats, for muscle contraction and proper development of bones.	Deficiency so far seen only in animals, with symptoms including sterility and abnormal fetuses, bone deformation, and muscle deformities.	Abundant in most foods, both plant and animal. Whole grains, legumes, and nuts are good sources.
Copper	Acts with iron to synthesize hemoglobin in red blood cells; necessary for glucose metabolism, formation of nerve walls and connective tissue.	In some infants fed cow's milk, a deficiency inhibits hemoglobin formation, causing anemia. Deficiencies in adults are unknown. Excess: in Wilson's disease, a rare metabolic-defect, there is abnormal storage in liver and other tissues. Can result in uremia, heart defects, hypertension, death.	In most foods. Organ meats, shellfish, nuts, dried beans and peas, and cocoa are good sources. (Like iron, it is absent from dairy products.)
Zinc	A component of insulin and enzymes important to digestion, protein metabolism, and synthesis of nucleic acids.	Deficiency is rare in the U.S.; retarded growth, even "dwarfism," retarded sexual development, anemia, poor wound healing. Excess: nausea, vomiting, diarrhea, fever.	Wheat germ and bran, whole grains, dried beans and peas, nuts, lean meats, fish, and poultry.
Fluorine	Normal component of teeth; prevents dental decay. May also be necessary with calcium and vitamin D to maintain strong bones and prevent demineralization in later life.	Deficiency results in tooth decay in young children, possibly osteoporosis in adults. Excess causes mottling of tooth enamel, deformed teeth and bones.	Water, either naturally or artificially fluoridated at a concentration of one part per million.
Chromium	Metabolism of glucose and protein, synthesis of fatty acids and cholesterol, insulin metabolism.	Poor use of glucose, perhaps caused by impaired insulin metabolism.	Corn oil, meats, whole grains.

requirements approach the highest level of any age after infancy. When a growing girl becomes pregnant, added nutritional requirements are imposed. A further complication may be imposed by the girl's nutritionally poor but typically teenage eating pattern.

A sample meal pattern that meets the needs of a healthy pregnant woman is shown in the accompanying table. The quantities or serving sizes consumed should be adjusted to fit individual requirements.

Infant Nutrition

In most developed societies, women have changed from a predominantly breast-feeding approach to a predominantly bottle-feeding society. In the past several years, the trend has been reversed slightly. Most manufacturers of infant food have taken the view that mother's milk and commercially prepared formulas based on cow's milk are very much the same biochemically and nutritionally. But it should be noted that the two have differences, however slight.

Advocates of breast feeding point out that human milk has been shown to be rich in host-resistant factors, which help the baby ward off illness. Breast feeding and an avoidance of premature introduction to semisolid foods, also may help to prevent food allergies in infancy.

Still, for some infants, breast feeding is unsuitable. Those with certain genetic backgrounds may be unable to tolerate human milk and may need special diets. In any case, when breast feeding is unsuccessful, infant formulas usually provide a suitable alternative.

Growth of the infant. A baby nearly triples the birth weight during the first year of life. The best guides to whether an infant is eating properly are growth charts. If the child is gaining at a steady rate along the expected path, there is no cause for concern.

Infant growth requires a relatively high intake of calories, protein, vitamins, and minerals. All of these needs are met by breast milk except vitamin D, which can be given simply and routinely.

Later, iron-rich foods such as infant cereals, meats, egg yolks, and greens can be introduced.

Water. Infants' water needs are relatively high, and in warm weather the requirement increases. Infants are particularly vulnerable to losses of water and salts through diarrhea and vomiting.

Nutrition in Childhood

The major nutritional problems of childhood include the development and maintenance of sound food habits for later life. It has been shown that failure to eat breakfast can lead to poor classroom performance. For older children and youths, nutrition education programs emphasize the importance of nutrition in life. The need for nutrition education for children and their families has been recognized as one of the important factors in establishing good lifelong eating habits.

Diet in the Middle Years

Many middle-aged persons take in too many calories, with food choices that are not always the wisest—too much fat, refined sugar, and alcohol. Lack of exercise and failure to develop habits to combat the ills of sedentary life also contribute.

The goal of nutrition in the middle years should be to develop dietary and living patterns that are conducive to a more active life associated with a sustained healthy work capacity, physical fitness, and the maintenance of a desirable weight for both men and women.

Diet in the Later Years

People who live longest, studies have shown, are those who follow a sensible diet lifelong and remain active in their later years. It is important to retain both as we grow older. Because the digestive and excretory processes slow down with age, many older persons eat fewer calories, which often makes it more difficult to obtain the right balance of nutrients; and illness and bodily changes may limit their activity. Although the "best" diet for older persons has not been determined (RDAs lump together all persons over the age of 51, which nutritionists consider misleading), meals high in fiber, low in fat, and with limited salt intake probably make sense. Older women should be sure to get plentiful amounts of calcium.

FOOD, EXERCISE, AND HEALTH

Years ago, nutritionists cautioned against such deficiency diseases as rickets, pellagra, and beriberi. Today, most nutritionists are faced with a problem far more pervasive: obesity.

IDEAL HEIGHT AND WEIGHT

This table, issued in 1983 by the Metropolitan Life Insurance Company, is based on weights of policyholders with fewest illnesses and longest lives. Heights were measured in shoes with 1-inch heels, and weights with 5 pounds of indoor clothing for men and 3 pounds for women. These figures represent population averages; your ideal weight may differ.

HEIGHT	MEN SMALL FRAME	MEDIUM FRAME	LARGE FRAME	WOMEN SMALL FRAME	MEDIUM FRAME	LARGE FRAME
4'10"				102–111	109–121	118–131
4'11"				103–113	111–123	120–134
5'0"				104–115	113–126	122–137
5'1"				106–118	115–129	125–140
5'2"	128–134	131–141	138–150	108–121	118–132	128–143
5'3"	130–136	133–143	140–153	111–124	121–135	131–147
5'4"	132–138	135–145	142–156	114–127	124–138	134–151
5'5"	134–140	137–148	144–160	117–130	127–141	137–155
5'6"	136–142	139–151	146–164	120–133	130–144	140–159
5'7"	138–145	142–154	149–168	123–136	133–147	143–163
5'8"	140–148	145–157	152–172	126–139	136–150	146–167
5'9"	142–151	148–160	155–176	129–142	139–153	149–170
5'10"	144–154	151–163	158–180	132–145	142–156	152–173
5'11"	146–157	154–166	161–184	135–148	145–159	155–176
6'0"	149–160	157–170	164–188	138–151	148–162	158–179
6'1"	152–164	160–174	168–192			
6'2"	155–168	164–178	172–197			
6'3"	158–172	167–182	176–202			
6'4"	162–176	171–187	181–207			

One definition of obesity is a weight that is 20 percent above the normal for a person's height (see the chart in this chapter). But a professional football player may exceed that measure by a wide margin, yet not carry an ounce of fat; so overweight is not synonymous with obesity. Another definition says that a person is obese when 20 percent or more of the body weight is fat. But that doesn't recognize that women have a naturally higher proportion of fat than men.

In the absence of a single accepted standard, many physicians use four yardsticks: (1) the height-weight charts; (2) the pinch-fold test to see how much excess flesh can be grasped between thumb and forefinger at the waistline or back; (3) the "eyeball test"—people who look fat to others are fat; (4) and the "mirror test"—people who look fat to themselves are fat.

By all these standards, Americans make up perhaps the fattest population in the history of the world, excluding certain South Seas islands where obesity is considered a mark of beauty. And this epidemic of obesity may account for our high incidence of diseases that obesity appears to be associated with—heart disease, still the nation's number-one killer, and diabetes among older persons.

As discussed in Chapter 1, "A Preventive Approach to Health," the combination of diet and exercise is central to sound weight control.

Water and exercise. Body temperature is regulated by water. As we exercise, we increase our body temperature, producing sweat. The evaporation of sweat cools the body, thus maintaining our normal temperature. This "cooling system" is hampered by temperatures in excess of 90 degrees or humidity in excess of 40 percent. Under these conditions, sweat is not evaporating, and therefore is not cooling the system efficiently.

Two serious problems can occur under these conditions—sunstroke and heat exhaustion. In order to prevent them, drink plenty of water before, during, and after exercise. Select clothing that allows air exchange between the skin and the air.

The other benefit of exercise. Many people who lead sedentary lives watch what they eat and still gain weight or remain overweight. When there is no program to burn off the excess, those unused calories turn to fat. Mealtime becomes one selection process after another in which the individual denies himself or herself a favorite food item because of its calorie content. We all have seen slender people who seem to have no trouble maintaining their weight even though they "eat like a horse." Only in unusual circumstances is this caused by natural or inherited tendencies.

This is not to recommend that you should go on a crash diet so that you can overindulge later. The yo-yo approach of fat to thin and back to fat again does more harm than good.

Eating Disorders

Although obesity is a major problem, some persons become so concerned about losing weight that they jeopardize their health.

Anorexia nervosa is a condition primarily found in young women who become obsessed with thinness. The victims are mostly white, adolescent, and from middle-class or wealthier families. They may begin to diet to lose only a few pounds, but then continue dieting, or even go without food, until they have lost as much as 30 percent of body weight. Yet they still consider themselves too fat. Often the compulsive fasting may be accompanied by compulsive exercise.

The condition may cause physical symptoms, including hair loss, low pulse rate, low body temperature, and constipation. Menstrual periods may stop completely or occur only intermittently; other endocrine functions may be disturbed.

The exact explanation for anorexia has not been determined. Some researchers believe that the early dieting causes or accentuates a disturbance in the hypothalamus area of the brain. The hypothalamus regulates the body's water balance, temperature, endocrine secretions, and sugar and fat metabolism, and is the location of the so-called appestat, which is believed to regulate the appetite.

Anorexics usually are treated with a combination of nutritional therapy, psychotherapy, and family counseling. In extreme cases, the patient may have to be hospitalized. The outlook is good if treatment begins early.

Bulimia affects people in a somewhat older age group, usually also female. Its victims go on food binges, eating voracious amounts and then forcing themselves to vomit immediately afterward, or purging themselves with laxatives. The binge-purge-binge cycle may go on for years and is hard to treat. The cause is not known, but an endocrine upset is suspected.

NUTRITION AND GOVERNMENT

Federal food programs. Even in a country as food-rich as the United States, many people cannot afford a wholesome diet. The federal government has therefore created various food programs that focus on high-risk populations. These programs include the school lunch program, the food stamp program, the WIC program (Supplemental Food for Women, Infants, and Children), and Meals on Wheels, which delivers hot, nutritious meals to shut-ins, the elderly, and the disabled.

Food monitoring. Since the Pure Food and Drug Act became law in 1906, the federal government has monitored the nation's food supply to see that foods and beverages are free of contamination. Today, federal laws are intended not only to protect us from impurities in foods, but also from advertising that may be misleading and potentially unsafe. In recent years, the government has enacted legislation that requires various kinds of food labeling.

Listing of ingredients. Government regulations called standards of identity define the composition of many foods, state which optional ingredients may be used, and specify which ingredients must be listed on the label. Examples of standardized foods are most canned fruits and vegetables, milk, cheeses, ice cream, breads, margarine, certain seafoods, sweeteners, and food dressings. Required or mandatory ingredients used in such standardized foods are exempt by law from label listings, although the Food and Drug Administration (FDA) has recommended that they be listed.

Earlier standards required that only a limited number of optional ingredients be listed because the special ingredients that could be used were named in the standard. Future standards can be expected to permit greater flexibility in the use of ingredients and, at the same time, require the listing of all optional ingredients. With the exception of certain spices, flavors, and colors, law requires the label to declare all ingredients in foods that are not standardized. Labels for all meat and poultry products, whether standardized or not, must list ingredients. Government regulations require that whenever ingredients are declared on the label, they must be listed in descending order of predominance by weight.

Nutrition labeling is partly a voluntary program. It becomes mandatory only when a processor makes a claim on the label or in advertising about the food's nutritional value, or when the food is enriched with any essential nutrients. The program applies to foods regulated by the Food and Drug Administration. That includes most foods except meat and poultry, which are regulated by the U.S. Department of Agriculture. The USDA also has approved the use of the same type of labeling on many processed meat and poultry products.

When a food label contains nutrition information, that information must be provided in a standard format that includes serving size and servings per container. For each serving, the label lists the calories and the protein, carbohydrates, and fat in grams, followed by protein and a minimum of seven specific vitamins and minerals in terms of the percentage of the U.S. Recommended Daily Allowances (RDAs). The quantities of other vitamins and minerals, sodium and potassium, cholesterol, and polyunsaturated and saturated fatty acids also may be included. The standardized way of presenting all this information is thought to be important to avoid confusing the consumer with multiple ways of expressing the same information.

Nutrition labeling can be of great importance to the consumer. It can help the cost-conscious shopper find the most nutritious product for the dollar and can help provide a well-rounded diet.

SIDE VIEW OF CEREAL BOX

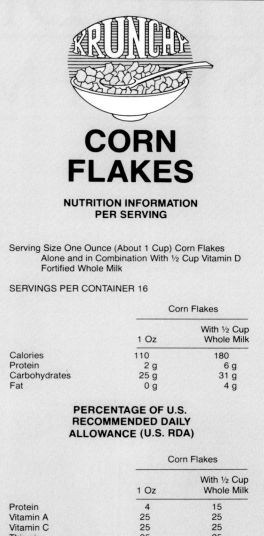

CORN FLAKES

NUTRITION INFORMATION PER SERVING

Serving Size One Ounce (About 1 Cup) Corn Flakes Alone and in Combination With ½ Cup Vitamin D Fortified Whole Milk

SERVINGS PER CONTAINER 16

	Corn Flakes	
	1 Oz	With ½ Cup Whole Milk
Calories	110	180
Protein	2 g	6 g
Carbohydrates	25 g	31 g
Fat	0 g	4 g

PERCENTAGE OF U.S. RECOMMENDED DAILY ALLOWANCE (U.S. RDA)

	Corn Flakes	
	1 Oz	With ½ Cup Whole Milk
Protein	4	15
Vitamin A	25	25
Vitamin C	25	25
Thiamine	25	25
Riboflavin	25	35
Niacin	25	25
Calcium	*	15
Iron	10	10
Vitamin D	10	25
Vitamin B	25	25
Folic Acid	25	25
Phosphorus	*	10
Magnesium	*	4
Copper	2	2

*Contains Less Than 2 Percent of the U.S. RDA of These Nutrients.

Ingredients Milled Corn, Sugar, Salt, Malt Flavoring, Sodium Ascorbate (C), Vitamin A Palmitate, Niacinamide, Ascorbic Acid (C), Iron Pyridoxine Hydrochloloride (B6), Thiamine Hydrochloride (B1), Riboflavin (B2), Folic Acid and Vitamin D7, BHA and BHT Added to Preserve Product Freshness

MADE BY KRUNCHY COMPANY PIONEER, IOWA 99999 USA

CHAPTER 22

THE DIGESTIVE SYSTEM

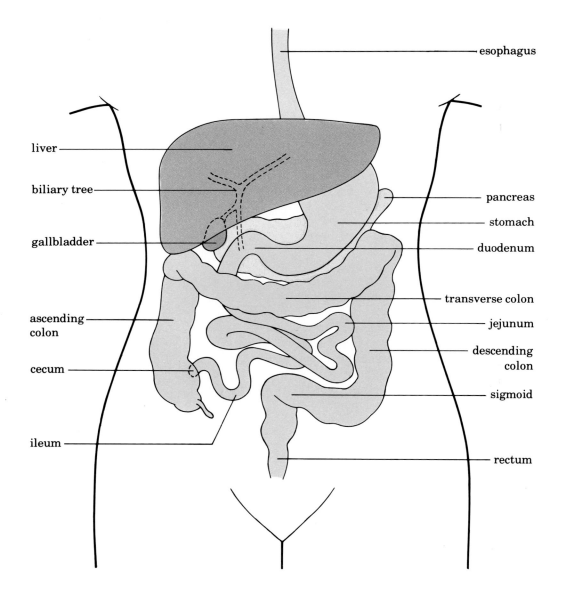

esophagus

liver

biliary tree

gallblader

pancreas

stomach

duodenum

transverse colon

ascending colon

jejunum

descending colon

cecum

sigmoid

ileum

rectum

Gastroenterologists, the medical specialists who study the digestive system and treat its disorders, usually classify the digestive system into two parts. They call the first part the tubular gut. The tubular gut can be thought of as a long, flexible tube that begins at the mouth and ends at the rectum. Its length is doubled and coiled back on itself, much the way you can coil or kink a garden hose, so that a great length is compressed into a limited space. Along the route, the tube assumes different shapes that we give different names. The small intestine is cylindrical and less than an inch in diameter in places. The stomach above it is shaped like a wine flask and can expand into a two-quart sack to do its job as a food reservoir.

THE DIGESTIVE SYSTEM

The organs of digestion are shown in an exploded view. The shaded portions represent the stomach and small and large intestines, which make up the tubular gut and deal with digestion and absorption. The unshaded areas are the liver and pancreas, where digestive enzymes and hormones are produced that help in the digestive process. Food is chewed into manageable pieces, then passes down the esophagus into the stomach, where it is exposed to acid, pepsin, and minor gastric enzymes. The food is churned into a pasty substance by the motor activity of the stomach wall. It moves into the duodenum, where bile from the liver and gallbladder and pancreatic juices from the pancreas assist in the chemical breakdown. Usable nutrients are absorbed through the walls of the small intestine. The remaining substances pass into the cecum. Water is squeezed out as the nutrients are transported through the colon and into the rectum. The remaining materials, about a quarter pound a day, then can be excreted.

The second part of the digestive system consists of the solid organs, the pancreas and the liver. Grouped with the liver are a set of small tubes (bile ducts) and a sack (the gallbladder). All play a prominent role in digestion and are linked to the system high in the tubular gut, where the digestive process begins. Their chemicals help break down food as it passes from the stomach through the intestinal tract. They have other duties as well.

The two parts of the digestive system are illustrated opposite and explained below left.

Most absorption of carbohydrates, proteins, and fats occurs in the jejunum and the first portion of the ileum. Substantial amounts of small intestine can be removed without greatly hampering absorption. The small intestine obviously has a large reserve capability. However, certain elements are absorbed only in a single area, and diseases in these areas can result in specific absorption problems. For example, vitamin B_{12} is absorbed only in the lowermost portion of the ileum. Extensive disease or surgical removal of the distal ileum can result in B_{12} deficiency anemia. Iron is absorbed primarily in the duodenum, and folic acid in the upper jejunum. Disease in these sites may cause failure of absorption of the these substances.

DIAGNOSING GASTRO-INTESTINAL DISORDERS

The years since 1960 have seen the development and widespread use of a large number of gastroenterological tests previously available in only a few research laboratories or not at all. Many of these involve endoscopy, a way of looking inside the body with the help of an optical device, which is described in Chapter 2, "Tests and Procedures." The specialist in gastrointestinal disorders frequently uses an endoscope to examine the upper intestinal tract (the esophagus, stomach, and duodenum) or the colon. Upper intestinal endoscopy sometimes is referred to as esophagogastroduodenoscopy, a tongue-twisting term that merely designates the organs examined. Examination of the colon by means of endoscopy is called (more simply) colonoscopy.

With attachments to the endoscope, the specialist also may retrieve bits of tissue for microscopic examination or remove polyps or small growths. A laser attachment, also described in Chapter 2, may be used to stanch internal bleeding.

The bile ducts and pancreas can be examined by another form of upper endoscopy, called endoscopic retrograde cholangiopancreatography, or ERCP. During an ERCP examination, a tiny tube, or catheter, is passed through the endoscope into the ampulla of Vater, the area of the duodenum where the pancreatic duct and bile duct empty. A contrasting dye is injected through the catheter, and X rays are taken. This is useful in diagnosing chronic inflammation of the pancreas, strictures and stones within the common bile duct, and certain tumors.

Peritoneoscopy (laparoscopy) allows direct examination of the abdominal organs and the thin membrane covering them. This is done by introducing a gas into the abdomen to separate the abdominal wall from the internal organs. A small magnifying device then can be inserted into the abdominal cavity through a small incision to observe the liver, spleen, exterior of the stomach, portions of the small and large bowel, and pelvic organs.

Esophageal motility study. By passing a suitable narrow tube into the esophagus, pressure waves can be recorded. This allows for the diagnosis of certain disorders of the esophagus, which the examining physician is unable to evaluate by any other means.

Liver biopsy. Obtaining a small fragment of tissue for biopsy frequently is important in diagnosing disorders of the liver. The tissue usually can be obtained by passing an extremely fine needle through the skin on the right side of the body.

Sigmoidoscopy (proctoscopy) uses a rigid tube introduced into the rectum to allow inspection of the lining cells of the rectosigmoid area. This is a common site for polyps and tumors. Sigmoidoscopy allows inspection of an area of relatively frequent disease easily and efficiently. Tissue for biopsies also may be obtained, and polyps often are removed.

Small bowel biopsy. A small catheter or flexible tube is swallowed by the patient and advanced through the esophagus, stomach, and duodenum. Small bowel mucosal tissue is obtained easily, without pain to the patient. Duodenal fluid also may be collected to examine for certain parasites.

Gastric analysis. Passing a catheter into the stomach to collect fluid allows measurement of stomach acid. Certain medications may be given intramuscularly or intravenously to stimulate acid production.

DISEASES OF THE DIGESTIVE SYSTEM

Gastrointestinal disorders range from a minor bellyache to more serious complaints.

The Esophagus

Hiatus hernia occurs when the lowest portion of the esophagus is located above the diaphragm and pulls the uppermost portion of the stomach with it. (Hernia is the term applied when any organ or part of an organ protrudes through the wall of the cavity that normally contains it.)

In some people, the displacement is quite small. It may come and go depending on body position, pressure on the abdominal wall, food within the stomach, and other factors. A hiatus hernia that moves is called a sliding hiatus hernia.

In past years, the simple diagnosis of a sliding hiatus hernia was considered sufficient to warrant surgery. This no longer is necessary. Many people with a sliding hiatus hernia complain of heartburn (pyrosis). However, it now is clear that heartburn is caused not by hernia, but by reflux into the esophagus of the stomach's contents, including potent hydrochloric acid.

Heartburn occurs because the enzyme pepsin and hydrochloric acid secreted by the stomach irritate the lining cells of the esophagus. When reflux bathes the esophagus in acid, most people feel a hot, burning sensation behind the breastbone. The burning sensation is sometimes accompanied by a hot, sour liquid in the back of the throat (water brash) and by chest pain. As might be expected, reflux into the esophagus is more likely to occur while lying down or bending over. Increased abdominal pressure, either because of overweight or the use of a tight belt or girdle, also helps to promote reflux. Chocolate, coffee, cola drinks, tobacco, and certain drugs all may make symptoms worse.

Practically everyone suffers from heartburn occasionally. The most effective treatment in most cases is simply to recognize and eliminate the

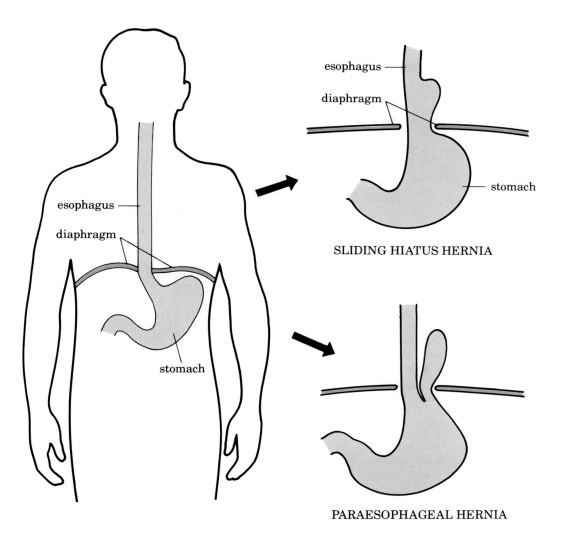

esophagus

diaphragm

stomach

SLIDING HIATUS HERNIA

esophagus

diaphragm

stomach

PARAESOPHAGEAL HERNIA

HIATUS HERNIA

Displacement of a portion of the stomach through the diaphragm is called hiatus hernia. In the drawing top left, the stomach, diaphragm, and esophagus are shown in their normal position. In a sliding hiatus hernia, the most common form, the lowermost portion of the esophagus has moved above the diaphragm, bringing a portion of the stomach up into the chest (top drawing). In the paraesophageal hernia (bottom drawing, right), the esophagus remains in normal place, but a part of the stomach has migrated through the hiatus to lodge beside it.

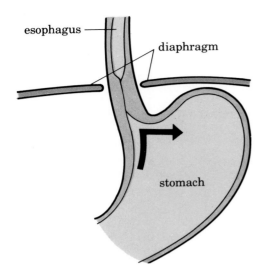

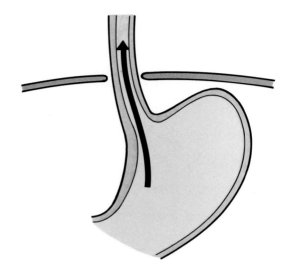

HEARTBURN

Reflux esophagitis, which is commonly known as heartburn, occurs because a weakened esophageal sphincter muscle cannot close sufficiently to prevent the stomach's contents from flowing back into the esophagus. Above, the normal *closed channel prevents backflow from the stomach. Above right, acid from the stomach easily gains entry into the esophagus, where it causes inflammation and burning.*

sources that trigger attacks. The overweight patient is encouraged to lose weight, the smoker is advised to give up tobacco, and chocolate is discontinued, along with cola drinks, coffee, and tea. Because symptoms often become worse soon after going to bed, the person is urged to elevate the head of the bed.

Antacids usually provide temporary relief. Occasionally, additional drugs are necessary. But some patients fail to benefit from any of these treatments and are candidates for surgical correction of the reflux problem. This usually involves bringing the lower esophageal sphincter down into the diaphragmatic hiatus, as illustrated in Chapter 33, "Understanding Your Operation."

Stricture is a localized area of narrowing. Most often, narrowing occurs in the lower esophageal area and stems from long-standing inflammation caused by reflux esophagitis. The principal symptom is a feeling that food is sticking in the throat. Indeed, many people can point to the exact location of the stricture. Strictures are a major concern because a physician must distinguish a benign peptic stricture from a narrowing caused by cancer.

The treatment of benign esophageal strictures most often is to enlarge or dilate the narrowed area. A variety of dilators are available. The most common are mercury-filled rubber tubes that are introduced in sequence, beginning with a small-diameter tube and gradually progressing to larger and larger tubes. Occasionally, dilation must be done in the operating room under general anesthesia, but most often it can be accomplished with the patient awake.

Esophageal varices, or dilated veins in the esophagus, resemble varicose veins in the legs. When they appear in the lower esophagus, they are a major threat because they may bleed massively and repeatedly.

Esophageal varices produce no symptoms until they bleed. The treatment of bleeding varices includes immediate hospitalization, blood transfusions, and attempts to stop the bleeding by medication and by directly plugging up the lower esophagus with a balloon (esophageal tamponade).

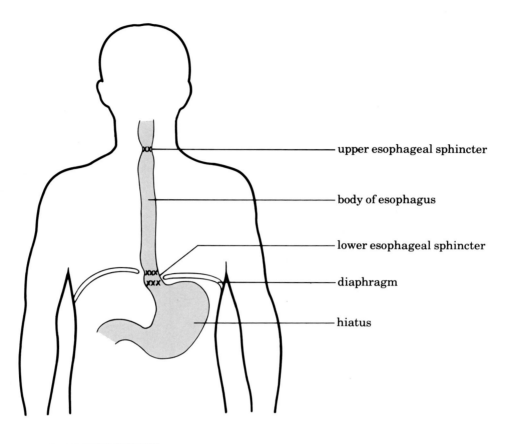

upper esophageal sphincter

body of esophagus

lower esophageal sphincter

diaphragm

hiatus

DOWN THE HATCH

The esophagus is a muscular tube that transports food from the mouth to the stomach. The upper esophageal sphincter opens to permit the passage of food, then closes to prevent swallowing air. The lower esophageal sphincter opens to allow food to enter the stomach and closes to prevent food from backing up into the esophagus again. The esophagus joins the stomach by passing through the hiatus in the diaphragm, the set of muscles that divides the chest and abdominal cavities.

Sometimes, a doctor using an endoscope can inject certain medicines directly into the area of bleeding to cause the blood to clot.

Tumors. Malignant tumors of the esophagus constitute about 4 percent of all fatal cancers in humans. Use of cigarettes and alcohol is known to be associated with esophageal cancer.

The most frequent symptoms of cancer of the esophagus are weight loss and swallowing difficulty. Such symptoms are not limited to cancer. The patient with esophageal cancer most often has less than a six-month history of food sticking, and often has no history of severe heartburn.

Cancers can occur anywhere in the esophagus, and treatment depends on their location. Cancers in the upper one-third of the esophagus are so close to other vital structures that surgery rarely is feasible. When the cancer involves the lower two-thirds of the esophagus and there is no evidence that it is widespread, surgery most often is undertaken. Unfortunately, the odds are poor for long-term survival.

SHAPE OF THE STOMACH

The stomach resembles an inverted wineskin, rounded at its upper end and tapering toward a neck (the pylorus). Joined with the esophagus through the hiatus opening in the diaphragm, the stomach lies in the upper portion of the abdominal opening. Food from the esophagus enters at the cardia and is stored in the fundus and upper body. Strong muscles in the walls of the body and antrum squeeze and knead the food as it moves toward the pylorus. The contents are then discharged at intervals into the duodenum.

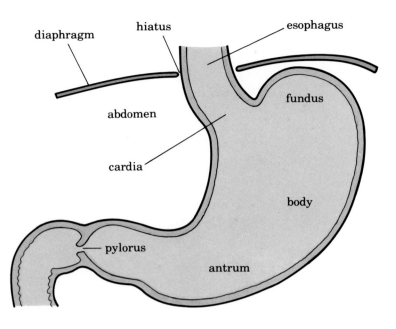

Motor Disturbances Of the Esophagus

Motor disturbances of the esophagus occur when the muscle is unable to perform its function (or performs it in irregular fashion) or when the nerves supplying the muscles are abnormal.

Achalasia is an unusual disorder characterized by failure of the lower esophageal sphincter muscles to relax. Normally, relaxation occurs during swallowing. In achalasia, however, relaxation does not occur.

Achalasia usually is slowly progressive. Earliest symptoms are vague, often nothing more dramatic than just slowness in eating. Gradually, the esophagus above the lower esophageal sphincter often dilates, sometimes to enormous proportions. Late in the course of the disease, the patient may have difficulty swallowing both liquids and solids, or may regurgitate when lying down.

Two forms of treatment are available. In pneumatic dilatation, a deflated balloon is placed in the narrowed esophagus, and then suddenly inflated under pressure, separating the thickened muscles. The other treatment is to separate the muscles surgically. There may be a higher risk of cancer in persons with long-standing, untreated achalasia.

Esophageal spasm generates multiple high-pressure waves at the same time in many different portions of the esophagus. Instead of the waves progressing in an orderly way from top to bottom, the entire esophagus is in spasm. The symptoms often are provoked by drinking very hot or very cold liquids. There is severe chest pain that closely mimics that of a heart attack. Treatment is to avoid substances that bring on spasm.

Esophageal diverticulum is an outpouching of the esophagus. One type may result from repeated forceful contractions of the esophagus, so-called pulsion diverticulum.

Inflammation of organs near the esophagus may push the esophagus out of normal position and cause a so-called traction diverticulum. Esophageal diverticula usually require no treatment, but if they produce symptoms, they may require surgical removal.

Webs are congenital, membranous bands that partially block the esophagus. Symptoms may not occur until adulthood, when food begins to stick in the throat. The disorder is treated by dilating the esophagus.

Esophageal atresia is a congenital failure of a portion of the esophagus to develop normally. It usually is diagnosed within the first hours or days of life. Atretic infants have a thread of fibrous tissue that connects normal portions of the esophagus. Surgery usually brings good results.

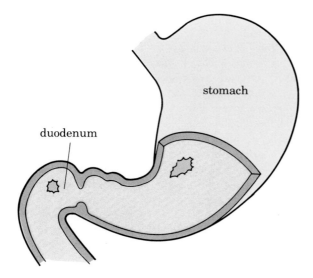

stomach

duodenum

ULCERS

Peptic ulcers may occur in the stomach, duodenum, or esophagus. Above, a gastric ulcer is shown in the stomach wall and a duodenal ulcer in a common location in the wall of the duodenum. Ulcers may erode the stomach or duodenal wall to various depths. Perforation enables contents to seep into the abdominal cavity.

The Stomach and Duodenum

Gastritis simply means inflammation of the stomach, commonly caused by ingestion of substances that break down the protective barriers of the stomach. Aspirin and alcohol are perhaps the most common offenders. Tobacco, and possibly coffee, also may contribute.

Acute gastritis may cause no symptoms, but when it does, it usually causes a burning, gnawing sensation in the upper abdomen. Since this pain is promptly relieved by antacids, milk, or food, it often is confused with ulcer disease. Occasionally, inflammation is so intense that the stomach lining is damaged. The person then may vomit blood (hematemesis) or pass it in the stool (melena).

Treatment of acute gastritis rests primarily on recognizing and avoiding precipitating causes. Antacids or drugs also may be prescribed.

The most common type of chronic gastritis is chronic atrophic gastritis. The normal furrows and ridges of the stomach are absent, with thinning of the membranes lining the stomach. The stomach may be unable to produce intrinsic factor, a substance essential for the normal absorption of vitamin B_{12}. The body's stores of B_{12} may be depleted, and a potentially serious form of anemia called pernicious anemia may occur. However, if recognized, pernicious anemia can be treated satisfactorily (see Chapter 7, "The Blood").

In less common chronic hypertrophic gastritis, the folds in the stomach are much more prominent than usual. There may be secretion of a protein-rich fluid into the stomach. Occasionally, excess acid is produced, and ulcer disease may result.

Patients with chronic gastritis often require no treatment. Pernicious anemia may be treated with injections of vitamin B_{12}.

Peptic ulcers. Ulcers are miniature excavations in the mucous membrane. They most often occur in the stomach (gastric ulcers) or duodenum (duodenal ulcers). About 80 percent of all ulcers are duodenal. Agents incriminated in the formation of gastric ulcers include aspirin and tobacco; cortisone, alcohol, indomethacin, phenylbutazone, and others. Folklore portrays the tense, hard-driving executive as ulcer-prone, but the link between personality and ulcers largely has been discredited.

Symptoms are burning, gnawing, and upper abdominal pain. The pain usually gets worse during fasting and improves after snacks or meals. It also is promptly relieved by antacids. The symptoms usually are periodic, with weeks or months of no symptoms interspersed with symptomatic periods. Some patients are awakened by pain in the night. Persons with gastric ulcers are more likely to have unusual symptoms than those with duodenal ulcers.

Occasionally, patients first are made aware of an ulcer by complications, including bleeding, intestinal obstruction (which will produce profuse vomiting), perforation (causing sudden, severe abdominal pain with nausea and vomiting), or penetration of the ulcer into a nearby structure such as the pancreas (producing severe abdominal pain, often back pain as well).

Avoidance of coffee, tobacco, alcohol, and aspirin usually is recommended. The use of bland diets, although still widespread, does not have proven value.

Cimetidine (brand name, Tagamet) is the most common drug prescribed for ulcer disease. Cimetidine and related compounds differ from antacids because they do not buffer acids. Instead, they turn off the acid-producing capability within the cells in the stomach. Cimetidine is potent and has been found to be remarkably free of serious side effects. It is of interest, however, that this class of drugs has not been shown to be superior to the regular use of a strong liquid antacid. The advantage of cimetidine lies in its convenience. It is easier to remember to take a single pill four times a day than to take antacids according to a complex schedule.

Follow-up of ulcer treatment is important. Ulcers in the duodenum almost always are benign. Occasionally, however, ulcers in the stomach are not the result of peptic ulcer disease but are ulcerations within a cancer. All gastric ulcers should heal within a certain time. If they don't, surgery probably will be necessary.

Surgery in ulcer disease. Although ulcer disease has declined in recent years, some persons still require surgery.

Perhaps the most common operation for duodenal ulcer is cutting the vagus nerve (vagotomy) to reduce the acid-producing potential in the stomach. However, the operation also reduces normal motor activity, so it often is necessary to combine the vagotomy with pyloroplasty, a procedure to promote drainage from the stomach. The combination is frequently referred to as "V and P."

Postgastrectomy syndromes. After surgery, the emptying of solid foods from the stomach may be slowed. Collections of food particles, called bezoars, may form. These may cause nausea or vomiting, or completely obstruct the stomach, so that additional surgery is required. Bezoars sometimes can be managed successfully, however, by drugs.

Some persons may complain following surgery of abdominal symptoms after meals, including abdominal bloating, sweating, nausea, diarrhea, and rapid heartbeat. This constellation of symptoms, called dumping syndrome, probably stems from the too-rapid emptying of liquids into the small intestine from the stomach. Hormonal changes may result as well. Persons with dumping syndrome must reduce fluid consumption with meals. Restriction of carbohydrates (particularly simple sugars) may help. For most, the symptoms of dumping syndrome resolve spontaneously.

Stomach cancer. The most common symptoms of stomach cancer are upper abdominal pain, loss of appetite, frequent fatigue, and weight loss. A physical examination may reveal a tumorous mass in the upper abdomen or in adjacent organs, such as the liver. An upper gastrointestinal X ray often discloses the tumor. Surgery can control bleeding, remove the obstruction, and relieve pain, but the cure rate is low. Even when the surgeon has removed all visible tumors, the likelihood of distant spread remains. Fortunately, the incidence of stomach cancer is declining.

Pyloric stenosis, narrowing of the pyloric opening, may be congenital or acquired. The congenital form usually is seen in male newborns (see Chapter 29, "Taking Care of Your Child"). Affected infants may vomit in projectile spurts, and often a hard mass can be felt in the upper abdomen. The pylorus must be opened surgically.

In adults, the pylorus often is narrowed as a result of scarring from prolonged, recurrent ulcer disease. Vomiting and weight loss are the most prominent symptoms. Although vigorous treatment with ulcer medications may reopen the narrowed area in some persons, surgery usually is required.

Marginal ulcer (anastomotic ulcer). The area where the stomach is sewn to the small intestine in the course of an ulcer operation is called an anastomosis. New ulcers may form in this area. Because of the deformity produced by surgery, the upper gastrointestinal X ray often fails to disclose these ulcers. Until recently, marginal ulcers were difficult to treat medically, and further surgery often was necessary. However, the drug cimetidine may permit more successful medical treatment.

THE LIVER

Although the liver is the largest organ inside the body, its importance does not lie in its size. Indeed, many people have survived after more than half of the liver has been removed. Total breakdown of the liver, however, is fatal. Moreover, the liver's functions are so myriad that disorders of the liver may manifest themselves in all parts of the body.

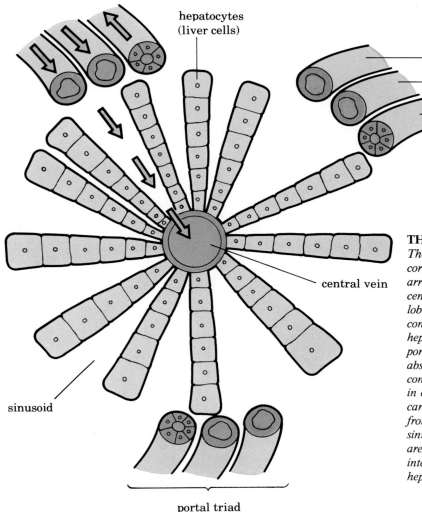

hepatocytes
(liver cells)

branch of the portal vein

branch of the hepatic artery

bile duct

central vein

sinusoid

portal triad

THE WORKING LIVER
The liver lobule is made up of stacks or cords of liver cells (hepatocytes) arranged in a radial fashion around a central vein. On the periphery of each lobule are several portal triads containing a bile duct, a branch of the hepatic artery, and a branch of the portal vein. Blood carrying nutrients absorbed from the intestinal tract is contained in the portal vein. Blood rich in oxygen from the heart and lungs is carried by the hepatic artery. Blood from both vessels courses through the sinusoids, where oxygen and nutrients are removed. The blood then empties into the central vein for return via the hepatic vein eventually to the heart.

Jaundice

Jaundice is caused by abnormal accumulation of the pigment bilirubin in the blood and body tissue. This yellow-brown substance, which is produced from breakdown of old blood cells, is metabolized by the liver and excreted into the bile to be passed out of the body via the intestinal tract. Bacterial action on bilirubin in the gut is what gives the stool its normal brown color. When bilirubin cannot be passed off by normal means, it accumulates in the liver and tissues throughout the body. The stool may become very pale, almost colorless, and a yellowish cast develops in the skin and in the whites of the eyes. This is why jaundice used to be referred to as "yellow jaundice."

Jaundice commonly occurs when a blockage of the bile duct causes a backup of bile and, thus, of bilirubin. But there are other causes as well. A severely inflamed or damaged liver may not be able to process the bilirubin delivered to it. Or, production of bilirubin by the rapid destruction of red blood cells may become excessive, and the capacity of the liver may be overwhelmed.

Jaundice caused by blockage of the bile ducts usually can be relieved by surgery, but other forms of jaundice do not benefit from (and may be harmed by) an operation. By endoscopy (see Chapter 2, "Tests and Procedures"), it now is possible to look at bile ducts to establish whether they are blocked without resorting to surgery. When successful, this procedure clearly discloses the bile ducts and can show the nature of any obstruction.

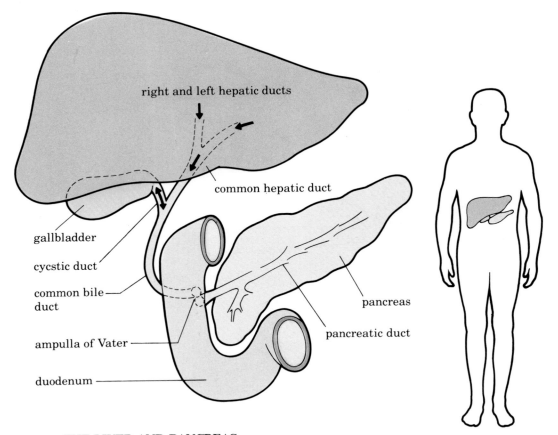

right and left hepatic ducts

common hepatic duct

gallbladder

cycstic duct

common bile duct

ampulla of Vater

duodenum

pancreas

pancreatic duct

THE LIVER AND PANCREAS
The liver, the gallbladder, and the pancreas occupy the upper abdomen. The liver is composed of four lobes, the largest being the right lobe. It is drained by a complex set of tubes. Bile flows from the liver via the right and left hepatic ducts into the common hepatic duct. Some of the bile is stored in the gallbladder through the cystic duct. The gallbladder contracts during meals and secretes bile through the common bile duct into the duodenum at the ampulla of Vater. The pancreatic duct, which joins the duodenum at the same place, drains secretions from the pancreas.

Hepatitis

Hepatitis means inflammation of the liver, which may be caused by toxins, drugs, radiation, or, most commonly, viral infection. The acute viral forms, some of which may occur in epidemics, are described in Chapter 32, "Infectious Diseases."

Chronic active hepatitis, unlike acute hepatitis, implies a long-term illness. Some cases are caused by drugs, some as a result of viral hepatitis, and some by post-transfusion hepatitis, but most have an unknown cause. Chronic active hepatitis may begin with a typical attack indistinguishable from acute viral hepatitis. In other cases, however, the illness begins gradually with a sense of fatigue, muscle or joint aches, nasal bleeding, easy bruising, or simply the gradual discoloration of jaun-

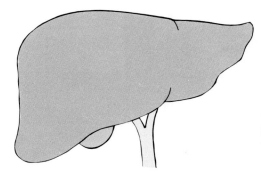
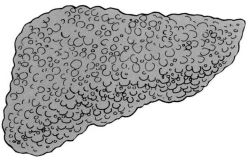

**NORMAL AND
ABNORMAL LIVERS**
The surface of a normal liver (left) is smooth. The most common type of cirrhosis of the liver (right) produces nodules of pinhead to bean size, giving a hobnailed appearance. The liver may be *enlarged or smaller than normal. An increase in fibrous tissue distorts the liver lobules and will obstruct the portal circulation.*

dice. The diagnosis often is delayed because of the mild, nondescript nature of the symptoms. The more severe cases are treated with cortisonelike drugs. The outcome frequently is favorable.

Alcohol and the Liver

Alcohol is one of the most common causes of severe liver injury in the United States. This does not mean that every social drinker suffers liver damage, because the liver can adjust well to moderate amounts of alcohol, and not all persons are equally susceptible.

The earliest liver change caused by alcohol produces no symptoms. Continued heavy drinking, however, can bring on inflammation of the liver tissue and death of some of the cells. This stage is called alcoholic hepatitis and does cause symptoms, primarily fever, jaundice, and abdominal pain. If the person stops drinking, the injury may be reversible. However, scarring of the liver (cirrhosis) may occur, even if drinking is stopped. Symptoms in this stage are fatigue, loss of energy, and swelling of the legs and abdomen.

Cirrhosis of the Liver

Although heavy use of alcohol is the leading cause of cirrhosis, there are many forms and causes of cirrhosis, which is characterized by extensive scarring within the liver substance. In addition, there are areas of liver tissue where cells have regenerated to replace those damaged by the disease. The anatomical arrangements of these cells is abnormal. The new arrangements, called regenerative nodules, function normally but block the normal pattern of blood flow through the liver.

Cirrhosis can produce a variety of symptoms. Salt retention occurs because the kidneys of a cirrhotic patient do not excrete salt properly. The usual result is swelling of the ankles and legs. Sometimes, the abdomen also swells. The treatment is to restrict the amount of dietary salt. Sometimes diuretic medications are given, too.

Portal hypertension usually becomes apparent when dilated veins at the lower end of the esophagus begin bleeding. Treatment generally is not undertaken until bleeding occurs. Surgery may be performed to shunt blood from the portal system into the general circulation, or medications may be injected to clot the vessels and stop bleeding.

Encephalopathy may be the principal problem in cirrhosis. The term means deranged function of the brain. In the patient with cirrhosis, this may take the form of memory loss, disorientation and confusion, or even coma. In all but the milder forms of this complication, some treatment is required, usually a low-protein diet and medications to decrease absorption of ammonia from the gut.

Certain forms of cirrhosis present their own pattern of symptoms and require special treatment.

Alcoholic cirrhosis, also known as micronodular cirrhosis or Laennec's cirrhosis, produces an irregular surface of the liver known as hobnail liver. Its cause, as the name implies, is a high consumption of alcohol over many years. The first step in treatment is to stop drinking, after which the doctor concentrates on managing the disease's complications.

Posthepatitic cirrhosis, or macronodular cirrhosis, is a form of progressive liver injury that occurs in a few people after a viral hepatitis attack. The condition usually is marked by gradual fluid accumulation. Victims also may have jaundice, abdominal pain, and other symptoms if inflammation and destruction continue. Treatment is similar to that for other forms of cirrhosis.

Primary biliary cirrhosis (cholangiolitic hepatitis) is a relatively rare form of liver disease, the cause of which is unknown. It is most common in women over 30. Cholestyramine often can control the itching. The disease often is fatal within five years.

Hemochromatosis (pigment cirrhosis) is a disease of iron overload (see Chapter 7, "The Blood"). Excessive amounts of iron are found not only in the liver but also in many other tissues, including the pancreas (diabetes), the heart (electrical abnormalities), or the gonads (impotence). The condition often runs in families. Treatment consists of removal of blood (phlebotomy), usually at weekly intervals.

Wilson's disease (hepatolenticular degeneration) is an inherited disease that usually strikes members of affected families between the ages of 10 and 25. It results from defective copper metabolism, associated with an inborn abnormality of the protein that normally binds copper. The metal accumulates not only in the liver but also in the brain, eyes, and other tissues. The victim may have neurological symptoms—bizarre behavior, slurred speech, staggering gait, and muscle contortion—or evidence of liver disease. Wilson's disease is progressive, but can be treated with D-penicillamine to remove the accumulated copper.

Liver Tumors

Tumors of the liver can be cystic (fluid-filled) or solid.

Solid tumors of the liver may be primary (arising within the liver) or secondary (spread to the liver from some other source). Benign primary tumors of the liver can arise spontaneously. However, it has become apparent that prolonged use of female hormones, including birth control pills, may lead to the formation of these benign tumors.

Hepatomas are malignant tumors originating in the liver. They usually arise in a previously scarred cirrhotic liver, but also may develop after other liver injury. Evidence suggests that the hepatitis B virus is important in the formation of these tumors. Persons with hemochromatosis or alcoholic cirrhosis also face higher risk of developing a hepatoma. When a hepatoma arises in a young person without underlying cirrhosis, surgical removal sometimes is attempted. In an older patient, this is seldom feasible.

Cancer in the liver frequently is spread from a source elsewhere, usually from the colon, lung, breast, stomach, or pancreas. When a secondary tumor is diagnosed in the liver, drug treatment generally is used.

THE BILIARY TREE

The biliary tree is another name for the bile ducts and the gallbladder. The bile ducts are conduits that carry bile from the liver to the intestinal tract. The gallbladder is the storage organ for bile.

Stone disease is the most common problem of the biliary tree. The formation of crystals or pellets can block the normal bile flow and cause acute pain. Gallstones and duct stones afflict an estimated 10 to 15 million Americans. More than 400,000 gallbladder removals are performed each year.

The stones themselves may be made up of a number of substances. The bulk are composed mainly or exclusively of cholesterol. A smaller number are made of calcium and bilirubin.

Many persons have gallstones without being aware of it. When a gallstone blocks the cystic

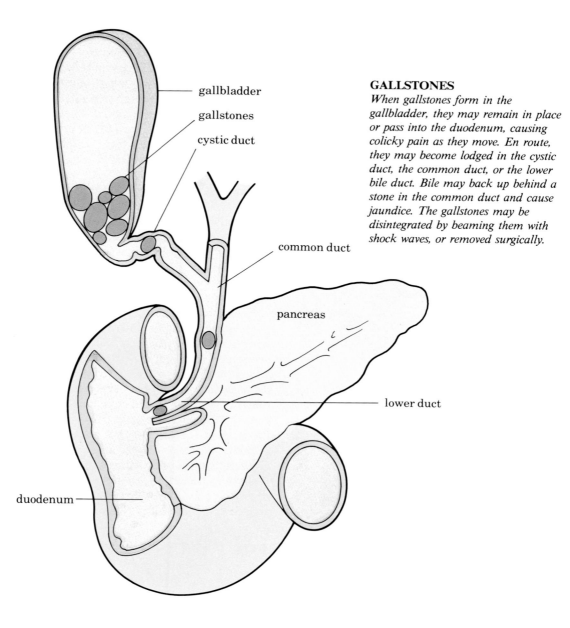

gallbladder

gallstones

cystic duct

common duct

pancreas

lower duct

duodenum

GALLSTONES
When gallstones form in the gallbladder, they may remain in place or pass into the duodenum, causing colicky pain as they move. En route, they may become lodged in the cystic duct, the common duct, or the lower bile duct. Bile may back up behind a stone in the common duct and cause jaundice. The gallstones may be disintegrated by beaming them with shock waves, or removed surgically.

duct, however, an attack of acute cholecystitis occurs and the pain can be memorable. Typically, it strikes suddenly with an acute, severe stab in the upper abdomen, usually under the lowest rib. Sometimes, it may be felt in the back, under the shoulder blade. The pain characteristically lasts two to 10 hours, and soreness may persist for several days afterward.

Some people have chronic cholecystitis. Often, their symptoms follow meals at a predictable interval. However, the notion that fatty foods are likely to provoke attacks probably is not true. Nor is fatty food intolerance a reliable symptom of gallbladder disease.

Some gallstones pass from the gallbladder but lodge in the common bile duct. The blockage may cause jaundice as well as the typical symptoms. Infection may arise in the backed-up bile, causing pain, fever, and chills.

Although the symptoms of gallbladder disease are characteristic, diagnosis usually is made by X ray. When typical symptoms are present and gallstones are verified, surgery is performed to remove the gallbladder (cholecystectomy) and explore the

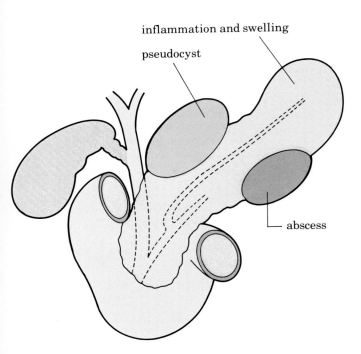

inflammation and swelling

pseudocyst

abscess

PANCREATITIS

Pancreatitis causes characteristic changes in the organ as well as complications. Uncomplicated acute pancreatitis is caused by escape of normal digestive enzymes, which then attack the pancreatic tissue and cause inflammation and swelling. Accumulations of uninfected fluid rich in pancreatic enzymes are called pseudocysts and often distort or obstruct nearby structures. Abscesses are accumulations of pus that may cause pain and fever. In chronic pancreatitis, diabetes mellitus and malabsorption also may occur.

common bile ducts if there is evidence of duct stones. A hotly debated question is what to do for a person who has stones but no symptoms. Surgery often is recommended for the younger person in good general health, but when stones are discovered in those over the age of 50 or those with underlying disease, surgery less often is recommended. Medication to dissolve the gallstones then may be considered.

A shock-wave treatment to dissolve stones without surgery (lithotripsy) was introduced in the 1980s. The patient lies on a table over a basin of warm water. High-energy ultrasound is beamed through the water at the body. The waves break

the stones into small fragments that are then passed off by the body. Lithotripsy is illustrated in Chapter 2, "Tests and Procedures."

Postcholecystectomy syndrome refers to abdominal pain that persists even after removal of the gallbladder. Occasionally, this pain represents a genuine bile duct disease. Most often, however, the pain probably comes from a different source. Not all abdominal pain occurring in patients with gallstones originates in gallbladder disease. Irritable bowel syndrome, for example, may be responsible. Thus, many persons labeled as having "postcholecystectomy syndrome" really are patients whose pain derives from other sources.

Cholangitis is a bacterial infection of the biliary tree. It most commonly occurs behind an obstruction in the duct. It is treated with antibiotics and surgery to clear the obstruction.

Sclerosing cholangitis is a chronic change in the bile ducts, resulting in a thickened ductal wall with areas of irregular narrowing. The change may occur after recurrent episodes of bacterial cholangitis. It also may be associated with certain bowel diseases, such as chronic ulcerative colitis. Symptoms are fever, chills, and pain. Surgery sometimes can relieve a local area of obstruction and decrease the incidence of infection, but there is no cure.

Stricture (narrowing) of the common duct usually results from prior surgery on the biliary tree. It also may occur as a result of stone disease. If not treated, it may cause chronic changes in the liver and ultimately cirrhosis. Surgery is the treatment.

THE PANCREAS

Disorders of the pancreas can arise from either of its two sets of functions. As an endocrine gland, it produces hormones, particularly insulin used in regulating blood sugar. Disorders in the hormone-producing cells can result in endocrine disease (see Chapter 18, "The Hormones and Endocrine Glands," and Chapter 19, "Diabetes Mellitus").

Pancreatitis

Pancreatitis (inflammation of the pancreas) may be classified as either acute or chronic. Acute pancreatitis means one or more attacks of inflammation of the pancreas, after which the organ returns to its normal function. Chronic pancreatitis, on the other hand, implies gradual deterioration of pancreatic function. Attacks of pain over the course of many years are associated with gradual destruction of the pancreas so that it can no longer perform its endocrine or enzyme-producing function. Diabetes and inability to absorb food nutrients are the end result of chronic pancreatitis.

Acute pancreatitis. Most attacks of acute pancreatitis are caused by gallbladder disease or by alcohol intake. The characteristic symptom is a severe stabbing pain in the upper abdomen, which then may move to the back. There may be sweating, fever, nausea, and vomiting, too. The first step in treating acute pancreatitis is to stop the use of alcohol, drugs, or other possibly harmful substances. Medications to reduce pain, intravenous fluids, and rest usually are prescribed. Sometimes a thin tube is placed through the nose and throat into the stomach to drain its contents. Surgery seldom is recommended.

Abscesses or cysts often form in the pancreas after an acute pancreatitis attack. Draining abscesses used to be quite difficult, but today their contents often can be sucked out with the guidance of ultrasound or a CT scan.

Chronic pancreatitis often begins with repeated attacks of abdominal pain diagnosed as acute pancreatitis. With gradual loss of pancreatic tissue, diabetes may occur. Serious disturbances of digestion may follow, and the person may lose weight, with increased amounts of fat and other nutrients in the stool. X ray of the abdomen may reveal multiple calcifications within the pancreas.

The treatment of chronic pancreatitis involves the avoidance of alcohol. Pain medications often are necessary. Surgery may help, particularly if there is a narrowed area or a stone in the pancreatic duct. Diabetes must be treated. Patients with chronic pancreatitis often continue to have symptoms and the long-term prognosis is poor.

Pancreatic Tumors

Insulinomas are benign tumors that contain insulin-secreting cells. Because insulin causes the blood sugar to fall, patients with insulinomas may have symptoms similar to diabetics who have been given too much insulin (causing an "insulin reaction"). Symptoms of nervousness, irritability, sweating, and rapid heartbeat may occur. Because the low blood sugar level stimulates the appetite, the person often gains weight. The treatment is surgical removal of the tumor.

Gastrinomas are tumors that secrete gastrin, a potent stimulator of acid output by the stomach. This produces severe ulcer disease that resists treatment. Patients have not only common ulcer symptoms, but complications such as hemorrhage, perforation, and obstruction.

Although many such tumors are single and benign, the majority are multiple and behave as malignant tumors of low virulence. Therefore, if a single tumor is suspected, surgery may be performed. Only about 15 to 20 percent of these tumors can be removed successfully by surgery, so many doctors instead remove the stomach. Because most gastrin-producing tumors, even malignant ones, spread very slowly, the patient may live many years in relatively good health. However, total removal of the stomach has become less common today. Patients are successfully managed with large doses of cimetidine, often in combination with other medications.

Cancer of the pancreas. Malignancies in the pancreas produce different symptoms, depending on their location. Cancers developing in the head of the pancreas may obstruct both the pancreatic duct and the bile duct, causing jaundice and thus leading to early discovery.

Pancreatic cancer occasionally arises in the ampulla of Vater, the point where the pancreatic duct and the bile duct enter the duodenum. The outlook for patients with tumors here is somewhat better than for patients with cancers elsewhere in the pancreas.

When the cancer originates in the body or tail of the pancreas, there ordinarily are no symptoms until the tumor has progressed too far to be operable. The first symptom usually is upper abdominal pain, which often radiates into the back. The patient may lose weight and develop diabetes. A profound change in mood, usually depression, is common. The increase in pancreatic cancer has not been matched by more successful treatment. Widespread use of ultrasound and CT scans has improved diagnosis but not survival.

THE SMALL INTESTINE

Afflictions of the small intestine range from congenital structural problems to progressive disease, and from mild symptoms to distressing ones.

Congenital atresia and stenosis. Occasionally, a section of the small bowel fails to develop into a tubular structure. A segment of fibrous cord develops instead. If the involved portion forms a tube that does not reach sufficient diameter to allow passage of foodstuffs, the narrowing is termed stenosis. The symptoms are those of intestinal obstruction: vomiting and a distended abdomen. The stenosis must be repaired surgically.

Meckel's diverticulum, an outpouching of the small intestine that produces a fingerlike pouch, is the most frequent congenital abnormality of the intestinal tract. It usually occurs near the junction of the small bowel and colon.

Ileus is a temporary inability of the small intestine to propel foodstuffs along its length so that absorption can take place. There are two types of ileus. Paralytic ileus occurs when any damage to the abdominal cavity or the nerves leading to the gut is severe enough to halt intestinal action. This may happen, for instance, immediately after surgery, when the bowel is silent. Paralytic ileus also may be caused by a perforation of the bowel or infection in the abdominal cavity. The treatment is to put the intestine at rest, stopping all food by mouth and draining the stomach with a tube passed through the nose. The underlying condition that caused the ileus must be treated as well.

Mechanical ileus (intestinal obstruction) occurs when blockage prevents the normal flow of intestinal contents. A common cause is an adhesive band that develops across the bowel. In an attempt to get beyond the obstructed segment, the intestine increases its propulsion activity with more forceful contraction of the intestinal walls. This causes severe abdominal pain. Later the abdomen enlarges and vomiting begins.

Other causes of mechanical small bowel obstruction include intussusception, a condition in which a portion of the small intestine telescopes within the adjacent portion of the intestine; volvulus, when a segment of bowel twists upon itself like a knot; and strictures, areas of narrowed bowel. The treatment of all three is surgical.

Hernias are protrusions of the small intestine through the abdominal wall. They include inguinal hernia (common in men), femoral hernia (common in women), and ventral hernia (through the abdomen's forward wall).

A reducible hernia is one in which the displaced portion of the intestine can be pushed back into normal position, usually with simple pressure of the fingers. An incarcerated hernia cannot be restored to its proper place. A strangulated hernia is an incarcerated hernia in which the blood supply to the intestine is pinched off by the narrowness of the opening. This dangerous condition is a medical emergency.

Inguinal hernia accounts for more than 80 percent of all hernias. The condition occurs when a loop of the bowel passes through the inguinal opening, the passageway through which the male spermatic cord passes to the scrotum. The cause usually is weakening of the abdominal muscles with age, but sometimes the opening has been widened by the strain of improper lifting or even a violent coughing attack. One or both sides may be affected. The hernia may develop gradually or arise suddenly.

Typically, an inguinal hernia shows itself with a bulge in the groin, accompanied by mild pain. An incarcerated hernia may cause bowel obstruction and greater pain. Even though an inguinal hernia may be reducible, elective surgery usually is recommended because of the danger of eventual incarceration and strangulation (see Chapter 33, "Understanding Your Operation"). However, an elderly patient may be satisfactorily treated with a truss, a garment to support the abdominal wall and keep the hernia reduced. Surgery also is recommended for femoral and many ventral hernias.

Regional enteritis (Crohn's disease) is a disease of unknown cause characterized by inflammation in the intestinal tract. It most commonly involves the distal ileum, the lowermost portion of the small intestine. The disease may occur primarily in the small bowel, primarily in the colon, or in both. Uncommonly, it may involve the esophagus, stomach, or duodenum.

Symptoms depend on the location of the inflammation and its complications. Indeed, it is not uncommon for a patient to have early symptoms of regional enteritis for many months or even years and be thought to have simple indigestion or irritable bowel syndrome. When the inflammation is in the distal ileum, the symptoms usually are crampy lower abdominal pain, diarrhea, and weight loss. Afflicted children may grow more slowly than normal and have fever, nausea, and vomiting.

Regional enteritis involves many systems of the body, so that symptoms and signs outside the intestinal tract may occur as well. They may include eye disease; canker sores; arthritis and muscle aches; red, raised, tender nodules on the skin of the legs; or even skin ulcers. Fissures, abscesses, or fistulae of the rectum are common. When the inflammation primarily affects the colon, diarrhea is common and frequently there is rectal bleeding.

Crohn's disease is treated with drugs of the cortisone family, such as prednisone, and with sulfasalazine if the colon is involved. The disease usually can be managed successfully with medication for a period of time, although a majority of patients eventually require one or more operations to remove affected portions of the bowel.

Malabsorption syndrome results from a number of diseases that prevent the small bowel from absorbing nutrients properly. The most striking symptoms usually result from an inability of the intestine to absorb fats. The cardinal symptom of fat malabsorption is the daily production of a large, bulky, foul-smelling stool. The stool usually is pale and very sticky. Oil globules may be seen in the toilet water. Patients who have had malabsorption for many months or years have weight loss (or failure to grow, in the case of children), easy bruising, weakness, and fatigue.

Several diseases of the small intestine may produce malabsorption syndrome. Celiac disease, also called nontropical sprue, usually is a disease of children, but also may occur in adults. It is caused by a sensitivity of the intestinal tract to gluten, a protein present in many grains, including wheat flour used in bread.

The child with celiac disease improves on a gluten-free diet, usually within weeks or months, but must follow the diet for an indefinite period, possibly for life. Extensive disease in the small bowel, such as regional enteritis, also may result in malabsorption.

Tumors of the small bowel are uncommon. Symptoms are obstruction and sometimes bleeding. A mass may be felt in the abdomen. The tumor usually is removed surgically.

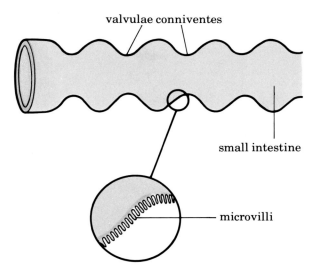

valvulae conniventes

small intestine

microvilli

THE COMPACT INTESTINE
The surface available for absorption in the small intestine is increased many times by the accordionlike folds of the intestinal walls, called valvulae conniventes, and the five million hairlike microvilli, shown above.

Carcinoid tumors are peculiar growths of the intestinal tract that frequently begin in the small bowel but also may occur in the appendix, cecum, or other areas. These tumors occasionally secrete hormones, most commonly serotonin. A benign carcinoid tumor is limited to the intestinal tract, and the serotonin is rapidly neutralized in the liver, so it produces no symptoms. Malignant carcinoid tumors may spread to the liver, and from there large amounts of serotonin may be released into the general circulation. This may produce a group of symptoms, including flushing, sweating, rapid heartbeat, and diarrhea. Antitumor drugs and other medications reduce the symptoms. Sometimes, all or most of the tumor can be removed surgically.

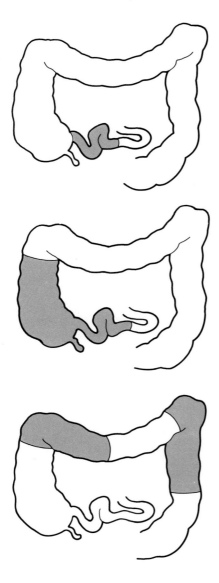

CROHN'S DISEASE
Regional enteritis, or Crohn's disease, may affect any part of the large or small intestine, and less commonly, the esophagus and stomach. Three common patterns of disease are shown here. Disease confined to the small intestine (enteritis) (top drawing) almost always involves the last portion of the ileum. Additional areas of the small intestine may be involved, sometimes with disease-free areas between. In the enterocolic variety (center drawing), both the small intestine and the colon are diseased. Colonic Crohn's disease may involve the entire colon, a segment, or multiple segments (bottom), but the small bowel is spared.

THE COLON

Like the small intestine, the colon is subject to disease throughout its length, malformations, and structural abnormalities. The more common malformations of the colon include imperforate anus and congenital megacolon.

● **Imperforate anus** may be a partial or complete blockage of the waste material's final passageway to the outside. It is discovered soon after birth. The infant may be unable to pass stools normally, and may have an enlarged abdomen and the crampy pain associated with colic. If the problem is only narrowing, daily dilatation may enlarge the rectum to the proper dimension. If the normal passage has not formed or is blocked, an operation will be necessary.

● **Congenital megacolon** (Hirschsprung's disease) occurs because of faulty development of the nerves that control the rectum (see Chapter 29, "Taking Care of Your Child"). Megacolon, too, usually becomes apparent shortly after birth, when the obstructed colon grows to giant proportions, swelling the abdomen. The condition can be corrected surgically.

Inflammatory Diseases Of the Colon

Appendicitis refers to an inflammation of the appendix, that unexplained blind loop of tissue suspended from the cecum. The inflammation may be caused by obstruction of the appendix, although there are other causes.

Appendicitis is rare before the age of 5 and seldom occurs after age 50. Typical symptoms are pain, nausea or vomiting, tenderness in the lower right portion of the abdomen, and fever. Often, the pain is felt first in the center of the abdomen, then shifts to the lower right portion after several hours. An important clue is sudden onset of symptoms in a person who previously was healthy.

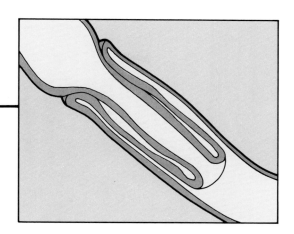

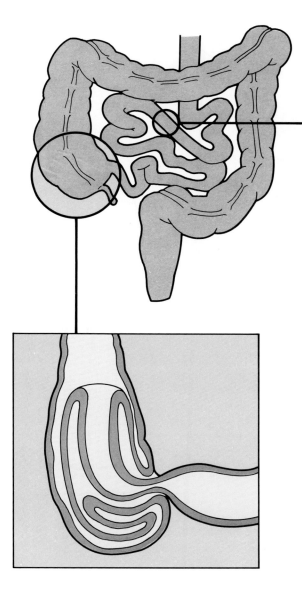

TELESCOPED BOWEL

Intussusception is a "telescoping" of a loop of bowel, somewhat like pushing the finger of a rubber glove into itself. The infolded segment may obstruct passage of the contents of the intestine and endanger the local blood supply. Symptoms usually include sharp, sudden abdominal pain, nausea, and vomiting. Immediate treatment is necessary. The top drawing shows a loop of small bowel telescoped into itself. At left, a loop of the ileum is telescoped into the cecum and ascending colon.

Prompt surgical intervention is necessary. It is important not to give the person food or laxatives, or to apply heat. Surgical removal of the inflamed appendix is a relatively simple procedure (see Chapter 33, "Understanding Your Operation").

Inflammatory bowel disease is a general term for inflammation of the lining cells of the colon. Causes include infection, types of dysentery, tuberculosis, gonorrhea, and certain parasites.

However, the most common forms of inflammatory bowel disease are those whose cause is unknown. There are two distinct types, Crohn's colitis (granulomatous colitis or regional enterocolitis) and ulcerative colitis. Crohn's colitis is the same basic disease as regional enteritis, except that it occurs in the colon.

Chronic ulcerative colitis is characterized by recurrent bouts of rectal bleeding usually associated with diarrhea. If disease is limited to a few centimeters of the rectum, it is termed ulcerative proctitis. More extensive disease may include the entire

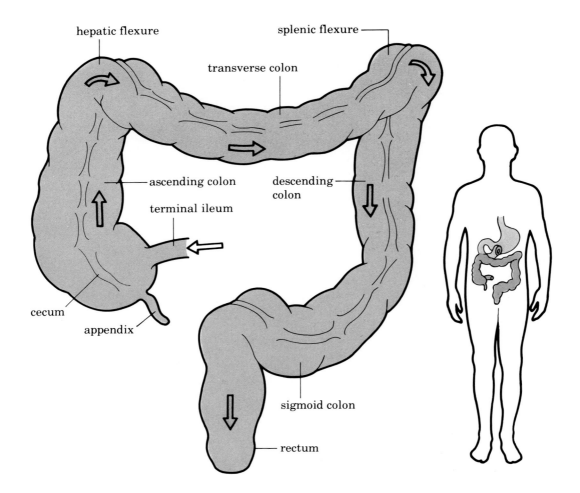

THE LARGE INTESTINE

The large intestine, or colon, forms a nearly rectangular shape around the perimeter of the abdomen. It begins where the ileum of the small intestine empties into the cecum. Contents then move upward (shown by arrows) through the ascending colon, make a 90-degree turn at the hepatic flexure, *travel across the transverse colon, turn again at the splenic flexure, and move through the descending colon to the S-shaped sigmoid colon to the rectum. En route, the quart of material from the small intestine is reduced and compacted to about one-fourth pound of daily stool.*

colon. The diagnosis usually is made by proctoscopic examination. In ulcerative colitis, the rectum almost always is involved. A colonoscope may be used to determine the extent of the disease and to assess the risk of cancer.

Some persons with proctitis can be treated with medicated enemas. When medication is needed, it usually is sulfasalazine. Cortisonelike drugs may be added.

Surgery ordinarily is considered in cases of toxic megacolon, when severe symptoms fail to respond to medical treatment, or in long-standing disease with precancerous changes. The entire colon then must be removed and the ileum attached to the skin (ileostomy) for emptying intestinal contents into a bag.

Toxic megacolon is an uncommon complication of ulcerative colitis. Patients with this disorder are very sick with fever, abdominal distension, and even mental changes. The abdomen is distended and X ray of the abdomen shows an enlarged colon. There is danger that the colon may perforate. If medication does not bring prompt improvement, surgery is undertaken.

A patient with severe and unresponsive symptoms but without megacolon is treated first with medications. If there is no improvement after several months, surgery usually is recommended.

Finally, surgery may be undertaken in some patients who have had their disease more than 10 years because the risk of colon cancer is increased, especially among those whose disease began in childhood and whose entire colon is involved.

Tumors of the Colon

Benign polyps make up the majority of tumors of the colon. These are localized overgrowths of tissue, often in or near the sigmoid colon. Some polyps have a fibrous stalk connecting the tumor with the colon. These are referred to as pedunculated polyps. Polyps usually cause no symptoms. The treatment of most polyps, whether they cause symptoms or not, is removal, because polyps occasionally may degenerate into cancer.

Most colonic polyps can be removed without an operation. The polyp is located by sigmoidoscope or colonoscope. A wire snare advanced through the scope is looped around the base (around the stalk if the polyp is pedunculated). Electrical current applied through the wire can cut through the tissue and simultaneously seal off any bleeding vessels. The severed polyp then is retrieved and examined for malignancy. There are a number of rare familial polyposis syndromes, where the polyps are widespread and the risk of cancer approaches 100 percent. The usual treatment for these patients is removal of the colon.

Malignant tumors. The cause of colon cancer, as with many cancers, is unknown. Some evidence suggests that the American diet plays an important role, but there is no reason to think that colon cancer has only one cause.

The location of colon cancer often determines its symptoms. Cecal cancers often produce only vague symptoms, such as weakness, weight loss,

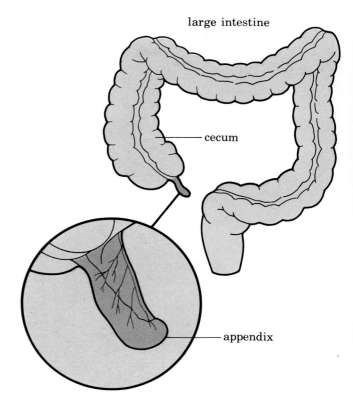

large intestine

cecum

appendix

APPENDICITIS
The vermiform appendix is a small, narrow, blind tube projecting from the cecum. A distended and inflamed appendix may rupture, release toxic contents, and cause peritonitis. The inflammation also may impair blood supply in the single artery serving the appendix. Gangrene may result. Although an inflamed appendix classically produces pain in the lower right abdomen, symptoms vary, especially in young persons. Do not give laxatives or painkillers to persons with abdominal pain.

and vague abdominal pain. They do not obstruct the flow of colonic contents because the contents are liquid and can pass through even a narrowed space with relative ease. Cecal cancers often bleed intermittently.

Colon cancers that occur in the sigmoid colon closer to the rectum are more likely to obstruct the passage of stool. They also are more likely to bleed, and therefore give earlier warning of their presence. Most cancers occur in the sigmoid or descending colon.

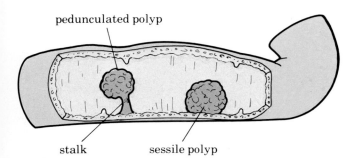

pedunculated polyp

stalk   sessile polyp

COLONIC POLYPS

Two types of polyps that may develop in the colon are called pedunculated if they have a stalk and sessile if they have no stalk. Differences in tissue seen under the microscope further divide them into adenomatous and villous. Some colonic polys apparently lead to the development of cancer. Large polyps are more dangerous than small ones, and villous polyps are more dangerous than adenomatous ones.

The treatment of most colon cancers is surgical. When the tumor is limited to the lining of the colon, the survival rate after surgery is 70 to 80 percent (without tumor recurrence) five years later. More extensive tumor invasion produces a much lower five-year survival rate. When the tumor occurs close to the rectum, the surgeon must remove the rectum as well as the tumor. This requires the patient to have a colostomy, in which a loop of bowel is brought through the skin of the abdomen. Stool passes through the loop and is collected in a bag for disposal. Most cancer that occurs higher up in the colon can be removed and the ends of the colon reattached. These patients will not require a colostomy and have normal bowel function afterward.

Other Colon and Rectal Disorders

Hemorrhoids are dilated veins that occur in the rectum. Hemorrhoids usually cause no symptoms and require no treatment. Occasionally, a blood clot or thrombosis develops in the hemorrhoid, but this usually is treated by a sitz bath (sitting in warm water with the legs out) or suppositories. Surgical removal of the thrombosed hemorrhoid occasionally is necessary. Surgery also may be performed if the ring of hemorrhoids becomes large and bulky. The other problem caused by hemorrhoids is bleeding. Repeated bleeding may be an indication for surgical treatment.

Irritable bowel syndrome is the most common diagnosis made in a gastroenterology clinic. The condition causes substantial suffering and loss of work, yet is poorly understood. Most often, the person complains of pain in the lower abdomen. There frequently is a pattern of disordered bowel movements. Some patients complain of constipation, others of diarrhea; most have alternating constipation and diarrhea.

The disorder often begins in late adolescence or early adulthood. Tension, anxiety, and worry may contribute, but it is not a "psychological disorder," because objective changes in colon activity can be found.

A surprising number of people with irritable bowel symptoms improve substantially when they learn that their pain does not represent cancer or some other feared disease. Often, a doctor will suggest that the patient follow a diet high in fiber, and may suggest that he or she supplement it by adding bran or other fiber. Drugs to quiet the bowel's spasms sometimes are prescribed.

Diverticulosis and diverticulitis. Diverticulosis means the presence of one or more diverticula in the colon. A diverticulum is an outpouching through a weakened area in the wall of the bowel. Such outpouchings are extremely common in people over age 50. In general, diverticula cause no symptoms, but occasionally, bleeding, infection, or inflammation may occur.

A person with a bleeding diverticulum develops sudden, copious, red rectal bleeding. The onset is so dramatic that he or she usually wastes no time in seeking medical attention. Treatment is to replace lost blood. If the bleeding does not stop spontaneously, surgery is necessary.

The infected diverticulum is referred to as diverticulitis. Diverticulitis begins as a rather abrupt onset of lower abdominal pain, a change in bowel habits (usually constipation), fever and sometimes chills, and sometimes rectal bleeding. Acute diverticulitis is treated with antibiotics. Fluids are given intravenously, and diet is restricted. After an acute episode, a high-fiber diet often is recommended.

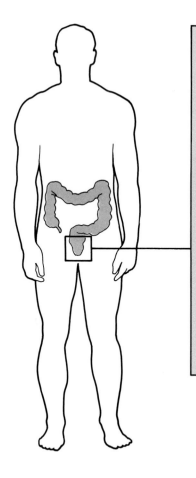

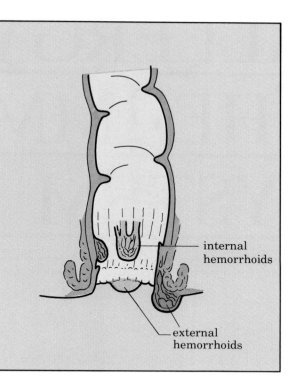

internal
hemorrhoids

external
hemorrhoids

HEMORRHOIDS
*The common condition of hemorrhoids
(piles) results from dilated veins in the
region of the anus. Internal
hemorrhoids originate fairly high in the
rectum. External hemorrhoids occur
outside the sphincter muscles that
control the outlet.*

Fistula. A fistula is an abnormal connection between adjacent structures. A rectal fistula usually forms between the skin around the rectum and the rectum itself. A symptom of a fistula is an abnormal drainage, often pus, but it also may resemble stool. The treatment is surgical to remove the connection.

Perirectal abscess usually begins with throbbing, constant pain around the rectal area. A tender mass may be found, either near or within the rectum. If the abscess is large, the person also may have fever. The abscess must be removed surgically.

Anal fissure is a tiny tear in the mucous membrane and skin at the anus. It is an extremely painful disorder, so there often is a conscious effort to avoid having a bowel movement. If the fissure has been present only a short time, the treatment generally includes pain medicine, warm sitz baths, and medicines to soften the stool. If the fissure has been present for some time, it may be necessary to repair it surgically.

Pruritus ani is not a disease but a symptom, and a common one. It is an intense itching sensation at the rectum. It is not caused by hemorrhoids. Most cases are of unknown cause. Relief usually is obtained by good (but not overly aggressive) anal hygiene. Pruritus ani is not a serious malady, but it certainly is a humbling one.

CHAPTER 23

ALLERGY AND THE IMMUNE SYSTEM

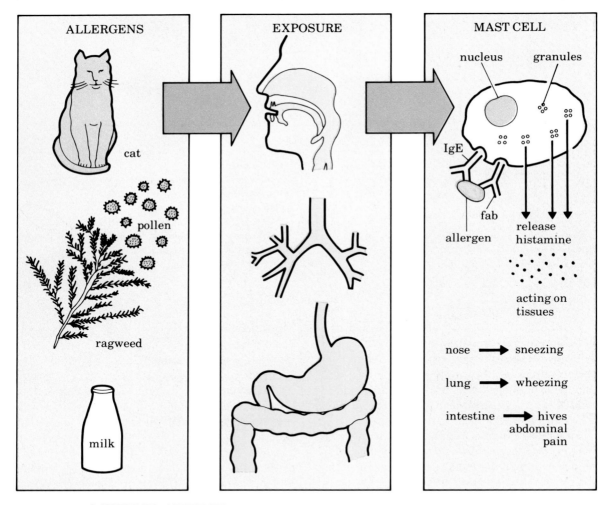

ALLERGENS

cat

pollen

ragweed

milk

EXPOSURE

MAST CELL

nucleus   granules

IgE

fab

allergen

release
histamine

acting on
tissues

nose → sneezing

lung → wheezing

intestine → hives
abdominal
pain

3 STEPS TO ALLERGY

The essentials of an allergic reaction occur in three steps. Allergens are substances that originate outside the body. Animal dander, plant pollens, and foods are examples. They usually enter the body through the nose and mouth, although some enter through the skin. They affect the mucous membranes of the nose, throat, and respiratory and digestive systems. When they combine with immunoglobin E (IgE), attached to the small mast cells in these areas, the cells release histamine and other substances that act on the tissues to produce symptoms such as sneezing, wheezing, and hives.

Allergies are harmful immunologic occurrences or diseases in which a person reacts abnormally to an everyday stimulus that would cause no problems in most other persons. Hay fever is an allergy; so is eczema; so is asthma. The abnormal immunologic reaction can affect many different systems of the body or all of them. Some allergies cause intestinal upsets, some cause skin rashes, and some cause breathing difficulties.

Immune responses normally protect us from infections caused by bacteria, fungi, parasites, and viruses, and from developing cancer. The immune system consists of protein molecules called immunoglobins (antibodies) that combine specifically with substances called antigens, the allergens that are foreign to the body. These antigens are present on the numerous infectious agents that enter the body through the skin and through the mucous membrane that lines the respiratory and gastrointestinal tracts. By combining with the antigens, the immunoglobins destroy them.

It is the immune system that is devastated by the tragic disease AIDS, or acquired immune deficiency syndrome.

Certain white blood cells called lymphocytes are the most important part of the immune system. There are two types of lymphocytes: B lymphocytes, which produce immunoglobins, the antibody proteins that combine with antigens; and T lymphocytes, which regulate production of antibodies and participate in immune reactions. They are the target of the AIDS virus, HIV (human immune-deficiency virus), and their destruction leaves the body vulnerable to potentially fatal infection. Another cell, the macrophage, also plays an important role in the immune system.

Each antibody has specific sites that recognize and combine only with a certain antigen. An immunoglobin (Ig) will react only with the antigen or allergen that fits into the sites. The production of antibodies in the presence of antigens is a complex one. Certain cells called phagocytes ingest the invader molecule and transfer information about its composition to the lymphocytes, which then produce antibodies to match it. These specialized cells not only attack the antigens but remain in the bloodstream to guard against future invasions.

The structure of the "body" portion determines how each antibody functions. Five types or classes of antibodies exist, each with a different body structure. They are designated IgG, IgA, IgM, IgD, and IgE. The functions of each class differ considerably.

IgG is the only type of antibody that can cross the human placenta from mother to fetus, and at birth the majority of a newborn infant's antibody proteins are provided by the mother's IgG.

IgA antibodies are transported to the external surfaces of the respiratory, gastrointestinal, and urinary tracts, and also into breast milk. IgA serves as the first line of defense against viruses.

IgM is the first antibody produced in response to infections or immunizations.

IgD's function is uncertain, but it may be involved with T lymphocytes in the control of antibody production.

IgE is the chief offender in the conditions we think of as allergies. It is responsible for hay fever, asthma, hives, eczema, and anaphylaxis.

Normally, antibodies are produced that react only with foreign or "nonself" antigens. However, antibodies to "self" (autoantibodies) can be produced that react with and injure the individual's own tissues. This is called an autoimmune disease.

IgE-TRIGGERED ALLERGIES

Just a small amount of IgE is present in blood plasma, one part per million. But that amount is extremely potent. The steps by which IgE triggers allergic symptoms are illustrated *opposite*.

When an allergen combines with its corresponding IgE antibody on the surface of a mast cell, the contents of the mast cell's granules are released. The histamine and other mediators cause nearby blood vessels to dilate and leak fluid through their walls. The result is swelling of tissues, increased mucous production, spasm of smooth muscles, itching, and an accumulation of inflammatory cells called eosinophils and neutrophils. Symptoms may be mild or severe, and vary with the location and extent of the allergen-IgE-mast-cell reaction.

Asthma

Allergic asthma occurs when certain inhaled antigens or allergens combine with IgE antibodies on mast cells in the lungs. The combination brings on attacks of airway obstruction, which is completely reversible but occurs repeatedly.

As explained in Chapter 10, "The Lungs," in normal breathing air is drawn through the nose or mouth and into the throat, then through the voice box (larynx) into the trachea, the large tube leading into the lung. The air then travels into smaller branching air tubes called bronchi. These tubes are surrounded by smooth muscle cells and glands that produce mucus. The bronchi end in clusters of air-filled sacs called alveoli, where the exchange of inhaled oxygen for carbon dioxide occurs.

During an asthmatic attack, the mediator released from mast cells causes spasm of the bronchial smooth muscle, narrowing the airways and limiting airflow. Excess mucous secretion further clogs the passages; the bronchial tubes become inflamed. Thus, the asthmatic wheezes because the passageways are not clear, coughs as he tries to clear them, and is short of breath because he cannot completely fill the alveoli.

In the majority of child asthmatics, IgE-mediated reactions are the major causes of the disease. By age 16, however, about half of children with allergic asthma become symptom-free spontaneously. Why this occurs is not understood. It may be related to a decreased exposure to allergens or to fewer respiratory virus infections.

Allergic asthma often is referred to as "extrinsic," meaning that its stimuli come from outside the body. In many adults, however, asthma more often appears to be related to chronic respiratory infections or exposure to nonspecific irritants such as fumes, strong odors, cold air, and ingestion of aspirin-containing drugs. These patients are said to have "intrinsic" (nonallergic) asthma.

Recognizing and preventing attacks. The telltale indication of asthma is its characteristic wheeze upon exhaling. Coughing, a tight or uncomfortable sensation in the chest, and shortness of breath also may indicate asthma, particularly if they occur in combination or after exercise. Asthma almost always is worse at night; repeated awakening between 2 a.m. and 4 a.m. almost always is a sure indication. Recognition of asthma is particularly important because steps to deal with it should be taken immediately.

Relief from asthma falls into two categories. First is avoidance of allergens such as animal dander, dust, or pollens. Respiratory irritants such as tobacco smoke, strong perfume, or cooking odors also should be avoided. The second step is use of medication. Extremely effective medications are available that can minimize bronchial muscle contraction and excess bronchial secretions.

Allergic Rhinitis (Hay Fever)

The most common IgE-mediated allergy is allergic rhinitis, popularly known as hay fever. Symptoms include congestion, swollen nasal membranes and obstructed breathing, itching and inflamed nostrils, and sneezing. Some persons have itching, watery eyes as well. The bouts occur either periodically (seasonal) or continuously (perennial) if there is a constant exposure to allergens.

As in other IgE-mediated allergies, the symptoms occur as chemicals are released from mast cells—in this case, in the nose.

Often, the symptoms of allergic rhinitis are mistakenly attributed to a "summer cold." But the difference is usually apparent. Typically, colds do not last more than a week and are accompanied by a painful, burning sensation in the nose and a thick yellow nasal discharge. The discharge of allergic rhinitis, in contrast, is clear and watery. Allergy and infection are not the only causes of nasal stuffiness, however. For example, congestion also occurs in the last months of pregnancy. It usually disappears after delivery. Overuse of decongestant nose drops and sprays also causes chemical irritation often mistakenly attributed to allergies.

Hives and Allergic Swelling (Urticaria and Angioedema)

Almost everyone has "broken out" in hives (urticaria) at some time. Hives occur primarily on the skin in the form of raised red welts that itch. Al-

DISTINGUISHING ALLERGIES FROM RESPIRATORY ILLNESS

	Allergic Rhinitis	Common Cold	Sinusitis	Bronchitis	Asthma*
Length of illness	Weeks or months, usually seasonal	At least 5–7 days; self-limiting	Days; months if not treated	1–2 weeks	Seasonal (allergic) to constant (non-allergic)
Cough	None, unless caused by post-nasal drip	Dry, hacking; mucus, if any, is clear	None	Severe; productive of purulent sputum	Plus wheezing and shortness of breath
Fever	None	Low-grade (if any)	Over 100°F; variable	Over 100°F; variable	None
Nasal discharge	Clear	Clear, copious	Purulent, thick, tenacious, yellow-green nasal discharge	No nasal discharge, discolored (purulent) sputum	No nasal discharge unless rhinitis is present; variable cough & sputum production
Pain	None	None, or headache and muscle ache at onset	Pain over involved sinuses	In chest, on coughing or drawing deep breath	Discomfort or tightness rather than pain in chest
Sore throat	None	Should be gone within 3 days	None	None	None
Other	Constant symptoms indicate allergen in the home or at work	1 to 3 episodes yearly common even in healthy persons	Sore throat may occur due to sinus drainage	Very common in cigarette smokers	Exercise and aspirin precipitate the episodes

*Consultation with your family physician is recommended.

though annoying, they seldom are life-threatening. Angioedema (allergic swelling) most often occurs beneath the skin, including the respiratory and gastrointestinal tract. In severe cases, swelling closes off the larynx, causing death.

There are several IgE-related causes of hives and angioedema, including penicillin, rubbing against a pollinating plant, being licked by animals, or being stung by insects. Food allergies also cause hives, although allergic persons usually are able to recognize the association without the help of a physician. Hives also occur in association with certain infections, such as the early phase of viral hepatitis.

Physical factors also induce hives. In these cases, IgE allergy is not involved. Pressure urticaria, for example, occurs when tight belts or brassiere straps cause histamine to be released from mast cells by simple pressure alone. The result is a

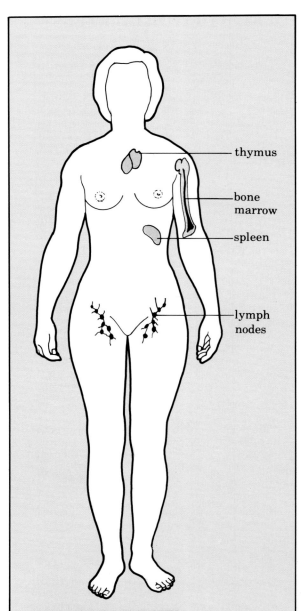

THE IMMUNE SYSTEM
Important elements of the immune system, which protects us against disease, are distributed throughout the body. Antibodies, which combine with invading substances and destroy them, are formed by highly differentiated lymphocytes called plasma cells, which originate in the bone marrow. T lymphocytes develop in the thymus gland under the breastbone. B lymphocytes are converted into plasma cells in the spleen. Both types of lymphocytes are stored in the lymph nodes.

line of raised welts precisely where the garment pressed.

Exposure to cold can cause an outbreak of angioedema. This can be a particularly serious problem if it occurs while swimming. The cold water can cause a massive release of histamine, causing an abrupt decrease in blood pressure.

Chronic urticaria (hives lasting over six weeks) can be a significant problem because of the appearance and bothersome itching. It often is difficult to identify the cause, but foods and drugs, especially aspirin, are always prime suspects. Emotional stress also may play a role. Hives appear to be aggravated by stress in some persons, and others apparently get hives only when stressed.

The most effective treatment for hives is to avoid the recognized factors that cause the symptoms. Antihistamines are effective in treating existing hives.

Eczema

The skin rash known as eczema (atopic dermatitis) affects 1 to 3 percent of the U.S. population. It is more common in infants and young children than adults.

The infantile form usually begins before 1 year of age with a reddened rash on the cheeks and ears, which then spreads to the backs of the arms and fronts of the legs. The skin problem frequently disappears about 1 year of age but may recur between the age of 3 and 5, when it is characterized by intense itching in the elbow and knee creases and on the sides of the neck. The intense itching induces scratching, which makes the rash worse and establishes a vicious itch-scratch cycle that is difficult to break.

The skin of eczema patients is easily irritated, so it is essential to minimize the use of strong soaps. The skin is characteristically dry, too. Thickening of the skin also develops after vigorous and prolonged scratching.

Scratching plays a central role in eczema. If it can be stopped or reduced, eczema will improve. If a child with eczema breaks an arm and a cast is applied, for example, the rash underneath will disappear. In children, it is important to keep fingernails trimmed to minimize the damage of scratching.

Anaphylaxis and Insect Stings

Anaphylaxis is the least common but most serious IgE-mediated allergy. It is a life-threatening emergency that requires prompt treatment. Symptoms begin within seconds to minutes after the sting of an insect or the ingestion of medications or foods that combine with IgE antibody on mast cells. There is a widespread, massive release of histamine. This results in leaky blood vessels throughout the body, with loss of blood volume, a fall in blood pressure, and, frequently, a disturbed heartbeat.

The most common cause of anaphylactic shock is reaction to penicillin; it accounts for the largest number of deaths. Fortunately, there are methods of testing for penicillin sensitivity, if it is suspected. A positive test allows another antibiotic to be substituted, or, if penicillin is the most effective drug available, close surveillance to be maintained.

Anaphylactic reactions to food most commonly involve shellfish. However, the person usually has an unmistakable first-exposure warning, and thus can avoid the offending dish thereafter.

The most dramatic cause of anaphylaxis is insect stings. About one in 200 persons in the United States has IgE antibody to stinging insects. At least 40 deaths a year are caused by insect stings in the United States.

There are two main groups of stinging insects: honeybees and bumblebees, which sting only when provoked, and vespids (wasps, hornets, and yellow jackets), which often sting without provocation. The yellow jacket is the most common source of dangerous stings.

First stings usually produce no symptoms except local discomfort and swelling at the site of the sting. These initial symptoms can be a warning, however. Subsequent stings by the same species of insect will lead to the generalized allergic symptoms. Thus, a susceptible person should take care to avoid insect stings. Outdoor activities should be engaged in with caution. Areas where insects have been seen should be avoided. Shoes, long pants, and shirts should be worn when walking in woods and fields. Gloves and a protective net to screen the neck and face should be used while gardening. Cosmetics, perfumes, and hair sprays should be avoided because their odors attract bees and vespids.

If an allergic person is stung, prompt treatment is essential. Persons known to be insect-allergic should carry emergency medication kits containing epinephrine (adrenalin) and antihistamine as well as an identification bracelet or necklace describing their allergy. The kits allow administration of adrenalin simply by pressing the dispenser

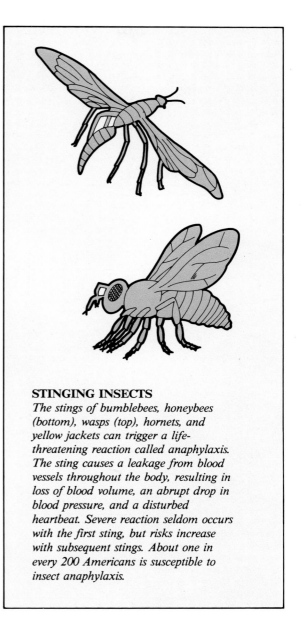

STINGING INSECTS
The stings of bumblebees, honeybees (bottom), wasps (top), hornets, and yellow jackets can trigger a life-threatening reaction called anaphylaxis. The sting causes a leakage from blood vessels throughout the body, resulting in loss of blood volume, an abrupt drop in blood pressure, and a disturbed heartbeat. Severe reaction seldom occurs with the first sting, but risks increase with subsequent stings. About one in every 200 Americans is susceptible to insect anaphylaxis.

against the side of the leg, without the necessity of injection.

Food Allergy

The onset of vomiting, diarrhea, abdominal pain, and particularly hives and angioedema after eating a specific food suggests an IgE-mediated allergy. Symptoms primarily arise in the digestive tract, where the food-allergen-IgE-antibody-mast-cell reaction is occurring. These usually develop within two hours after eating.

Some allergists believe that breast-fed babies have fewer allergies than bottle-fed babies, appar-

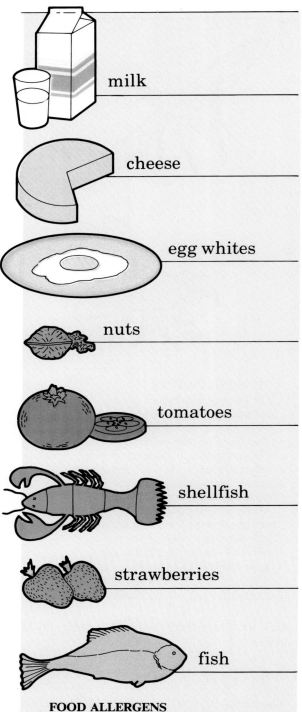

milk

cheese

egg whites

nuts

tomatoes

shellfish

strawberries

fish

FOOD ALLERGENS
Many foods can cause allergies, which usually are manifested by outbreaks of hives and abdominal pain. The foods illustrated above commonly trigger symptoms. Most persons are allergic to only a few foods, and it seldom is necessary to buy special foods or follow a severely restrictive diet.

ently because the mother's milk confers a protective effect. There is disagreement about this finding. It is known, though, that a nursing infant can react with allergy to foods the mother eats while nursing.

ALLERGENS

What are allergens, those mysterious substances that can cause the body to react in so many different ways? A variety of ordinary substances fall into this category, and they enter the body by many different routes. Allergens are swallowed, inhaled, injected, or applied directly to the skin. They are in the air we breathe, the ground we walk on, the animals and plants around us, the medicines we take, and the food we eat.

Food

Virtually any food has the potential to cause an allergic reaction. Those frequently blamed include cow's milk and other dairy products, such as ice cream and cheese; egg whites; pipped fruits such as tomatoes and strawberries; beef; nuts of various kinds; fish and shellfish, especially shrimp and lobster. Wheat often is said to cause allergic reactions, but only rarely is responsible.

Identifying the food causing the allergic symptoms often is easy. Because the symptoms occur within such a short time, the most recent foods eaten are obviously suspect. The presence of IgE antibody to that particular food usually can be confirmed by a skin or RAST test described below.

Avoiding the food in the future, however, may be more of a problem than identifying it. Many foods are used in recipes where one might not expect to find them. Shrimp, for instance, is used in small amounts in Chinese dishes and in certain soups. It is easy to avoid whole milk, butter, and ice cream, but milk also turns up in such foods as margarine and packaged luncheon meats. Cooking odors also can provoke allergic reactions.

The allergy is never to the entire food, but to some natural chemical within it, or to some chemical produced in the breakdown of foods in the gastrointestinal system. In these cases, it may be even more difficult to identify the offender. When the allergen is not obvious, some physicians suggest keeping a food diary in which all foods eaten over a given period are recorded in an attempt to

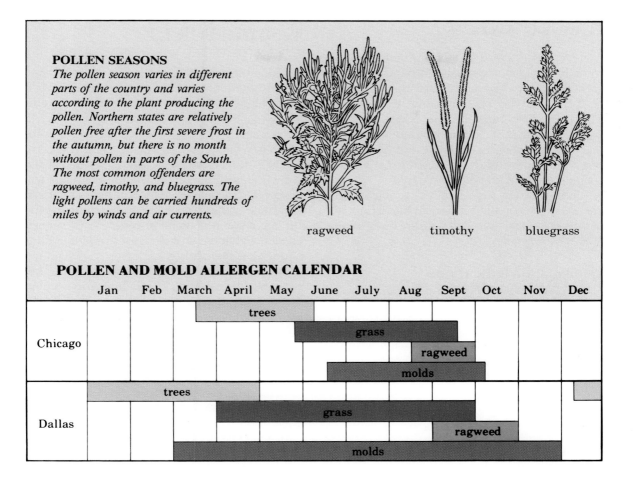

POLLEN SEASONS

The pollen season varies in different parts of the country and varies according to the plant producing the pollen. Northern states are relatively pollen free after the first severe frost in the autumn, but there is no month without pollen in parts of the South. The most common offenders are ragweed, timothy, and bluegrass. The light pollens can be carried hundreds of miles by winds and air currents.

ragweed   timothy   bluegrass

POLLEN AND MOLD ALLERGEN CALENDAR

	Jan	Feb	March	April	May	June	July	Aug	Sept	Oct	Nov	Dec
Chicago			trees			grass			ragweed			
								molds				
Dallas		trees			grass					ragweed		
				molds								

establish a pattern that will identify the cause. An elimination diet also can be used. In this diet, suspected foods gradually are added to the person's menu one at a time until symptoms occur. Elimination diets are particularly useful in identifying the source of allergies in small children, whose diets can be controlled more easily.

Pollens

Pollens are small microscopic grains that are the male germ cells of plants and are essential for plant fertilization. Not all pollens cause IgE allergies, but trees, grass, and weeds, which are pollinated by the wind, produce large amounts of pollen, which is small, light, and easily transported in the air. Thus, ragweed pollen has been detected hundreds of miles out in the Atlantic Ocean. A single ragweed plant can produce a million grains of pollen a day.

There is a relatively constant pollinating season for each species of tree, grass, and weed, depending on climate, as shown in the pollen and mold calendar above. The individual's symptoms develop only when the particular pollen that reacts with his or her IgE is in the air.

Molds

Molds, which grow on plants, foods, and other living matter, produce large amounts of spores even smaller than pollens. In northern states, spores begin to appear in May and increase through June and July. In the South, molds are present throughout the year.

Molds are more likely to cause allergic asthma than pollens, which more often produce eye and nasal symptoms. The smaller size of the mold spores allows easier entrance into the lungs. Indoors, molds may cause year-round allergic symptoms. They may proliferate in air conditioners or in office carpeting after shampooing. Individuals who develop respiratory symptoms while mowing grass more often have allergy to mold spores, which grow on grass, than to grass pollen.

Household Allergens

House dust is a mixture of a large number of potentially allergenic materials. Mold spores, food particles, insects, hair and dander from household pets, and decaying organic matter from pillows, mattresses, toys, furniture, and fibers are often found in house dust. Recently, it has been shown that a living organism, the house dust mite, also is present in house dust. It is believed to be the most common cause of house dust allergy.

When pets are kept indoors, a considerable amount of dander and hair is distributed throughout the household. Cats and dogs are major causes of allergic symptoms.

Drugs and Medications

The ancient proverb "One man's medicine is another man's poison" is illustrated strikingly by the fact that 10 to 20 percent of patients experience some type of adverse drug reaction while hospitalized. IgE-mediated reactions to penicillin are frequent, but other medications also cause reactions.

WHO GETS ALLERGIES?

Several factors appear to determine who carries IgE sensitivity and who does not. First, an inherited predisposition usually is present. Between 60 and 70 percent of infants whose parents both have a history of IgE allergies will develop some allergic symptom before 2 years of age.

The second obvious factor is exposure to the specific allergen that stimulates IgE antibody formation. This exposure begins immediately after birth in the form of foods and airborne allergens such as house dust and animal hair and dander. Viral respiratory infection also may play a role, especially in the development of allergic asthma. The exact role is controversial and still under investigation. However, the first episode of wheezing in an infant very often begins during a viral infection, usually diagnosed as asthmatic bronchitis. It is important to emphasize that IgE production does not persist without continued exposure to allergens. If the allergens are removed, the chain of events leading to symptoms can be interrupted.

TESTING FOR IgE

The presence of intermittent or seasonal nasal or chest symptoms strongly suggests the possibility of allergic rhinitis or asthma. Confirmation usually is done by allergy skin testing, in which a minute amount of the suspected allergen is introduced into the superficial skin by a puncture or an injection. If IgE antibody is present, a raised, itchy, red wheal or hive resembling a mosquito bite will appear within minutes. The skin test is the most rapid and sensitive method of detecting specific IgE antibody. It is useful in pollen, mold, animal dander, and house dust allergies, and also in diagnosing penicillin allergy.

Recently, tests have been developed that use serum for the detection of IgE antibodies without the necessity of skin testing. These depend on the use of a highly sensitive radioimmunoassay procedure called RAST (radioallergosorbent test), which measures the amount of IgE to specific allergens in test tubes. This procedure sometimes is indicated in small children in whom skin testing is difficult or in persons with extensive skin rash. It also is used to monitor changes in IgE antibody levels during treatment.

It should be emphasized, however, that the best clues come from an extensive patient history as interpreted by a knowledgeable physician.

PREVENTION AND TREATMENT OF IgE ALLERGIES

Avoidance. The first and most important step in treatment is to minimize exposure to the offending allergens. This often is the easiest, usually the least expensive, sometimes the most effective, and always the safest treatment. Avoiding allergens in the home is the best way to improve symptoms in patients with IgE allergies to house dust, animal danders, and feathers.

It is impossible to avoid exposure to pollens and molds in the atmosphere. Exposure can be reduced, however, by removing weeds around the home and by keeping doors and windows closed as much as possible. Home air conditioners are beneficial because doors and windows can be kept closed, preventing the entrance of airborne pollens and molds. Forced-air heating systems that recirculate the air increase the amount of dust, molds, and animal hair and dander in the air, so it is important to vacuum the air ducts thoroughly before use in the fall, and to install and change frequently the filters in the furnace. Special mattress and pillow covers protect against house dust mites, often found in the bedroom.

Pets should not be permitted in the house and particularly not in the allergic person's bedroom. Animal hair and dander will persist in the home for weeks to months after the pet is removed so that immediate benefits may not be obvious. The pet should never be allowed back in the house just because improvement has not occurred.

Medications. Antihistamines are effective in allergic rhinitis and hives because most of the symptoms are directly related to the action of histamine in the nose and skin. Different types of antihistamines are available. The newer, nonsedating antihistamines cause fewer side effects than earlier products.

Prescription drugs that relieve the spasm of bronchial smooth muscle in asthmatics include theophylline and adrenalinlike medications, which are effective for as long as 12 hours when taken by mouth. These drugs are more effective in preventing asthmatic symptoms than in reversing symptoms already present, however.

Corticosteroid or cortisonelike medications are effective antiallergic drugs but have significant side effects if used in large doses and for prolonged periods. The drug cromolyn, available in three forms, also is a major antiallergic drug.

The overuse of aerosol spray medications for allergic rhinitis or asthma can aggravate nasal and lung symptoms by irritating the tissues. Overzealous advertisements encourage the use of these nonprescription drugs, which in some cases perpetuate rather than relieve the problem.

Emotional factors. Although emotional stress frequently can aggravate allergic symptoms, emotions almost never are the sole cause of allergic rhinitis or asthma. There is no firm evidence that a particular personality type is predisposed to eczema or asthma, nor that asthmatic patients have more emotional problems than nonasthmatics.

Immunotherapy. For those with significant, persistent allergic symptoms, the physician may suggest a program of hyposensitization or immunotherapy, better known as "allergy shots." This consists of injecting increasing amounts of the allergen to which the patient has high IgE antibody levels as shown by skin tests and symptoms. Initially, a minute amount of allergen is injected, then a gradually increased dose at intervals of several days to a week.

Immunotherapy should be used only in conjunction with avoidance and preventive medications. Benefits are not apparent until after six to 12 months of treatment. It has been shown conclusively that the majority of persons receiving immunotherapy for ragweed hay fever have significantly fewer symptoms and require less medication. Immunotherapy with purified venoms is particularly effective in preventing the severe life-threatening reactions in persons allergic to insect stings.

OTHER ALLERGIC DISEASES

Although most allergic reactions can be attributed to IgE antibody, the other immunoglobins sometimes are responsible.

Hypersensitivity Pneumonia

Many people are exposed to high concentrations of dusts from organic material at work or in the home. The particles are six times smaller than most plant pollens, so they can be drawn deeply into the tiny air spaces of the lung. When exposure continues for long periods, IgG antibody and specific T lymphocytes are produced. They interact with the dust allergen and cause inflammation.

Symptoms of hypersensitivity pneumonia are delayed until six or more hours after exposure. The person who has previously felt and breathed well develops chills, a cough, shortness of breath, and fever. The symptoms closely resemble those of infectious or bacterial pneumonia and a chest X ray may show shadows in the lungs. The patient may even be hospitalized and treated with antibiotics. Within a day or two, symptoms begin to disappear, seeming to confirm that an infection was present. However, on return to the dusty environment, symptoms recur. With repeated episodes, a progressive, irreversible loss of lung function occurs.

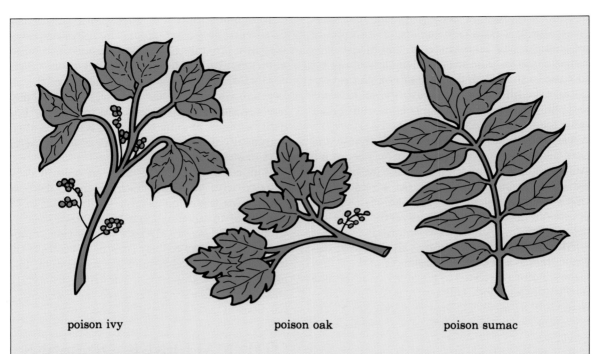

poison ivy   poison oak   poison sumac

Poisonous Plants

Plants of the Rhus family, shown above, can cause a severe allergic dermatitis, or skin rash. The offending agent is a plant oil, urushiol, found in the plant sap. Contact with leaves or branches can trigger the rash, itching and blistering within hours after exposure. The rash may be spread to other parts of the body by oil on the fingers. The eyelids are especially vulnerable. Sometimes the oil may be carried on the fur of pets, or on clothing. At least seven out of 10 Americans are sensitive to the plant oils; those who claim to be immune frequently are affected on repeated exposure.

As shown, the three plants have distinctive appearances. Poison ivy, the most common, grows as a vine or bush and is characterized by notched leaves in groups of three. It is found in most parts of the U.S. Poison oak, with groups of three leaves resembling oak leaves, grows primarily in the West. Poison sumac, with seven to 13 paired leaves per stalk, is a southern plant.

After exposure to any of the plants, the skin should be washed thoroughly to remove oils. Cool, wet compresses or calamine lotion feel soothing; antihistamines may relieve itching. In severe cases, corticosteroids may be prescribed.

Immunotherapy, to build up tolerance by gradual exposure to increasing doses of plant extract, sometimes is suggested for outdoor workers, but is not always successful. The "best" cure is prevention, by recognizing and avoiding the plants.

Hypersensitivity pneumonia has been recognized for 50 years in farmers who handle spoiled or moldy hay. Recently, similar symptoms have been observed among workers in office buildings where the central air conditioning system is contaminated with molds. This type of hypersensitivity pneumonia has been called "Monday morning fever," because persons feel well on weekends but experience renewed symptoms on returning to the contaminated office environment. Homemakers also can develop hypersensitivity pneumonia when home humidifiers attached to the furnace or hot air heating system are turned on without being thoroughly cleaned.

Skin Rashes (Allergic Contact Dermatitis) and Cosmetics

Allergic contact dermatitis, or skin rash, is more common than any other allergic reaction. Allergic contact dermatitis, as well as irritant dermatitis, which does not involve an allergic reaction, is described in Chapter 9, "The Skin." In the allergic form, the outbreak of redness, small raised papules, and blisters occurs because small chemical allergens called haptens, which do not induce an allergic reaction by themselves, combine with skin proteins and become allergenic. The reaction is delayed, occurring up to a day after exposure to the chemical, compared to the immediate reactions caused by IgE. Many chemicals or haptens are capable of inducing this reaction. Cosmetics are often a source. Medications and perfumes often cause contact sensitivity.

After the first exposure to the offending chemical, allergic sensitization develops over seven to 10 days. On reexposure, a blistering rash develops at the sites of contact. The sensitizing potential of the chemical depends on its ability to combine with skin proteins, the concentration of chemical touching the skin, and the area of skin contacted. The length of contact also is important. Contact on injured skin is much more likely to cause sensitization than on normal skin.

It is important to discover which chemical substance is causing allergic contact dermatitis. This can be done by careful history and by patch testing. Patch testing is done by applying a small nonirritating amount of the suspected chemical to a gauze bandage and attaching it to normal skin on the back or arm. In 24 to 48 hours, the patch is removed. If the person is sensitive to the chemical, a localized reddened spot of varying intensity will be present. The best treatment is to minimize or completely avoid the allergenic chemical. For instance, nickel jewelry is a common cause of sensitivity, but it is relatively easy to avoid earrings, bracelets, rings, and necklaces containing nickel. Avoidance is more difficult in occupational exposures. Rubber sensitivity is caused by chemicals added to natural rubber gum. Because rubber is so widely used in industry, it may be necessary for a worker to change jobs.

Extensive contact dermatitis may require the use of cortisonelike drugs by mouth. Locally applied cortisone ointments are among the few medications that can be used safely for rashes of any sort without running the risk of causing contact sensitivity.

AUTOIMMUNE DISEASES

Autoimmune diseases are produced by harmful immunologic reactions to the body's own tissues. These "allergic to self" diseases can be life-threatening or associated with chronic severe symptoms. They may attack any part or organ system of the body, including the blood, connective tissue, thyroid, and nervous system.

It is important to recognize that the autoimmune or autoallergic reaction is against normal tissues. There is considerable evidence that the normal, protective immune response can recognize early changes in cells that may develop into malignant tumors. This type of response to altered tissue, called "immune surveillance," is an important defense mechanism against cancer. It also appears that very early in life and in the elderly, the peak ages of cancers and leukemias, there is a relative deficiency of immunity, allowing these cancers to arise.

Major autoimmune diseases are described in chapters relating to the specific organ system affected. They include Rh disease in the newborn (erythroblastosis) and autoimmune hemolytic anemia, discussed in Chapter 28, "Pregnancy and Childbirth"; hyperthyroidism, in Chapter 18, "The Hormones and Endocrine Glands"; myasthenia gravis, in Chapter 11, "The Brain and Nervous System"; and systemic lupus erythematosus, or SLE, in Chapter 17, "Arthritis and Related Diseases."

CHAPTER 24

THE KIDNEYS AND URINARY SYSTEM

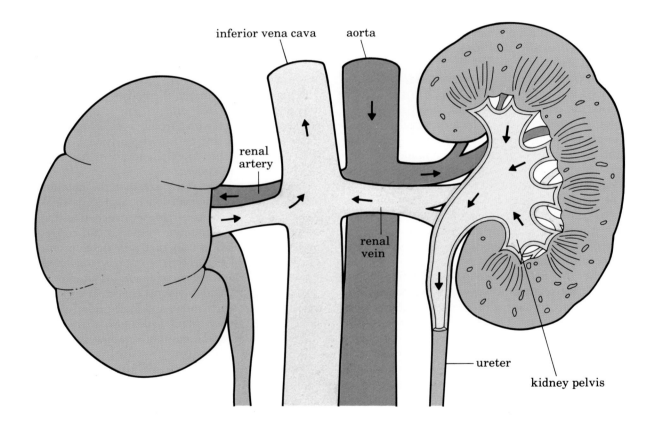

THE KIDNEYS IN ACTION

About 400 gallons of blood flow through the kidneys each day, arriving via the renal artery and leaving via the renal vein. The black arrows show the blood pathways. As shown in the cutaway drawing, the delicate workings of the kidneys filter materials from the blood and concentrate about 1½ quarts of urine daily. Urine is collected in the kidney pelvis and passes down the ureter to the bladder.

We all know the kidney's method for ridding the body of waste. Urine, a supersaturated solution of salts, is formed in the kidneys, drop by drop. It is funneled down a tiny conduit called the ureter, then into a storage organ called the bladder, and finally, when a half pint or more has been collected, it is carried outside the body via another conduit, the urethra. The organs that transport urine out of the body are known as the urinary system.

A LOOK AT THE KIDNEYS

The kidneys are a pair of maroon-colored, bean-shaped organs, each weighing about half a pound. They are so distinctive in shape that if we describe a swimming pool or sofa as kidney-shaped, listeners know immediately what we mean. Located behind the abdominal cavity, they lie at the base of the rib cage. The right kidney is a little higher than the left. It rests just beneath the liver, and the left kidney rests beneath the spleen.

Renal arteries connect the kidney directly to the aorta, the main artery of the body, and bring its blood supply. After blood has passed through the kidneys, it returns to circulation through renal veins linked to the vena cava, the body's main vein. As urine is formed in a kidney, it flows into the renal pelvis, a funnel-shaped structure that covers the small ducts leading from the kidney. Each pelvis is connected to a ureter, which feeds into the bladder.

Removal of one kidney leaves function virtually intact. The remaining kidney slowly enlarges to compensate for the loss of its partner. Even when up to 90 percent of function in both kidneys has been destroyed by disease, the kidneys still can maintain normal blood volume and adjust the composition of body fluids to sustain life. In fact, some persons are born with a solitary kidney and the fact is never realized until the absence is disclosed by X ray or autopsy.

The Collecting System

The urine collecting system operates on the principle of gravity and is simplicity itself. After the clear fluid has been manufactured by the tubules, it flows into a series of microscopic collecting ducts that merge into several funnel-shaped structures, the papillae, then into cuplike calyces, which feed into larger calyces until finally all pour their products into a large single cavity, the kidney pelvis. The pelvis is partly inside and partly outside the kidney and is drained by two tubelike ureters, one for each kidney. The pressure of the urine and the force of gravity carry the urine down the ureters into the bladder.

The bladder is a storage organ. It is elastic, built of a strong network of muscle fibers that allow the wall to stretch as urine collects. The outlet at the base is surrounded by sphincter muscles that tighten like purse strings and keep the liquid from escaping until it can be disposed of. That occurs when nerves within the walls send signals to the spinal cord and brain that the bladder is ready to be emptied. Messages relayed back to the bladder stimulate the organ to contract and simultaneously relax the purse-string muscles. The urethra, the final passage out of the body, is relatively short in women—1 to 2 inches long—but measures 8 to 9 inches in men.

The Kidney Hormones

In addition to their other duties, the kidneys produce three hormones that are released into the bloodstream and regulate other body functions.

Renin is a large protein that acts as a catalyst to activate another protein, angiotensin, which is made in the liver. In one of the body's feedback systems, angiotensin then acts on the cells of the adrenal cortex to produce another hormone, aldosterone, which "tells" the kidneys to retain salt and water. Thus, the kidney senses when the body is threatened by excess loss of fluid or blood, and releases renin to warn the body. Aldosterone returns the message to hold back salt and water to protect the blood volume.

Erythropoietin is sent by the kidney through the blood to the bone marrow. There it stimulates the production of red blood cells.

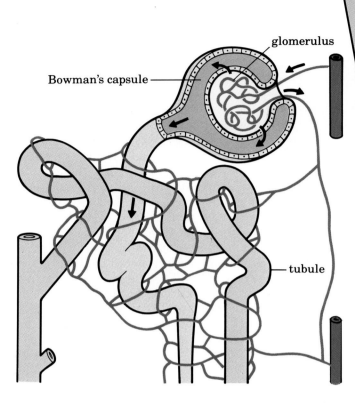

glomerulus

Bowman's capsule

tubule

Bowman's capsule

Henle's loop

collecting tubule

THE FILTRATION PLANT

The kidney's filtration system has three basic elements: the cup-shaped Bowman's capsule, the glomerulus, which is a tufted network of capillaries within the capsule, and the convoluted tubule. Blood arrives via the capillaries and is filtered through their walls and into the space between the double walls of the capsule. The filtrate then passes down the tubule, where most of the water and some other substances are reabsorbed and the remainder is concentrated as urine. Arrows show the direction of flow. After filtration, the blood returns to circulation.

WHERE URINE FORMS

The urine-forming unit of the kidney is the nephron, shown greatly enlarged (top). A kidney in miniature, its major features are the Bowman's capsule, the convoluted tubules, and Henle's loop, which doubles the length of the filtering areas, and the collecting tubule. The drawing above shows the location of the nephron in the curved outer portion of the kidney. There are about 1 million nephrons in each kidney. A network of capillaries encircles each nephron, allowing excess fluid, electrolytes, and nutrients that have been filtered through the glomerulus to return to the blood.

Vitamin D, the "sunshine vitamin," normally is manufactured in the skin or provided in the diet. But kidney action transforms it into an enormously more potent form. The "enhanced" vitamin helps control absorption of calcium from the digestive system and the laying down of calcium in the bones.

In severe kidney disease, calcium often is lost in the urine and phosphate retained. Blood levels are low in calcium and high in phosphate. The body responds by releasing a hormone from the parathyroid gland in the neck, which mobilizes calcium from the bones.

Congenital Abnormalities

Like teeth and fingerprints, kidneys are highly individual. Probably no two persons in the world have kidneys exactly alike.

Horseshoe kidney is one of the more common abnormalities. The two kidneys are linked across the top or bottom into a single mass of tissue in the shape of a capital U. Sometimes the bridge between the two does not contain functioning tissue. Sometimes the two kidneys act as one.

Double ureters also are relatively common. Instead of the customary single ureter draining each kidney, some persons have duplicates on one or both sides. This usually is harmless.

Ectopic kidney ("out of normal place") occurs because the fat pad that normally surrounds and protects the kidneys is missing, allowing one or both to move out of position. Sometimes both are found on the same side of the body. The malformation may cause a kink in the ureter, damming the urine behind it and leading to swelling.

Solitary kidney, which is a single kidney from birth or two kidneys fused so that they function as one, may go unnoticed for years, but a solitary kidney leaves the person without a spare. The existence of a solitary kidney is important to know before a kidney operation, because the patient cannot count on an extra kidney to take over.

Polycystic kidneys develop before birth. The kidneys contain hundreds of tiny blisterlike cysts that collect fluid and have no outlet. In children, polycystic kidneys may fill to enormous size and may be felt in the abdomen. Sometimes the cysts rupture and bleed. The condition, which has a tendency to "run in families," is slowly progressive and can lead to gradual kidney failure.

Vesico-ureteral reflux is the name given to backflow of urine into the ureters instead of into the urethra during urination. It is common in

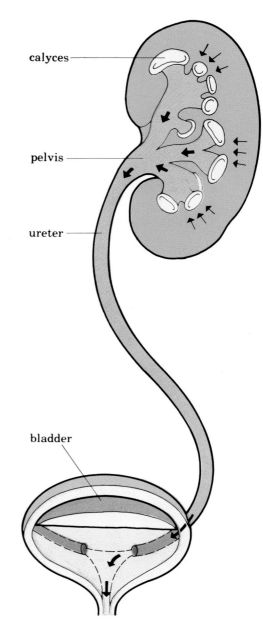

COLLECTION OF URINE
The system for collecting urine is shown in the cross section. The cuplike calyces receive urine from the nephrons (suggested by small black arrows). The pelvis extends partly outside the kidney and funnels urine into the ureter and to the bladder, which stores it temporarily.

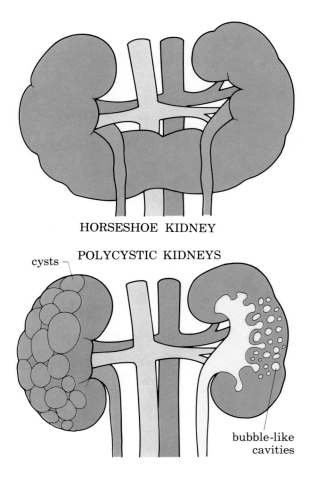

HORSESHOE KIDNEY

POLYCYSTIC KIDNEYS

cysts

bubble-like
cavities

KIDNEY MALFORMATIONS
*Kidney malformations are not
uncommon. At top is a horseshoe
kidney, so-called because the kidneys
are joined in the shape of the letter U.
Below, polycystic kidneys are covered
with blisterlike cysts and have bubble-
like cavities inside. Because of the
kidneys' great reserve capacity, many
persons live all their lives with a
malformation and never become
aware of it.*

young children, tending to disappear with age. If
not outgrown or corrected, the condition can
cause pressure damage to the kidney called reflux
nephropathy.

Urethral valves, which are bits of membrane-
like tissue growing from the lining of the urethra,
may obstruct the flow of urine in young boys. The
tissue can be removed surgically.

Tests and Instruments

Techniques for studying the functions of the
kidney and visualizing the urinary tract have been
developed extensively in recent years.

Urinalysis. Urine is readily obtained and easily
studied in the laboratory. From a clean specimen
of about two to three ounces, most standard tests
for kidney disease can be performed.

Small amounts of protein are always present in
urine. Their presence is referred to as proteinuria
or sometimes as albuminuria because the principal
blood protein in urine is albumin. The finding of
small amounts is not alarming. Most nephrologists
do not consider protein in the urine to be abnormal
unless one or more grams are excreted in a day.

Small amounts of glucose also are found in the
urine of healthy persons. An excess of glucose, a
condition called glycosuria, may be a sign of diabetes, but also may result from severely damaged
kidneys.

Victims of severe kidney disease often cannot
produce a concentrated urine. The amount of salt
is slight relative to the amount of water. A person
who drinks large amounts of fluids also excretes a
highly dilute urine to rid the body of excess water.
Therefore, measurement of specific gravity is
meaningful only when the amount of fluids consumed beforehand is known.

Blood or pus in the urine is abnormal and calls
for investigation. During menstruation, there may
be some mixing of menses with urine. Women
should always inform their physician if they are
menstruating when a urine sample is given.

When urine is cooled below body temperature,
crystals form and the fluid becomes cloudy. This is
normal and no cause for alarm. Crystals tend to
obscure blood and pus cells so that fresh urine
must be examined to see them clearly under the
microscope.

Because bacteria are picked up by the stream as
it passes over the external tissues, their presence in
urine does not necessarily signify infection. Only
when large numbers of bacteria are found in freshly obtained urine in several consecutive tests does
one have "significant bacteriuria."

The nitrite test allows persons to test for urinary tract infection at home. The test is based on the principle that small amounts of nitrate from the diet are excreted in the urine. When nitrate is exposed to large numbers of bacteria for about six to eight hours, nitrite is formed and will produce a pink color when mixed with the chemicals impregnated onto filter paper in the test strip. When the strip is moistened with or dipped into the urine, the color changes within a few seconds if nitrite is present. A first morning voided urine sample must be used because it represents urine that has incubated in the bladder overnight.

Properly used, the nitrite test has a 70 percent chance of detecting infection. If performed on three consecutive days, the odds rise to 90 percent.

Blood tests and timed urine collections are used together as measures of kidney function to determine the efficiency of the remaining nephrons. The test usually measures amounts of urea or creatinine, the products of protein and muscle breakdown. Sometimes inulin, a sugar polymer, is measured for even more accurate determination.

X rays. The kidneys often can be outlined on X rays of the abdomen. They can be seen best by intravenous pyelogram. In this test, a radiopaque dye is injected into the veins, then is rapidly excreted by the kidneys. X rays every few minutes show the kidney shape, the collection of dye in the pelvis, ureters, and bladder. Doctors can even determine whether the bladder empties properly by waiting until it is filled with dye, then X-raying after voiding to see whether dye is left behind.

If kidneys are too severely damaged to excrete dye from the blood, dye can be introduced into the bladder and the ureters via a catheter.

A **renal arteriogram** is used to examine the blood vessels of the kidney. Radiopaque dye is injected into the aorta near the renal arteries by threading a fine catheter through the arterial circuit. An arteriogram is particularly useful for determining blood flow in the kidney and visualizing tumors or cysts.

A catheter is a rubber or plastic tube used to drain urine from the bladder, relieve obstructions, or inject dye and measure resistance to passage. It also can be used to test for residual urine. Catheters sometimes carry bacteria with them into the bladder, but they may be lifesaving if they relieve obstruction or permit emptying of bladders that are poorly controlled because of disease of the spinal cord.

A cystoscope is a lighted, flexible, tubelike instrument with a magnifying lens that can be inserted through the urethra into the bladder to allow the urologist to inspect the bladder visually. The urologist thus can detect points of bleeding, tumors, or bladder stones. About the diameter of a fine pencil, the cystoscope often is equipped with tiny attachments that can lift out small stones, burn off tumors, or snip bits of prostate to relieve obstruction.

Drugs

Many drugs can alter the blood supply to the kidney or enhance the flow of urine. Those that promote urine production are called diuretics, and in their simplest form are known as osmotic diuretics. They draw water with them when excreted by the kidney. The most common examples are urea and mannitol, a compound similar to the sugar glucose that the body does not metabolize.

Other drugs directly alter the function of the tubules. Spironolactone, for instance, limits the action of the hormone aldosterone, causing excretion of sodium and water and retention of potassium. Mercurial diuretics, very rarely used today, interfere with reabsorption of sodium and chloride by the kidney. Acetazoleamide interferes with exchange of bicarbonate and chloride in the kidney and produces an alkaline urine. Thiazide, ethacrynic acid, and furosemide, all commonly used, are known as high-ceiling diuretics because they produce the greatest increase in loss of water and sodium of any known diuretics. Excessive use can lead to dehydration and low body stores of sodium and potassium.

DISEASES OF THE KIDNEY

Kidney diseases often are classified according to the portion of the kidney that suffers the most damage, either the glomerulus or the tubules. Actually, many diseases involve both the glomerulus and tubules and are grouped as glomerulonephritis, or "Bright's disease."

The nephrotic syndrome of childhood, also known as minimal glomerular disease or lipoid nephrosis, is the most common disease affecting the glomerular tissue only. Many of the victims of the disease are under 4 years old. The cause is unknown. Unlike many other forms of kidney disease, there is no inflammation of the kidney and no abnormal findings can be seen under the microscope. The disease is characterized by leakage of blood protein into the urine.

Sometimes, the first symptoms are puffiness around the eyes, or difficulty putting on the child's shoes. Or, there may be large amounts of foam in the urine. Later, the small body, particularly the abdomen, may be swollen with fluid. In addition, the disease liberates fats into the blood, so that the serum becomes milky instead of crystal clear. Droplets of fat in the shape of a Maltese cross appear in the urine.

Fortunately, childhood nephrosis often disappears spontaneously or can be treated effectively with corticosteroids or other drugs. Nephrosis can leave the young kidney damaged, however, and it can recur.

Most diseases that progressively damage the kidney and ultimately lead to kidney failure are forms of glomerulonephritis. The cause is not understood. In some cases, the inflammation seems to result from an immune reaction in which the body mistakenly attacks its own tissue. Antibodies produced by the immune system form a complex with antigens that damages the glomerular membrane and allows protein to leak through.

Acute glomerulonephritis is self-limiting in 95 percent of cases. More common in children than adults, it usually begins with blood in the urine, puffiness in the cheeks and face as fluids are retained, and a sharp rise in blood pressure. Acute glomerulonephritis usually disappears even without treatment, although hospitalization may be required to provide a special diet and to monitor blood pressure.

Chronic glomerulonephritis refers to long-standing, persistent inflammatory kidney disease. Most cases are of unknown cause, although the immune reaction likely is implicated here, too. The disease can occur at any age, but is more common in adults. Because it develops slowly in most cases, the disease usually is not detected until the person begins to complain of feeling weak, has aches in the region of the kidney, or is found to have high blood pressure. Blood studies reveal anemia and increased concentrations of urea and creatinine. The urine may contain large amounts of protein and red blood cells.

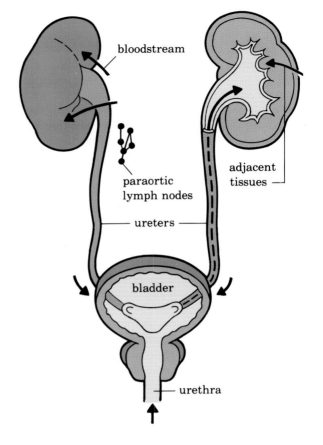

KIDNEY INFECTIONS
Kidney infections arrive via various routes, ascending from the bladder and ureters, from adjacent tissues, from the bloodstream, and from the lymphatic system. Bladder inflammation (cystitis) usually is caused by bacteria migrating up the urethra (lower arrow) and may be confined to the bladder.

The rate of progression of chronic glomerulonephritis varies. Some people may have the disease for five to 10 years without needing kidney dialysis. Others deteriorate in a few weeks or months. Although some persons can be treated, most who eventually require dialysis or kidney transplant have had their kidneys destroyed by these diseases.

Alport's syndrome is an inherited form of glomerulonephritis. It often is accompanied by deafness and also may affect the eyes.

Interstitial nephritis refers to any condition that produces inflammation and damage to the kidney tubules and the spaces between them. Among the causes are overuse of analgesic medicines and allergy to such drugs as penicillin and sulfonamides.

Infections of the Kidney And Urinary Tract

Because urine ordinarily is sterile until it is passed through the urethra, bacterial growth in the urine is abnormal. But it is by no means uncommon. At any time, about 1 percent of the girls in the preschool and school years have asymptomatic bacteriuria, or silent growth of bacteria in the urine. Thereafter, the frequency increases by about 1 percent for each 10 years of life. About one-third of all women will acquire asymptomatic bacteria during their lifetimes.

Although not generally alarming, bacterial infections of the urinary system can be distinctively painful and unpleasant.

Cystitis (inflammation of the bladder) may be produced by drugs, radiation, or foreign objects, as well as by bacterial infections. Regardless of the cause, the symptoms are often the same: burning on urination, frequent urination, pain in the lower abdomen over the bladder, and cloudy, sometimes bloody, urine. In bacterial infections, pus cells and bacteria may be seen when urinary sediment is examined under the microscope. Many antibiotics are available to treat bacterial bladder infections.

Urethritis refers to inflammation of the urethra, also from a variety of causes, including (but by no means limited to) gonorrhea or other venereal organisms. As with cystitis, urination is painful and sometimes pus is passed. Bacterial cases can be treated with antibiotics.

Pyelonephritis, a bacterial infection of the kidney, causes fever and pain over the kidneys, below the ribs; the person may become acutely ill. Urine contains pus cells and bacteria. Some people have both cystitis and acute pyelonephritis at the same time. Most cases of acute pyelonephritis improve gradually, but antibiotics hasten healing.

Chronic pyelonephritis indicates either a continued, smoldering infection of the kidney (active)

Bed-wetting

Our culture places great importance on the privacy of urination and defecation. Parents are pleased by children who are toilet trained early and distressed by those who can't control their urinary or bowel movements. The child (or grandparent) who wets the bed is considered difficult and troublesome.

Enuresis, urinary incontinence, is a common condition of childhood. It appears to run in families, and is surprisingly widespread. One study indicated that 20 percent of 6-year-olds and 10 percent of 7-year-olds had never experienced a full month without an episode of bed-wetting. Even one in twenty 12-year-olds had not had a dry month. The bed wetters were about equally divided between boys and girls.

A majority of children are reliably dry at night by the age of 4. The remainder gain nighttime control as they grow older. A few are successfully nighttime trained, then relapse and wet their beds again. A psychological upset (such as the birth of a brother or sister) or a urinary infection may be the explanation for these secondary cases. Physical abnormalities rarely play a part if the child can control the bladder during the day.

The specific cause of bed-wetting is not known. The child usually has a normal-size bladder. Because it appears to run in families, one possible explanation is congenital delayed maturation of nerves controlling the bladder. Some, but not all, bed wetters visit the bathroom more often during the day.

Remedies are not wholly satisfactory because the cause is not known. Most stress decreasing the anxiety of parents and children through counseling. Limiting fluids at bedtime may help, as can bladder-training exercises and rewarding success.

Alarm systems work for some children. A pad-and-buzzer method consists of two layers of foil or wire mesh separated by a layer of cloth and connected by wires to a battery and bell or buzzer. Wetting on the cloth completes the circuit, sounds the alarm, and wakes the child. The repeated association of bed-wetting and being rudely awakened is said to condition children to greater bladder control usually within two to 10 weeks.

or simply old scars of healed infection (inactive). In severe cases, large portions of the kidney may be destroyed and the infection may even spread to the tissues surrounding the kidney. Many severe chronic or recurrent pyelonephritis cases occur in persons with diabetes, kidney stones, or obstruction of urinary flow. Their cases may lead to end-stage kidney failure.

Sources and symptoms. The source of bacteria in presumably sterile urine is something of a mystery. Bacteria probably are introduced in small numbers into the female bladder periodically (no one knows how often) and rapidly shed by the urine stream during voiding. The event is not detectable because urine passed through the urethra always picks up a few bacteria, and tests cannot determine where the bacteria originated. Sexual intercourse and methods of wiping the genitalia after voiding are thought by some to be important means of introducing bacteria into the bladder, but this has been difficult to document scientifically. Furthermore, urinary infections are common in sexually inactive schoolgirls and more common in elderly women than in sexually active females.

Urinary tract infections produce many of the same symptoms of painful and frequent urination as vaginal and venereal infections and often are confused with them. The infections are quite distinct, however, and there is no evidence that the bacteria that cause urinary tract infections can be transmitted to a partner during intercourse.

Kidney and Bladder Stones

Urinary stones generally are categorized by their primary location either as renal (kidney) stones, technically called nephrolithiasis or renal calculus, or bladder stones. These hard bits of crystalline material precipitated into the urine may obstruct the flow of urine from the kidney and cause kidney damage. More often, stones lodge temporarily in one or both of the ureters and produce severe pain and blood in the urine. Or they serve as location for persistent infection of the urinary tract.

Kidney and bladder stones may be divided into several distinct types, based on their chemical composition. Treatment varies according to their makeup.

Calcium-containing stones account for about two-thirds of stone cases in the United States. They generally are composed of calcium oxalate or calcium oxalate mixed with calcium phosphate. Why calcium oxalate stones develop is not known in most cases. Some occur in persons with elevated calcium levels in blood or urine, but the reasons for elevation are not known, either. "Stone making" seems to run in families. There is no clear link to diet, but persons who regularly drink three or more quarts of milk a day, take megadoses of more than 300 units of vitamin D daily, or use large quantities of bicarbonate of soda run a higher risk.

Struvite or infection-induced stones make up about 15 percent of all cases of kidney stones. They are composed of magnesium ammonium phosphate and occur mainly in patients with chronic urinary tract infections containing urea-splitting bacteria. The stone may grow so large that it fills the entire renal pelvis, forming an antlerlike shape that gives it the name "staghorn" calculus. The growth eventually may fill the pelvis and obstruct the kidney completely.

Many victims of infection-induced stones are invalids who require long-term use of a catheter to drain the bladder. Other cases are associated with structural abnormalities of the urinary tract.

Uric acid and cystine stones make up about 10 percent of all cases. Uric acid stones result from gout; cystine stones from a hereditary disease that interferes with the handling of an amino acid in proteins.

Many persons pass tiny stones and are never aware of it. Others are notified by blood in the urine or by painful urination as gritty bits of sand pass along the urethra. The pain of kidney colic can be excruciating and unforgettable. It occurs when a stone enters one of the ureters and works its way down, gouging as it goes. The pain is felt sometimes in the back, sometimes in the pelvic area, and may be accompanied by nausea, vomiting, chills, and fever.

Treatment of stones. Because the treatment differs by type of stone, a person may be directed to attempt to collect a sample by urinating through a fine strainer. The stones then can be given to a physician for analysis.

Stones containing uric acid may indicate that the person has gout, requiring treatment with alkali, high fluid intake, and drugs such as allopurinol. In contrast, calcium oxalate stones call for antacids that bind calcium and phosphate, or the drug hydrochlorothiazide, which cuts down the amount of calcium excreted into the urine. This prophylactic method inhibits stone formation.

Extracorporeal shock-wave lithotripsy (ESWL), described in Chapter 2, "Tests and Pro-

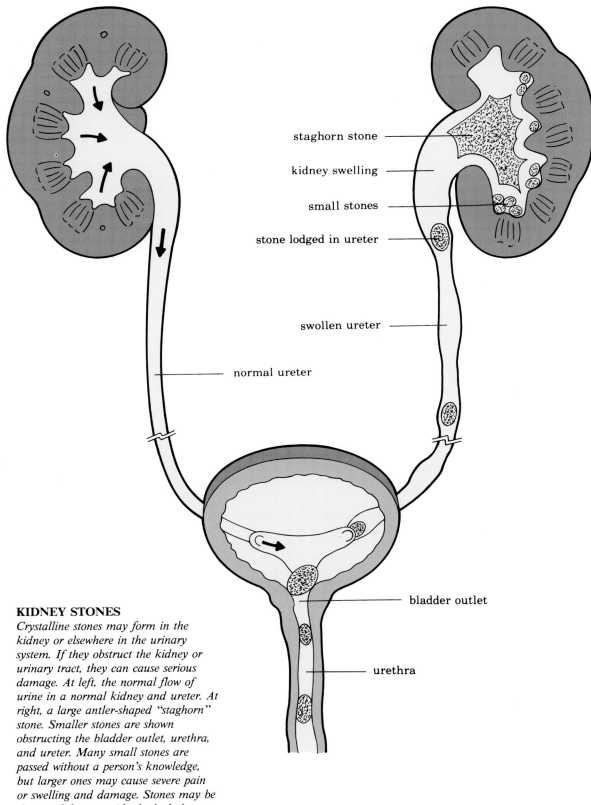

staghorn stone

kidney swelling

small stones

stone lodged in ureter

swollen ureter

normal ureter

bladder outlet

urethra

KIDNEY STONES

Crystalline stones may form in the kidney or elsewhere in the urinary system. If they obstruct the kidney or urinary tract, they can cause serious damage. At left, the normal flow of urine in a normal kidney and ureter. At right, a large antler-shaped "staghorn" stone. Smaller stones are shown obstructing the bladder outlet, urethra, and ureter. Many small stones are passed without a person's knowledge, but larger ones may cause severe pain or swelling and damage. Stones may be destroyed from outside the body by beaming them with shock waves.

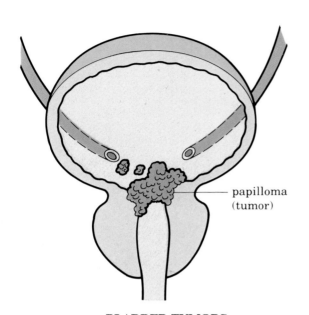

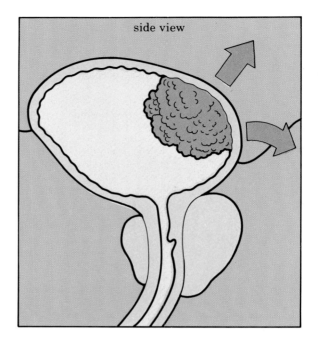

side view

papilloma
(tumor)

BLADDER TUMORS
*Bladder tumors frequently reveal
themselves by bloody or cloudy urine. At
left, a papilloma tumor completely
blocks the entrance to the urethra. At
right, a malignant tumor on the rear*

*wall of the bladder does not interfere
with urinary outflow. Unless detected
and removed early, malignancies may
spread via the lymphatic system to
nearby tissues.*

cedures," has come into widespread use for treatment of calcium stones, especially small ones. In this procedure, the person lies on a table over a basin, while high-intensity shock waves are passed through the water. Focused on the stone, the shocks cause the crystals to disintegrate and be flushed away. When stones measure less than 3 centimeters, a single painless treatment usually is successful. Hospitalization seldom is longer than two days.

With larger or infection-induced stones, multiple ESWL treatments may be necessary, especially if stones are of the staghorn type. If the stones still cannot be destroyed, they may have to be removed surgically. The kidney must be split, the stone removed, and the organ sewn together.

Large bladder stones that cannot be passed and cause pain, bleeding, or obstruction usually are treated by inserting a special cystoscope into the bladder to crush them. Fragments are then flushed away. Unfortunately, some persons are chronic "stone makers" and have recurrent episodes of stone disease.

Tumors of the Kidney And Urinary System

The major tumors of the urinary system occur in the kidney, bladder, and prostate. In addition, the kidney is a common site to which other tumors spread. Fortunately, cancers of the genitourinary system have a much more hopeful outlook than other cancers. For instance, nearly 70 percent of persons whose kidney cancer is detected early survive five years or more.

Kidney cancer. Wilms' tumor is one of the most common forms of cancer in children under 5 years of age and accounts for about one-fourth of all childhood cancers. Because of its origin early in development, most Wilms' tumors occur in children under age 2, and rarely after age 5.

The tendency to develop Wilms' tumor appears to be inherited. Fortunately, Wilms' tumor responds well to treatment. Radiation therapy and chemotherapy have achieved an 80 percent two-year disease-free survival rate, even when the cancer is widespread on discovery.

Renal carcinoma, the most common adult form of kidney cancer, strikes more men than women, usually between ages 45 and 60. The cancer may first show itself with confusing symptoms such as unexplained fever, a high white blood count, weight loss, and fatigue. Blood in the urine and flank pain are late symptoms.

Kidney cancer usually develops in a single kidney. If the cancer is detected before it has spread to nearby organs, the diseased kidney can be removed surgically. The other kidney takes over function and chances of recovery are relatively high. If the cancer is widely spread before discovery, chances of successful treatment are slim.

Bladder cancer accounts for about 6 percent of male cancers in the United States and 2 percent of female cancers. In certain geographical areas and in certain occupations, however, these percentages are much higher. Workers exposed to aniline and other dyes used in the textile, paint, and rubber industries, and residents of certain industrial areas, show an increased rate of bladder cancer. The disease also appears linked to cigarette smoking.

Bladder tumors arise mostly in the cells lining the urine collecting system. Apparently, the bladder is a particular target because urine is stored there, increasing the bladder's exposure to potential cancer-inducing substances in urine.

Bladder tumors tend to bleed and may give early warning of their presence before the disease has invaded the bladder wall or spread to regional lymph nodes; it usually is not a highly malignant cancer and may spread slowly. Localized tumors often can be cut or burned out by a cystoscope inserted through the urethra. Even if the cancer has progressed into the organ wall, it often may be treated successfully by removing a segment of the wall. In more severe cases, the entire organ may be removed surgically.

Prostate cancer is described in Chapter 25, "The Male Reproductive System."

Injury

The kidneys are well protected and are much less likely than the liver or spleen to be damaged during injury to the abdomen. In a violent impact, however, the kidney may be torn and bleed profusely. Blood pours into the capsule, pooling in surrounding tissues and back muscles, a condition called a retroperitoneal hematoma.

The condition is not limited to injury or wound victims, however. Patients taking anticoagulant drugs or who have a tendency to bleed because of low blood platelets or hemophilia also develop hematomas, not always easily recognized because the

kidneys are located so deep into the body. Massive bleeding into the urine can produce blood clots that obstruct the flow of urine. More often, however, kidney injuries result in only slow bleeding.

The bladder and urethra also may be torn during injury to the pelvic bones in severe crush injuries. This requires prompt measures to redirect the flow of urine by placing tubes into the ureters or the kidney pelvis.

Diseases That Affect the Kidney

Generalized diseases in the body often damage the kidneys or choose these vulnerable and important organs as a particular target.

Hypertension presents a special threat to the kidneys because proper blood pressure is crucial to their filtering action. Consistent, heightened pressure can cause severe and lasting damage to the delicate membranes of the glomerulus. Fortunately, hypertension usually can be detected readily and is a correctable disease.

Toxemia of pregnancy, a form of hypertension, is less common today than in the past. It can be controlled by restricting salt and taking other measures to lower blood pressure.

Diabetes, particularly when it has been present for many years, may damage the glomeruli of the kidney by thickening the membranes. This condition allows blood protein to leak out of the blood vessels into the urine.

Gout disrupts the kidney in several ways. Crystals of gout-induced uric acid may form in the cells of the tubules or the space between them, causing irritation and disturbing function. Crystals may form in the channels of the tubules, or uric acid stones may dam the ureters and block flow. Flushing the kidneys with water or using medications that reduce acid production or neutralize it with alkali lowers the risk.

Arteriosclerosis affects blood vessels throughout the body, but is a particular threat to the small capillaries of the kidney (see Chapter 6, "Blood Vessel Disorders").

Kidney Dialysis

Dialysis is required when the kidneys no longer are able to filter all the wastes from the blood. The wastes accumulate in the body and can lead to damage and ultimately to death if not corrected. If

THE ARTIFICIAL KIDNEY

The principles of an artificial kidney, which purifies blood outside the body, are shown in this schematic drawing. Blood is pumped from the patient's arm into a network of cellophane tubes that are bathed in a solution of electrolytes at exactly the concentration desired in the blood. Substances are exchanged through the microscopic pores of the cellophane. The purified blood is then returned to the body through a large vein.

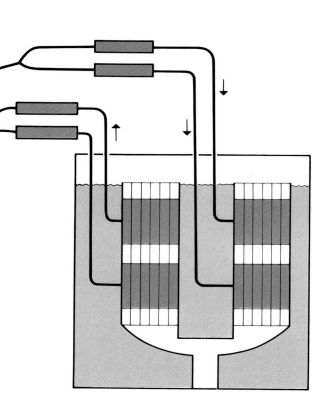

the condition is temporary, resulting from acute illness or injury, dialysis is needed only until the kidney recovers, which usually occurs swiftly. More often, it is a result of gradual, long-term destruction of the kidney by disease.

Hemodialysis is what most people mean when they speak of the "artificial kidney." It refers to a machine that purifies the blood outside the body. Blood is pumped from an artery into a vast length or series of tiny hollow fibers, against a counter-flow of dialysis solution. Waste molecules are washed away as they are diluted by the dialysis, while desired electrolytes pass into blood. Excess water is removed by raising the resistance to blood flow in the circuit. The blood then is returned to the body via a large vein.

Long-term hemodialysis patients usually are fitted with a shunt (see illustration) in the forearm, tying into an artery and a vein. This simplifies

connecting them to the system at each visit. During dialysis, they are given an anticoagulant such as heparin to prevent the blood from clotting. The anticoagulant is neutralized afterward by prot-amine to return clotting to normal.

The first artificial kidney was invented in the 1950s by Willem Kolff, a Dutch physician. It has undergone steady revision and improvement since. The original model was about the size of a small bathtub. The most common model, smaller than a human fist, contains 20,000 fibers and can be used in the patient's home.

Peritoneal dialysis uses the thin membranes of the abdominal cavity to substitute for the filtering membranes of the kidney. A solution similar to that used in hemodialysis is fed into the abdomen by force of gravity, draining through a long plastic tube from a large bottle suspended over the patient. The fluid bathes the surface membranes of the abdomen, exchanges waste molecules for the electrolytes in the solution, then drains off into an outflow bottle placed on the floor. The process is repeated until blood composition has reached proper levels. Excess water is removed by increasing glucose in the fluid, so that it draws water out of the body into the outflow bottle.

Like hemodialysis, peritoneal dialysis has become simpler and more automated since it was first devised. Regular dialysis patients now wear a special adapter or plastic plug in the abdominal wall so that a needle need not be threaded through the abdomen on each dialysis visit. Bottles can be hooked up so that a fresh bottle of fluid is tapped automatically each time another has been used and the waste drained away.

Both dialysis processes require about six to eight hours and must be performed two to four times a week, depending on the condition of the patient's kidneys. Some persons require close supervision at a hospital center, but thousands of others now perform either peritoneal dialysis or hemodialysis at home. A network of dialysis centers around the country trains patients and families to perform dialysis, including how to monitor blood levels and administer drugs if necessary.

Kidney Transplant

For young people with end-stage kidney disease, and for older ones who face long-term treatment on the artificial kidney and who do not have other major diseases, a replacement kidney donated by another person is the ultimate hope. Kidney transplant has become the most common of all organ transplant operations. More than 10,000 persons per year are returned to full, active life-styles after receiving a new kidney.

The most successful transplants are from one identical twin to another. Close relatives are the next best choice, and many relatives have willingly donated a kidney to a loved one. Most donated kidneys, however, come from persons who have died suddenly, often in accidents, and who have willed the organs or whose survivors have agreed to the donation.

As in other organ transplants, kidney transplant is a delicate procedure, calling for skill and speed (for surgical details, see Chapter 33, "Understanding Your Operation"). Donor and recipient must be carefully matched by tissue and blood type. The donated kidney must be removed rapidly, within minutes of death, and kept alive in special solutions until it can be installed in place.

The introduction of the drug cyclosporin, which suppresses the body's immune system and blocks rejection of the transplanted organ, has dramatically increased the success rate for kidney transplants. Even patients in their 70s now may receive a new kidney. More than 90 percent of patients who receive a new kidney from a close relative are restored to healthy kidney function, and the figure is almost as high for those who receive donated kidneys. Even those who are less successful may return to dialysis.

Keeping the Kidneys Healthy

Although there are many over-the-counter nostrums purporting to promote good health by flushing out the kidneys and urinary system, these vital organs usually require no special medicines or attention. The system of urine production and disposal works automatically if there is an adequate daily intake of water, nutrients, and salt. For most persons, that means about two to three quarts of fluid a day and about two grams of salt. The amount varies with temperature, exertion, illness, thirst, and desire for salt.

Normal blood pressure is important to the health of kidneys. Hypertension can severely damage the delicate capillaries, so it is important to keep close watch on blood pressure and to treat it promptly and effectively when detected.

Overuse of aspirin and other pain relievers also can harm the kidneys. These drugs should be used sparingly. Large amounts of bicarbonate of soda or antacid may lead to calcium deposits in the kidneys. Their use, too, should be minimized.

Severe blood loss from injury elsewhere in the body or shock leading to a drop in blood pressure can harm the kidneys by causing them to shut down their blood flow and depriving the cells of the kidney of their blood supply. Structural damage to the kidney and acute kidney failure can result. First-aid measures in the event of injury or accident should deal with shock first in order to prevent the complication of kidney failure.

Diarrhea and vomiting rob the body of salts and water. If they are not replaced, kidney shutdown may follow. No matter how bad you feel, it is important to take plenty of fluids in the event of illness. Because the functional reserve of the kidney tends to diminish with age, the need is particularly acute in older people.

CHAPTER 25

THE MALE REPRODUCTIVE SYSTEM

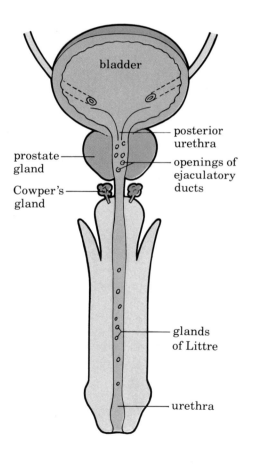

bladder

prostate gland

Cowper's gland

posterior urethra

openings of ejaculatory ducts

glands of Littre

urethra

The male reproductive system is closely involved with the urinary system. The male urethra is about nine inches long, running the full length of the penis. It carries off urine, but is also the passageway through which the male reproductive materials travel en route to their possible union with those of the female.

THE MALE ORGANS
The male reproductive and urinary organs are closely related. The urethra, through which urine passes, extends from the bladder to the meatus. The prostate gland surrounds the urethra. The ejaculatory ducts open into the posterior urethra. Cowper's glands and the Littre's glands secrete fluid into the anterior urethra to lubricate and help the sperm during intercourse. Sperm are manufactured in the testes and transported through the vas deferens, illustrated on page 316.

Disorders or abnormalities of both the male reproductive and urinary systems are treated by urologists or urologic surgeons. The entire system is sometimes spoken of as the genitourinary system. The most prominent parts of that system include the prostate gland, through which the urethra passes and which, along with the seminal vesicles, produces much of the seminal fluids; the testes (male sex glands), where spermatozoa and male hormones are produced; the vas deferens, which conveys spermatozoa to the urethra for ejaculation; the penis; and the scrotum, the sac containing the testes.

THE MALE URETHRA

For purposes of description, the continuous male urethra is divided into two anatomic areas. The portion that begins at the bladder outlet and runs through the prostate gland is referred to as the posterior or prostatic urethra. The remainder is called the anterior urethra and is located primarily in the shaft of the penis. The posterior urethra contains openings through which the ducts of the surrounding prostate gland empty secretions. These secretions are carried away during urination. Also located within the male urethra are the openings of the ejaculatory ducts, which carry spermatozoa from the testes to the urethra to be carried to the outside. Spermatozoa are the male cells that unite with the female egg. The anterior urethra also includes certain small glands, the so-called Littre's glands, which help keep the urethra lubricated, particularly during sexual intercourse. The two Cowper's glands also secrete a lubricating fluid,and empty into the anterior urethra.

Defects and Narrowings Of the Urethra

A stricture, which is an abnormal narrowing of the passageway of the posterior urethra, can be present at birth (congenital), or it can occur later in life.

Hypospadias is a failure of the urethra to close on what is considered the underside of the penis. It is like an open trough or a tube with large openings. The sphincter muscles that control urination function normally and the person is able to contain his urine. However, the troughlike external opening interferes with the normal delivery of the urinary system and with the transport of semen to the outside. The defect can be corrected surgically, usually early in childhood.

Epispadias is less common. A portion of the upper side of the urethra remains open, as a slit or a roofless channel running a short distance from the end of the penis. Sometimes the opening begins and ends at the base of the penis. In that case, normal sexual intercourse and delivery of semen is not possible. Malformation of the bladder's sphincter muscles prevents the person from controlling urination. A urologic surgeon can restore urinary control and form a new tube.

Injuries

Injuries to the male urethra are serious for two reasons. First, the urethra is rich in blood vessels, which are subject to recurrent engorgement and changes in size during sexual excitement. Injury can cause severe hemorrhage, pooling of blood under the surface, and extensive blood loss. Injury also breaks the urinary pipeline, permitting urine to seep into the surrounding tissues where it can cause inflammation and other damage.

If the injury is in the posterior urethral region, urine can seep into the area between the anus and scrotum or into the tissues around the bladder. The presence of the urine may not be obvious on initial physical examination. Posterior seepage can create a serious situation rapidly unless drainage and repair are carried out.

Anterior seepage is usually recognized quickly because there are no sphincter muscles to hold back the blood or other fluids, and bleeding is

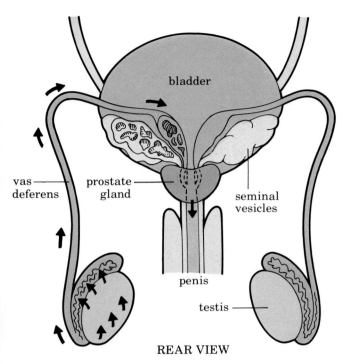

bladder

vas deferens

prostate gland

seminal vesicles

penis

testis

REAR VIEW

MALE REPRODUCTIVE ORGANS

The system for delivery of spermatozoa into the urethra is outlined in this rear view. Spermatozoa are manufactured and stored in the testes, pass through the vas deferens, and are mixed with secretions from the seminal vesicles and prostate gland before being ejaculated into the urethra.

almost constant. When the man voids, an alarming swelling of the penis and scrotum occurs. Early repair of such tears or cuts or traumatic damage is achieved by sidetracking the urine to bypass the injury until the conduit is reconstructed.

Strictures

Symptoms of stricture, or urethral narrowing, are general slowing of urinary flow, a desire to urinate frequently, and, occasionally, dribbling at the end of urination. The same symptoms, however, are produced by prostate enlargement or obstruction at the bladder neck.

Among the underlying causes of urethral strictures are physical and chemical injuries, birth defects, and inflammations. There are three common areas of stricture. One is at the bladder neck, usually as a result of an operation near the junction of the posterior urethra and the bladder. This can result from a transurethral resection of the prostate gland. The second common area is the bulbous urethra, where the anterior urethra begins. The third common area is the meatus or external opening. Strictures can be corrected surgically, or can be dilated with instruments called bougies, or urethral sounds. These instruments include both rigid and flexible materials designed to pass by the area of narrowing and permit careful expansion of it by progressive dilation with lubrication applied.

THE PROSTATE GLAND

This accessory male sex gland is closely associated with the lower urinary tract. The posterior or prostatic urethra forms a channel through the prostate gland. The urethra's wall contains muscles that hold urine in the bladder until it is ready to be expelled. The prostate has openings through which its own secretions are emptied into the urethra and carried away during urination or during the sexual act.

The prostatic and seminal vesicle secretions supply substances necessary to maintain spermatozoa in their long course through the female genital tract. These secretions contain acid-base substances, sugar, and other nutrients.

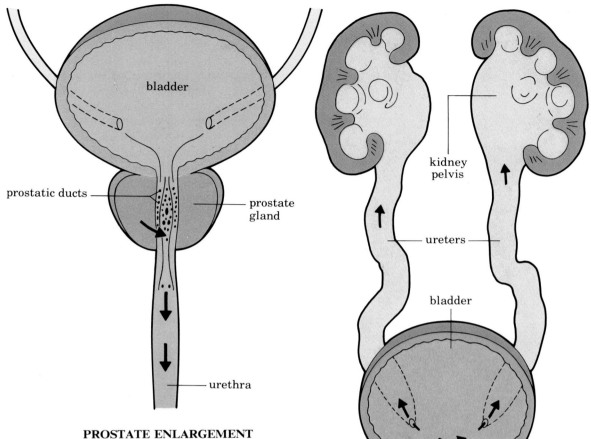

PROSTATE ENLARGEMENT
An enlarged prostate can cause serious damage to the upper urinary tract by obstructing the flow of urine. The drawing above shows the normal ureters, bladder, and urethra. At right, an enlarged prostate compresses the bladder outlet. If the obstruction is not relieved, the bladder dilates and weakens. Backed-up urine enlarges and weakens the ureters and can dilate the kidney pelvis. Continued pressure can severely damage the kidney tissue.

Diseases of the prostate gland are very common and can be serious. Congenital abnormalities of the prostate are extremely rare unless they are associated with other abnormalities.

Examining the Prostate

Examination of the prostate has a special diagnostic function. The patient is generally asked to bend over with hands on knees or to support himself on a chair or table. The doctor inserts a lubricated, rubber-gloved index finger into the rectum.

By feeling the prostate through the rectum, the doctor can tell a good deal about its condition. The doctor's sense of touch will detect whether the prostate is firm, or soft and boggy, or stony hard, or hard in a few areas, all significant findings.

A complete prostate examination usually includes a prostatic massage to obtain prostatic secretions for study later. A few strokes during the

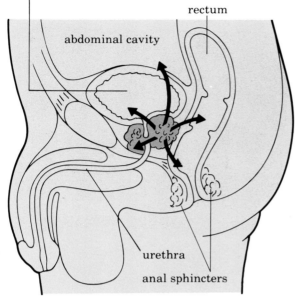

PROSTATE CANCER
The arrows show how prostate cancer spreads. Organs and structures that may be invaded are the abdominal cavity, rectum, bladder, anal sphincters, and urethra. Early prostate cancer causes few symptoms, so a physician's examination is the best method of detection.

rectal examination expel secretions from the prostate through the urethra. The secretions are then collected on a glass slide, a cover slide applied, and studied under the light microscope. If pus is found, it may indicate an infection. Other elements also help in the diagnosis. Prostatic massage is useful to empty the prostate and to relieve congestion.

Urine specimens (usually three) are obtained. If the first specimen contains pus or bacteria but the next two are clear, infection probably is limited to the urethra. If all three specimens in the so-called "three-glass test" show infection, the site of the infection can be in the bladder or the kidneys.

Prostatitis

Infections of the prostate gland (prostatitis) in younger men usually are caused by organisms such as those of gonorrhea, which is described in Chapter 32, "Infectious Diseases." In these cases, the infection travels up the urethra to the prostate, then spreads beyond it. In older men, prostatitis usually is nonspecific and nongonorrheal. Prostatic infections also can be blood-borne from infection elsewhere in the body.

Acute bacterial prostatitis is encountered less frequently since the modern era of antibiotics. Symptoms are acute: high fever plus an urge and frequent need to urinate. There may be blood in the urine at the beginning and end of urination. Sitting may be uncomfortable because of pain in the genital area.

Chronic bacterial prostatitis is seldom accompanied by fever. Urination is frequent, both day and night, and urine may be cloudy or contain blood. Usually there is no history of acute prostatitis. Respiratory infections or abscessed teeth may be contributing factors.

Prostatitis is treated essentially the same way as infection elsewhere in the body: establish good drainage, remove the source of infection, and destroy the infecting organisms.

Benign Prostatic Enlargement

In medical language a benign tumor is one that is not cancerous and does not invade other parts of the body. Symptoms of a benign tumor, however, can be anything but benign in the patient's estimation. This usually is true of tumors of the prostate. This condition is a result of an overgrowth (hypertrophy) of the prostate gland associated with aging. It is estimated that two-thirds of the men between 60 and 70 have some degree of prostatic enlargement.

The outstanding symptom of prostatic enlargement is urinary obstruction caused by narrowing of the urethra. There is an increased frequency of urination, especially at night. The urinary stream may be slow to start, less forceful, decreased in caliber, and end in dribbling.

Operation. There are four standard techniques of prostatectomy for relief of this benign condition. Three are considered "open" procedures in which the area is approached through an outside incision. The fourth, which employs a route through the urethra, is called transurethral resection. The open techniques are termed suprapubic prostatectomy, retropubic prostatectomy, and perineal prostatectomy, although the procedures are not in truth prostatectomies, but rather removal of the overgrown portion of the prostate gland. The prostate capsule and its remaining components are generally left behind.

In selected cases the transurethral resection of the prostate gland is a safe and acceptable alternative to the so-called open operations. Since it is accomplished without an incision, some doctors believe the transurethral resection is superior because the length of stay in the hospital and degree of discomfort to the patient may be less.

Prostatic Cancer

Prostate cancer is the second most common cancer to afflict the American male. An estimated 20 percent or more of all men over 60 have prostatic cancer in some form. Prostate cancer, however, is a relatively slow-growing cancer of low virulence. In contrast to benign prostatic hypertrophy, which at an early phase can produce evidence of urinary obstruction, prostatic cancer is unlikely to provide early symptoms. The cancer often is present for some time without being suspected.

Prostatic cancer in its early stages can be suspected as the result of a routine rectal examination. The presence of a stony-hard area in the prostate will arouse suspicion. Conditions such as prostatic stones and certain chronic infections are difficult to distinguish from cancer by rectal examination alone, so it is necessary to remove a small piece of prostatic tissue (biopsy) from the suspicious area for study under the microscope.

The American Cancer Society recommends that every man over age 50 have a rectal examination annually. If a suspicious area is detected in the prostate, an early biopsy can be obtained. When prostate cancer is recognized early and treated by surgery or radiation, the cure rate is high.

New methods of radiotherapy for prostate cancer involve insertion of radioactive isotopes such as iodine or gold. Proponents believe these methods are as effective as surgery or external radiation.

Hormones. For more than 30 years doctors have known that prostate cancer is susceptible to hormones that influence its natural course. Male sex hormones are believed to have an accelerating effect on the growth of prostatic cancer. For a variety of reasons, female hormones (diethylstilbestrol [DES] or its derivatives) have an opposite effect. Prostate cancer patients sometimes benefit from the administration of so-called female sex hormones or from removal of the male hormone effect by castration (removal of both testes). No patient is ever cured by such hormone treatment, but the growth of the tumor can be controlled or limited for months, perhaps even years.

THE TESTES

Hormone-producing interstitial cells of the testes, also known as the cells of Leydig, are independent of the organ's spermatozoa-producing department. Tumors of these cells are extremely rare. Changes in the part of the testes that forms the spermatozoa also are relatively rare and usually are associated with various forms of intersex.

Undescended testis or cryptorchidism is a condition in which one or both testes fail to descend into the scrotum from the abdomen, where the organs grow during fetal development. The defect may be genetic and congenital, it may be mechanical, or endocrine factors may interfere. If only one testis is involved, the defect probably is mechanical, but if both are involved the underlying problem may be hormonal, such as a poorly functioning pituitary gland. Sometimes, improving function by administering pituitary extracts will ease the testicle into its proper position. If surgery is needed, doctors generally agree that the operation should be done before age 5 and certainly before the onset of puberty.

Tumors of the testicle are highly malignant and can occur at any age, but are most common between ages 20 and 40. Any mass in the testicle, especially if not associated with fever, should be suspected of malignancy. Treatment is extensive surgical excision and, depending on the type of tumor, irradiation or other therapy.

Removal of the tumor is achieved through an incision in the groin. The clamped spermatic cord and the testis are then carefully removed. Depending on the stage and appearance of the tumor, additional treatment may be given. In some cases

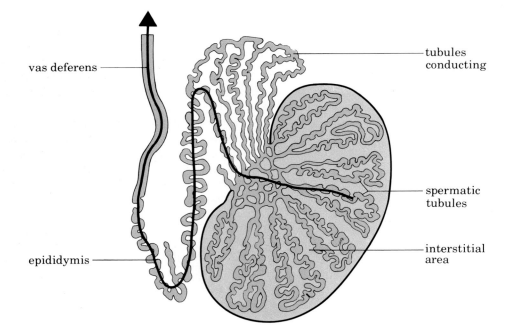

vas deferens

epididymis

tubules
conducting

spermatic
tubules

interstitial
area

THE TESTES

This is a cross section of a testis, the gland that produces spermatozoa and male hormones. Sperm are produced in the spermatic tubules, and hormones are produced in the interstitial area. The conducting tubules are part of the

epididymis, a portion of the seminal duct lying upon and behind the testis. The vas deferens leads to the urethra. The path of the spermatozoa is indicated by arrows.

the lymph nodes that drain from the testis and pass through the back part of the body cavity also are removed.

Hydrocele is an accumulation of fluid in the scrotum and cystic dilation of the coverings of the testes. The swelling is obvious, varies in size, and can be painful. Hydrocele frequently is associated with hernia. Spermatocele is a similar cyst involving the sperm-conducting apparatus. The treatment is removal, if indicated by the patient's symptoms.

IMPOTENCE

Increasing levels of sexual awareness and the development of satisfactory penile prostheses for impotence are factors that have increased the number of patients who come to doctors for diagnosis and treatment of sexual problems. Impotence, something seldom talked about in an earlier era, now can often be treated.

Normal erections can be expected if there is an anatomically normal penis, adequate arterial blood flow, and intact nerve supplies. If no physical cause for impotence is apparent, a careful interview with the patient and preferably his sexual partner in a professional setting might reveal a psychological explanation. Some physicians use a sexual function questionnaire. One important question the doctor usually asks is whether the failure to achieve erection is situational, occurring under some circumstances but not others.

Medications or diseases can cause impotence. Medicine for high blood pressure can interfere with the ability to achieve erections because of the effects on penile nerves or penile blood pressure. Other causes can be diabetes mellitus, hyperthyroidism, alcoholism, or the use of tranquilizers or antidepressants.

Because implantation of a penile prosthesis is the most common surgical cure for impotence, it is important to determine the sexual partner's attitude about prosthetic surgery. The implantation usually is preceded by a series of tests for physical abnormalities of the penis. Tests also will be made for interference with the penile blood supply and other conditions that might interfere with intercourse or with satisfactory implantation of a prosthesis.

Some implants are of a rigid or semiflexible nature. Others include an inflatable device and connecting tube that can be implanted under the skin, then inflated or deflated by pressure on the inflate/deflate mechanism. This mechanism is connected to the inflatable device by a surgical procedure and the control button and operative system placed under the skin in the pubic area.

INFERTILITY

Semen analysis in the study of infertility or in routine endocrine surveys sometimes reveals a very low sperm count. The sperm under microscopic inspection may be of unusually poor quality or show lack of movement, or may be completely absent. In cases of poor sperm counts without evidence of endocrine problems, the administration of small doses of the hormones testosterone or chorionic gonadotropin can be helpful. Other forms of male infertility have been attributed to a so-called slackening of gonadal function. In men there is no true, identifiable counterpart of the menopause, although it has been documented on occasion in some men. This is characterized as a symptom of loss of self-confidence and associated behavior, poor memory, insomnia, loss of libido, apprehension, and nervousness. Occasional cases respond to testosterone therapy. Among men who have low sperm counts and difficulty in conception, it is not uncommon to find a varicocele, which is a varicose vein of the spermatic cord. Removal of such varicose lesions, which are usually localized, can lead to recovery of sperm count levels and successful conception.

VASECTOMY

Surgical interruption of the vas deferens, which normally carries sperm from the testes to the urethra, has become an increasingly popular method of contraception. It is frequently performed under local anesthetic in a physician's office or clinic. The operation consists of a small incision on either side of the groin. The vas is then lifted forward and

severed and the two ends are cauterized to seal them off, or sometimes tied with ligatures. The healing process is said not to be painful, and sexual performance ordinarily does not suffer. For a period of weeks afterward, however, it is necessary to use another form of contraception until all sperm are cleared from the vas.

Although regarded as minor surgery, the procedure is not without problems. These include bleeding or inflammation at the site of surgery. In some cases, the operation fails to obstruct the passage of sperm, or the passageway later reopens, resulting in pregnancy.

More recently, some men who had vasectomies have sought to have fertility restored by having the severed vas reunited surgically, or reanastomosed. Many of these procedures have failed because of the inability to open the passageway. A few surgeons have reported success on a limited number of patients. The success may be improved by the introduction of microsurgery techniques that allow the tiny canals to be rejoined under enormous magnification.

CIRCUMCISION

Shortly after birth, many males throughout the world undergo what is termed prophylactic circumcision to remove some of the foreskin on the penis. For some, the procedure has both a medical and a religious significance, and is sometimes performed according to strict ritual. Medically, hygiene usually is given as a reason for circumcision. It also is said that the incidence of cervical cancer is lower in women whose sex partners have been circumcised. These contentions are disputed, however, and the medical value of circumcision is a matter of debate. The position of the American Academy of Pediatrics is that infant circumcision is not required medically.

Circumcision in an adult sometimes is performed for medical reasons, including the avoidance of infection, the presence of conditions that make infection likely (such as diabetes), or a history of irritation. Another reason is to avoid cancer of the glans of the penis, because most cases of penile cancer worldwide are found in uncircumcised men. In adult circumcision, extra care must be taken to avoid postoperative pain and blood loss. The operation is performed under local, spinal, or general anesthesia. There is no evidence that adult circumcision affects potency.

CHAPTER 26

THE FEMALE REPRODUCTIVE SYSTEM

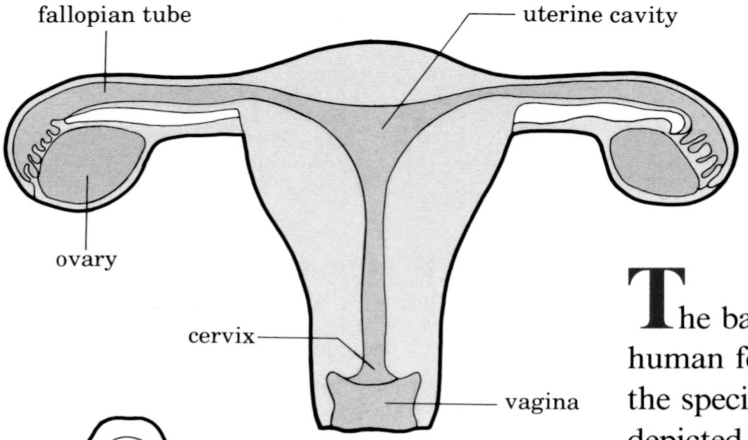

fallopian tube — uterine cavity

ovary

cervix

vagina

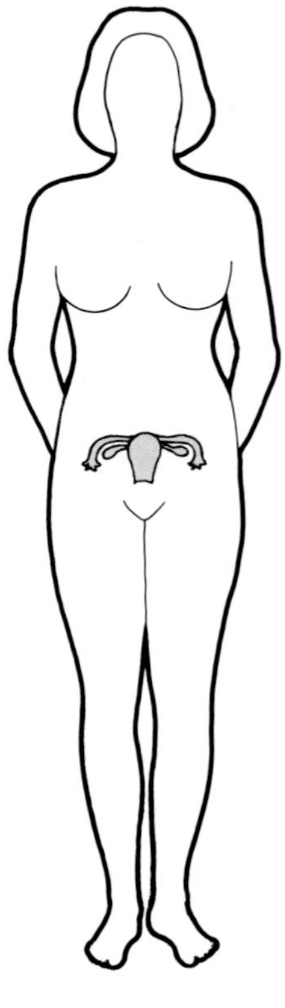

REPRODUCTIVE ORGANS
The female internal reproductive organs are located in the pelvic area of the lower abdomen (drawing at left). The normal structures are shown in cross section. In addition to reproduction, the ovaries produce hormones responsible for breast development, genital maturation, hair distribution, and redistribution of body fat.

The basic organs that distinguish human female from male and enable the species to reproduce itself are depicted in the illustration here. Although the organs are located in the pelvic area, their functions are orchestrated by the pituitary gland beneath the brain. The pituitary, in turn, is directed by the hypothalamus in the brain above it. The role of the endocrine system in reproduction is described in Chapter 18, "The Hormones and Endocrine Glands."

The female reproductive organs, as shown, are the ovaries, uterus, fallopian tubes, vagina, and external genitalia. Briefly, the ovaries store and nourish the eggs (ova) and produce the female hormones estrogen and progesterone; the fallopian tubes are the passageways through which the ovum travels en route to possible fertilization by the male sperm; the uterus, with its lining, the endometrium, provides a bed for the egg if fertilization occurs and nourishes the pregnancy through the subsequent nine months; and the vagina, or birth canal, is the entry through which sperm reach the ovum and the outlet through which a baby passes at birth.

Conception and pregnancy are described in Chapter 28, "Pregnancy and Childbirth."

NORMAL PUBERTY

By age 12, most females begin the physical and behavioral transition from childhood to adolescence. Puberty is characterized by a series of changes, such as a sudden spurt in the rate of growth, maturation of the breasts (thelarche), the appearance of secondary sexual hair in the armpits and pubic area (pubarche), and the first menstruation (menarche).

Breast development begins with darkening around the nipple at about 11 years. Pubic hair growth begins about age 11 and usually reaches adult quantity by age 14. The first menstrual period occurs any time from ages 9 through 17. If a girl has not had a menstrual period by age 16, she should seek medical attention.

MENSTRUATION

Menstruation is a cyclical discharge of blood, secreted fluids, and degenerated tissue from the uterus. A menstrual cycle, calculated from the first day of one menstrual episode to the first day of the next, is usually 28 days, but varies from 24 to 32 days, both among individuals and from period to period. Blood flow usually lasts three to seven days, with an average total blood loss of about one ounce per period. Menstrual periods usually occur each month (except during pregnancy) through the age of about 50.

The degenerated tissue in the menstrual substances is shed from the lining of the uterus and, in effect, represents a failed pregnancy. As a result of a timed series of events directed by the endocrine system, normally, once a month the ovaries develop one or more eggs from the woman's storehouse of several hundred thousand, preparatory to potential fertilization. Female hormones nourish the egg and also act on the endometrium to prepare a

bed to receive it. If fertilization does not occur, however, the tissue around the ovulation site undergoes degeneration, the hormone levels in the blood fall, and the lining of the uterus is shed.

Menstruation requires normal body functions, a normal pituitary gland, a responsive ovary, and a normal uterus. Defects in any of these can prevent the start of menstruation or cause menstrual periods to stop, even if they have been regular.

Absence of Menstruation (Amenorrhea)

Vaginal causes. The most common reasons menstruation fails to begin in an otherwise normally developed female are abnormalities of the vagina and uterus. These abnormalities range from an imperforate hymen—the hymen is the piece of tissue that narrows the opening of the vagina—to incomplete development of the uterus. The hymen varies greatly in form, but it is rarely completely closed. It also can be opened surgically, allowing trapped menstrual blood to escape.

Uterus. The absence of the uterus or of a portion of the vagina is rare, but when it does occur, the vagina ends as a blind pouch. The woman does not have menstrual periods, but usually can have normal sexual relations. Sometimes a dilator may be used to enlarge the vagina.

Ovaries. Because the ovaries produce estrogen and progesterone, failure of these organs to develop means that the shedding of the lining of the uterus (menstruation) does not take place. Women with this condition also lack breast development and other secondary sexual development.

Gonadotropins are substances that stimulate the gonads, or reproductive glands, such as the ovaries. Two pituitary gonadotropins, known as FSH and LH, are integral to the menstrual process. A low production level of these hormones can result in an absence of menstruation. The condition may be a result of chronic disease, such as diabetes mellitus, but most often arises from a disturbance of the pituitary or the hypothalamus. Amenorrhea is frequently associated with extreme weight loss, and is common in female runners who carry very little fat on their bodies, and in anorexics, who are obsessed with thinness. (See Chapter 21, "Nutrition.")

Irregular Uterine Bleeding

Bleeding without ovulation. Young women often have irregular bleeding when they first menstruate, because the early cycles are not ovulatory

HORMONE LEVELS DURING MENSTRUAL CYCLE

A cyclical series of endocrine events controls ovulation, menstruation, and conception. At the beginning of the cycle, follicle-stimulating hormone (FSH) is secreted by the pituitary gland. Under its stimulation, an ovum (egg) matures and estrogen is secreted. Estrogen inhibits the flow of FSH but triggers a secondary pituitary hormone, luteinizing hormone (LH), which causes ovulation, the release of the egg for possible fertilization. Cells around the ovulation site then secrete the hormone progesterone, which enhances the preparation of the uterine lining for implantation of the fertilized ovum. If conception does not occur, estrogen and progesterone levels fall and menstruation takes place.

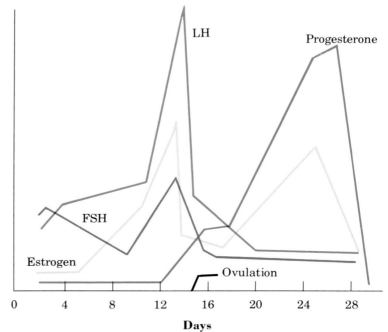

cycles. Irregular bleeding often disappears as ovulatory cycles ensue, except in cases of anemia.

Ovulatory bleeding. There may be spotting or slight bleeding at the time of ovulation, which occurs about 14 to 16 days before a menstrual period, due to a slight decrease of estrogen. The spotting lasts one or two days.

Spotting before menstruation. A menstrual period may be preceded by several days of spotting because of decreased hormonal levels and consequent irregular shedding of the lining of the uterus. These cycles may persist for several months before subsiding or reverting to normal cycles.

Bleeding without ovulation, mid-cycle bleeding, and irregular shedding are termed dysfunctional uterine bleeding. Profuse cyclic or irregular menstrual bleeding can also be a sign of a pathologic condition and should be investigated. In older women, abnormal bleeding before or after menopause should be investigated.

Menopause

Signs and symptoms. The menopause begins when ovulation stops. The average age is 51. Afterward, irregular menstrual periods and times of lack of menstrual periods are not unusual. Next comes a decrease in the production and secretion

of estrogen, accompanied by signs and symptoms of the deficit in the organs dependent upon estrogen, such as the uterus, cervix, vagina, and breasts. Most characteristic of the postmenopausal period are hot flashes and shrinking (atrophy) of the genital organs. Symptoms such as inability to sleep, irritability, or depression, considered by many women to be part of the menopause, are much more difficult to attribute to reduction of estrogen.

The vasomotor symptoms that affect the blood vessels and produce hot flashes and sweats trouble as many as 60 percent of menopausal women. Estrogen deficiency also causes a gradual reduction and eventual loss of the thickness of the vaginal wall. The result is increasing dryness in the vagina. When the deficiency is severe, there is vaginal irritation, itching, and sometimes pain during intercourse.

Osteoporosis is an age-related loss of bone mass that can occur in both men and women, but is commonly associated with the menopause. Its causes and treatments are described in Chapter 16, "The Bones and Muscles."

Estrogen replacement therapy (ERT) for the postmenopausal woman is beneficial for relieving involuntary hot flashes, sweats, and symptoms attributed to atrophy of the vagina. ERT also is beneficial for stabilizing osteoporosis. The usual regimen calls for the postmenopausal woman to take prescribed doses of estrogen daily to offset the physical changes of menopause; often the regimen is cyclical, with the woman taking estrogen for three weeks, then abstaining for a week. ERT also is prescribed for women after hysterectomy, because they no longer produce their own estrogen. At one time, ERT was used cautiously because studies indicated it increased the risk of endometrial cancer. Risks do rise somewhat, but studies have shown that other risks (such as the risk of hip fracture from osteoporosis) outweigh them.

INFECTIONS

Infections of the female reproductive tract involve both the external and the internal genitalia, and they are among the most common gynecological complaints.

External Infections

Vulvitis. Most of the time, inflammation of the vulva results from profuse vaginal discharge caused by vaginal infection. However, a primary infection of the vulva called vulvitis can occur secondary to a herpes virus infection (described in Chapter 32, "Infectious Diseases"). Fortunately, treatment with the topical drug acyclovir can relieve painful first attacks and decrease the frequency and severity of recurrences.

Vaginitis. The most common forms of vaginitis, which means infection of the vagina, are yeast or monilial vaginitis, trichomonas vaginalis vaginitis, and Gardnerella vaginitis. All produce irritation of the external genitalia, itching, frequent urination, and occasional pain when urinating or during intercourse.

Yeast vaginitis. Yeast or monilial vaginitis is caused by a fungus known as *Candida albicans.* The infection also is known as candidiasis or moniliasis. It occurs during pregnancy, and also among women who take oral contraceptives. Yeast vaginitis also can follow treatment with broad-spectrum antibiotics. The treatment requires insertion of suppositories or cream in the vagina.

Trichomonas vaginalis vaginitis. Infection with the *Trichomonas vaginalis* usually causes vaginal discharge, irritation of the vulva, itching, and pain during intercourse. The most effective treatment is metronidazole (Flagyl), an oral medication requiring a physician's prescription. Because trichomonads can be harbored in the male urinary

tract and be retransmitted during intercourse, it is recommended that sexual partners seek medical attention and therapy simultaneously.

Gardnerella vaginitis produces less severe itching and burning. Flagyl applied topically is the preferred treatment.

Internal Infections

Cervicitis is an inflammation of the cervix. The red and irregular surface around the cervical opening resembles that caused by some cancers, so an examination is important to rule out a malignancy. Usual treatment of chronic cervicitis is application of antibiotic vaginal cream.

Gonorrhea is one of the most common sexually transmitted (venereal) diseases (see Chapter 32, "Infectious Diseases"). It infects the internal genital tract organs—the uterus, fallopian tubes, and ovaries. As many as 80 percent of the women who contract the disease have no symptoms; others urinate frequently or experience pain while urinating. As the infection advances to the uterus and fallopian tubes, the woman may have abdominal pain with fever. Prompt antibiotic treatment brings a return to normal temperature and clears the abdominal signs. But resulting adhesions in the fallopian tube can cause infertility.

Chlamydia is a recently identified sexually transmitted disease that appears to be even more common that gonorrhea. A symptom may be a green, purulent vaginal discharge, but often the infection is "silent" even though there is significant inflammation of the pelvic organs. Most cases are discovered during routine gynecological examinations. Undetected chlamydia can lead to infertility, or, in the event of conception, to infection of the newborn during birth. The infection can be treated with the antibiotics tetracycline and doxycycline.

DISORDERS OF
THE REPRODUCTIVE ORGANS

Pelvic Relaxation

Pelvic relaxation results from a weakening of the supporting tissues of the bladder, the upper walls of the vagina, the uterus, and the rectum. The organ or part of the organ then can move out of normal position or alignment and create a sense of pressure in the vagina, or feel as if a structure is protruding from the vagina. Other symptoms include pelvic pain and inability to control urination.

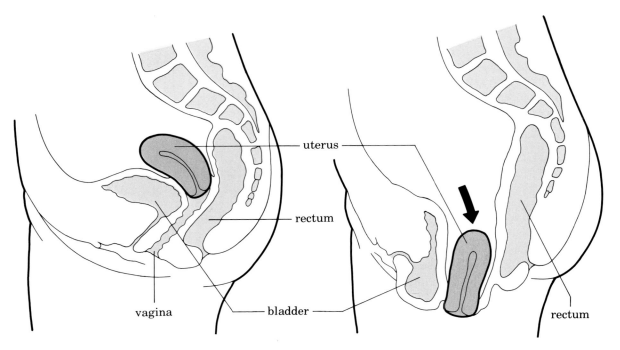

uterus

rectum

vagina — bladder

rectum

PROLAPSE

Prolapse occurs when the supporting ligaments of the uterus are injured or stretched, often as tissues lose their elasticity with age. The left drawing shows a uterus in normal position. In the drawing at right the uterus has prolapsed into the vagina. The condition can be so severe that the entire uterus protrudes beyond the vagina, causing discomfort and inflammation. The condition is usually repaired surgically, but sometimes a supporting device is inserted in the vagina.

Uterine prolapse. Uterine prolapse occurs when the supporting ligaments of the uterus are stretched or injured and permit the uterus to descend into the vagina. The prolapse can be so severe that the entire uterus protrudes beyond the vaginal opening. The bladder frequently prolapses, too. Uterine prolapse can be treated with a pessary, a supporting device inserted in the vagina to hold the uterus in place, or surgical removal of the uterus.

Vaginal wall relaxation. Relaxation of the front wall of the vagina results in cystocele and urethrocele, a bulging of the bladder and the urethra. Symptoms consist of a bearing-down sensation and protrusion of the organs outside the

vagina. There may be a loss of urine during coughing, sneezing, or laughing. Some women must wear protective clothing. Surgery can relieve the symptoms in most cases.

Relaxation of the back wall of the vagina creates a protrusion of the rectum into the vagina, called a rectocele. A minimal amount of rectocele usually does not produce symptoms, but a considerable protrusion pushes the bowel into the herniated sac. Simultaneous surgical repair of the front and back walls of the vagina usually corrects a cystocele, urethrocele, or rectocele.

Endometriosis

Endometriosis is a disease in which tissue from the lining of the uterus implants outside the uterus on the pelvic structures, usually on the ovaries. The displaced tissue responds to all the hormonal variations of the menstrual cycle, just as the endometrium inside the uterus does. The disease apparently occurs when endometrial fragments of the uterus flow backward up through the fallopian tubes to implant and grow. The disorder occurs most often in women between 20 and 35 years of age. Although endometriosis has been discovered in many women who did not have significant symptoms, endometriosis can cause severe pain during menstrual periods (dysmenorrhea) and pain during intercourse (dyspareunia). Infertility sometimes leads a patient to see a physician.

Therapy is often aimed at relieving the symptoms yet conserving the organs necessary for childbearing. Combinations of estrogens and progestogen may be used to suppress ovulation, thereby creating a pseudopregnancy that allows the endometrial glands to atrophy. Conservative surgery may be performed to remove endometrial implants and adhesions. Radical surgery to remove the ovaries is done only in women who are beyond the childbearing age or when the disease is severe and has not responded to treatment.

Ovarian Cysts

An ovarian cyst is a closed cavity or sac. Some are fluid-filled, some are in a semifluid state, and others are solid. Cysts are usually small. They occur in women of all ages, and produce symptoms only when they create pressure on other organ systems. A cyst can become large enough to increase the size of the abdomen before it is noticed. An ovarian cyst is not painful unless it twists or ruptures and hemorrhages into the abdominal cavity. Any twisting or bleeding of an ovarian cyst must be treated immediately. Ovarian cysts are usually removed surgically.

Cancer of the Reproductive Tract

Cancer of the cervix is the most common cancer of the reproductive tract. The earliest recognizable indication is dysplasia, a change in the superficial cells of the covering (epithelium) of the cervix. Theoretically, if dysplasia remains untreated, it will progress into preinvasive cancer of the cervix. When the cancer progresses past the preinvasive stage by spreading from the site of origin to invade the tissue beneath the epithelium, it is called invasive cancer. Dysplasia or preinvasive cancer of the cervix usually does not cause symptoms and frequently the diagnosis is suspected by a positive Pap test obtained during a routine examination. The Pap test is highly successful in detecting the cancer and allows treatment at a stage when cure is certain.

Removal of preinvasive cancer is done by an operation or by cryosurgery. In a young woman, a cone biopsy of the cervix or cryosurgery is recommended. For the patient who is beyond childbearing years or who considers her family complete, the selected treatment may be hysterectomy. The cure rate of preinvasive cancer of the cervix is virtually 100 percent.

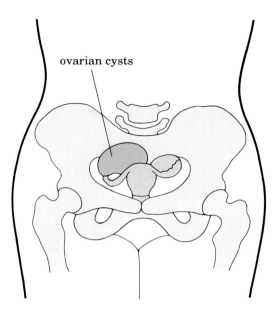

ovarian cysts

OVARIAN ENLARGEMENT
An enlargement of an ovary can be cystic, filled with fluid, or solid. It may cause no symptoms until it is large enough to press on adjacent organs, as in the drawing above, or until it is twisting or bleeding, in which case it must be removed surgically.

Symptoms of invasive carcinoma of the cervix include irregular bleeding, bleeding after intercourse, pain, and weight loss. A woman who experiences irregular spotting should seek medical attention immediately because the possibility of curing invasive carcinoma decreases markedly in advanced stages.

Cancer of the uterus. About three-fourths of all cases of endometrial cancer (cancer of the lining of the uterus) are found in women beyond the menopause. The average age of occurrence is between 50 and 60. Because the primary symptom is bleeding, any bleeding in a woman who is past the menopause should be investigated thoroughly. The diagnosis is made by obtaining tissue from the inside of the uterus by dilation of the cervix and curettage of the endometrium or by taking a biopsy of the endometrium. The treatment is removal of the uterus, fallopian tubes, and ovaries. Radiotherapy may follow. The outlook is favorable.

Cancer of the ovary is the fourth leading cause of death from cancer among American women. About 60 percent of all malignant ovarian tumors occur in women 40 to 60 years old, 20 percent in women under 40, and the remainder in women over 60. But many women have advanced disease before they seek medical help for the first time. Treatment involves drug therapy, X-ray therapy, or surgery. The basic operation is a total abdominal hysterectomy with removal of the fallopian tubes and ovaries. If the disease is extensive, the surgery is often followed by X-ray therapy and drug therapies.

INFERTILITY

Infertility presents a problem for 10 percent of married couples. Conception depends upon normal female ovarian function, meaning that ovulation must occur. The hormones from the ovary must prepare the uterus so that if fertilization occurs, the fertilized egg can implant in the uterine lining and grow. The male must deposit a sufficient number of motile spermatozoa in the vagina because the sperm have to migrate through the cervix and the uterus to the fallopian tubes before fertilization can take place. In the course of a fertility evaluation, all of these aspects are examined.

A general history and physical examination of the woman should be accomplished. A semen analysis is done on the male partner to see if he has enough motile spermatozoa. Whether ovulation occurs on a regular basis can be determined by keeping a chart of the woman's basal body temperature (which will rise slightly at ovulation), by sampling the lining of the uterus, or by hormone assays. A hysterosalpingogram can be performed to be sure there are no abnormalities of the uterus. If tubal disease has blocked the tubes, surgery may be necessary. If ovulation is not occurring, drugs are available to induce it. If the natural hormones are not of sufficient levels to prepare the lining of the uterus, hormonal therapy is prescribed.

CONTRACEPTION

Methods of avoiding pregnancy have been used for centuries. Although breast feeding reduces the risk of pregnancy and is a method that has been used historically, it is not highly effective. Oral contraceptives and intrauterine devices are newer methods of family planning. The use of a contraceptive reduces the statistical probability of pregnancy, but the range of effectiveness is wide and varies from less than one pregnancy in 100 women

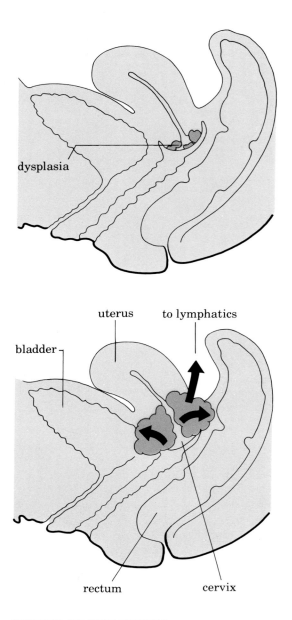

CANCER OF THE CERVIX
The most common cancer of the female reproductive tract is cancer of the cervix. It can be cured if detected early. The first indication is likely to be a distinct change of cell structure, called dysplasia, at the cervical opening (upper drawing). The cells are obtained and tested by Pap smear. Although not all dysplasias become cancerous, if not identified and treated, they can progress to become invasive cancer, which spreads to nearby structures (lower drawing) and may be too far advanced for cure.

per year with oral contraceptives to between 10 and 40 pregnancies in 100 women per year using the rhythm method. It is estimated that if 100 women were to have regular intercourse for one year with no form of contraception, 80 to 90 of them would become pregnant, most in the first three months.

The Rhythm Method

During the menstrual cycle, there are days of absolute infertility, days in which the woman is potentially fertile, and days when pregnancy is unlikely but possible. A number of procedures have been devised to help identify the time of maximum fertility so intercourse can be avoided to decrease the likelihood of pregnancy.

The best way for a woman to determine her infertile period is to record the durations of 12 cycles. A cycle is determined from the first day of one menstrual period to the first day of the next. Ovulation occurs 14 to 16 days before the next menstrual cycle. Allowing for about 72 hours of survival time for both the ovum and the sperm, the unsafe time for intercourse is between 11 and 18 days before the next period begins. To allow for variation in cycle length, the first unsafe day is determined by subtracting 18 from the number of days of the shortest of the last 12 cycles. The last unsafe day is determined by subtracting 11 from the number of days in the longest cycle. If the shortest of the last 12 cycles is 23 days, and the longest is 33 days, then the calculation is 23 minus 18, which equals 5; and 33 minus 11, which equals 22. Thus, conception is considered possible from day 5 up to and including day 22.

The rhythm method sometimes is coupled with methods to identify the time of ovulation more precisely. One way is to chart basal body temperature, which rises when ovulation occurs. Another is to monitor changes in the body, including a marked increase in the volume of mucus secreted by the cervix. Both improve the effectiveness of the rhythm method.

Condoms

The condom, or rubber prophylactic, is one of the common contraceptive methods. It can be effective if used properly. Failures are recorded at five pregnancies per 100 woman-years when used correctly. The condom has the advantage of being

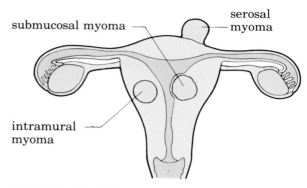

FIBROID TUMORS
Benign tumors of the uterus, known as fibroid tumors or myomas, afflict 20 percent of women over 35. They develop on the exterior surface of the uterus, in which case they are called subserosal myomas, beneath the mucous lining of the uterus (submucosal myoma), or within the uterine wall (intramural myoma). Myomas frequently produce no symptoms, but if they cause abnormal bleeding or press on other organs, surgical removal is often necessary.

widely available, and it decreases the likelihood of transmitting venereal disease. Its use is particularly important in combating the spread of AIDS. The condom is put on the penis when full erection occurs and before the penis enters the vagina. Following intercourse, it may be necessary to hold the condom in place when the penis is removed from the vagina so the condom does not slip off. Using a chemical spermicide in the vagina as well as in the condom further lessens the chance of pregnancy.

Barrier Methods: Diaphragms

The diaphragm is a rubber cup attached to a circular metal ring, which must be fitted for a woman by a physician. It is positioned in the vagina so that it covers the cervix. A spermicidal jelly or cream is placed within the diaphragm so that there is both a mechanical and a chemical barrier. When used diligently, the diaphragm has an effectiveness in the range of 2 to 15 pregnancies per 100 woman-years. Although reliable and without serious side effects, the diaphragm does require a high degree of motivation. It must be inserted in the vagina before intercourse and remain there for at least six to eight hours thereafter.

Preparations that kill sperm are available as foams, creams, jellies, and vaginal suppositories. They work in two ways: First, the inert chemical base that holds the spermicide acts as a barrier to the entry of the sperm into the cervix. Second, the agent contains a spermicidal chemical that immobilizes and kills the sperm. The failure rate of using spermicidal preparations alone, without a diaphragm, can be as low as five pregnancies per 100 woman-years for motivated users.

Intrauterine Devices (IUDs)

Intrauterine devices (IUDs) are usually made of steel and plastic. The sizes, shapes, and types of IUDs vary. Some have copper wire wound around them and some contain a hormonal material. They are inserted into the uterus by a physician and normally remain there until removed or expelled.

How IUDs work is not completely known. It is now believed that in humans the intrauterine device creates an environment in the uterus that is not conducive to early growth of the embryo or interferes with the sperm as they pass through the uterus to fertilize the ovum in the fallopian tube. The theoretical effectiveness of most IUDs is one to two pregnancies per 100 woman-years. Once the device is inserted, the patient needs no other form of contraception. If an IUD is tolerated well for several months, subsequent expulsion or removal because of pain or bleeding is markedly decreased. However, as many as 20 to 30 percent of users discontinue within the first year.

The IUD is inserted during menstruation to reduce discomfort, but most women experience cramping for a short time. The device should not be used if the woman is pregnant, has abnormal bleeding, or has pelvic infection in the uterus or fallopian tubes. Infection in the vagina usually does not rule out IUD use. Some physicians will not prescribe an IUD for a woman who has never given birth, primarily because of the increased pain and increased frequency of expulsion. Side effects that occur with intrauterine devices include bleeding, usually at the time of insertion. IUDs usually do not cause a change in the menstrual cycle. However, there may be occasional bleeding between periods. Most expulsions occur in the first three months after insertion.

Complications from use of the intrauterine device include perforation of the uterus and pelvic inflammatory disease. Perforation commonly occurs at the time of insertion. The likelihood of perforation depends on the skill of the inserter and the type of device. Pelvic inflammatory disease (bacte-

rial infection of the reproductive organs) occurs in about 2 percent of the users. Although most cases are mild, some can be severe enough to cause infertility.

Oral Contraceptives

Hormonal contraception ("the pill") is the most widely used form of contraception. Most hormonal contraceptive preparations consist of estrogens and progestogens, which are synthetic derivatives of estrogen and progesterone. The combinations vary. The optimum dosage for each woman is the lowest amount of each hormone that will produce the desired effect.

Pills are normally prescribed for 20, 21, or 22 days in a row. The woman takes one each day, then abstains for seven days. Pills are often packaged in reminder packets, with one for each prescribed day and vitamin or iron tablets for the "off days." During the seven days a woman is not taking the contraceptive pill, she normally has withdrawal bleeding.

Contraceptive pills act by altering the neuroendocrine system that controls the hypothalamic-pituitary-ovarian relationship, thus inhibiting ovulation. They also induce change in the reproductive tract by making the cervical mucus thick and tenacious so that it prevents sperm migration, and they affect the endometrium and tubal function in a way that is detrimental to conception. If ovulation occurs—and it can in the presence of a low-dosage pill—pregnancy rarely results because the reproductive tract is unfavorable for sperm migration and ovum transport.

The theoretical effectiveness of using the combined pill is 100 percent, with a failure rate of only 0.1 pregnancy per 100 woman-years. When patient errors are included, however, the effectiveness becomes approximately five pregnancies per 100 woman-years. The failure rates are attributed to women forgetting to take the pills regularly or discontinuing them before they institute another method of contraception.

"Morning-After" Pills

The administration of estrogens after intercourse interferes with pregnancy. The estrogens must be taken shortly after intercourse, before the fertilized egg implants in the uterine wall. Large doses of estrogen, usually in the form of diethylstilbestrol (DES), are given daily for five days, beginning within 24 to 36 hours after intercourse. Some women experience nausea, vomiting, and possible

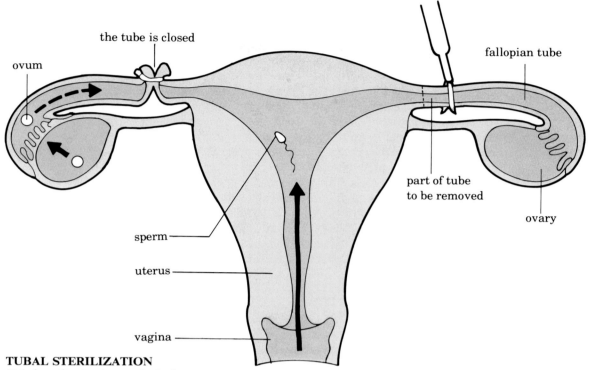

the tube is closed

ovum

fallopian tube

part of tube
to be removed

ovary

sperm

uterus

vagina

TUBAL STERILIZATION

Tubal sterilization is a method of severing or closing off the fallopian tube so that sperm and ovum cannot unite. In the laparoscopic method, shown here, two small incisions are made in the abdomen to allow insertion of the laparoscope, which is a sighting device, and an instrument to cut or cauterize the tube. A section of tube is usually removed and the ends sealed.

disturbances of the menstrual cycle. The "morning-after" administration of estrogens is considered an emergency measure, not a routine method of contraception.

STERILIZATION

Sterilization as a means of fertility control is the most popular form of contraception for couples over 35 years of age who have achieved their desired number of children. In either sex, the objective is to prevent egg and sperm from uniting by interrupting their route permanently.

Vaginal total sterilization is begun by making an incision in the vagina to the rear of the cervix and into the pelvic cavity. The fallopian tubes are viewed through the incision, then grasped and tied with sutures, and a portion is removed. In most instances, this procedure is done under general anesthesia and requires a 48-hour hospital stay.

Postpartum sterilization. Immediately after a woman has had a child, the uterus is enlarged and a postpartum tubal sterilization can be carried out quickly and easily. The procedure is usually performed through a small abdominal incision just below the navel. The incision is usually 2 to 4 centimeters (about 1½ inches) in length. The most common technique removes a portion of the fallopian tubes, after which the remaining section is closed with sutures.

Minilaparotomy is sterilization performed through a small abdominal incision in a nonpregnant woman. It is done under general or local anesthesia. An incision of 3 to 4 centimeters is made just above the pubic area. An instrument is placed in the uterus to elevate it and to view the fallopian tubes. The tubes are then closed off in the same manner as in postpartum sterilization. With local anesthesia, the woman can be discharged the same day.

Laparoscopic tubal sterilization can be done in an outpatient facility. A laparoscope is a long cylindrical instrument with a lens and a light system. It is less than ½ inch in diameter, about the size of a pencil.

The surgeon inserts a needle into the abdominal cavity through a small incision below the navel. Through this needle, carbon dioxide or nitrous oxide gas is introduced. The gas raises the abdominal wall, and allows the insertion of a sharp instrument, known as a trocar, and a cannula. The trocar is then removed and the laparoscope is inserted through the hollow cannula, allowing the surgeon to observe the abdominal organs. Frequently, a third incision is made above the pubic hairline so that another instrument can be inserted to grasp each fallopian tube separately and close it off, or occlude it. Occlusion can be accomplished by placing a tight band around each tube, or by cauterizing (burning) a midsection of each tube. The gas then is allowed to escape from the abdominal cavity, the laparoscope is removed, and the incisions are sutured.

INDUCED ABORTION

Induced abortion, the deliberate interruption of a pregnancy, can be brought about in several ways.

A low-risk pregnancy is one in which the woman is healthy and has been pregnant fewer than 12 weeks from the first day of her last menstrual period. The procedure usually requires only a short outpatient visit, and is associated with a low rate of complications or death. Abortion during this first trimester is performed under local, spinal, or general anesthesia. Local anesthesia, or paracervical block, is preferred and consists of injecting an anesthetic in each side of the cervix. Additional pain medication or a tranquilizer is sometimes administered as well.

The technique is similar to dilatation and curettage, which involves viewing of the cervix, followed by gradual dilatation through the use of dilators increasing in size. Once the cervix is dilated, a hollow cannula or tube is inserted in the uterus, and the contents of the uterus are removed through vacuum aspiration. The entire procedure takes about 15 minutes.

In some instances, the removal of the tissue is performed with special forceps and a curette.

A high-risk pregnancy is one in which a woman is in her second trimester, meaning she is between 12 and 24 weeks pregnant.

The techniques used in most instances after the 12th week involve amniocentesis. This is the act of inserting a needle through the outer wall of the abdomen into the amniotic sac, or the bag of wa-

ters (see Chapter 28, "Pregnancy and Childbirth"). A drug is then instilled that produces uterine contractions and results in a spontaneous abortion (delivery of the fetus and placenta) in 12 to 36 hours. In addition to increased risk, the disadvantage of this technique is that the woman consciously experiences the labor and expelling of the fetus. In about one in four cases, this method results in an incomplete delivery of the placenta and curettage must be performed to remove it. Another pregnancy termination technique is the use of a suppository or drug that is placed in the vagina and is absorbed through the vaginal mucosa. It, too, induces labor contractions that result in the delivery of the fetus and the placenta. The suppository method has the same disadvantages as amniocentesis, those of undergoing labor and risking incomplete abortion, which could necessitate curettage to remove the retained placenta. However, it is easier to administer.

The chance of complications for the high-risk group rises rapidly as the stage of the pregnancy advances. The immediate risks are perforation of the uterus, laceration of the cervix, or hemorrhage. Complications that occur within one week of the procedure include infection and hemorrhage. The risk of these complications is as high as 20 to 25 percent when the pregnancy is between 12 and 20 weeks and less than 5 percent for first-trimester abortions. An abortion of a pregnancy less than 12 weeks from the last menstrual period is surgically much easier, emotionally much easier, and much safer for the patient.

OPERATIONS

Operations Through the Vagina

Dilatation and curettage. Cervical dilatation and uterine curettage (D&C) is done to diagnose abnormal uterine bleeding and, in some instances, to control hemorrhage. It also is used following incomplete abortion or to obtain a tissue sample for biopsy. D&C is one of the most commonly performed gynecologic operations.

This procedure can be done under local anesthesia. The position of the uterus is identified by inserting a probe through the cervix to the uterus. Dilators are inserted into the cervical canal and gradually increased in diameter until a long-handled metal scraping instrument called a curette can be inserted into the cavity of the uterus. The curette is a rather firm instrument that has a spoon-shaped loop at one end for removing tissue.

Cervical biopsy involves taking a small amount of tissue from the cervix to confirm or rule out the possibility of cancer. The procedure usually is conducted when a woman has a positive Pap smear or when a growth or lesion can be identified. The tissue is sent to a pathologist for analysis.

Cauterization and cryosurgery. Cauterization of the cervix is performed to relieve chronic infection of the cervix or the cervical glands. Although cauterization usually is done with a hot probe or a caustic substance, it is not necessary to anesthetize the patient. After cauterization, the infected tissue degenerates and is replaced by healthy tissue. An alternative is cryosurgery, which involves freezing the tissue.

Vaginal hysterectomy. Removal of the uterus through the vagina (vaginal hysterectomy) is recommended when the uterus is associated with uterovaginal prolapse, or vaginal wall relaxation. Vaginal hysterectomies are generally reserved for benign circumstances, although some operations for cancer of the cervix can be performed safely through the vaginal canal.

The technique of removing the uterus begins with incision of the vaginal mucosa. The attachments of the uterus are then divided and sutured. Next, the bladder and the anterior wall are displaced, and an opening is made into the peritoneal cavity at a point between the uterus and the rectum. Then, the uterus is removed, the peritoneal cavity is closed, and the vaginal mucosa is closed. The procedure is done under general or regional anesthesia.

Operations Through the Abdomen

Abdominal operations can be performed through either a vertical or a transverse (side-to-side) incision in the skin. Vertical incisions usually are located in the midline and extend from the navel to slightly above the pubic hairline.

Transverse incisions usually begin in the line of skin cleavage just above the pubic hair. The transverse incision is carried through the skin, the fatty layers, and some of the coverings of the muscle. A transverse incision produces a negligible scar, which is preferred by most women, but the incision can be a disadvantage to the surgeon because it limits exposure of the organs.

Abdominal hysterectomy. Abdominal removal of the uterus is chosen over a vaginal hysterectomy if there is a questionable malignancy, if abdominal exploration is suggested, if the uterus is excessively large, if the woman has a history of inflammatory disease, if severe adhesions are suspected, or if an ovarian cyst could be malignant.

Reasons for hysterectomy include uterine myoma (fibroids), cancer of the body of the uterus, cancer of the ovary, and chronic inflammation or infection of the fallopian tubes. Ovaries are not routinely removed from young women who still have ovarian function.

Myomectomy. For women who are young and wish to bear children, myomectomy—removal of the uterine fibroids—is preferred over removal of the entire uterus. This is usually done through the abdominal route and requires incising fibroids located in the uterine wall, shelling them from the area, and repairing the uterine wall.

Salpingectomy, the removal of a fallopian tube, is performed when there is an ectopic (tubal) pregnancy (see Chapter 28, "Pregnancy and Childbirth"), when there is an infection in the fallopian tube, when the tube has become a fluid-filled sac, or combined with oophorectomy or hysterectomy.

The most common reason for removal of a fallopian tube is tubal pregnancy. If the tube is unruptured, an attempt is made to remove the pregnancy without disturbing or removing the tube. If the tube is ruptured, it is removed.

Ovarian cystectomy. In cases where there is a benign cyst of the ovary, the cyst can be shelled out of the ovary, leaving the ovarian tissue in place. Frequently, the ovary regains normal function.

Oophorectomy. A persistent tumor in the pelvis that is suspected of being ovarian in origin is a reason for oophorectomy, the abdominal removal of an ovary. It is recommended if the tumor is benign.

CHAPTER 27

CANCER OF THE BREAST

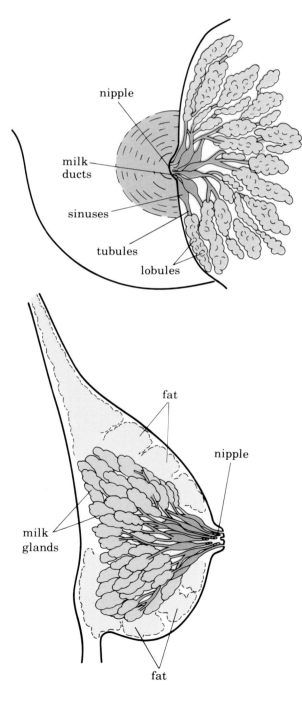

The normal breast is a complex structure of glands that respond to stimulation by various hormones, particularly in relationship to reproduction and nourishment of an infant. It originates before birth from a special bandlike thickening of tissue, extending from under the arm to the groin region. This is known as the milk line. From birth until the approach of puberty, the breast changes very little. Near the onset of puberty, the breast enlarges due to an increase in glands, ducts, and fat.

After a girl begins to menstruate, a change in the breast takes place with each period. During the premenstrual phase, the blood supply and the size of the glands increase. In the post-menstrual phase, the glands become smaller and the breast remains inactive until the next premenstrual phase.

BREAST STRUCTURES
The basic structures of the breast are shown in horizontal and vertical cross section. The lobules are clusters of microscopic sacs, or alveoli. Their milk gland cells secrete milk for breast-feeding. The alveoli empty into small ducts that form larger ducts and then connect to the 15 to 20 main ducts converging at the nipple. The vertical view shows how fibrous tissue is interspersed throughout the breast to provide support. Most breast cancers arise in the cells lining the ducts.

The breast is in its most active form during pregnancy. It visibly enlarges after the second month. The duct system develops during the first six months, and the glands develop during the last three months. This increased activity continues throughout the nursing period.

Structure

The structure of the breast is illustrated in this chapter. The gland cells are the primary component. They are arranged to form microscopic sacs called alveoli, which secrete milk for breast-feeding. The alveoli are arranged in clusters called lobules, which empty their contents into a duct or small canal. Small ducts join to form larger ducts, and eventually lead to the main ducts, of which there are about 15 to 20 converging at the nipple.

Interspersed around the glands and ducts and between the lobules is a fibrous tissue that supports the breast.

Lymphatics. Lymph vessels are channels that carry exchange fluid and by-products from cellular activity, cast-off cells, bacteria, and other matter from the body for reprocessing. The lymphatic fluid that contains this material flows into lymph nodes. The lymph nodes draining the breast are found in the axilla (underarm area), the infraclavicular and supraclavicular fossa (hollow around the collarbone), and the internal mammary region (along blood vessels beneath the breastbone).

Nonmalignant Breast Abnormalities

The breast is very responsive to hormonal changes. The hormones affect not only the glandular tissue but the fibrous tissue as well. Thus, it is not uncommon for either glandular tissue or fibrous tissue to become more prominent, producing a lump in the breast. Indeed, mammary dysplasia, also known as fibrocystic disease, is probably the most common breast abnormality.

Glandular tissue can proliferate or become cystic, producing abnormal lumps. These lumps are not malignant, and usually do not represent any threat to a woman's health. However, they often are difficult to distinguish from malignant tumors.

BREAST CANCER

The term "cancer" applies to an abnormal growth of cells that can invade surrounding tissues. These cells also have the property of being able to travel via the lymphatic fluid or blood to distant parts of the body and can start new colonies there.

Breast cancers start predominantly in the cells lining the ducts and less commonly in the cells lining the alveoli. Breast cancer spreads predominantly in three ways: local extension, lymphatics, and blood vessels.

Initially, cancer grows by local extension. As the cancer cells break through the membrane surrounding the duct or lobules, they gain access to the connective and supportive tissue of the breast. Frequently these cancer cells enter the lymphatic channels and/or the blood vessels, and are transported to the regional lymph nodes or to more distant organs of the body.

The lymph nodes most frequently involved are the underarm (axillary) nodes and, less commonly, the supraclavicular nodes above the clavicle bone or the internal mammary nodes. The pattern of spread is not wholly predictable. Sometimes the cancer seems to spread only to these nearby nodes to progress no farther. In other cases the cancer may spread to more distant sites very early in the course of the disease.

The other structural system that can be invaded directly is the blood vessels. If cancer cells grow into blood vessels, they gain access to the bloodstream, so that they can move to other parts of the body. The growth of cancer cells in a site of the body distant from the original cancer is termed "distant metastasis." When cancer is confined to its site of origin, it is spoken of as "local"; when it has spread to adjoining tissue, it is described as regional. Breast cancers also are classified as Stages I, II, or III, or as invasive or noninvasive.

There is considerable variation in the tendency for breast cancer to spread. Some cancers grow slowly and reach tremendous size without ever spreading to lymph nodes or to distant sites. On the other hand, some breast cancers, even though small, are very aggressive in their ability to spread. As a general rule, however, the smaller the breast cancer when it is discovered and treated, the less chance the cancer has to spread beyond the breast.

There is a special category of breast cancer called "in situ" or "intraductal" that is recognizable under microscope as a cancer, but the cells have not spread beyond their origins in the normal confines of the duct or lobule. Fine-screen mammography has made these tumors much more easily detected than in the past. These noninvasive cancers are highly likely to be cured by current methods of treatment.

Tests for cancer. One of the major aids in determining whether a lump is benign or malignant is a radiographic tool known as a mammogram. A mammogram is an X ray of the breast from several views, as illustrated in Chapter 2, "Tests and Procedures." The combination of physical examination with mammography can produce a high degree of accuracy in determining whether a lump is benign or malignant. However, even in the best of situations, these tools can be wrong about 10 percent of the time.

If both the physical examination and the mammogram suggest a breast cancer, a biopsy will be needed to confirm the diagnosis. This sampling of tissue usually is performed on an outpatient basis, under local anesthesia.

Sometimes the doctor may seek further information by using ultrasound, which uses reflected high-frequency sound waves to map the inside of the breast. It sometimes is used to distinguish between cystic and solid masses and thus to help identify benign or malignant tumors.

If a malignancy is confirmed, additional tests may be recommended to evaluate the possibility of distant spread. Among the more useful and frequently employed examinations are: chest X ray, serum enzyme levels (blood test), blood count, and bone scan (use of mildly radioactive materials to take pictures of bone activity). Even with all of the tests available and the use of the most accurate of techniques, the majority of distant growths can be detected only when they are fairly large (more than ½ inch in diameter).

Who Is at Risk?

A woman's risk of breast cancer normally begins in the late 20s and steadily increases through the remainder of her life. Statistically, her lifetime risk is estimated at 7 to 10 percent.

The most important factor associated with a higher risk of breast cancer is a family history of the disease, especially if a mother or sister was affected. The highest risk occurs where two or more close maternal relatives have had breast cancer. A strong family history of breast cancer also points to possible development of breast cancer at an earlier age. If maternal relatives have been affected before menopause, the risk also is increased.

Women with previously treated breast cancer are at higher risk for development of a second breast cancer in the opposite breast, especially if there is a history of bilateral cancer in their mothers and sisters.

Weaker risk factors include obesity, lack of pregnancies or pregnancies late in life, and an unusually long menstrual life. The high-fat American diet also has been implicated, but its role is controversial. Other suspected factors, such as use of estrogens or birth control pills, have not been shown to be associated with an increased risk.

Treatment

The treatment for breast cancer is determined individually. The best course in each case depends on the size and location of the cancer, whether multiple sites are involved, whether the nodes are affected, the health and age of the patient, and various clinical findings. In general, the question is whether or not the woman can be treated safely without loss of her breast. An unknown frequently is whether, or where, the cancer has spread.

The three main types of treatment are surgery, radiation, and chemotherapy. Depending upon the individual patient, these types of treatment may be used singly or in combination.

Surgery. Total mastectomy, sometimes called modified radical mastectomy, is the most common surgical procedure. Total mastectomy removes all breast tissue, but leaves undisturbed the underlying pectoral muscles. In earlier years, surgeons removed the muscles, too, as well as all the adjacent lymph nodes, a procedure known as the Halsted radical mastectomy. Repeated studies have shown that the survival rates are about the same for total or radical mastectomy so that the more drastic procedure is not considered necessary. Radical mastectomy is still performed occasionally, however, if circumstances appear to warrant it.

In total mastectomy, the lymph nodes in the armpit are dissected in a separate incision to determine whether the cancer has spread beyond regional involvement. Nodes, however, are not automatically removed as they are in the Halsted operation.

Total mastectomy with or without removal of the axillary nodes frequently is followed by a course of radiation treatment.

Another surgical procedure is called wide excision, sometimes nicknamed "lumpectomy." In this operation, the tumor itself is removed, along with bordering tissue that appears to be tumor-free. The remainder of the breast and the muscles are left intact. Often, wide excision is combined with a six- to eight-week course of radiation. Some doctors believe that wide excision should be confined to smaller tumors.

Comparative studies of women who have had wide excision, wide excision plus radiotherapy, and total mastectomy show approximately equal survival rates. However, some doctors consider current experience too brief to make a final judgment on which of these procedures is the most beneficial.

The ability of mammography to detect in-situ cancers smaller than 1 centimeter has raised the question of how or whether to treat them. The controversy was heightened when Nancy Reagan, then First Lady, was found to have a tiny in-situ cancer and opted for total mastectomy. Most doctors believe that only the growth should be removed, but others declare that total mastectomy is a 100 percent cure.

Radiation. X-ray therapy on the breast area may be performed as a primary form of treatment or as a follow-up to surgery. When the cancer is localized, very small, and of a common type (Stage I), the outcome of radiation versus surgery is about the same. Even Stage II (regionalized) cancers less than 4 centimeters in size may be treated satisfactorily with radiation only. When radiation is used following mastectomy, it is focused on the lymph node areas, and also is used for residual cancer.

Six weeks of radiation is about the normal course of treatment, whether primary or adjuvant. The dose is standard for most common presentations. Following radiation, the breast may increase in size and weight because of accumulated fluid, but after about a year becomes softer and smaller.

Chemotherapy has come to play an increasingly important role in breast cancer management. At the time of initial treatment, it is not always possible to detect all distant spread of cancer. Chemotherapy or hormone therapy, following initial treatment, aims to track down and destroy these very small distant metastases.

The question of which patients should receive adjuvant, or followup, therapy, still is debated. Most doctors agree that premenopausal women whose cancer has been detected in the nodes should undergo adjuvant therapy. Chemotherapy for these women is the more established method of treatment. The most commonly used medications are cytoxin, methotrexate, and 5-fluoracil (5-FU). The appropriate treatment is less clear for postmenopausal women with positive nodes. The possible therapies include chemotherapy with the drugs listed above or hormonal therapy using tamoxifen.

For pre- and postmenopausal women whose nodes show no involvement at the time of initial treatment, information still is preliminary. It is known that a certain percentage of the node-negative women will have a relapse, or outbreak of cancer elsewhere in the body, within five years. However, these women cannot be identified with certainty at the time of initial treatment. Thus, many of them are being treated with chemotherapy or tamoxifen, and this therapy appears to lower the relapse rate. (However, some doctors say that the costs of medication are high, the proper duration of treatment is unknown, and it is unclear which women will benefit and which will not.)

BREAST RECONSTRUCTION

For many women who have had a total mastectomy, it is possible to reconstruct a breastlike form by implanting a liquid-filled sac under the skin in the breast area. The resulting implant has the contour and feel of a normal breast. The implant may be performed at the time of the initial surgery, or at a later date. Immediate reconstruction saves performing a second operation. The question of reconstruction should be planned with the doctor before surgery.

Many women may prefer a prosthesis, an artificial breast worn inside the bra. Thanks to a wide variety of prosthetic materials, most women can achieve a natural appearance after surgery.

An operation called a subcutaneous mastectomy sometimes is performed to remove unaffected breast tissue and replace it with an implant. This procedure is not a form of cancer treatment. It may be done in a high-risk woman who has had one breast removed and hopes to reduce the risks of involvement of the other breast. Because not all tissue is removed, however, the risks are not lowered to zero.

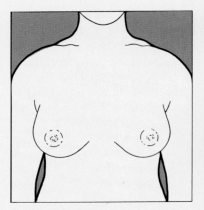 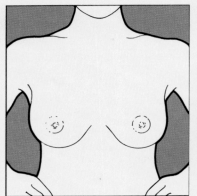 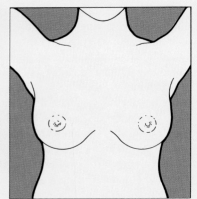

**BREAST
SELF-EXAMINATION**
Look into a mirror with both arms relaxed at your side. Compare the breasts for size, color, and position. Note any ulceration, scaling, discharge, nipple changes, skin puckering, or shrinkage.

Place your hands on your waist and press inward. Turn from side to side and note any of the changes mentioned earlier.

Place your hands behind your head, pressing firmly. Turn from side to side and again look for any changes. Relax your hands at your sides. You are now ready to feel the breasts.

YOU AND BREAST CANCER

Monthly self-examinations, as illustrated in this chapter, can detect breast cancer at early stages when there is less risk of regional or distant spread. Localized cancer is treated more easily with a higher chance of success.

When breast cancer is found, a woman always should discuss the particulars of the disease (and its spread, if any) with her physician. In addition, she should learn about and discuss the doctor's recommendations and the treatment alternatives.

You are the most important person in discovering a breast cancer. Approximately 90 percent of all breast cancers are found by women themselves. Often the discoveries are accidental, occurring when you brush your hand across the breast and touch a lump, or discover a change in breast texture while showering, or notice a dimpling of the skin of the breast while dressing. More early breast cancers are found when women regularly examine their breasts. Self-examination plus regular professional examination and mammography are the best weapons against breast cancer.

It is not difficult to understand why self-examination is so important. You can examine yourself much more frequently than a professional examiner. Most important, repeated examination allows you to become so familiar with the textures and contours of your breast that early changes quickly come to your attention.

Breast self-examination should be done with a relaxed attitude. Keep in mind that your breast normally may be somewhat lumpy. Do not become alarmed if you feel a distinct lump. Most breast lumps are benign. Many women have benign lumps that rise and subside with the menstrual cycle.

If you should discover a lump, a thickening, a dimple, a discharge, or any other change in feel or appearance, bring it to the attention of your physician for further evaluation. Even though most lumps are benign, abnormalities should be promptly evaluated. Unnecessary delay only defeats the advantages of careful self-examination.

When a physician examines your breast, he or she either will tell you that the lump is not suspicious and that you should continue with your own self-examinations and periodic clinical checks, or the doctor will consider the lump suspicious enough to perform additional tests.

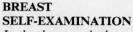

**BREAST
SELF-EXAMINATION**
*In the shower or bath, run a wet
soapy hand down one breast from
the collarbone to the nipple, feeling
for any lumps or thickening or
changes from previous examinations. Repeat the process on the
opposite breast.*

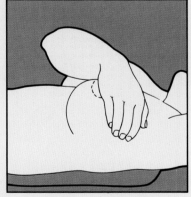

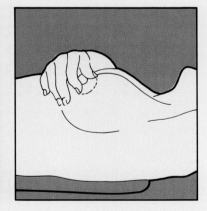

*After bathing, lie down. Place a
pillow beneath your left shoulder
and place your left hand behind
your head. Use the palm of your
right to examine the left breast.
Gently move it in a circular motion
around the entire breast. A small
amount of lotion or oil will make
your fingers more sensitive to the
feel of the breast.*

*Then, move your fingers in toward
the nipple and repeat the circular
motion. Do this until the entire
breast is covered. Notice the firm
ridge of tissue in the lower portion
of the breast.*

*Gently squeeze the nipple between
your thumb and index finger. Look
for any discharge. Gently depress
the nipple to check for a lump
beneath the nipple area. Repeat this
process on the other breast.*

CHAPTER 28

PREGNANCY AND CHILDBIRTH

The overall objective of every pregnancy is simple: a healthy mother and a healthy baby. For the mother, that means maintaining or improving her physical and emotional health, reducing complications through prompt identification and treatment, and improving standards of care for the labor and delivery process.

For children, the goals of care are reduction of mortality during birth and the early days of life, and the reduction of birth defects. A comprehensive prenatal program of medical and educational care is needed to provide the most service for mother and child.

The woman who suspects she is pregnant should schedule a visit to an obstetrician after she has missed a second menstrual period. Most doctors like to begin care when the woman is about eight weeks pregnant. By then, the symptoms of pregnancy usually are recognizable, but it still is early enough to outline a full program of care. Visits to the obstetrician after the first are commonly scheduled at one-month intervals until the woman is 32 weeks pregnant, then at two-week intervals for a month, and then weekly thereafter.

MOTHER AND CHILD
The mother and her developing fetus are closely interlocked throughout the nine months of pregnancy. The arrows show how the blood vessels of the mother's uterus carry nourishment and oxygen from her body into the placenta, then through the umbilical cord to reach the developing baby. The reverse set of arrows traces the path of the baby's wastes, which are disposed of through the mother's body. Fingerlike villi (center) help transport substances through the placenta. The so-called placental barrier helps remove substances that might harm the developing child.

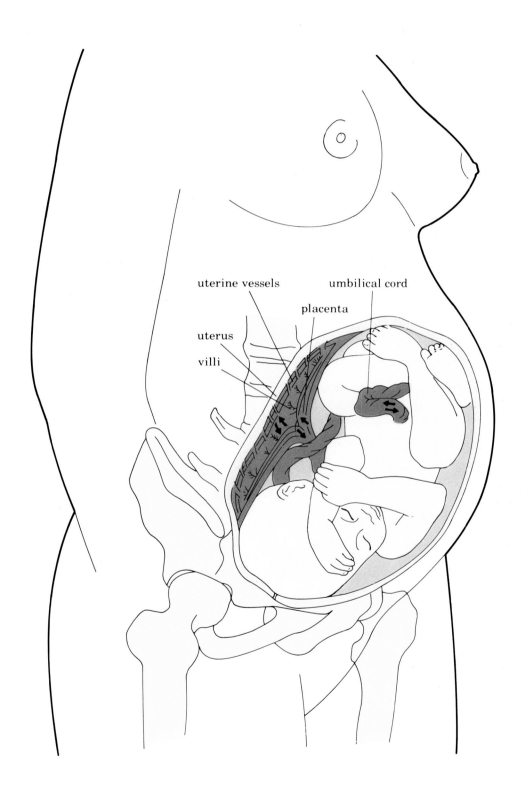

SYMPTOMS OF PREGNANCY

How does a woman know when she is pregnant? In a healthy woman who previously has menstruated regularly, a delayed period is the best indicator. Because of the usual variation in menstrual cycle length, however, this sign is not always reliable until the anticipated menstrual period is 10 to 14 days overdue. When a second period is missed, the probability becomes much stronger.

Other early signs of pregnancy include:

Nausea and vomiting. The first clue commonly is "morning sickness," which often begins in the early part of the day and subsides by afternoon. Some doctors believe that nausea results from a direct hormonal change brought about by the pregnancy; others believe that the gastrointestinal tract is affected by changes in sugar metabolism. The problem usually subsides spontaneously after 12 to 14 weeks.

Breast changes. Another early indication of pregnancy is an increase in breast size and weight. The increase is more pronounced than the increase before a regular menstrual period. The breasts may become tender, and the glands around the nipple area may enlarge. The pink-brown area around the nipple (the areola) also darkens.

Fatigue. Many women find that they tire easily and lack pep during very early pregnancy. The decreased energy levels may be related to increased circulating levels of progesterone, a hormone produced by the placenta.

Urinary disturbances. Direct pressure from an enlarging uterus and congestion of the blood vessels within the pelvis create an almost constant sensation of bladder fullness and lead to frequent urination, even in the middle of the night. This symptom, too, usually subsides after four to five months, but may recur near term.

Physical findings. A physician usually can diagnose pregnancy two to three weeks after the first missed menstrual period by physical signs alone.

Enlargement of the uterus is detectable as early as six weeks in a woman pregnant for the first time, and usually no later than eight weeks in women who have had previous pregnancies.

In the past, the detection of fetal heart tones was a relatively late physical finding. Today, small ultrasonic stethoscopes called Doppler units detect the heart tones much earlier. These battery-powered devices beam high-frequency sound waves into the uterus and trace their echoes. They pick up heart tones as early as nine or 10 weeks.

Pregnancy Tests

Unless a woman needs to know definitely and early, for job or other reasons, a pregnancy test is not absolutely necessary. Testing today is swift, accurate, and inexpensive, however, and can even be conducted, relatively reliably, at home.

Hormonal tests. Most of the new urinary pregnancy tests are designed to detect human chorionic gonadotropin (HCG) in a sample of morning urine. HCG is a hormone secreted by placental tissue that rapidly enters the mother's circulation after conception. The individual test methods vary in their sensitivity. Almost all of the tests will detect a pregnancy 10 to 14 days after the missed menstrual period, and a few are capable of doing so even before a period has been missed. Most home pregnancy tests use a dipstick that turns color in the presence of HCG. They are considered less sensitive than lab tests.

Regardless of the type of test, the first morning sample of urine is preferable because it usually is more concentrated. The concentration can be enhanced by minimizing fluids the night before.

Blood tests. A test using a blood sample rather than a urine sample measures even the most minute concentrations of HCG. This analysis, called a beta subunit HCG determination, detects pregnancy just a few days after conception. It is especially useful in suspected cases of ectopic pregnancy (pregnancy outside the uterus), medical complications, or unwanted pregnancy.

Ultrasound. Diagnostic ultrasound involves transmitting low-energy, high-frequency sound waves into the patient's abdomen and displaying the returned echoes as a two-dimensional image on a television screen. Ultrasound also may be used intermittently during pregnancy to monitor fetal development.

The echoes from the amniotic sac form a distinctive circle or ring that can be seen as early as four to five weeks after the last menstrual period or two to three weeks after conception. Echoes representing the fetus can be seen at six weeks.

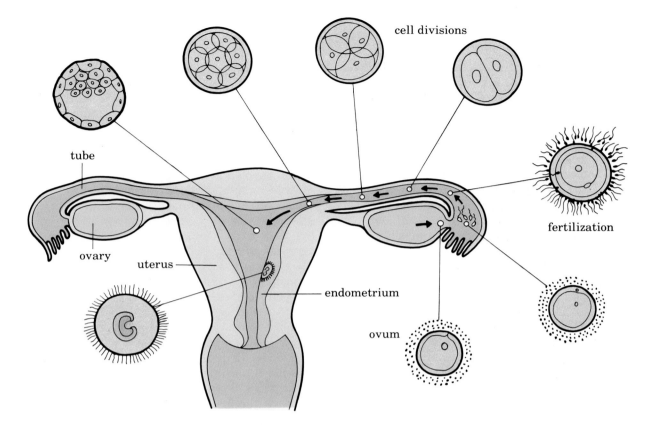

cell divisions

tube

ovary

uterus

endometrium

ovum

fertilization

FERTILIZATION AND IMPLANTATION

The sequence of ovulation, fertilization, and implantation of the fertilized egg is a multistep process. It begins when the ovary releases a ripened ovum (egg) from its follicle. If the ovum encounters spermatozoa in the fimbrial end of the tube, fertilization occurs. The male and female cells unite into a single cell, *which then undergoes a series of divisions during a three- or four-day descent down the tube. The cell cluster, now called a morula, then floats free in the uterine cavity for several days before it embeds itself in the endometrium, the lining of the uterus, which nourishes it.*

PHYSICAL CHANGES
IN PREGNANCY

Changes in the uterus. The most dramatic physical changes in pregnancy involve the uterus. The weight of uterine muscle increases tenfold, and the capacity of the uterine cavity increases more than 500-fold. The enlargement is possible because muscle fibers become longer and thinner, and numerous new muscle fibers are formed. Supporting ligaments are stretched significantly as the organ expands.

The blood flow to the uterus increases, too. To accommodate the growing demands, the blood flow must increase from one-half ounce per minute in early pregnancy to more than one pint per minute when birth is near.

Cervical changes. Changes in the cervix accompany those of the uterus. As the pregnancy advances, the muscle fibers of the cervix are stretched up into the lower portion of the body of the uterus. This makes the cervix shorter and thinner in preparation for labor. The cervix also rolls

Fetal Development

If you could peer inside the uterus a month after conception, you would hardly believe that the tiny bit of tissue before your eyes could grow into a breathing, squalling baby. The diminutive figure measures only ¼ inch long—less than the length of a newborn's fingernail—and weighs perhaps 1/100 of an ounce. You would see no human face, no arms, no legs—just a small rudimentary tail.

Yet the most complex and vital organs already are forming. The month-old fetus has a microscopic brain, a threadlike spinal cord, and a crude nervous system. A U-shaped tube two millimeters long forms the heart and is pumping blood through primitive arteries. Another tube leading from the mouth is a rudimentary digestive tract, and a bulge midway in its length marks the spot where the stomach will develop.

A month later, there is no mistaking the human characteristics. Eyes, a nose, mouth, and ears give it a decidedly human countenance. Arms and legs have developed, complete with fingers, toes, elbows, and knees. Sex organs have become apparent, although it is still difficult to distinguish male from female. And the fetus has grown. It now measures a full inch from head to heel and weighs 1/30 of an ounce.

At the end of the third month, the baby is three inches long and weighs a full ounce. Fingernails and toenails show, and the buds of baby teeth appear in the jawbone. An observer can detect the presence or absence of a uterus. A rudimentary kidney excretes waste into the amniotic fluid. The fetus moves, but too slightly for the mother to feel.

At four months, nearly all vital organs are formed, yet the fetus is not ready to live alone. It is now about 6½ inches long and weighs about four ounces. Fine hair covers the body, and a few hairs appear on the head. More active now, the baby wiggles tiny arms and legs. Using an amplified stethoscope, the doctor can hear the fetal heartbeat—a rapid 140 beats per minute, faster than that of the mother.

By five months, the fetus has developed hair, eyebrows and lashes, and even facial expressions. The father can hear the fetal heartbeat by placing an ear against the mother's abdomen. And the fetus now moves vigorously and frequently; the mother can "feel life." The baby is now nearly a foot long and weighs almost a pound and a half.

At six months, the fetus is 15 inches long, weighs two and a half pounds, and is growing rapidly. For the first time, the fetus looks like a miniature human being. The skin is covered with fuzz and a creamy substance called vernix caseosa ("cheesy varnish"), a ⅛-inch-thick layer that protects the skin from the fluid environment.

At seven months, the fetus is 16½ inches long and weighs four pounds. Development now is mainly a process of fine-tuning, getting ready for independent existence. The intricate biochemistry governing many bodily functions begins to evolve; production starts on the body's 20,000 enzymes. The nerve cells mature and the fetus fattens.

During the last two months, the fetus gains a half pound per week, accumulating layers of fat to increase its ability to survive in the outside world. At eight months, the fetus weighs six pounds; at full term, it weighs seven and a half pounds.

The last organs to be fine-tuned are the lungs. Even though the child appears fully mature, the respiratory system is not ready. The lungs cannot function until acted upon by chemicals that are among the last to be produced. Some doctors believe normal birth can begin only when the fetal respiratory system has completed this maturation.

Prior to the end of the seventh month, an infant has only an outside chance to survive if born prematurely. The chances increase with each additional day or week in the womb. Despite an old belief that a seven-month-old baby has a better chance to live than an eight-month-old baby, no evidence confirms that notion. However, at eight months, the chances of survival are nearly as good as if the baby had completed the full term of pregnancy.

out and softens, becomes pliable, and sometimes bleeds on contact. Mucous glands are stimulated by the hormonal influence of the pregnancy and often give rise to an excessive vaginal discharge.

Skin. Increased hormone levels cause darkening of the nipples and genitalia, and "stretch marks" (stria) on the skin of the abdomen. Skin conditions such as acne often improve.

Metabolic changes and weight gain. The average woman gains 24 pounds during the nine-month period. Of this amount, 19 pounds are accounted for by the pregnancy itself: the fetus, about 7½ pounds; the placenta, 1 pound; the amniotic fluid, 2 pounds; added weight of uterus, 2½ pounds; increased weight of breasts, 2 pounds; and increased blood volume, 4 pounds. The rest of the weight represents accumulated fats and fluids retained by the body but that normally will be lost after birth. It is important that the woman gain at least this amount, because restricting weight gain can result in a baby of low birth weight, which poses a greater risk of complications. Gains of up to 35 pounds are considered normal.

Hormonal changes of pregnancy produce dramatic changes in water metabolism. This means that the woman's tissues retain more water. The functional capacity of the kidneys appears to increase during pregnancy, primarily because of an increase in the rate of blood flow.

Protein metabolism is changed to allow an accumulation of amino acids, the building blocks for fetal growth and development. (Increased protein requirements in pregnancy and lactation are discussed in Chapter 21, "Nutrition.")

Carbohydrate and insulin metabolism. Some women develop diabetes during the course of pregnancy, known as gestational diabetes, then revert to a normal state of sugar tolerance after the delivery. For patients already known to be diabetic, the additional stress of pregnancy requires stringent dietary control as well as an increase in the daily dosage of insulin. Gestational diabetes is discussed in Chapter 19, "Diabetes Mellitus."

Cardiovascular system. Although the volume of the heart enlarges only 10 percent during pregnancy, the heart pumps as much as 40 percent more blood than in a nonpregnant woman. Each stroke of the heart pushes out more blood, and the heart rate itself increases. These changes are necessary to supply the increasing demands of the growing fetus.

Respiration. The total capacity of the lungs is not significantly changed by pregnancy, but the rising diaphragm, pushed upward by the expanding uterus, can squeeze the lungs. Consequently, the mother feels short of breath, especially during the eighth month. The condition ordinarily subsides in the last few days before delivery.

Gastrointestinal tract. Besides the nausea and vomiting of early pregnancy, the stomach and intestines are significantly compressed by the enlarging uterus. Constipation is common, as the movement of food through the gastrointestinal tract slows. Reflux of the stomach acid into the esophagus often causes heartburn.

Musculoskeletal system. The increased weight of the pregnancy tends to shift the center of gravity forward. The curve of the spine compensates to shift the weight back, causing a characteristic swayback stance. These changes can produce discomforts ranging from dull aches to sharp pains in the back, pelvis, and legs.

Emotions. Mild emotional upsets are common in pregnancy and should be understood as a part of adaptation to motherhood. It must be remembered that the father is by no means immune to the emotional impact.

COMMON PROBLEMS IN PREGNANCY

Because pregnancy is not an illness, the overwhelming majority of women carry on with their normal lives virtually throughout the nine-month period. Most, however, have minor discomforts and complaints.

"Morning sickness." Nausea and vomiting, often the first clues that a woman is pregnant, may persist in mild form throughout the early part of pregnancy. The symptoms usually can be controlled by minor changes in diet. Dried fruit or crackers, particularly in the morning, help to coat the stomach. It may help to eat six or seven small meals rather than three large ones. A hurried schedule or emotional pressure can increase nausea, and "taking things easy" sometimes calms the queasiness. If nausea and vomiting are severe or become so frequent that no food is retained, the physician should be informed.

Constipation, common in early pregnancy, usually can be corrected by drinking plenty of fluids. Bran cereals also are helpful. Mild laxatives will not harm the fetus in any way.

Heartburn, a hot aching sensation just below the breastbone, is common during later pregnancy, as stomach acids back up and irritate the sensitive lining of the lower esophagus. Highly seasoned foods accentuate the problem, as do late-night dinners, because acid refluxes more easily when a woman is lying down. Milk or over-the-counter antacids usually are helpful. Using pillows to elevate the head also helps.

Gas. Gas production in the bowels increases during pregnancy, often resulting in excessive belching or passage of gas. Foods such as baked beans, chili, cabbage, and cauliflower are best avoided during later pregnancy.

Diarrhea also results from bowel changes associated with pregnancy. The problem usually subsides spontaneously. During episodes of diarrhea, liquids or bland foods are advisable. If the problem persists, over-the-counter preparations of kaolin-pectin may be used safely.

Hemorrhoids, large swollen veins that emerge around the anus and cause considerable discomfort, stem from the increased back pressure created by the large pregnant uterus. They can be aggravated by constipation. The discomfort usually can be relieved by topical preparations.

Fatigue. Especially in early pregnancy, a woman is likely to tire easily and feel sleepy. She is not able to tolerate as much exercise as before pregnancy. Her need for more rest should be taken into account when planning recreation or work.

Backache. In the early months, backache is likely to be related to stretching of the ligaments that support the uterus. In later months, it often results from the stress on the spine by the enlarging abdomen.

Most pregnant women prefer firm, straight chairs. A firm mattress provides sleeping support.

Simple exercises of abdominal and back muscles help decrease back pain. Hot baths and aspirin also are helpful.

Light-headedness. Episodes of light-headedness or even fainting result from hormone-induced relaxation of the blood vessels, which then become less responsive to changes in posture.

A pregnant woman should rise from bed gradually and use caution in getting up abruptly from a chair. Pregnant women are particularly prone to faint after emerging from a whirlpool, sauna, or very hot tub bath. Exposures to high heat conditions should be restricted.

Insomnia. Anxiety, combined with physical discomforts, may make it difficult for a pregnant woman to fall asleep. Avoiding late-night meals, exercising daily, and reassurance from her family or physician sometimes are all that is needed. A glass of milk before retiring sometimes is helpful.

Varicose veins. The pregnant uterus may significantly impair the return blood flow from the legs toward the heart, causing the superficial veins in the legs or groin to swell. Some women also develop pain and tenderness in these vessels, a condition called varicose veins (see Chapter 6, "Blood Vessel Disorders").

Varicose veins seldom are a problem in a first pregnancy, but the risk increases as subsequent pregnancies further weaken the vein walls. The tendency appears to be inherited. Sufficient bed rest and sitting with the legs elevated are the most important precautions. A woman who must be on her feet should wear support stockings.

If a vein becomes tender, swollen, or inflamed, or if severe pain develops, the physician should be informed immediately. Inflammation of the vein (phlebitis) must be treated promptly.

Varicose veins usually subside six to eight weeks after delivery. Surgery rarely is necessary during pregnancy.

Vaginitis. Inflammation of the vagina and external genitalia is somewhat more common during pregnancy because of altered hormonal balance. Although monilia or yeast infection is the most common type of vaginitis, the physician should be consulted for a proper diagnosis and treatment. Most vaginitis is easily correctable.

PERSONAL CARE
AND HYGIENE

Nutrition. For each fetus, there is a genetically determined ideal weight that can be achieved only if the mother consumes adequate protein and calories in her diet during pregnancy. This is especially important for the woman who enters pregnancy at less than her ideal body weight, the woman who has poor nutritional status, or the woman who gains weight inadequately during pregnancy. In addition to adequate protein and caloric intake, certain vitamins and minerals must be increased during pregnancy. The most notable are iron and folic acid, which, in addition to dietary sources, can be obtained in capsule form or are included in certain multivitamin preparations.

In the woman whose prepregnancy diet is adequate, the additional requirements of pregnancy can be completely met by the addition of one quart of milk per day to the diet. A balanced diet that includes citrus fruit or orange juice, eggs, meat, fish, bread, vegetables, and potatoes in addition to eight ounces of milk at each meal should ensure adequate nutrients for both the mother and the developing child.

A recommended diet for pregnant women is shown in Chapter 21, "Nutrition."

A woman's pattern of weight gain is a good indicator of her nutritional status. She should gain about 10 pounds during the first 20 weeks, then three-quarters of a pound to a pound each week thereafter. The gain should be steady, as shown in the illustrations in this chapter. Women who gain at a substantially lower rate face an increased risk of problems with fetal development, as do those who gain considerably more rapidly.

Strictly vegetarian diets that exclude dairy products, or fad diets that markedly restrict essential nutrients (such as protein, iron, or certain vitamins or minerals), are hazardous during pregnancy.

Women who are planning to breast-feed require a weight gain of four to seven pounds more than the recommended average gain of 24 pounds. This extra weight is for fat stores that help the initiation and maintenance of lactation.

Prepared Childbirth

A variety of childbirth preparation classes are provided in almost every community. Although several formats are offered—Lamaze, Bradley, Childbirth Education Association (CEA), and Leboyer—the factual content of most parent education programs is similar. The differences are philosophical.

Most obstetricians strongly advise that both parents take these classes to prepare for labor and delivery. They are offered as part of the hospital's prenatal service, or by a local Y, by adult education centers, or by community colleges. There usually are six classes, beginning about the seventh month of pregnancy. The classes are taught in groups of 20 by a trained childbirth education instructor.

Classes usually include information on pregnancy, labor and delivery, the postpartum period, and introduction to parenting. Most classes stress an understanding of the physical and hormonal changes of pregnancy, body conditioning exercises, relaxation and breathing techniques, birth mechanisms, and the role of support personnel in the delivery process. Information is provided on the stages of labor, medications, and potential complications of childbirth.

Initially, the goal of childbirth education was to minimize the pain associated with labor and delivery. Today, however, childbirth education also seeks to improve the quality of the childbearing experience.

MOTHER'S WEIGHT GAIN

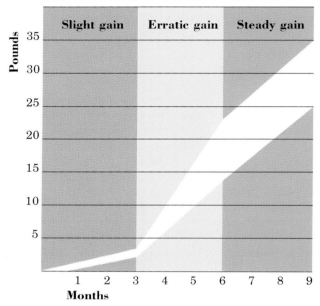

WEIGHT GAIN

The pregnant woman should gain at least 25 pounds during pregnancy, but the rate of gain is more important than the amount. As the bottom line of the chart shows, she should gain about 10 pounds during the first 20 weeks, then about three-quarters of a pound a week until delivery. Women who gain at a lower or high rate run a higher risk of birth complications. A sudden spurt in weight is a danger signal, indicating that the body is retaining fluid.

Exercise. Regular exercise is important in pregnancy. Many women choose daily routine calisthenics. Walking, swimming, golf, and tennis provide equally good exercise, as long as all are carried out in moderation. About an hour a day of exercise is desirable.

Pregnancy exerts an adverse influence on neuromuscular coordination, so sports requiring a high degree of reflex coordination, such as waterskiing, snow skiing, diving, and ice skating, should be avoided or restricted. Aerobic exercises are fine for women who performed them before pregnancy, but probably should be tempered in duration and vigor in late pregnancy.

Travel. Travel, including air travel, has almost no detrimental effect on pregnancy. The only major drawback is the tendency for blood to pool in the lower extremities during prolonged sitting. A pregnant woman should stop or get up to stretch every one to two hours.

In the last few weeks of pregnancy, long trips should be avoided, if possible, because an early labor might find the woman in unfamiliar surroundings or without access to obstetrical care.

Many women continue to drive an automobile virtually throughout pregnancy, and there is no reason not to do so if it can be done comfortably.

Smoking during pregnancy has harmful effects. Infants born to smoking mothers are significantly smaller than those born to nonsmokers, and the reduction in average birth weight appears to be directly proportional to the number of cigarettes smoked per day. The long-term effect on the child still is under study.

Alcohol. In recent years, the damaging effects of maternal drinking on the fetus (fetal alcohol syndrome) have been recognized and widely publicized. Infants born to mothers who drink regularly (two or more drinks per day) have an increased chance for mental and motor retardation. The severity of the fetal alcohol syndrome appears to be directly proportional to the amount of alcohol consumed. However, there appears to be little harm to either mother or fetus in an occasional drink or glass of wine.

Medications. Most obstetricians try to limit medications given a mother, but feel that those necessary for health or comfort can be used without adverse fetal effects. There is no reason for a woman to deny herself two aspirin when she has a severe headache, nor refrain from the use of antihistamines for a severe cold. Obviously, it is advisable that the patient discuss any and all of these medications with her physician and abide by her physician's recommendations.

NORMAL BIRTH
At the end of "transition" labor, the baby's head emerges from the birth canal, gently assisted by the obstetrician's hands. Most babies are born facing toward the floor. The obstetrician will rotate the baby's head slightly to ease the passage of the shoulders through the opening.

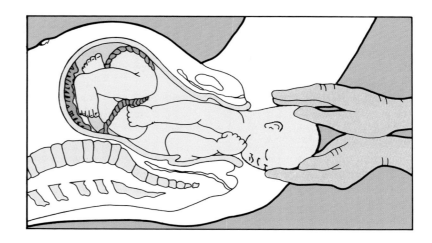

LABOR AND DELIVERY

The average length of a normal pregnancy is between 38 and 42 weeks (from the first day of the last normal menstrual period).

There are three possible indications that labor is approaching. Not all women experience all three, although some experience them without being aware of it. They can appear in any sequence.

Contractions of the uterus. Irregular, infrequent tightenings of the uterine muscle generally increase in frequency and duration as term approaches and often are mistaken for early labor. These contractions are relatively painless and sometimes are experienced as backache or merely increased pressure.

As labor begins, contractions are felt more intensely and may occur at regular intervals. The first sensation may be a mild backache, followed by a slight abdominal cramp. Initial contractions usually last for 10 to 20 seconds and come 20 to 30 minutes apart. The interval gradually narrows, and the duration and intensity increase.

The onset of contractions may dislodge the plug of mucus that has closed off the uterus during pregnancy. There is a scant amount of bleeding, often so slight that it goes unnoticed. This phenomenon is called "show." Labor may begin shortly afterward.

About 10 percent of women experience premature rupture of the amniotic membranes. This means that the "bag of waters" surrounding the baby has broken before the start of active labor. Depending on the size and location of the break, there may be a gush or a trickle of fluid from the vagina. In most women near term, labor can be expected to begin within 24 hours.

Although all three signs are considered normal, any heavy bleeding or leakage of any large quantity of fluid through the vagina should be reported immediately to the physician. Most patients are asked to come to the hospital when there has been any significant bleeding, leakage of fluid, or regular contractions at intervals of five minutes or less.

Labor Progress

Labor is the start of regular contractions of the uterus that produce a change in the cervix. For the woman having her first child, active labor can range from six to 14 hours or more. For subsequent pregnancies, however, labor generally is shorter, ranging from three to 10 hours. Prolonged labor can be detrimental to both mother and child. On the other hand, labors lasting only one to two hours are equally undesirable and are associated with a higher incidence of fetal distress.

Labor Assessment

When a woman arrives at the hospital or clinic in suspected labor, a general physical examination is performed. The medical team's first step is an abdominal and pelvic examination to assess the progress of the labor. The following is what the medical team looks for.

Presentation. The doctor or nurse must determine whether the baby is arriving headfirst or bottom first. Rarely, the fetus tries to deliver shoulder first, face first, or brow first. Labor then may be obstructed.

Dilation refers to the diameter of the opening of the cervix. The size is recorded in centimeters ranging from 0 to 10 (0 to 4 inches). Because the average fetal head measures 9.5 centimeters in diameter at term, the opening must dilate to 10 centimeters to allow for easy passage. The first few centimeters of dilation usually require more time than the last several centimeters.

Effacement. Before labor, the cervix measures more than an inch in length and is said to be uneffaced. Before labor or during the early phase of active labor, the cervix continues to thin out and shorten, a process called effacement. The cervix that is completely effaced may range from several millimeters in thickness to the thickness of tissue paper. The position of the cervix in the pelvis and its general consistency also are important. Obviously, a softened cervix will efface and dilate more rapidly than a firm one.

Station is the term used to designate how far the fetal head has descended within the pelvis. A pair of bony landmarks called the ischial spines represent the plane of the midpelvis. When the leading part of the baby's head has reached the midpelvis, the patient is said to be at station zero. This means that the widest portion of the baby's head has successfully negotiated the inlet to the pelvis. Further descent is referred to as plus centimeters. Station plus 3 or plus 4 means that the head is visible in the vagina and the baby is ready for imminent delivery.

Position. Even if the baby appears headfirst, the doctor or nurse usually determines whether the baby is facing forward or backward because this is directly related to successful progress in labor.

In some instances, it is not possible in the preliminary examination to determine whether active labor is under way. If the labor is false, the woman may be discharged, often with a mild sedative to help her rest.

In cases of active labor, the woman generally is transferred to a private labor room with a trained obstetrical nurse or resident physician in attendance. An external or internal electronic fetal monitor, described below, often is attached to follow the progress of labor.

Stages of Labor

Labor commonly is classified into three and sometimes four stages, although in fact they are a continuous series of events.

The first stage begins with dilation of the cervix and ends when it has become fully dilated. This is the longest stage of labor. For women having their first baby, labor often proceeds no more rapidly than a centimeter of dilation per hour. In subsequent pregnancies, the cervix usually dilates faster.

During the first stage, the intensity of contractions gradually increases. Under this pressure, the membranes containing the amniotic fluid may rupture. If they do not, the doctor may suggest rupturing them artificially in hopes of accelerating the delivery.

The second stage begins with full or complete dilation of the cervix and ends with delivery of the infant. For first pregnancies, this stage requires from 30 minutes to two hours; for subsequent pregnancies, a few minutes to an hour. During this time, the baby's head must travel another three to five centimeters to pass through the birth canal. If difficulty occurs during descent, the doctor may have to intervene, either through use of forceps or by cesarean section.

The third stage of labor begins with the birth of the infant and ends with the delivery of the placenta or afterbirth. The placenta usually is passed spontaneously within several minutes of delivery. If the placenta is retained a half hour or more, the obstetrician may need to remove it under a brief general anesthetic.

Fourth stage. The first hour after delivery is regarded by some to be a "fourth stage of labor." Vital signs, especially the blood pressure, must be recorded frequently and the amount of bleeding must be carefully recorded. One of the most common problems encountered during this time is atony, or relaxation of the uterus, which may bring on increased bleeding. The doctor or nurse can massage the uterus through the abdomen or give hormonal medications.

Delivery

A woman who previously has borne children is taken to the delivery room at or before full dilation of the cervix according to how fast her labor is progressing. Most first-time mothers remain in the labor room until the baby's head is visible at the entrance of the vagina.

Most mothers are placed on their backs on the delivery table, with the legs in metal stirrups for support. This position allows the greatest flexibility for the obstetrician to assist delivery. The genital area is cleansed with a local antiseptic, and the legs, abdomen, and buttocks are covered with sterile drapes.

When delivery is imminent, most women will benefit from an episiotomy. This is an incision in the outer part of the vagina extending toward the anus. It allows more room for an easy delivery. In addition to reducing pressure on the fetal head, episiotomy helps prevent stretching and tearing of the muscles. It also decreases the incidence of bowel and bladder problems caused by lack of vaginal support in later life.

At birth, most babies arrive facing rearward. As the head emerges, the mother often is asked to refrain from pushing or to pant like a puppy to allow greater control of the delivery process. The head usually rotates left or right as the shoulders make their way through the maternal pelvis. A gush of amniotic fluid or blood then occurs. Infants who are born facing forward may require assisted rotation with use of forceps.

After the delivery, the newborn's nose and mouth are gently suctioned and the baby is dried briskly with gauze sponges or cloth towels. If there is no difficulty, the infant can be placed on the mother's abdomen while the cord is clamped and cut. The infant then is swaddled in warm blankets and cradled in the mother's arms or placed nude in an infant warmer beside the delivery table.

The newborn infant must have a thorough physical examination. The eyes, ears, nose, palate, heart, lungs, and abdomen are carefully examined. Birth defects are sought and ruled out. A tube is passed into the stomach, and the rectum is checked to assure that the gastrointestinal tract is open. Commonly, a blood sample is taken from the umbilical cord.

The infant is weighed, and the length and head circumference are measured. Silver nitrate or an antibiotic is applied to the baby's eyes to prevent infection.

ELECTRONIC FETAL MONITORING

Although the overwhelming majority of infants today are delivered safely and without handicap, the first and second stages of labor represent the most hazardous period in a person's entire life. Close surveillance during labor and delivery is essential to the delivery of a healthy baby. That surveillance is now carried out electronically in most hospitals.

Electronic fetal monitoring provides continuous and instantaneous display of the fetal heartbeat and measures each interval from one fetal heartbeat to the next. The electronic fetal monitor also provides a graphic display of uterine contractions. All are important indicators of the baby's health. There are two simple methods of electronic fetal monitoring. Two belts are placed over the mother's abdomen to record fetal heart rate and uterine contractions. When labor is well established after rupture of membranes, a tiny lead can be applied directly to the fetal scalp, and a small plastic tube is inserted past the cervix to measure the duration and intensity of uterine contractions. Although the belt method is cumbersome and imposes certain restrictions on the mother's movement, neither method carries any significant risk or discomfort to the mother or baby.

Fetal scalp sampling. The direct sampling of blood from the fetal scalp allows the concentration of oxygen and carbon dioxide to be measured directly. Oxygen lack also causes a buildup of acid in the fetal bloodstream, detectable by a fetal scalp blood sample.

COMPLICATIONS OF LABOR AND DELIVERY

Induction of labor. In certain high-risk obstetrical conditions, it may be necessary or desirable to deliver the infant before labor starts spontaneously. Labor is induced by artificially rupturing the membranes, by inserting a small plastic instrument through the vagina and cervix. This can be done without discomfort to the mother or jeopardy to the infant. Near term, this procedure alone can bring on labor in 70 to 80 percent of patients.

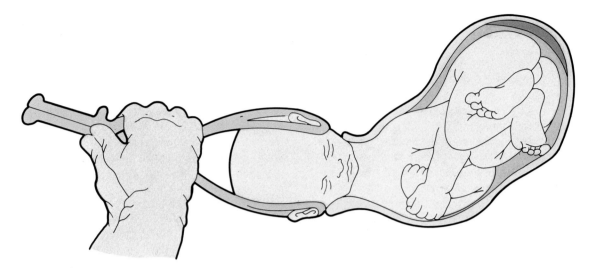

FORCEPS DELIVERY
Metal instruments called obstetrical forceps sometimes are used to deliver the baby's head without injuring the baby or mother. Various types of forceps are used for different problems of *delivery, but all consist of two curved blades that are inserted separately, then joined by a lock. In practice, the forceps delivery usually is performed with the baby facing the floor.*

Another method of induction involves the use of oxytocin, a pituitary hormone that stimulates the uterus to contract in rhythmic fashion. Small amounts of oxytocin can be administered by a controlled intravenous drip into a vein. When properly administered and monitored, oxytocin-induced labor carries little additional risk over that of spontaneous or natural labor.

Arrest of labor. Infrequently, labor progress stops during the active phase of cervical dilation. This occurs because the baby's head is too large for the size of the pelvis. X-ray measurements of the bony pelvis sometimes are necessary. If no disproportion is shown, the doctor can augment the labor by rupturing the membranes or by stimulating the uterus with oxytocin. If these methods are not effective, cesarean delivery may be necessary.

Rh sensitization. RH disease (erythroblastosis fetalis) is a condition caused by breakdown and destruction of fetal red blood cells by antibodies from the mother. The condition occurs only in Rh-negative women who bear Rh-positive infants and is described in Chapter 7, "The Blood."

Breech delivery. In about 4 percent of deliveries, the infant appears buttocks first, a so-called breech delivery. The incidence is higher in premature births.

Breech vaginal delivery carries increased risk factors for mother and infant. In the frank breech configuration, the baby's legs are extended and the feet are tucked up beside the ears. This position is most favorable for vaginal delivery. In a complete breech position, the knees are flexed and the infant is literally sitting with feet over the cervix. The incomplete breech position refers to the appearance of one or both feet at the entrance to the vagina, with the buttocks high above the pelvis. The infant is literally standing up. This presents the highest risk for vaginal delivery because of the increased opportunity for kinking the umbilical cord and the decreased effectiveness of a foot or leg in dilating the cervical opening.

The time of labor in breech presentations ordinarily is longer than in a headfirst delivery. General obstetrical practice is to leave the membranes intact as long as possible to dilate the cervix more effectively. Once the cervix is fully dilated, the second stage is prolonged in an effort to bring the buttocks down.

As the buttocks emerge from the vagina, an episiotomy is performed. Then the obstetrician gently guides the delivery of the shoulders. Delivery of the head is accomplished manually or by using special forceps designed for the purpose.

Forceps delivery. When the position of the baby or ineffective labor makes spontaneous delivery difficult, the doctor uses curved stainless steel instruments called forceps to assist. Most forceps have a cup-shaped blade to precisely fit the head's contours, and are shaped to traverse the mother's pelvis safely. A skilled obstetrician often can bring about delivery in difficult cases with greater ease and safety than a spontaneous birth.

A number of different types of forceps are used. Special forceps assist the baby from the outlet when the mother is too tired to push. Others are designed for application in midpelvis and are especially helpful in rotating a fetus who is in poor position for delivery. Forceps are particularly useful if there is fetal heart rate distress, massive bleeding, or meconium (green stool) staining.

When the second stage of labor is progressing poorly, most obstetricians consider using forceps. If the instruments cannot be applied easily or there is difficulty in extracting the fetal head, the procedure is abandoned and cesarean delivery is selected as the safer alternative.

Forceps deliveries generally are classified into low- and mid-forceps procedures. Low forceps are used when the leading part of the baby's head is visible at the vaginal opening. The most common reason for their use is maternal fatigue. Low forceps also are useful in achieving better control over a delivery, and routinely are used in the delivery of premature infants.

Mid forceps most commonly are used to rotate the fetal head to a normal position for delivery. If the baby's head is turned, it may fail to descend properly through the mother's pelvis, and delivery is obstructed.

Cesarean section. Delivery by cesarean section is far more common today than in the past. In some hospitals, cesarean births account for 20 to 25 percent of all deliveries. Repeat cesarean deliveries make up much of this total. In a first labor, the most common reason for cesarean delivery is cephalopelvic disproportion, which means that the infant is too large or the pelvis is too small for a safe vaginal delivery. Although measurement of the maternal pelvis usually is carried out in early pregnancy, it often is impossible to confirm cephalopelvic disproportion until a trial of labor ends in a failure of labor to progress. The second most

common reason for cesarean birth is fetal distress. However, the reasons for cesarean delivery are relative rather than absolute. Many hospitals require a second opinion before a first cesarean delivery is performed.

The operation is performed by incising the skin and fatty tissue, then the fascia or tough connective tissue. The lining of the abdominal cavity (peritoneum) is entered, and the uterus is exposed. The skin incision is made vertically from a point below the navel to a point just above the pubic bone, or a slightly curved incision is made from side to side just above the pubic hairline.

The lining of the uterus is incised crosswise in the lower part of the uterus just above the bladder. The bladder is pushed downward to avoid injury. An incision is made in the muscular wall of the uterus just above the bladder and extended from side to side. After the bag of waters has been ruptured, the infant is carefully delivered by hand or by forceps through the incision. The placenta is removed manually, and the uterus is closed by a locking suture in either two or three layers.

Most patients experience significant abdominal discomfort after the procedure, but pain usually can be controlled with medications the first few days. The usual hospital stay is four to five days.

Although the risk of cesarean delivery increases slightly with each procedure, there is no limit to the number a woman can undergo.

PREGNANCY
COMPLICATIONS

Miscarriage. Between 10 and 15 percent of all pregnancies end in miscarriage. The majority occur early, sometimes before the woman is even aware she is pregnant. However, loss of pregnancy can occur at any time in the second trimester.

Most mothers experience a mild degree of cramping during the first trimester. Severe cramping, especially when associated with vaginal spotting or bleeding, must be considered a threat to miscarry and should be reported to the doctor at once. Several terms are applied to different types of early miscarriage. *Incomplete abortion* means that the products of the pregnancy have been partially expelled through the cervix. In an *inevitable abortion,* no tissue is passed, but bleeding and cramping

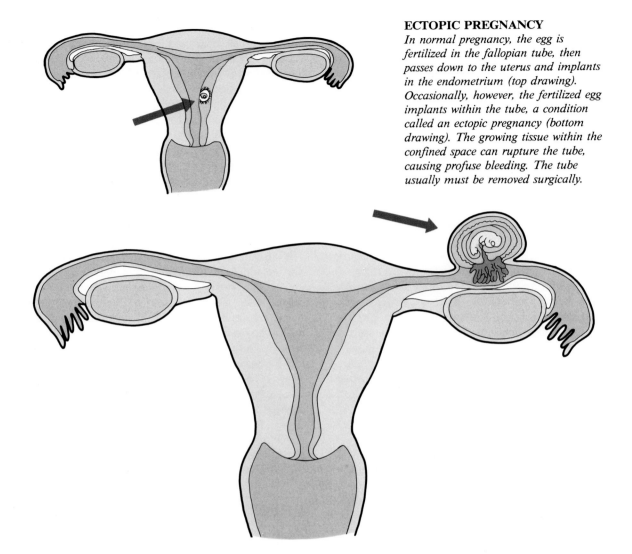

ECTOPIC PREGNANCY
In normal pregnancy, the egg is fertilized in the fallopian tube, then passes down to the uterus and implants in the endometrium (top drawing). Occasionally, however, the fertilized egg implants within the tube, a condition called an ectopic pregnancy (bottom drawing). The growing tissue within the confined space can rupture the tube, causing profuse bleeding. The tube usually must be removed surgically.

are so great that they rule out continuation of the pregnancy. The term *missed abortion* refers to a halt of uterine growth in the absence of bleeding, cramping, or passage of tissue. Whether miscarriage is inevitable, incomplete, or missed, a dilatation and curettage (D&C), a minor operation (see Chapter 26, "The Female Reproductive System"), almost always is necessary.

Ectopic pregnancy. In rare cases, the fertilized ovum implants in the wall of the fallopian tube itself. As the pregnancy enlarges, the tube ruptures, causing profuse bleeding into the abdomen. Symptoms of ectopic pregnancy vary, but usually include pain (often limited to one side) and irregular vaginal bleeding.

Pelvic examination may reveal a lump or mass beside the uterus. Diagnostic ultrasound can visualize the mass. Despite these methods, diagnosis of ectopic pregnancy often remains inconclusive, and a surgical procedure known as laparoscopy, described in Chapter 2, "Tests and Procedures," must be performed. In rare instances, it is possible to attempt to salvage the damaged tube, but the complication rate for bleeding, infection, and recurrent ectopic pregnancy is high.

Women who have had pelvic inflammatory disease, major pelvic or bowel surgery, or previous ectopic pregnancy face an increased risk.

Placental problems. Any bleeding during the second or third trimester must be considered abnormal, whether spotting or bright flow.

Placenta previa results when the pregnancy is implanted low in the uterine wall. As the pregnancy develops, the outlet of the uterus can become completely covered by the placenta (central placenta previa), thus blocking the safe passage of the fetus. In marginal placenta previa, the uterine outlet is partly blocked. In either case, bleeding may result as early as 24 to 26 weeks.

Although the bleeding usually is painless, immediate hospitalization and bed rest is mandatory. If bleeding is profuse, premature delivery by cesarean section is necessary.

Abruptio placentae. Premature detachment of the normal implanted placenta from the uterine wall occurs in about one in 200 pregnancies. The term *abruptio* is reserved for severe degrees of separation involving half the surface area of the placenta. Immediate cesarean section is the only hope for saving the baby.

Premature labor. In the United States today, premature labor is the leading cause of death, ranking higher than heart disease, cancer, or stroke. Almost one in 10 infants born today is significantly premature—less than 37 weeks gestational age or weighing less than 5½ pounds.

Even though all organ systems are present in the premature newborn, the majority are not mature enough for full function. This is especially true of the lungs, where the tiny air sacs lack stability and tend to collapse. The result is known as respiratory distress syndrome and usually requires mechanical support of breathing with a respirator.

With improved techniques and equipment, however, an intensive neonatal-care nursery can help infants to survive even as early as 25 or 26 weeks. Such infants are best delivered at a medical facility capable of providing immediate intensive obstetrical and newborn care. Many patients who appear likely to deliver prematurely need to be transferred to such a hospital if the local facility is inadequate. Where premature labor is exceedingly rapid, delivery occurs unexpectedly and necessitates infant transport in an incubator.

Medications also are available to dramatically suppress uterine contractions. The majority of labors can be stopped through specific action on the muscle cells of the uterus, averting premature delivery. Or, a cortisonelike drug may be administered to the mother prenatally to stimulate and mature the premature fetal lung. Although not effective in all patients, the medication has been shown to benefit most infants from 26 to 35 weeks and has no major maternal or fetal side effects.

If premature labor cannot be halted or there are maternal reasons why labor cannot be stopped, careful electronic fetal surveillance is required. The premature fetus is much more susceptible to the stresses of labor than a full-term baby. Vaginal delivery usually is accomplished with forceps to protect the delicate head from the sudden compression and decompression associated with its emergence from the vagina.

Preeclampsia and eclampsia. These two conditions, once called toxemia, still are not completely understood. Preeclampsia is a condition in the latter half of pregnancy characterized by hypertension; swelling of the feet, hands, legs, or face; and the appearance of protein in the urine. Without prompt medical intervention, the condition progresses to eclampsia, characterized by convulsions and a state of coma. Preeclampsia and eclampsia are a significant threat to both mother and infant.

The only cure for these conditions is delivery of the infant. The first step in management is absolute bed rest. If the hypertension is mild, delivery can be delayed from a few days to several weeks to allow the fetus to mature. Although the woman can be given a mild sedative for comfort, no medication has been shown to be effective in curing the condition, and diuretic medications sometimes impede the circulation of blood through the placenta.

Although preeclampsia and eclampsia are most common in young women having a first baby, the condition can appear in any pregnancy, regardless of age or number of children.

Multiple births. Twins occur in the United States about once in every 93 pregnancies, and triplets occur once in 8,500.

Multiple gestation immediately shifts any pregnancy to a high-risk category. There is a markedly increased risk of premature birth. There also is an increased incidence of labor difficulties, and the necessity for cesarean delivery is increased. Nonetheless, a healthy outcome can be expected.

Identical twins originate from an early division of a single fertilized ovum. Such twins are identical in sex and physical appearance, and carry the same genetic information in their chromosomes.

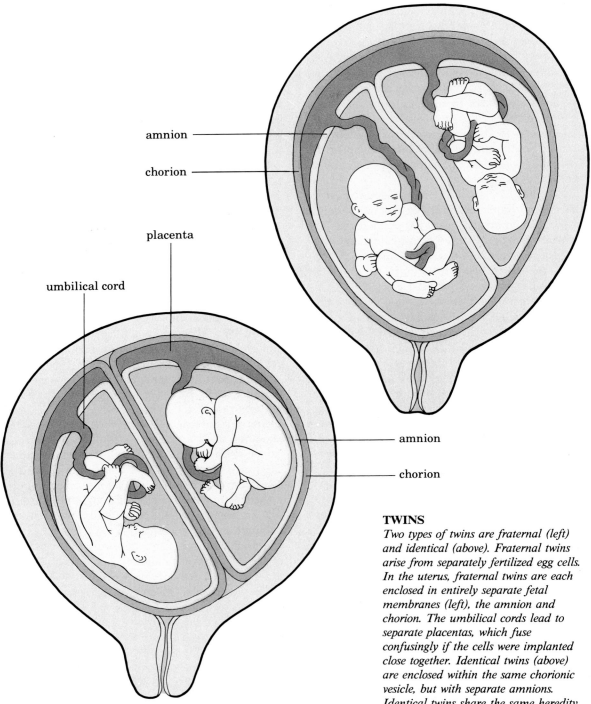

amnion

chorion

placenta

umbilical cord

amnion

chorion

TWINS

Two types of twins are fraternal (left) and identical (above). Fraternal twins arise from separately fertilized egg cells. In the uterus, fraternal twins are each enclosed in entirely separate fetal membranes (left), the amnion and chorion. The umbilical cords lead to separate placentas, which fuse confusingly if the cells were implanted close together. Identical twins (above) are enclosed within the same chorionic vesicle, but with separate amnions. Identical twins share the same heredity package, are always of the same sex, and closely resemble each other. Fraternal twins are more common. They have different genetic makeups and are not always the same sex.

Fraternal twins originate from two separate ova fertilized by two separate spermatozoa. These implant separately in the uterus, and growth and development occur independently, even though the twins may share a common fused placenta. Fraternal twins are not necessarily of the same sex.

Statistically, about two-thirds of all twin pairs are fraternal and one-third are identical.

Twins most often are diagnosed by rapid uterine enlargement. The diagnosis is easily confirmed by diagnostic ultrasound, even as early as the ninth or 10th week of pregnancy.

MEDICAL RISK FACTORS IN PREGNANCY

Maternal age. The greatest pregnancy risk is seen in mothers at each end of the reproductive age spectrum. Teenage mothers face increased risk of miscarriage, prematurity, and ineffective labor patterns resulting in an increased incidence of cesarean birth. Mothers in their 30s and 40s are at risk for these same problems and are more prone to deliver infants with genetic defects.

Maternal weight. Patients with a prepregnancy weight of less than 100 pounds or greater than 200 pounds also face greater risk of prematurity, retardation of fetal growth within the uterus, and irregular, ineffective labor patterns. Nutritional or dietary consultation is particularly important for women in this category to aid fetal growth.

Diabetes. A number of pregnant women develop gestational diabetes, described earlier in this chapter and in Chapter 19, "Diabetes Mellitus."

A woman with diabetes should consult her internist, obstetrician, and nutritional counselor before conception if possible, and certainly as soon as pregnancy is suspected.

Hypertension. Retarded fetal growth, immaturity, partial separation of the placenta, and fetal distress during labor increase in patients with hypertension. During the pregnancy, the diastolic blood pressure should be held between 85 and 100. Medications can lower the mother's blood pressure while sparing the circulation to the uterus and the placenta.

Thyroid disease. Patients who have markedly excessive or insufficient thyroid hormone function rarely become pregnant. Women with a low thyroid function who are maintained on thyroid preparations generally must increase dosage to compensate for the demands of pregnancy.

Cardiac disease. Women with a history of rheumatic fever or congenital heart defects face increased risk during pregnancy. As the blood volume increases, the strain on the heart and lungs can be enough to cause congestive heart failure.

Infectious disease. Rubella, cytomegalovirus, toxoplasmosis, and encephalitis are associated with an increased risk of fetal death or genetic handicaps. For most short-term viral and bacterial infections, risk to the baby is not dramatically increased. Urinary tract infections, especially infections of the kidney itself, carry an increased risk of premature labor.

AFTER THE DELIVERY

The six-week period after delivery is known as puerperium. During this time, the hormonal changes associated with pregnancy subside, and the organ systems of the body slowly return to the prepregnancy level. The majority of these changes are complete after six weeks, when most obstetricians schedule a checkup visit for the mother.

Bleeding. Most patients continue to bleed lightly for three to six weeks or more after delivery. Generally, the vaginal flow (lochia) changes from dark red to dark brown and finally to an almost clear mucuslike substance. Heavy flow with bright red bleeding or large clots should be reported to the physician immediately. Cramping also should subside gradually.

Bowel habits. Constipation is common after delivery, and a woman would be wise to increase her daily fluid intake as well as the roughage in her diet. She should not hesitate to use a mild laxative whenever necessary.

Exercise. An exercise program can be started on a gradual basis the first few days after vaginal delivery. Women who have delivered by cesarean section should delay for about two weeks or as instructed by their physician. The obstetrician may suggest special exercises for tightening the muscles of the pelvic floor and for preventing subsequent problems with bowel or bladder function.

Rest. A decrease in energy levels is the rule rather than the exception for a woman who has just delivered a baby. Fatigue is even more pronounced in the patient recovering from cesarean birth. The new mother should allow at least an hour or two during the day for a short nap or a period of uninterrupted rest with her feet elevated.

CHAPTER 29

TAKING CARE OF YOUR CHILD

Most children are well most of the time. Most problems that do arise can be thought of as normal processes. In only a few instances do serious complications occur. The challenge to parents and physicians is to recognize the difference between normal processes and complications, to learn not to worry needlessly about those that will clear with no specific therapy, and to avoid harmful interventions and anxiety. A good motto for parents is the prayer: "God give me the serenity to accept those things that cannot be changed, the courage (and knowledge) to change those things that can be changed, and the wisdom to know the difference."

NORMAL PROCESSES THAT OFTEN CAUSE CONCERN

Feeding

In proportion to their life span, humans have the longest period of childhood of any species. This presumably is to allow for growth and maturation of the brain. The infant must grow from about seven pounds at birth to 21 to 28 pounds at 1 year old (a threefold to fourfold increase) and only to 120 to 180 pounds by maturity over the next 20 years. The absolute growth of 14 to 21 pounds in the first year rarely is exceeded in any other year.

"Breast is best" refers to the fact that breast milk by itself meets this incredible growth requirement for the first three or four months of an infant's life, and nearly completely meets it for the first six to eight months.

Breast feeding has the advantage of providing all known nutritional requirements and probably some we do not know about. One exception is vitamin D, which often is given as a supplement to breast milk. In nature, enough vitamin D was produced in the skin through interaction between hormones and sunlight. But with clothing, northern climate, and indoor living, production sometimes is not sufficient. Even without supplemental vitamin D, however, few children show signs of deficiency. Breast feeding is clean, provides protection against many infections, and can be provided easily as needed. And the breast always is ready for the irregular hunger or sucking needs, whereas even bottled formula requires some preparation.

Breast milk also is less likely to cause allergy and may result in less obesity later in life. Just as important, the physical contact between a breast-feeding mother and a nursing baby promotes bonding, an important first step in normal human development. Although difficult to define, indicators of bonding in newborns include fondling, kissing, cuddling, and prolonged gazing. There is debate over when it occurs. Some argue that the first few hours are crucial, but humans probably have much greater flexibility than that. If circumstances do not permit contact in the first few hours, parents can make up for it later.

Yet none of the nutritional or psychological advantages of breast-feeding are absolute. All can be compensated for if you decide to feed a formula. Most parents who bottle-feed infants now use prepared formula, which has protein altered to be more like human milk, fat content modified, and various trace elements. And bottle-feeding has the advantage that the father can help feed the baby.

Techniques of feeding. The baby should be put on the breast as soon as possible after delivery. The first feedings will yield a substance called colostrum rather than true milk, but colostrum is an important source of antibodies to protect the baby against infections. True milk will not "come in" until three to five days after birth. The baby will lose weight until then, but the weight loss is normal and no cause for worry.

Babies vary in the amount they take at a feeding. Breast-fed babies stop feeding naturally when satisfied, but parents of bottle-fed babies sometimes become concerned when the child takes less than expected. Merely because the doctor has prescribed five ounces at a feeding does not mean that the baby will take this amount each time. Let the baby be the guide.

"Solid foods" for babies are soft purees. They usually are started at about three to four months. There is no need to give a baby any foods except milk until that time. An exception is orange juice, which can be started at three to four weeks.

When solids are begun, single-grain cereals such as rice or barley are the usual first choice. The first serving usually is about one or two teaspoons mixed with either formula or breast milk. The quantity can be increased gradually. A few foods then may be added to the baby's diet every two to three weeks. A common sequence is fruits, then vegetables, then meats. After nine to 12 months, babies can eat small mashed-up portions of whatever you eat. From six to nine months, the baby can learn to drink from a cup and then can be switched to whole cow's milk and weaned from the breast to bottle, although some mothers prefer to continue to offer the breast.

Feeding and growth after the first year. In the second year, the incredible weight gain of the first 12 months slows and the baby's food intake diminishes. Most children appear chubby at 1 year old, then gradually slim down until at 4 to 6 years they appear skinny. During this process, they eat much less avidly. In early adolescence, girls, in particular, may appear fat again.

Parents often are more concerned about irregular eating patterns and junk foods among adolescents. Little is known about the long-term effects, but in the short term, if the child is not gaining more than expected or is not losing weight, there is little evidence that irregular eating schedules or junk foods are harmful.

Growth in Infancy

Physical growth has two dimensions: height and weight. Individual babies have different rates of growth but these rates usually are steady. That's another way of saying some babies grow faster than others. Doctors find it useful to plot height (really length in infants, because it is measured lying down) and weight on charts that express various normal rates. A child growing steadily according to the growth curve is perfectly normal, even though he or she may be considerably smaller than another child the same age.

Body proportions change remarkably from birth to maturity. Legs are short in proportion to trunk at birth, and the head is large compared to the rest of the body. Despite the head's size at birth, it has a lot of growing to do, mostly in the first year of life. A head that grows too quickly or too slowly demands a thorough medical checkup.

Growth only can be meaningful when compared over time, and when height and weight are studied together. There is nothing intrinsically more healthy about a child far larger than his peers than a child who is smaller. Heredity is the main determinant. Unfortunately, because Americans tend to feel that bigger is better, parents of a smaller child may become worried. Steady growth is one of the best signs of good health, no matter what the percentile.

Overweight usually becomes apparent in adolescence and persists into adult life. It has become a major problem in the Western world. There are no simple answers, however, to prevention or treatment of obesity in children. Heredity plays a role, as well as too many calories or not enough exercise. It is wise to encourage adolescents to exercise,

CHILD DEVELOPMENT LANDMARKS

MONTH	NORMAL VARIATION	ACCOMPLISHMENT	
1	2 weeks	Smiles	
2	2 weeks	Coos	
3	2 weeks	Holds head up	
4	3 weeks	Grasps object	
5	3 weeks	Rolls from back to front	
6	3 weeks	Sits alone	
7	3 weeks	Crawls	
8	3 weeks	Uses pincer grasp	

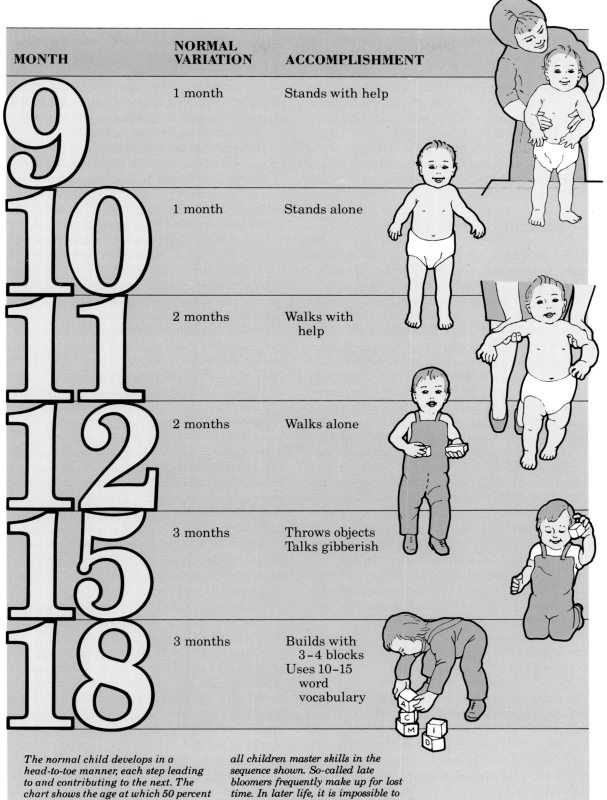

MONTH	NORMAL VARIATION	ACCOMPLISHMENT
9	1 month	Stands with help
10	1 month	Stands alone
11	2 months	Walks with help
12	2 months	Walks alone
15	3 months	Throws objects Talks gibberish
18	3 months	Builds with 3–4 blocks Uses 10–15 word vocabulary

The normal child develops in a head-to-toe manner, each step leading to and contributing to the next. The chart shows the age at which 50 percent of normal children master the skill pictured, but range can be wide and not all children master skills in the sequence shown. So-called late bloomers frequently make up for lost time. In later life, it is impossible to recognize which individuals developed early and which did not.

and to maintain examples at home of balanced, regular, and moderate-calorie meals. So-called glandular troubles (too little thyroid hormone) do not cause obesity. Successful weight loss or obesity prevention almost always is the result of individual, family, and peer interaction. Peer group weight-reduction programs for adolescents and adults have been successful, but rapid weight loss should be avoided.

Sometimes, adolescent girls literally starve themselves in a quest for thinness. This condition, which can have serious consequences, is discussed in Chapter 21, "Nutrition."

Adolescent Growth

Adolescence is a time when every boy and girl feels different and is very sensitive to the differences. It is quite natural that slightly earlier or later growth spurt or puberty will cause anxiety.

Girls start their growth about two years before boys, and there has been a trend to increasingly early onset of puberty in both sexes over the past 100 years, probably due to better nutrition.

As early as age 8, girls may begin to have breast enlargement, although 10 to 12 years is more common. The first menstrual period usually occurs two years later. On average, girls in the United States begin to menstruate at 12.4 years today.

In boys, no similar dramatic event announces the arrival of puberty. However, from 10 to 14 years, growth of the penis, pubic hair, underarm, chest, and facial hair, and muscle mass occur. In rare cases, a girl's increase in height to 6 feet or more worries parents and the girl a great deal. Such growth can be stopped with female sex hormones, but such therapy rarely is needed and must be supervised carefully by a physician (see Chapter 18, "The Hormones and Endocrine Glands").

Late onset of puberty is a major social problem for both boys and girls. While sex hormones can expedite the customary sex changes, they rarely are needed and can have harmful side effects. The best advice for adolescents who fail to start puberty as soon as their peers, or who feel too tall, too short, too big, or too little, is to see a doctor to be sure that no treatable disease is responsible, then to accept that size differences are normal and one of the things that make humans so interesting. For rare forms of growth failure due to abnormalities of the pituitary gland, synthetic growth hormone now is available.

Development: A Wholistic Approach

Growth is increase in size; development is increase in complexity of function. Mostly, that means neurological and psychological function, and most of our measures of development in children are expressed in neurological or psychological ways—walking, talking, or thinking.

The process of development. Development proceeds in a head-to-toe sequence. The first parts of the nervous system to increase complexity of functioning are the brain and the cranial nerves.

The first evidence of a new skill in a baby is the ability to smile. The bonding process that starts at birth is then cemented. Each new stage is exciting to watch, but is just as much an interaction with the baby's environment as the first smile. The chart in this chapter lists easily observed developmental tasks of the first 18 months and the average age when they are accomplished.

A delay in development that occurs early in life is likely to be more profound and have greater consequences than delays that occur later. Thus, a physician will test the baby's development at each visit to assess progress.

Common Developmental Concerns

A number of symptoms that often concern parents should be considered separately from disease because they are variations of normal development and rarely, if ever, lead to any persistent problem.

Constipation is a condition of excessively hard stools with difficulty of passage, sometimes leading to rectal pain. It is not defined by the frequency of stools. The importance of a daily bowel movement has been overemphasized in the past. Consistency of the stool, not frequency, is the criterion.

Children are frequently constipated after an acute illness because they drink and eat less and thus have fewer fluids. Others are chronically constipated as a result of a diet containing little fiber or an all-milk diet. Usually, all that is necessary to relieve constipation is to add fruits and vegetables to the diet. Laxatives, suppositories, or enemas should be avoided. Great difficulty in passing stools that is unrelieved by adding fruit to the diet should be brought to the attention of a physician.

A common problem is constipation related to toilet training (see below). Some children rebel against the compulsory or threatening environment, hold in their stool, and finally produce a large and hard stool. The stool is hard because the water it normally contains has been reabsorbed by the bowel. Passage may cause a small, painful fissure in the rectum, which sets up a cycle of further stool withholding, pain, and more fissures. If this problem occurs, see your physician.

Toilet training is an important stage of development that can be exhausting for both parent and child. Fortunately, the conflicts rarely have any lasting effects.

Bowel training normally comes before bladder training, usually about the middle of the second year. Most children have a reflex some 20 minutes after eating that stimulates their bowels to move. They usually give some indication—grunting, straining—that the reflex is occurring. When the parents recognize the sign, the child can then be placed on the potty chair.

It seems best to use a small, freestanding potty chair rather than a seat attached to a full-size toilet, because the height and flushing action frighten some children. The child should be left on the chair for five to 10 minutes at most, then removed if there is no result. Don't scold, push, wheedle or coax, or show that the child can irritate you by withholding the bowel movement.

Bowel training occurs at a time when children normally are going through what is called "the terrible twos." Problems arise if parents allow the normal 2-year-old struggle for independence to carry over to bowel training.

Bladder training usually occurs after bowel control has been achieved. When a child indicates that he or she is about to urinate by moving about or holding the genitals, or at regular intervals after meals, help him or her to the potty. However, if urination does not occur, don't get upset, even if the child urinates immediately after you have buttoned his or her clothing. Most children achieve daytime urine control by 3 or 4 years, although there is wide variation among individual children. Nighttime bladder control takes longer. The bladder needs to be large enough to store the urine produced overnight. About 10 percent of children do not achieve nighttime dryness by age 6.

Bed-wetting or enuresis is a troublesome issue that occurs at some time in most children (see Chapter 24, "The Kidneys and Urinary System"). A child who previously has been dry often may regress to bed-wetting after an illness, after moving to a new home, or after the arrival of a baby in the family. Some extra time and attention for the child are all that is needed for this temporary setback.

Allergy, diabetes, abnormalities or infections of the urinary tract, or serious psychiatric problems sometimes are held responsible for persistent bed-wetting. These are doubtful explanations in the absence of other symptoms. Bed-wetting is a developmental problem, like late walking or talking. The majority of otherwise normal children who are bed wetters pass through this developmental problem without signs of other difficulties. But the tolerance of a mother who has to change a wet bed morning after morning is limited, and the sense of insecurity provoked in a child explains why parents seek any solution and doctors are willing to try anything to help.

Treatment is not necessary until age 5 or 6. Restricting fluids before bedtime and using a reward system (stars on a chart, praise, or other rewards) for dry nights may help. Some parents awaken the child after two to three hours, or set an alarm for the child. Mild medications and alarm systems can be prescribed by your doctor.

Temper tantrums. Under stress of being refused, punished, or frustrated, the child will appear to lose control with stamping, shouting behavior. Tantrums usually cease by age 4 or 5. Firmness, consistency of punishment, and isolating the child until the attack subsides are useful.

Colic, characterized by prolonged crying, usually at night, is common in babies during the first three months of life. The causes are not known, but colicky babies usually are healthy otherwise. There is no way to tell whether the baby is in pain, although many may draw up their legs, turn red in the face, and sometimes strain as if about to have a bowel movement. Sucking seems to be more of a need than actual hunger. A pacifier, swaddling, feeding, burping, rocking, or carrying may help. Some doctors prescribe medication, although there is little evidence that it does much good other than to reassure the parents. The condition seldom persists beyond the first six months.

Cradle cap appears as a thick scaling or crusted patch on the scalp. The cause is unknown. It is not related to frequency of bathing. It probably stems from oil glands of the scalp that are not developed fully (see Chapter 9, "The Skin"). Cradle cap is treated by removing the scab or crusts by softening them with baby oil or petroleum jelly, gently combing out the scales with a fine-tooth baby comb, then shampooing daily. The condition clears completely with time.

Diaper rash is caused by the irritant effect of urine-soaked diapers on the baby's sensitive skin. Changing diapers often, leaving the baby "open to the air," and using talc, cornstarch, or baby pow-

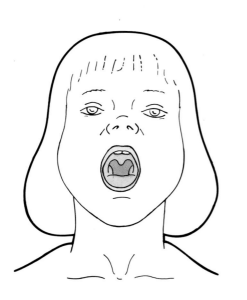

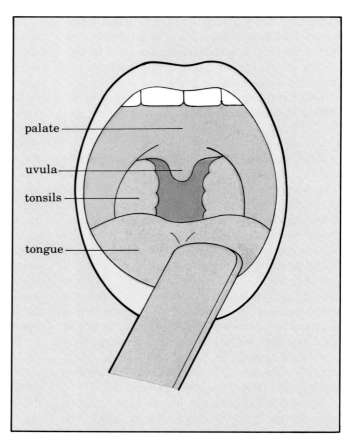

palate

uvula

tonsils

tongue

ENLARGED TONSILS

Swollen and inflamed tonsils in the throat can readily be seen, especially when the child's tongue is depressed (right drawing). The enlargement usually occurs during and after periods of infection, because tonsils are part of the body's system for fighting disease.

Sometimes the tonsils themselves become infected. Bouts of "tonsillitis" usually decline as the child grows older, and removal of the tonsils and adenoids, which are related tissue at the back of the nasal passages, is less common than in the past.

ders all help (but be sure the baby doesn't inhale the talc). Occasionally, the raw wounds of the rash become infected with bacteria, in which case antibiotic ointments and soaks may be needed.

Teething usually begins about six months of age and proceeds until the 20 primary teeth are in place, generally by age 2 years (see Chapter 20, "The Teeth and Oral Health"). Some children are cranky during teething, but this normal process does not cause fever, convulsions, or other problems previously attributed to it. Rather, the teething child is simultaneously being exposed to common infections, which are the cause of the fever and irritability. Because teething goes on almost continuously from 6 to 24 months, infections and teething sometimes are bound to coincide. Rubbing the gums with a finger or providing

teething biscuits, a chilled rubber ring, or plastic teething devices that can be filled with water and chilled in the refrigerator is all that is needed.

Thrush is a mild fungus infection of the mouth that is described in Chapter 9, "The Skin."

Tonsils and adenoids. Most parents do not think of tonsil and adenoid conditions as normal processes. Yet most alleged disorders of these organs really are normal, and removing them by operation, previously the most common surgical procedure in the United States, is less commonly recommended today (see Chapter 15, "Ear, Nose, and Throat," and Chapter 33, "Understanding Your Operation"). All children have large tonsils and adenoids as part of their normal development, because these bits of lymphatic tissue play a key role in defense against infections. Because the preschool and school-age child is repeatedly exposed to strange bacteria and viruses, the tonsils and adenoids frequently are enlarged and may become infected. But removal merely for frequent throat infections is not needed and will not reduce the frequency of infections. As children grow older, the number of infections drops.

With antibiotics, few children have complications of tonsillar infection. Only when tonsils and adenoids are so large that they obstruct breathing is removal indicated.

Sleep disturbances in children are common. Infants vary in when they begin to sleep through the night. Usually it occurs around six to eight weeks (to the great relief of their parents). During the second year of life, many children resist going to bed or awaken during the night. It can be safely stated that no child ever suffered from sleep deprivation at this age, although parents surely have. It is advisable to establish a quiet routine for bedtime and a firm deadline for going, with no wavering response to requests for "one more drink of water." Similarly, when a child awakens in the night, go to the bedside once to assure yourself that everything is in order, then firmly ignore the crying after that.

It also is important to recognize that children vary in the amount of sleep they need, just as they vary in other ways.

COMMON PROBLEMS

It is useful for parents to realize that temporary disruptions such as diarrhea, vomiting, and respiratory infections are common, affecting virtually every child at some time in life. They rarely have any long-term consequences. Parents need to understand how to manage these temporary upsets, yet be aware of the rare instances when they should seek advice from a physician.

Diarrhea

Development occurs in the biochemical reactions of the body as well as in the nervous system. For instance, kidney function at birth is quite different than it is later, because the newborn's kidneys do not concentrate urine (do not conserve water) as much as those of adults. This enables the baby to lose some of the water present at birth. Infants have a larger proportion of their body composed of water (nearly 80 percent) than at any other time in life. But if a baby develops diarrhea in the first weeks of life, he or she has greater trouble conserving water as a result.

Preparation of Children For Hospitalization

When hospitalization is planned, children should be fully prepared so they avoid psychological trauma that may lead to night fears afterward and even delay recovery. Children aged 1 to 5 fear separation from home and familiar surroundings most, while 5- to 10-year-olds fear the trauma of surgery and tests. Most hospitals now permit a parent to stay with a young child to minimize this trauma. Many hospitals also offer day surgery. The child is admitted to the hopsital in the morning, the operation is performed, and the child is sent home later in the day when the anesthesia has worn off. Recovery occurs at home and separation trauma is avoided.

Telling the child a few days before hospitalization what to expect, reading from one of the many excellent books available to prepare children for hospitalization (ask your doctor for suggestions), staying with your child in the hospital, and providing recreation programs (often called child-life programs) in the hospital have been shown to prevent the potentially harmful effects.

A baby also has a much smaller margin of safety in water needs and water reserves. If water intake is diminished or if the water loss is increased by vomiting or diarrhea, the infant can quickly become dehydrated. The smaller the baby, the greater the danger.

However, it recently has been shown that oral rehydration therapy, which uses a solution of water with salts and sugar, promotes water absorption and maintains fluid and electrolyte balance. Should the diarrhea not subside with simple fluids, the doctor may prescribe rehydration, which makes hospitalization unnecessary.

All babies get diarrhea occasionally. Most instances in the United States are caused by common viruses, for which there is no specific treatment. The main requirement is to supply fluids until the infection has run its course. Commonly used treatments such as paregoric or kaolin and pectin are of no value, and may harmfully lull the parent into believing that the condition is being treated, while neglecting the needed fluids.

Most children with diarrhea can take small amounts of fluid. Ginger ale (with the fizz out), apple juice, or weak tea is good. A baby up to 2 years of age needs two and a half to three ounces of fluid per pound of body weight each 24 hours. Watching the behavior or vigor of the baby, the urine output, and weight are all important in treatment and evaluation of the baby with diarrhea. If the baby loses weight, decreases urine output, or becomes listless, or if there is bloody diarrhea, a physician should be called.

Breast-fed babies often have very soft, yellow stools. This is not diarrhea. A green stool is important only because it signifies more rapid passage of the stool, before the green bile has had a chance to be changed to brown or yellow. It is the water loss, not the color of the stool, that is important.

Vomiting

Vomiting in infants and children is most commonly caused by bacterial infections, sometimes with diarrhea, or ear or general viral infections. If vomiting begins suddenly in a previously healthy child who remains alert and who has not had a head injury, the treatment is to withhold everything by mouth until vomiting stops and for one to three hours thereafter. Then, give small amounts of clear fluid every 20 minutes, starting with one-half tablespoon and gradually increasing to one-half ounce. The frequency then can be decreased and amounts increased. Almost all children with simple infectious causes of vomiting will respond in 24 to 36 hours. In babies under one month, or when vomiting is accompanied by drowsiness or abdominal pain, a physician should be called.

Fever

Babies inherit antibodies from the mother against most infections, but the immunity ends by four to six months of age. For the next 10 years, children develop their immunity by acquiring infections. Each child must have about 10 to 12 common infections per year for the first 10 years of life. The cardinal symptom is fever, a marked increase in body temperature above the "normal" reading of 98.6 degrees Fahrenheit.

When fever occurs, many parents give acetaminophen, an aspirin substitute, the amount dependent on age, to return the temperature toward normal. This makes the child comfortable and soothes parental fear of a complication of high fever unique to children—a febrile convulsion or fit, described later in this chapter. Actually, acetaminophen is unlikely to prevent convulsions, which seem to be related to how quickly a fever has risen, rather than to its actual height. Still, convulsions, even brief ones, are worrying to all.

If the child is active, is taking fluids well, and (for older children) does not complain of headache or muscle ache, medications are not recommended. Artificially suppressing fever actually may prolong the illness, and make it difficult to assess the child's recovery. It is much more important to determine whether there are uncommon symptoms or complications. Even with a temperature of 103 to 104 degrees, a child who is alert and eating well is rarely seriously ill.

Treatment of fever. Aspirin previously was the main medical treatment for fever, but in children it now has been associated with a rare but serious complication called Reye syndrome. Therefore, most physicians instead recommend acetaminophen, in liquid or tablet form. Children's-dose strength should be used for anyone under 5 years of age. If the child is under 1 year of age, consult your physician for dosage.

The best treatment of most fever is time. Suppositories, alcohol or water sponging, enemas, and other time-honored ways of lowering fever are not very effective and a few are dangerous. Of the old methods, the best is to place the child who is old enough to sit without support into a tub of tepid water and gently sponge the entire body. This treatment will reduce fever and promote comfort.

Upper Respiratory Infections

The common cold is familiar to all. Its symptoms can include the well-known runny nose, slight fever, headache, muscle ache, and slight cough. There still is no known treatment. The accompanying nasal congestion, which may produce noisy, somewhat difficult breathing in small babies, is best treated with an infant nasal aspirator, a small rubber bulb to remove the secretions by suction. Nose drops and oral decongestants are widely used but are unwise in babies under six months of age.

Upper respiratory infections may lead to ear infections or pneumonia if air passages become obstructed and elimination of bacteria is decreased. In some children with allergies, ear infection may be associated with wheezing and may be the first clue to what later becomes asthma.

Bronchiolitis is a common viral infection in babies, usually those under 2 years of age. The signs are wheezing (like asthma), coughing, and slight fever. Rarely, children will become fatigued as a result of the labored breathing and require hospitalization for oxygen and even breathing assistance. A good home remedy resembles that for croup, described below.

Common Contagious Diseases

Most "childhood diseases" have been eliminated by widespread immunization, but a few persist.

Chicken pox (technically called varicella) is contracted by all children at some point, although in a few instances the encounter may be delayed until young adulthood. A vaccine has been developed but is not yet in general use. The incubation period for chicken pox is 12 to 19 days after exposure. Symptoms are fever (usually mild) and headache, followed in a day or two by the characteristic rash that starts as a small red spot, rapidly progressing to a pinhead-size blister that turns to a scab in three or four days. The amount of rash varies in different children. The blisters are itchy, and secondary infections occur as a result of scratching. Any commercial preparation of calamine lotion or an antihistamine may reduce the itch. The disease usually ends in a week.

Roseola occurs largely in children six months to 2 years, starting with a high fever and irritability. After three to five days, the fever drops to normal, and in a few hours, there is a characteristic rash—pink flat spots, especially on the trunk. This rash rarely lasts longer than 24 hours. Treatment consists only of the methods to reduce fever.

Common Misconceptions About Infections

Colds, sore throat, and diarrhea do *not* result from getting wet or chilled, although other stressful events do reduce resistance in some children. All are caused by germs, mainly common viruses. In addition to cases in which symptoms make the illness evident, many more children carry the germs but show no signs or symptoms. Most immunity, in fact, comes from these asymptomatic infections. Thus, when your child has a mild upper respiratory infection but otherwise feels well, you can send him or her to school, for he or she poses no greater risk to others than the many asymptomatic children carrying the same germ. The same situation holds in reverse. There is no point in keeping your child home to prevent exposure to children with one of these common infections. Your child is as likely to catch a cold from an asymptomatic playmate as from one who has symptoms.

Conjunctivitis ("pink eye") is inflammation of the whites of the eye and the eyelids. It may accompany one of the viral diseases described above, it may be the only symptom of a virus infection, or it may result from an allergy, foreign body, or bacteria (see Chapter 14, "The Eyes"). Itching is common in allergy-caused conjunctivitis but not in the other cases. Bacterial conjunctivitis usually causes more pus. Treatment of common viral conjunctivitis usually is not necessary. Mild eye washes may bring comfort, but if pain or pus is present, consult a physician.

IMMUNIZATION SCHEDULE FOR CHILDREN

Making sure your child is immunized against the most common childhood diseases—diphtheria, tetanus, pertussis (whooping cough), polio, measles, mumps, and rubella (German measles)—is very important. Because there are risks associated with immunization, as well as with the failure to immunize a child, you should discuss this subject with your doctor. The following immunization schedule is recommended by the American Academy of Pediatrics. Because immunization recommendations change from time to time, it is important to check with your child's doctor about the most current schedule. If your child is ill when an immunization is scheduled, tell the doctor. The immunization may have to be postponed until the child has recovered from the illness.

2 months	DPT, oral polio
4 months	DPT, oral polio
6 months	DPT (oral polio optional)
12 months	TB test
15 months	measles, mumps, rubella (one injection)
18 months	DPT, polio boosters, Hib conjugate
4–6 years	DPT, polio boosters
14–16 years	tetanus, diphtheria

Immunizations. With the exception of sanitation and pure food, immunizations have produced more improvement in the health of children in the past 100 years than any other scientific advance, and are important for every child. A timetable of immunizations is shown in the chart above.

Recently, concern has grown about possible side effects from pertussis (whooping cough) vaccine, which usually is given in combination with the vaccines against diphtheria and tetanus in a shot called DPT. It is true that the pertussis component of DPT can cause a reaction, most commonly mild fever, crying, irritability, or soreness at the injection site. Very infrequently, in about one in 300,000 cases, brain damage can result. Although this risk is real, the risk from the disease itself is far greater. Prior to immunization, about one in 20 victims of whooping cough died.

Meanwhile, a safer and more effective pertussis vaccine is expected to be licensed in the near future. The American Academy of Pediatrics and the federal Centers for Disease Control strongly urge parents to continue the standard immunization schedule.

In addition to DPT, polio vaccine, especially the live-virus type, may cause a mild reaction. If the child is uncomfortable after an immunization, acetaminophen can be given, and you should inform your physician before the next dose.

SERIOUS ACUTE ILLNESSES

Most acute childhood illnesses are self-limiting, cause no long-term consequences, and require no treatment. A few acute illnesses, mostly infections, do not follow this rule. They require prompt diagnosis and treatment, which may be lifesaving.

Croup is marked by noisy breathing when inhaling (in contrast to asthma or bronchiolitis, which involve wheezing during exhaling). Most cases are caused by an acute infection that causes swelling in and around the larynx. As the larynx grows, croup becomes less common. Cases are rare after age 5.

Some children have repeated attacks without much fever or other signs of a cold or infection. Treatment with steam then usually is sufficient. Take the child into the bathroom, turn on the hot shower, sit, and hold the child. The comfort of being held reduces anxiety and helps lower the need for air. If the croup does not subside in half an hour with steam or mist, if it increases in intensity, or if it is associated with fever of more than 103 degrees or with drooling, go immediately to a hospital emergency room. Children with severe croup sometimes require lifesaving measures.

Pneumonia still is a common disease of children, but most often is caused by bacteria and can be treated successfully with antibiotics at home.

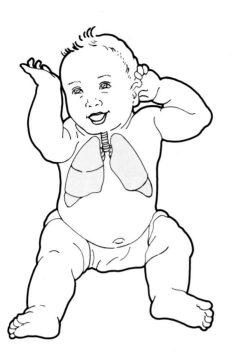

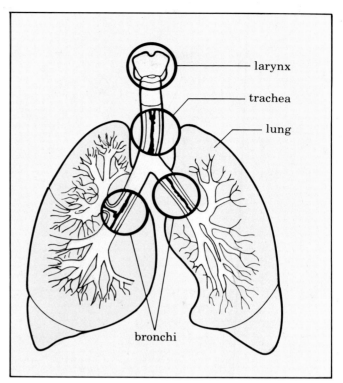

CROUP

Noisy breathing and a ringing cough are characteristic of croup, which results from a swelling in and around the larynx. It usually is caused by an acute infection. Secretions of thick mucus also can clog the larynx, bronchi, and trachea and further obstruct air passage to and from the lungs. Croup may be accompanied by high fever. Mild cases may be relieved by steam inhalation or a cold-mist vaporizer, but severe croup is a medical emergency and victims should be taken to a hospital emergency department immediately.

Even viral pneumonias, which do not respond to these drugs, rarely cause serious illness. Symptoms include fever, cough, and rapid breathing. In small babies, the cough may be absent and only a grunting breathing present. Older children may produce sputum, which sometimes is rusty or blood-tinged. If these symptoms are present, call your physician.

Meningitis is an inflammation of the membranes surrounding the brain and spinal cord (see Chapter 11, "The Brain and Nervous System"). Early symptoms are difficult to distinguish from those of a self-limiting infection. Most cases occur between ages six months and 4 to 5 years. In addition to fever and vomiting, indications include lethargy or unresponsiveness, poor color, stiff neck, a rash (which occurs only with one type), or convulsions. These symptoms are an emergency warranting a prompt call to your doctor.

Meningitis can be treated successfully today if diagnosed promptly. If allowed to continue untreated, it has severe consequences. Occasionally, meningitis occurs in epidemics in schools, and antibiotics may be prescribed as a preventive measure. The most common type of meningitis in young children is caused by the *Hemophilus influenzae* bacterium. It now can be prevented by immunization.

Streptococcal sore throat. Virtually all children are exposed to the common "strep" germ, and most will have several bouts of strep infection while growing up. There are dozens of different strains of "strep." Infection with any of them produces immunity only to that particular strain. Regardless of strain, symptoms are similar: fever, severe sore throat, difficulty swallowing, and swollen lymph glands in the neck. There also may be vomiting and abdominal pain. Certain strains produce a rash. This variety is called scarlet fever.

Untreated cases of strep throat occasionally may lead, about two weeks afterward, to rheumatic fever, which can result in heart damage. Treatment with antibiotics almost always prevents this.

If your child has a sore throat, your doctor may want to take a throat culture to confirm the presence of the bacterium. Penicillin must be given for 10 days to adequately eliminate the germ.

Ear infections (otitis) and chronic fluid in the middle ear (serous otitis media), which are common problems of preschool children, are described in Chapter 15, "Ear, Nose, and Throat."

Acute problems of the newborn. The major problems of the newborn result from premature birth. Control of temperature is difficult, and handling of infections is inefficient. Therefore, premature babies are placed in incubators to stabilize body temperature, and to protect them from infections. They often must be fed by tube or intravenously. Respiratory distress syndrome (RDS), caused by immaturity of the lungs, is the most life-threatening problem of small newborns. The baby cannot absorb oxygen and rid the body of carbon dioxide adequately. Breathing is rapid, and the baby may die from exhaustion and lack of oxygen. Treatment of this condition has improved so much, however, that the majority of babies weighing less than two pounds at birth can be saved.

Usually, the baby's breathing is assisted by placing a tiny tube in the trachea. Blood oxygen, carbon dioxide, and sugar are carefully monitored, and any metabolic abnormalities are treated.

Babies with respiratory distress syndrome usually breathe normally in three to five days. Most develop normally, although a few have persistent lung disease. Because respiratory distress syndrome is the largest single cause of death in all of childhood, prevention and effective treatment are leading to a continued decrease in infant mortality.

Thanks to improved methods of feeding premature babies, and the advances in treatment and prevention of respiratory and infectious diseases of the newborn, the outlook for even very tiny preemies now is very good.

CHRONIC DISEASE

Pediatrics, until recently, was consumed with the burden of acute illness. Now that many of the more serious acute illnesses can be controlled or prevented, chronic disease, defined as any illness that lasts three months or more, has become a major focus of pediatric care.

Asthma, the most common chronic physical disease of childhood, affects 3 to 5 percent of all children. Asthma is characterized by attacks of wheezing brought on by obstruction of the small air passages of the lung. The causes include allergy to pollens, dusts, or fumes; cold air; emotions; infections; and, occasionally, other agents. Some cases are of unknown cause. Severity varies from mild, occasional attacks to severe, frequent ones. Many treatments, including drugs, avoidance of allergens, and desensitization, can help most asthmatic children lead fully active lives. (See Chapter 10, "The Lungs," and Chapter 23, "Allergy and the Immune System.")

Birthmarks are common and result from enlargement of blood vessels in the skin or from extra pigment in the skin.

Hemangiomas, or strawberry marks, are not present at birth, but appear after the first two to four weeks of life. They are caused by a collection of small blood vessels in the skin. Hemangiomas all shrink with time, lose their color, and disappear. Treatment by surgery, X ray, or dry ice produces more scars than if time is allowed to eradicate the lesion. Another common type of hemangioma ("stork bite") is a light salmon pink flat patch, common on the forehead or the back of the neck. These, too, disappear without treatment.

Moles are permanent pigmented spots on the skin (see Chapter 9, "The Skin"). If they are large and occur in highly visible areas, moles can be removed by surgery or covered with cosmetics.

Port wine stains are a special type of birthmark with purple stain and small blood vessels on the skin. They may occur anywhere on the body, but the most disfiguring are those on the face. In older children and young adults, some stains may be removed by laser treatments. Other stains are covered cosmetically or with a neutral tattoo.

Convulsions are frightening. Nearly 5 percent of children have one convulsion (also called a seizure or fit) by the age of 5. Most follow a high or sudden fever and are called febrile convulsions. The child suddenly loses consciousness, rolls up his or her eyes, then twitches all over rhythmically. The episode is followed by a general relaxation and apparently deep sleep. The convulsion may be over in a few seconds or may persist for several minutes.

Almost all convulsions cease by themselves. Reducing fever will not help in the acute stage.

A few children tend to have recurrent seizures with high fever until they are 4 or 5 years old.

Some physicians prescribe an anticonvulsant drug such as phenobarbital, but others consider the side effects (hyperactivity and reduced attentiveness) more dangerous than the small risk of recurrence. A single febrile seizure in an otherwise healthy child seldom produces harm in the long run.

Cystic fibrosis (CF) is one of the more common inherited conditions, occurring in about one in 1,000 children. Cystic fibrosis affects mucous glands in the body, producing thick secretions, which block small airways, resulting in chronic infection, coughing, wheezing, and shortness of breath. There often are intestinal symptoms as well. Cystic fibrosis and its treatment is described in Chapter 10, "The Lungs."

Diabetes mellitus in children is different from that in adults (see Chapter 19, "Diabetes Mellitus"). Known as Type I or juvenile diabetes, the disease occurs because the body cannot produce enough of the hormone insulin to regulate sugar balance. Symptoms, which occur suddenly, are thirst, frequent and copious urination, and weight loss despite increased appetite. Acute complications include accumulation of acids in the body (acidosis); long-term complications, occurring after many years, include hardening of the arteries, diminished kidney function, and visual problems. Injections of insulin can control symptoms. A full description of therapies is found in Chapter 19.

Heart defects and heart disease in children cause great anxiety among parents, but serious heart disease is quite uncommon. Congenital heart defects can be diagnosed with great precision, and many can be corrected completely by surgery. Younger children and babies usually show some symptoms. Some babies are blue (cyanotic) because venous blood from the right side of the heart mixes with arterial blood from the left, the result of an opening between the two sides. Other symptoms are easy fatigue shown by slow or interrupted feedings, and rapid breathing. Treatment with digitalis to strengthen the heart muscle, diuretics to remove excess fluid, and surgery have saved the lives of many such children.

The major acquired heart disease in children is rheumatic heart disease, a complication of rheumatic fever. The symptoms and signs are fever, joint pains or arthritis, involuntary jerky movements called chorea, and heart disease. Rheumatic fever usually follows a streptococcal infection. With prompt treatment of "strep throat" and pre-vention of second attacks of rheumatic fever by daily penicillin therapy, the heart damage and the heart failure that formerly were consequences of rheumatic fever have been almost totally prevented. The consequences and treatment of rheumatic heart disease in adults are discussed in Chapter 5, "The Heart and Circulation."

Heart murmur. As many as 40 percent of children have a heart murmur sometime during childhood. Most are of little consequence. Murmurs stem from turbulence in the flow of blood, much like the noise made by rapids in a river. Abnormal heart valves can cause murmurs because they create turbulence in the blood flow inside the heart. Most functional (innocent) murmurs arise outside the heart because of slight turbulence in the flow of blood through veins, and are less noticeable as children grow. A physician usually distinguishes between functional and organic heart murmurs by their location, timing, and character.

Hernias are small openings in the abdominal wall with ballooning of a bit of intestine through the opening.

Umbilical hernias occur at the navel and are common in babies. They may range in size from the diameter of a small pencil to as big as a finger. Umbilical hernias almost never cause harm. As the abdominal muscles become stronger, the hernias close by themselves.

Inguinal hernias occur in the groin. They may occur at any time in life. If the intestine cannot be pushed back into place (reduced), the hernia may strangulate as the blood supply to the intestine in the sac is pinched off. A hernia operation, even in the very young, is simple and effective.

Hydrocele is a collection of fluid in the scrotum. It may look like a hernia and in some instances is associated with a hernia. In infants with only a hydrocele, no treatment is necessary.

Intussusception, seen in children under age 2, occurs when one part of the intestine telescopes into another. The blood supply of the internal portion may be cut off, leading to gangrene.

Symptoms occur suddenly, with crying, repeated attacks of abdominal cramps, vomiting, and blood in the stool (often appearing as "currant jelly"). This is an acute emergency. Many hospitals now are able to reduce the bowel with manipulation under fluoroscope with barium in the large bowel. At times, surgery is necessary.

Pyloric stenosis stems from enlargement of the circular muscle at the end of the stomach, which obstructs the passage of food. It occurs mainly during the first two months of life. The major symptom is vomiting after feeding, often so forcefully that the material spurts several inches. A doctor usually can feel the mass of muscle. A simple operation to cut the enlarged muscle fibers cures the condition.

Skin rashes are common in children. Many result from acute general infections, such as roseola, described above. Others are short-term, ranging from tiny spots to generalized red rashes and even to hives. Still others, such as eczema, recurrent hives, scabies, and lice, are more chronic (see Chapter 9, "The Skin").

Intellectual Development Problems

In the past, many parents felt as stigmatized by a retarded child as by one with venereal disease. But few children are so severely retarded that they cannot become self-sufficient adults. The causes of severe retardation are many, but all are quite rare. Blood tests on newborns can diagnose some problems soon after birth, allowing treatment to forestall retardation. Other problems, such as the chromosome abnormalities causing Down syndrome, can be diagnosed by analyzing fluid from the uterus during pregnancy (amniocentesis).

Much more common are the milder forms of retardation, which are more of a handicap during school years, when ability to memorize is important. Most children with mild retardation grow up able to function effectively in the workplace.

If your child is not developing as you believe he or she should, it is important to have further tests performed to determine the amount of delay and the most likely cause, and to set up a program of help.

Failure in school or learning problems are sometimes the first evidence of developmental difficulties. Understanding of this field has developed rapidly. It is important to recognize that failure in school is not necessarily caused by low IQ. Dyslexia (inability to read), hyperactivity syndrome, attention deficit, and emotional disturbance are some of the terms used for various causes.

Hyperactivity, with its usual accompanying symptom of school learning difficulty, may affect as many as 5 to 15 percent of children in grade school. The majority are boys. The characteristics include normal (or higher) intelligence but poor school performance, disorders of attention (short span and distractible), impulsiveness, and several types of specific problems with reading, spelling, arithmetic, or coordination. Diagnosis and management should be done by a team that includes the child's physician, school representatives, and specific therapists for reading or emotional upsets.

Hyperactivity and learning problems are a specific problem mainly in relation to schooling. Many of these children, once they pass this hurdle, do well during the rest of their lives.

PREVENTION: KEEPING CHILDREN HEALTHY

Accidents are the leading cause of death among children who have successfully passed the first month of life. The causes vary by age. Burns, falls, and poisonings are major causes in the preschool period, and drowning and motor vehicle accidents (both as a pedestrian and rider) are major causes during school ages. In adolescence, motor vehicle accidents (including motorcycles) are by far the major cause of death and serious injury.

There generally are two approaches to accident prevention. One is to make the environment safe, and the other is to teach children to practice safe habits of living. By far, the first approach has been most successful to date. Examples are child-resistant caps on medicines and household poisons, grilles on windows of buildings to prevent falls, flame retardant nightwear, and motorcycle helmets. Many states now require automobile safety seats for babies and young children, and the use of seat belts for older children.

The chart opposite includes a list of common accidents and accepted preventive measures by age group. Each age has its own risks and its own priority for prevention.

Life-Style to Promote Health

Medical care for illness has limited effectiveness. The ways we live, eat, exercise, handle stress, and use alcohol and tobacco are important in determining how healthy we are as adults. "A Preventive Approach to Health" is outlined in Chapter 1. Its principles apply to children as well as to adults and should be taught by word and precept in the family.

KEEPING CHILDREN SAFE

Typical Accidents	Normal Behavior Characteristics	Precautions
First Year		
Falls, inhalation of foreign objects, poisonings, burns, drownings	After several months of age can squirm and roll, and later creeps and pulls self erect. Places anything and everything in mouth. Helpless in water.	Do not leave alone on tables, from which falls can occur. Keep crib sides up. Keep small objects and harmful substances out of reach. Do not leave alone in tub of water.
Second Year		
Falls, drowning, motor vehicles, ingestion of poisonous substances, burns	Able to roam about in erect posture, goes up and down stairs, has great curiosity, puts almost anything in mouth, helpless in water.	Keep screens in windows. Place gate at top of stairs. Cover unused electrical outlets. Keep cords out of easy reach. Keep in enclosed space when outdoors and not in company of an adult. Keep medicine, household poisons, and small sharp objects out of sight and reach. Keep handles of pots and pans on stove out of reach, and containers of hot foods away from edge of table. Protect from water in tub and pools.
2 to 4 Years		
Falls, drowning, motor vehicles, ingestion of poisonous substances, burns	Able to open doors, runs and climbs, can ride tricycle, investigates closets and drawers, plays with mechanical gadgets, can throw ball and other objects.	Keep doors locked when there is a danger of falls. Place screen or guards in windows. Teach about watching for automobiles in driveways and in streets. Keep firearms locked up. Keep knives, electrical equipment out of reach. Teach about risks of throwing sharp objects and about danger of following ball into the street.
School Age		
Falls, drowning, burns, pedestrian auto accidents	Adventuresome	Safe school playgrounds, supervised swimming pools, helmets and leg and arm pads for skateboarding, play off streets.
Adolescent		
Auto accidents, falls	Peer pressure, athletic drive	Seat belt use, safe driving, no driving with alcohol, supervised sports in age appropriate competition, use of helmets for motorcycles and bicycles.

CHAPTER 30

EMOTIONAL AND MENTAL HEALTH

When a person is psychologically healthy, he or she enjoys an inner sense of well-being and an ability to function well in the world. A healthy person can cope with the problems of everyday living, feel emotion, love others, work successfully, play with enjoyment, and be reasonably optimistic about the future. When stress comes along, he or she can react flexibly, according to the needs of the situation, not in an inflexible, rigid way. Psychological health enables a person to balance his or her own interests and needs for self-expression with responsibilities to family and community.

THE ORIGINS OF EMOTIONS AND BEHAVIOR

Why do we feel the way we feel? What makes us behave the way we behave? Those who study the subject conclude that a complex interweaving of psychological, biological, and social factors determines each individual's pattern of feelings and behavior. The process begins early in life, even before birth.

Psychological Factors

A long-standing psychological explanation for behavior is based on the ideas of unconscious conflict. According to this theory, we all enter life with a certain set of basic drives and wishes. These include the drive to have what we want when we want it, to experience pleasure rather than pain, to be unconditionally approved and supported, and to be angry and retaliate when we are frustrated or deprived. Some psychologists would include the sexual drive, and others would include aggression. We also develop an inner sense of prohibition against these drives and wishes, producing potential for conflict. Because everyone has a similar set of drives, society has established taboos and regulations to make for order, further increasing the likelihood of a clash. That is why we all must learn to control our feelings, to delay gratification, and in general, to follow the rules instead of the drives. Because this is a compromise solution, the price paid by everyone is the potential for conflict, which generally remains unconscious. The psychologically healthy person is one who can work out ways to balance several conflicting pulls.

Another ingredient in healthy psychological growth is freedom from truly excessive stress or deprivation. A child whose life situation is too disadvantaged and whose minimal survival needs are not met may not develop healthy ways of coping with life. (Some children, however, have a combination of perceptions, ingenuity, talents, and resources that enables them to rise above an early life of unfortunate circumstances.)

The interaction between a child and the most significant caretaking person (in our culture, usually the mother) is another major determinant of early development. The ideal caretaker embodies qualities that facilitate optimum psychological growth in the child. These include three abilities: to strike a balance between unqualified loving and limit-setting, to encourage the development of innate skills and talents, and to gradually help the child enter and master the larger world of the community while still providing his or her basic needs for nurture, attachment, and closeness within the family. Parents obviously are less effective if they are immature and self-centered, depressed, chronically resentful of the burden of the child, obsessed with their own occupation, or more seriously emotionally ill. Marital strain, open quarreling, and a general atmosphere of unhappiness and discontent also can take their toll on a child's development.

Relatives, neighbors, teachers, and siblings can compensate for parental deficiencies and other deprivations. This wider network always is necessary to broaden a child's perspective and to serve as models in adapting to life situations.

According to these notions of personality development, basic habits are learned early. If learning has been faulty, the resulting habits can be self-destructive and impede further learning. But in advantageous circumstances, early self-destructive habits can be modified and replaced by better ones, even after adolescence.

Social Factors

A person's mental health and social environment are intricately interwoven. Abnormal behavior as well as overt psychiatric symptoms can be brought on or changed by social and cultural conditions. Undesirable circumstances (low social class, poverty, sexism, racism, discrimination, and lack of family support) correlate with poor psychological adjustment (stress, anxiety, depression, role confusion, a sense of helplessness, and failure to achieve potential). The fact that these frequently occur together does not necessarily mean that one always causes the other. Many mentally ill persons have never experienced these adverse conditions.

Overall, there is a direct relationship between economic position and mental health. Greater numbers of poor people suffer from more serious psychological disorders, especially psychoses, addictions, and alcoholism. A sense of hopelessness and a perception of inability to improve one's life undoubtedly contribute to psychological problems. Still, many people respond to social instability and precarious life situations creatively and constructively, so the poor are not inevitably vulnerable to psychological problems, nor are the rich immune.

Second-class status can be a powerful determinant of how people adjust. Our society defines "nonwhites" as inferior. If there are no strong countervailing family traditions or personal resources to draw upon, a nonwhite child may grow up with a poorly formed identity or sense of self, and low self-esteem. Our society remains pervaded by institutional racism, with its systematic barriers to the acquisition of power by nonwhites. Reactions to such limitations can be lowered self-esteem, rage, chronic stress, and anxiety.

Social attitudes and institutions communicate the same message of inferiority to women. As more women have begun to work outside the home in recent years, they have come into closer contact with overt discrimination. This problem has been compounded by the expectation that employed women also will handle the full burden of responsibility for child-rearing and running a household. Society's acceptance of role change for women has been slow. For many women, this period of transition and upheaval frequently brings frustration, guilt, a sense of inadequacy, and particularly lowered self-esteem.

The full-time mother who does not work outside the home runs different risks. Her self-esteem may be too dependent on the success of her children and her husband. She also faces a paradoxical situation. Having fulfilled the idealized role of full-time mother, she nevertheless receives a major portion of blame if her child does not develop well. Even if she enjoys her role, she sometimes fears that employed women will scorn her.

The social institution of the family has a powerful impact upon all of its members. The extended family—a network of aunts, uncles, grandparents, cousins, close friends, and neighbors—is an invaluable resource for development and growth. The recent decline of the extended family has been accompanied by the predominance of the nuclear family—two parents and their children—that is relatively isolated from the informal presence of relatives and others. Also, divorce and single-parent households have come to be much more acceptable social patterns. Households composed of several adults and children have been shown to be as effective as the husband-wife nuclear family in fostering psychological growth in children. A full understanding of the effects of changing household patterns on mental health remains incomplete, however.

Evidence does exist that social change of any kind produces strain for all involved. We also know that individuals with more supportive social contacts, such as marriage, frequent visits with relatives and friends, church participation, and group participation, tend to live longer, experience fewer illnesses, and cope better with minor and major life stresses.

Biological Factors

The body regulates itself through a vast network of interdependent biological systems that operate with chemical and electrical responses to signals from the environment or other body systems. Automatic feedback allows these systems to work together for smooth functioning physically, emotionally, and behaviorally. Each system is regulated much as a thermostat regulates temperature in a room. Malfunction of any of these regulating mechanisms can lead to an exaggeration or a deficit in chemical and electrical events in the body. Automatic smooth function then is disrupted. The brain is the organ in closest touch with the environment. It also is the major organ regulating the responses of other body systems. Sophisticated and delicate research techniques now make it possible to measure changes in brain function so that brain activity can be experimentally altered and then correlated with behavior. Resulting theories propose that electrical and chemical abnormalities in brain function contribute significantly to psychiatric illnesses and other disorders of feeling and behavior.

The brain is composed of billions of cells called neurons (see Chapter 11, "The Brain and Nervous System"). The circuit construction of the brain consists of an astronomical number of connections among these neurons. The neurons communicate bits of information to one another by transferring minuscule amounts of chemicals (neurotransmitters) across tiny spaces (synapses) between the cells. The transfer occurs because an impulse is generated in certain specialized parts of the cell. The information passed from cell to cell in this system is the physical basis for thinking, moving, perceiving, remembering, and virtually every other human psychological dimension.

For human beings to function best, nerve cells and circuits must develop normally and be maintained in good working order. Scientists cannot yet even begin to visualize how prenatal events or factors of early childhood such as maternal attention or hours spent watching television can influence the development of the brain systems that control behavior and feelings. Fortunately, there is increasing evidence that injured child and adult brains can compensate for impairments and learn new ways to accomplish lost functions. But a full scientific understanding of the biological bases of psychiatric illness is a hope for the future.

In explaining individual qualities and tendencies, the ancient division between heredity (that with which one is born) and environment (that which is shaped by upbringing and life experience) is as significant today as it has been for centuries. Preliminary studies indicate that the basis of individual temperament may be partially genetically determined. Each person has relatively fixed and enduring personality traits and predictable emotional and behavioral responses to life situations.

Clearly then, the quality of the relationship between an infant and parent is not determined entirely by the parents' personality or "parenting ability." A parent will respond quite differently to a naturally quiet, receptive, predictable baby than to an irritable, jittery, unsmiling one. This is an example of the complex interplay between heredity and environment and the difficulty of isolating biological and psychological factors.

Many psychiatric abnormalities presumably involve an inherited predisposition. They include schizophrenia, manic-depressive disease, certain other types of depression, obsessive-compulsive personality disorder, and phobic personality disorder, all of which are discussed later.

DISORDERS OF EMOTION AND BEHAVIOR

Development and Adjustment

Personality development begins early but continues beyond childhood. The personality can grow and mature throughout the adult years. Each new stage of life necessitates coping with a different set of "crises." At each level, we must reexamine our sense of identity (who we are), interpersonal relationships, career and other goals, values, and perspective on life and death.

When a person moves from childhood through adolescence to adulthood, the time comes to alter the image of parents as all-knowing guides and ever-available sources of support, to acquire adult values and ethics, to solidify gender identity, and to make vocational choices. In early adulthood, one must go on to explore alternatives in many areas, making decisions about career, marriage, parenthood, and life-style. Those who make these transitions in their early twenties are in the position, by their mid-thirties, to reassess whether the earlier decisions are appropriate for their current life. Commitments are reexamined and are either altered or strengthened.

Middle life typically is characterized either by achievement of stability, with continuing productivity and contributions to the future, or by stagnation. For both men and women, many important changes in biological function occur. Inevitable experiences require significant adjustment. They include the success or failure of career and other activities, illness and death of parents, and independence of children. There is an increasing awareness of the passing of generations.

The later years also can be marked by difficult circumstances—the waning of intellectual and physical capacities, the loss of a spouse, declining energy and activity, occupational retirement, a decreasing sense of usefulness, and impending death.

Some stress may accompany each of these transitions. Because stress normally contributes to the continuing development and growth of the personality, management of these transitional states brings the opportunity to move toward either more effective or more disorganized functioning. In the process of adapting to change, we can learn more innovative problem-solving techniques and develop more creative and mature modes of coping. Or, if the necessary adjustment is greater than the person can accomplish, adaptation fails, and inappropriate, less-mature styles reemerge. Occasionally, severe and long-standing emotional disorders can result. The actual outcome depends on the stability of the person's personality, the extent of his or her social support network, and the presence of circumstances of deprivation. But it is probably safe to say that almost everyone who goes through the transitional phases of life experiences some degree of stress.

Adjustment disorder is the psychiatric term for poor response of short duration to these transitional stresses. The severity of the maladjustment can range from mild anxiety to serious physical or emotional symptoms. An adolescent who was too dependent on his parents as a child may develop physical illness on leaving for college, so that departure is postponed. An intelligent, competent woman who neglected her own personal development after marriage to stay home may begin to experience anxiety attacks after the birth of a third child.

All these situations also may involve underlying psychiatric problems. But the symptoms that develop at the time of the life-stage transition can be considered a separate disorder if the person soon returns to his or her previous behavior after the milestone is passed.

The diagnosis of adjustment disorder also applies to a poor response to inordinate stress in other situations. Again, the symptoms can be mild to severe, but recede as the situation improves. A man who dropped out of high school, drifts from job to job, and has no stable, intimate relationship may experience the symptoms of a classical depression when fired by his employer if he has no savings and is refused state aid. But if his financial status is stabilized, he returns to his own characteristic level of functioning. Clearly, the man has long-standing problems of psychological maladjustment, but his depression is a separate, temporary disorder, induced by the situation and abated with elimination of the stress.

Divorce, severe marital discord, serious illness, lawsuits, and other life crises also can precipitate adjustment disorders. But these problems of living usually do not become chronically disabling, unless a sufficiently supportive environment is lacking, or the personality is not sufficiently flexible.

Character Disturbances And Neuroses

Everyone has a fairly constant personality style—predictable ways of perceiving the world and coping with opportunities, challenges, and misfortunes. Different individuals tend to be anxious, compulsive, depressed, passive and dependent, withdrawn, given to physical complaints, or flighty. This is simply "the way they are." Under stress, these modes of behavior or particular coping styles become exaggerated, but remain simply extreme forms of the individual's usual traits.

In some persons, however, the collection of traits is so pronounced that it interferes with normal functioning. People whose persistent behavior patterns fit this description fall into one of two categories, usually classified as personality, or character, disorders or neuroses.

Personality disorders range from mild to severe. When the disorder is mild, the person's behavior resembles normal functioning. A person with a moderate disorder usually is viewed as eccentric. Severe disorders can be genuinely disabling. The significant feature of a personality disorder is that the persons seldom are made uncomfortable by its existence. Their behavior is not accompanied by anxiety, unlike neurotics, and they do not view themselves as ill. In fact, they may deny that the behavior pattern exists. If they admit that it does exist, they may deny that it is abnormal. For this reason, they seldom respond well to psychotherapy.

Obsessive-compulsive personalities are perfectionistic and competitive. They are preoccupied with punctuality, orderliness, cleanliness, and doing things just right. Commonly, these persons engage in repetitive rituals, like incessantly checking gas jets, or always touching or arranging objects in a certain, unvarying order. Obsessive-compulsive people crave work, whether exalted or trivial. They are ambitious, and need to control everything. Often they cannot express feelings, and, indeed, may even lack the ability to experience them.

Passive-aggressive personalities express anger in disguised ways. Procrastination, stubbornness, inefficiency, "forgetting," and negativism characterize these people. While appearing to comply, they, in fact, manage subtly to defy authority. By seeming to be helpless and needy, they provocatively manipulate the surroundings toward their own needs.

Hysterical or histrionic personalities are emotionally overreactive and dramatic. They need to be the center of attention and are preoccupied with their appearance and the impression they make on people. They may seem to be sexually preoccupied, but they simply wish to be taken care of and treated as special.

Schizoid personalities are loners. They have few friends and little social life. They are shy, reclusive, and avoid intimacy. They seem aloof, cold, detached, and sometimes bland.

Antisocial personalities are impulsive, untrustworthy, and irresponsible toward persons and property. Some, such as the confidence man, are experts at mobilizing people and manipulating them to their own ends. They transgress rules and regulations, but they experience little guilt and do not respond to punishment. They do not appear to distinguish right from wrong.

The cause of personality disorders is poorly understood. There is some evidence that genetically determined traits may contribute. Faulty learning patterns and defective problem-solving techniques may be involved, too.

Grossly disturbed family settings tend to produce individuals with personality disorders more often than do smoothly functioning families. The former include families in which one parent controls and dominates, families in which the child is scapegoated so parents can avoid facing marital difficulties, and settings in which the child is taught that the world is not to be trusted, or that other people must be outsmarted and cheated if one is to get ahead. Undoubtedly, the role of social and economic deprivation also is important. But even the best environment does not guarantee the best outcome in some cases.

Neuroses are defined by specific, persistent patterns of responses to life events. Unlike those with character disorders, however, people with neuroses experience uncomfortable symptoms. Psychiatrists and psychologists classify them into three main groups, but many people have neurotic difficulties that fail to fit into any of these formal categories.

Anxiety neurosis. Anxiety in response to an unpleasant memory or the anticipation of an unpleasant experience is common, normal, and necessary. But a diffuse feeling of anxiety not related to a specific cause is not normal. This state, known as free-floating anxiety, is characterized by a sense of dread or panic and a feeling that something terrible is about to happen. Physical symptoms are common—tensed muscles, chest pain, fast heart rate, abdominal cramps, and light-headedness. The attacks may come several times daily to once every few months. Anxiety neurosis sometimes shows a strong family history. Some people have intermittent, incapacitating "panic attacks" that appear unrelated to precipitating events or to behavior at other times, and some specialists believe these may have a congenital, neurological basis.

Phobic neurosis is characterized by irrational fear in the presence of or anticipation of harmless objects or situations. Phobic persons may fear insects, enclosed spaces, open spaces, high places, or driving in an automobile. Phobias can develop suddenly or gradually, and can appear intermittently or so continuously that the person is virtually incapacitated.

Phobics are aware that their fears are irrational, yet the sensations of panic or losing control are so intolerable that the precipitating situations or objects must be avoided at all costs, and they develop elaborate measures to ward them off. A person with a phobic fear of water may walk several blocks out of his way to avoid passing a building with a fountain in the lobby.

Obsessive-compulsive neurosis, unlike the obsessive-compulsive personality disorder, is characterized by conscious anxiety at the time of the obsessive thoughts and compulsive acts. Patients with this disorder can be severely disabled. A typical obsession is the persistent intrusion of an unwanted thought or urge over which the person has no control. Intrusive swear words, sexual images, or something as simple as a fragment of a song are common. The person then is unable to concentrate on anything else or even to hold a conversation.

Compulsive rituals vary from simple actions to complex behavioral patterns. One of the most common compulsive rituals, repeated hand washing, usually is associated with overwhelming fear of dirt and contaminants. The practice can lead to inflammation or even ulceration of the hands and arms. Often the normal activities of living are impeded because the ritual occupies so much time.

Psychosis

Psychosis is not a specific clinical diagnosis, but rather a descriptive term. It denotes significant or serious loss of contact with reality. The current definition of psychosis roughly corresponds to such earlier terms as "madness" or "lunacy."

Schizophrenic patients appear psychotic only during the periods in which symptoms are severe, although symptoms may continue in a less noticeable form during periods of remission. Patients with mania, depression, paranoid states, and organic brain syndromes can be intermittently psychotic. Many diseases, injuries, and drug reactions can produce temporary psychological illness of psychotic proportions.

Schizophrenia

Schizophrenias are a group of diseases that are among the most severe and disabling of mental illnesses. These diseases are characterized by disorders of thinking, perception, feeling, behavior, and social relationships.

A schizophrenic's thinking tends to be illogical or controlled by a private logic that others do not understand. Connections between one thought and the next are not apparent, and rapid shifts in content occur. Thoughts may come very slowly and with great difficulty, or may seem to be interrupted suddenly. The capacity for abstract thinking frequently is impaired. Schizophrenics may experience delusions, strongly held false beliefs that cannot be changed despite reason or evidence to the contrary. They may be certain that others control them or their thoughts, or that they are being harassed, followed, or tortured. The most common schizophrenic perceptual distortions are auditory hallucinations, in which the person "hears" a voice talking to or about him.

The expression of feelings in schizophrenia tends to be reduced in intensity and frequency. Emotional response is shallow, and the experience of pleasure is rare. He or she may react inappropriately, such as laughing on hearing sad news.

Schizophrenics have difficulty establishing close relationships, and tend to withdraw into a world of their own. The range of isolation includes simple shyness to total reclusiveness. As the condition gradually worsens, patients may ignore personal cleanliness, appearance, and social decorum, and may assume bizarre habits and life-styles.

Most specialists now agree that schizophrenia actually is several different diseases. Some patients pursue a relentless downhill course. They experience frequent psychotic episodes, with general personality deterioration between episodes. Other patients have intermittent psychotic periods, but function fairly normally between those periods. They do not deteriorate with time. About one-fourth recover permanently, however, and another one-fourth have long-lasting periods of recovery.

There are many theories about the cause of schizophrenia. Heredity undoubtedly plays an important predisposing role. Current research implicates a genetic component in as many as 40 percent of cases. One actively pursued avenue of research blames an upset in the brain's neurotransmitters, the chemicals that carry messages between cells. The significance of psychological and social factors—parent-child interaction, family relationships, and environmental stress—has not been reliably assessed. But there is no doubt that biological, psychological, and social factors interact in complex ways.

Affective (Mood) Disorders

What specialists call "affective" disorders are those characterized by disturbances of mood.

Depression. Virtually everyone experiences occasional periods of depression, usually precipitated by a stressful event. The most predictable depression is grief following the loss of a loved one. These depressions are appropriate and usually short-lived, and they are only mildly and temporarily disruptive of normal activities and enjoyment.

The psychiatric disorder known as depression is more serious, involving changes in mood, perception and thinking, and bodily function. One-fifth of Americans are said to have an episode of depression at some time in their lives; it is the psychiatric disorder for which most people seek help. The person feels sad, discouraged, and sometimes irritable. Crying spells are frequent. He or she may be beset by inappropriate feelings of guilt, a decreased sense of self-worth, helplessness, hopelessness, and a loss of interest in and pleasure from usual activities. The most frequent changes in body function are decreased appetite, weight loss, constipation, and sleep disturbances (usually early awakening). Thinking is slowed, and is characterized by difficulty in concentrating and by indecisiveness. Thoughts of suicide are common, and all too frequently are acted upon.

One form of depression seems to involve no perception of depressed mood by the patient. Rather, he or she describes only a physical problem, related to any organ system, for which no cause can be found. This form of "masked" depression is particularly common in the elderly.

Depression actually may be several distinct diseases resembling one another but characterized by different causes, courses, and degrees of responsiveness to treatment.

Depressions triggered by an event may actually differ from those apparently unrelated to any specific happening, some specialists believe. A given experience can have great significance to one person and very little to someone else. The meaning of the event or loss to the individual seems to be the important factor. Another group of patients has a depressive disease with episodes appearing "to come out of the blue."

Mania is characterized by a general speeding up of most functions. The person's mood is elevated, expansive, fluctuating, or irritable. Speech is rapid; rhyming and punning are common. Thinking is easily distracted, with rapid shifting from one topic to another. The need for sleep is markedly reduced, energy level is very high, and self-esteem is inflated. Mania is usually a recurrent disease.

Manic-depressive disease is characterized by intermittent episodes of both mania and depression. (The American Psychiatric Association now officially uses the classification "Major Affective Disorder, Bipolar" for mania and manic-depressive disease, and "Major Affective Disorder, Depression" for depression.)

Evidence indicates that at least some forms of affective disorders probably run in families. A higher incidence also has been demonstrated in persons or families with a history of alcoholism. Scientists have noted changes in the chemical functioning of the brain that point toward a biological basis for some depressions and for mania. There is some evidence for a genetic marker for certain forms of the disease.

Suicide is the most serious outcome of depression and mania. Between 5 and 15 percent of depressed patients succeed in killing themselves. Although they frequently make explicit reference to their suicidal impulses, families and physicians tend to minimize them. Subtle clues include talking about taking a long trip, suddenly making a will and putting affairs in order, and preoccupation with death or with suicide of a friend.

Family and friends should be alert for depression and suicidal thinking in persons who are isolated and alone, who have experienced a recent loss, or who are chronically ill.

LIFE EVENTS AND STRESS

Rank	Life Event	Mean Value
1	Death of spouse	100
2	Divorce	73
3	Marital separation	65
4	Jail term	63
5	Death of close family member	63
6	Personal injury or illness	53
7	Marriage	50
8	Fired at work	47
9	Marital reconciliation	45
10	Retirement	45
11	Change in health of family member	44
12	Pregnancy	40
13	Sex difficulties	39
14	Gain of new family member	39
15	Business adjustment	39
16	Change in financial state	38
17	Death of close friend	37
18	Change to different line of work	36
19	Change in number of arguments with spouse	35
20	Mortgage over $10,000	31
21	Foreclosure of mortgage or loan	30
22	Change in responsibilities at work	29
23	Son or daughter leaving home	29
24	Trouble with in-laws	29
25	Outstanding personal achievement	28
26	Wife begins or stops work	26
27	Beginning or ending of school	26
28	Change in living conditions	25
29	Revision of personal habits	24
30	Trouble with boss	23
31	Change in work hours or conditions	20
32	Change in residence	20
33	Change in schools	20
34	Change in recreation	19
35	Change in church activities	19
36	Change in social activities	18
37	Mortgage or loan less than $10,000	17
38	Change in sleeping habits	16
39	Change in number of family get-togethers	15
40	Change in eating habits	15
41	Vacation	13
42	Christmas	12
43	Minor violations of the law	11

The stress events can trigger medical illness. Some are more likely to do so than others. The Social Readjustment Rating Scale, compiled by Drs. Thomas Holmes and Richard Rahe of the University of Washington, rates 43 events in terms of their impact on health. The effects of these are cumulative—the more such events experienced in a single year, the greater the likelihood that the person will become ill. A total of 150 to 199 points in a year on this scale carries moderate risk of health problems. Accumulating 200 to 299 points carries medium risk, and 300 points or more brings severe risk. Although many events are "positive," it is the experience of change that provides the stress.

Disorders with Prominent Physical Symptoms

Stress. Stress is a way of describing what happens to an organism that must cope with change. Psychological and physiological mechanisms aim to maintain stability while simultaneously adjusting to stressful events in the environment.

Some people cope; others do not. Response depends on a variety of factors: how the demand of the situation is perceived, habit, early life experiences, temperament, personality and the range of coping responses, the capacity to learn new habits, and the social support system.

However, it seems that any disruption of the steady state takes its toll on the human body and psyche. The simple experience of normal life events, positive and negative, has a cumulative effect on physiological and psychological health even when a person adapts well. The greater the magnitude and number of life changes during a given period, the greater the likelihood a person will develop physical and psychiatric symptoms. Individuals who experience two to three times the expected number of life changes in a year are at much greater than average risk of developing a fatal heart attack within a year or two of the changes, for instance.

Psychophysiological disorders. According to one theory, psychophysiological disorders are the physical expression of emotional states kept out of awareness. The person is unaware of the psychological upset and instead develops a backache, headache, nausea, or other physical symptoms. The person presumably cannot tolerate an unpleasant emotion, yet is unable to alter circumstances to eliminate the source of stress. As a result, a physical symptom develops rather than a phobia or a compulsion.

A specific event appears to act as a trigger. A patient may be admonished by an employer or experience a rejection (actual or perceived) from an important or respected person. Or it may be the anniversary of a death or other significant loss. The reaction to the event could be rage, helplessness, or loss of self-esteem, but the ultimate response is pain, diarrhea, or chest tightness.

Repeated occurrence of the same pattern can result in exaggerated and sustained physiological changes. Traditionally, asthma, ulcerative colitis, peptic ulcer, essential hypertension, and some skin diseases have at times been referred to as "psychosomatic" diseases.

Hypochondriasis. "Hypochondriac" is a term commonly applied to people who have many longstanding physical complaints. Hypochondriasis superficially can resemble a psychophysiological disorder but is very different in origin and response. True hypochondriacs are characterized by a remarkable preoccupation with physical symptoms, actually organizing their lives around their presumed illness. The more a doctor attempts to reassure them, the worse they feel.

It is clear that hypochondriacs genuinely suffer, yet the reasons they experience pain and remain so preoccupied with their symptoms are not clear.

Hypochondriasis seems to be a face-saving device for people who want to be taken care of. The "physical" illness also serves as a ticket of admission to doctor and hospital care, and a legitimate reason for being dependent on others and being unable to carry out responsibilities.

Organic disease. Many physical illnesses masquerade as psychiatric disorders, with emotional symptoms among the most noticeable features. Between 10 and 30 percent of patients admitted to psychiatric clinics have a physical illness that accounts for their psychiatric distress.

Disease of virtually every organ and metabolic system can have psychological symptoms. Anyone who experiences emotional or behavioral changes should have a thorough physical evaluation before assuming a psychiatric cause is responsible for the symptoms.

Disorders of Aging

Organic brain syndromes are characterized by the gradual onset of disordered thinking, perception, and behavior. Persons lose recent memory, forget names, and become disoriented. These symptoms once were categorized as senility and an inevitable consequence of growing older. They now are often recognized as evidence of Alzheimer's disease, an untreatable neurological disorder described in Chapter 11, "The Brain and Nervous System."

However, many treatable conditions also may account for these symptoms. They include heart failure, low blood sugar, thyroid disease, and poor nutrition, as well as side effects of certain prescription and nonprescription drugs. Psychological stress also may induce the condition temporarily.

Depression. Mild to serious depression in the elderly often shows the classical clinical symptoms described earlier. Very commonly, though, the depression is masked, presenting itself in the form of multiple physical complaints or vague physical decline. These masked depressions can cause the patient to withdraw, which in turn can lead to malnutrition, vitamin deficiency, and dehydration.

The most seriously misdiagnosed depression of the elderly mimics Alzheimer's disease. Memory loss, forgetfulness, and confusion actually are signs of depression in these cases. Most depression of the elderly responds to treatment, but depression must be identified before it can be treated. Sadly, many cases are neglected because they are incorrectly diagnosed as untreatable.

Sexual Dysfunction

Sexual dysfunction often has an emotional basis. Both physical and psychological causes of sexual problems are discussed in Chapter 25, "The Male Reproductive System," and Chapter 26, "The Female Reproductive System."

PSYCHIATRIC TREATMENT

Perhaps as many as 200 treatments for psychiatric disorders have been given names and called therapies.

Psychological Therapies

Psychological therapies aim to modify undesirable personal characteristics—feelings, attitudes, responses, and behaviors.

Psychoanalysis. In psychoanalysis, patient and analyst work together to understand how troublesome feelings and behaviors relate to earlier life events. The goal is to rework unconscious conflicts. Previous response patterns are changed and symptoms are relieved because core components of the personality are changed. Psychoanalysis requires several sessions weekly and lasts from two to five years or more.

Insight therapy aims at understanding and eliminating certain psychological conflicts in order to bring about symptom relief. Attention is directed toward current interpersonal difficulties. Therapy takes place one to three times weekly, and lasts one or two weeks to several years.

Relationship therapy tries to help a relatively immature or underdeveloped personality to grow. Patient and physician focus on new techniques of problem solving. Family contacts and medication are employed as necessary. Relationship therapy tends to be shorter than other forms of therapy.

Supportive therapy does not aim at major symptom relief. Rather, the goal is to provide support during difficult and stressful situations and to help a patient "return to normal."

Behavioral Therapy

The theory of behavioral therapy is that maladaptive responses are undesirable habits that have been learned over a period of time, and that new and more adaptive habits can be learned to replace them. The reasons for the symptoms are less important.

Each response or symptom is described by the patient as explicitly and objectively as possible. What else was happening at the time is noted, too. The patient may keep a careful diary, detailing each occasion of response and the surrounding events. Once the connection between events and response becomes clear, an attempt is made to learn new ways of reacting.

These techniques have had some success in the treatment of phobias, severe obsessions and compulsions, intense anxiety states, and sexual dysfunction. The techniques frequently are employed for treating addictive disorders such as alcoholism, drug abuse, obesity, and smoking.

Biofeedback attempts to train the mind to control bodily reactions, such as regulating blood pressure, for instance. Biofeedback has shown some success in the amelioration of symptoms that are based on stress.

Group Therapy

Group therapy encompasses a wide range of treatment rationales and goals.

Supportive or counseling groups aim to maintain and strengthen healthy parts of an individual personality. Participants focus on the skills of interacting with others, and on conscious problems of living.

In general, anyone who can benefit from individual therapy also can benefit from group sessions. Patients with all types of neuroses respond well, but particularly those who have difficulty dealing with others, who are competitive, or who feel uncomfortable in close relationships.

Marital Therapy

Marital therapy aims to help relatively stable couples who have conflicts with emotional, sexual, social, financial, or child-rearing problems. This form of treatment has become more important in recent years, with change in the family, more open relationships and alternatives to marriage, and the decline in previously supportive institutions, such as the extended family and the church.

The goal of marital therapy is to help the individual partners as well as the couple as a unit, because the relationship itself can maintain and worsen individual problems, but it can succeed only if both partners have a genuine motivation to explore and change the relationship. If one participates only to please or pacify the other, results usually are poor. However, even if divorce is the eventual outcome, therapy often can reduce vindictiveness and unhappiness.

Family Therapy

Family therapy focuses not only on the individual's personality and past development but also on each person as a member of the family. Emphasis is on understanding how individual behavior originates in the family's needs and expectations, and how the behavior then feeds back into the family to further influence the interactions.

Drug Treatment

Treatment of psychiatric disorders has been revolutionized by the introduction and widespread use of effective medications.

Antipsychotic agents can be effective in treating some aspects of schizophrenia, severe manic-depressive illness, psychotic depressions, and paranoid states. The drugs reduce agitation and calm the person's emotions. They also diminish hyperactivity, disturbances of thinking, hallucinations, and delusions. Secondarily, withdrawal and social isolation are lessened.

Drugs cannot change unfavorable life situations, but they can reduce their impact. However, all of these drugs interact extensively with other kinds of medication, and careful medical monitoring is essential.

Antidepressant drugs are quite successful for some patients, especially those whose depressions cause difficulties of sleeping and eating, constipation, and slow movement. Patients who have intermittent recurrent depression and who respond to medication often continue to take the drug for some time after the symptoms have subsided to avoid a relapse.

Some depressed persons experience only partial improvement of their symptoms. Patients with low-grade continuous depression actually respond better to psychotherapy than drugs. For patients who do respond to antidepressants, a combination of drugs and psychotherapy often is used.

Tricyclic antidepressants are the most commonly used of these drugs. They must be administered for approximately three weeks to produce a change in mood. Side effects include sedation, dry mouth, constipation, and blurred vision. In the elderly, tricyclic antidepressants may have cardiac and urinary side effects. The antidepressants are continued in decreasing dosages for several months after the symptoms have subsided to ensure complete remission.

For very severe depressions of psychotic proportion, both antipsychotic agents and antidepressants are administered simultaneously during the first few weeks. Antidepressant medications also have been shown to be effective for some phobias and for anxiety states with panic attacks.

Lithium is the drug that is most effective for the treatment of mania and bipolar illness. It usually controls the acute episode within two weeks. Continued indefinitely, lithium can prevent future manic episodes or reduce their intensity and length. There is some indication that lithium also may help to prevent future episodes of depression in some patients with manic-depressive disease, and perhaps in some cases of recurrent depressive disease as well. Side effects include light-headedness, dizziness, sleepiness, staggering and numbness, and nausea and vomiting.

Antianxiety agents (tranquilizers) are the most commonly used prescription drugs of any type. Although most doctors and patients use these drugs wisely, overuse continues to be a matter of public concern.

When a patient reports nervousness to a doctor, both parties frequently find it easier to use a pill than to investigate the source of anxiety. Patients who are temporarily under unusual stress are frequently given a drug. So are those with mild character disorders that lead to a response of anxiety to the normal stresses of life. In actual fact, these people probably could control and reduce their anxiety simply by taking some time with their doctor to explore and understand the circumstances causing the upset, and then planning ways to deal with it.

Some patients improve simply because they are taking a pill and are in contact with a caring authority figure, the doctor. So the actual benefits of these drugs are difficult to measure. When correctly used, however, they can alleviate symptoms quickly, enabling the patient to adapt and learn alternative approaches to a problem.

Hospitalization

The number of persons hospitalized for psychiatric treatment has decreased dramatically in recent years. Hospitalization today is reserved primarily for short-term treatment of acute episodes of psychiatric illness. For chronic illnesses, intermittent hospitalization in combination with drug treatment after discharge results in shorter hospital stays and fewer episodes of rehospitalization. Nevertheless, certain patients with disorders difficult to treat, primarily schizophrenics, may require long-term or frequent hospitalization.

CHAPTER 31

CANCER

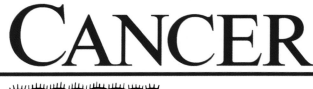

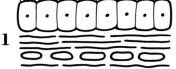

1

NORMAL LINING
OF A LUNG AND BRONCHUS

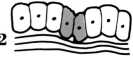

2

METAPLASIA
(changes)

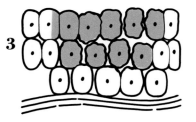

3

CARCINOMA-IN-SITU
(no penetration)

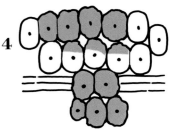

4

INVASIVE CANCER

THE PROGRESSION OF CANCER

*Cancer has six stages of development.
Drawing No. 1 shows the normal lining
of the small tube of the lung: a single
layer of cells with a brushlike border
(cilia) on a connective tissue base called
a basement membrane. Drawing No. 2
shows chronic injury to the cells from
smoking. They are disorganized, have
lost their cilia, and are piled up in more
than one layer in some places. This
stage is called metaplasia. In drawing
No. 3 the cells are visibly changed, with
many layers piled up, but have not
penetrated the basement membrane.
This stage is called carcinoma-in-situ.
In drawing No. 4 the abnormal cells
have broken through the basement
membrane into underlying tissue, the
stage known as invasive cancer. Drawing
No. 5 shows the stage called regional
metastasis. The cancer has reached the
lymph channel, and a colony has been
established in a lymph node. In drawing
No. 6 the bloodstream has carried
cancer cells to the brain and liver. This
final stage is called distant metastasis.*

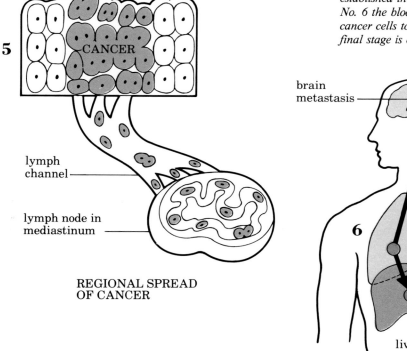

5   CANCER

lymph
channel

lymph node in
mediastinum

REGIONAL SPREAD
OF CANCER

brain
metastasis

6

liver
metastasis

DISTANT SPREAD OF CANCER

Cancer is not a single disease, but more than 100 different diseases with a common characteristic: abnormal growth, division, and proliferation of cells, which spread from their site of origin to other parts of the body, invading and destroying normal organs and tissues as they spread.

Cancer can arise in any part of the body. Earlier chapters have discussed specific forms of cancer (lung cancer in Chapter 10, "The Lungs," and leukemia in Chapter 7, "The Blood").

In all its forms, cancer is the second leading cause of death in the United States, trailing only heart disease. In recent years, there have been well over 900,000 new cases of cancer annually (excluding skin cancer) and nearly 500,000 deaths. However, cancer is by no means inevitably fatal, if recognized promptly and treated effectively. The percentage of cancer victims who survive five years after diagnosis—the relative survival rate—is estimated at 49 percent.

Cancer occurs most frequently among older people. More Americans live longer, surviving to the age at which cancer has always been most prevalent. When the figures are adjusted to reflect this shift, it can be seen that incidence and death from most forms of cancer have changed little. Some exceptions are the tragic increase in lung cancer, particularly among men, and more recently among women, and the steady decrease in stomach cancer in both sexes.

WHAT IS CANCER?

Cancer is an abnormality of body cells that have escaped from the body's controlled behavior patterns. How and why this escape occurs is one of science's major mysteries. It could be caused by a loss of "repressor" substances that presumably limit the activities of normal cells. Or it could be caused by the introduction of some outside substance such as a virus. It might be that a virus already present is activated by some other event.

The transformation of normal cells to cancer cells resembles a mutation, the sudden permanent change in cell composition caused by some force from outside that affects the cell. The altered cell then must survive and divide successfully to form a mass of abnormal cells. Possibly this progression is promoted by the addition of other substances or stimuli not in themselves cancer-producing, or by a drop in the defense mechanisms that normally protect the body against change. There is evidence that the abnormal cells sometimes reverse their behavior and return to normal, so the process may not be inevitably and invariably one-directional.

A mass of cells growing rapidly and independently and no longer contributing to normal organ function is called a tumor, or neoplasm. Not all tumors are cancerous. Some, which grow within a capsule and do not recur after removal, are called benign, although this does not mean they are always harmless. If they occur in vital organs or where there is limited space for expansion, such as within the skull, benign tumors can be life-threatening. Cancer, however, is said to be malignant because it always carries a capacity to kill.

Cancer's spread, called metastasis, is its distinctive and dangerous feature. As cancer cells multiply and grow, they invade the channels of the lymphatic system, or may penetrate blood vessels. The bloodstream or lymphatic system carries the cells to distant parts of the body, so that secondary colonies (metastases) may be established elsewhere. Because "curing" cancer means removing every last cancerous cell, a metastasized cancer is difficult, though not impossible, to eradicate.

We usually speak of three stages of cancer: (1) localized, when the cancer is limited to its original site; (2) regional, when it has reached adjacent organs or nearby lymph nodes; and (3) distant, or disseminated, when the cancer cells have been carried to other parts of the body.

THE CAUSES OF CANCER

Although hundreds of chemicals have been reported to produce cancers in experimental animals, only about two dozen have been verified as causes of cancer in man. Three are of general importance: (1) tobacco smoke products, especially cigarettes, which produce chemicals called polycyclic aromatic hydrocarbons; (2) asbestos, especially combined with smoking; and (3) excessive use of estrogens, the female sex hormones.

Tobacco smoking has caused widespread lung cancer and is associated with cancer of the mouth and esophagus, especially when combined with heavy drinking. Estrogens have been implicated in cancer of the uterus in women. Asbestos induces a high rate of cancer among those who work with it, especially if they also are smokers.

Among the industrial carcinogens, aromatic amines—used by dye manufacturers and by other industries—produce bladder cancer. Vinyl chloride induces a rare type of liver cancer among heavily exposed workers.

X rays or other forms of ionizing radiation can induce leukemia, thyroid cancer, and when the source is radium or plutonium, cancer of the bone. Sunlight induces skin cancer in people of light complexion (see Chapter 9, "The Skin").

Viruses have been demonstrated to cause certain uncommon forms of leukemia and lymphoma as well as several other forms of cancer. The Epstein-Barr virus is associated with a jaw cancer among African children, as well as cancer of the nasopharynx among southern Chinese. The hepatitis B virus is associated with liver cancer, and the human papilloma virus (HSV2) is associated with cancer of the cervix.

Cancer-causing (oncogenic) viruses consist of DNA or RNA, the nucleic acids that are the components of the genetic mechanism of all forms of life. In some way, these viruses become part of the structure of the cell, altering it in such a way that it has cancerous properties. It also has been demonstrated that such viruses may be present in the cell, yet latent and undetectable until aroused to activity by some precipitating event.

REACTIONS TO CANCER

Cancer, like any disease, occurs when some outside stimulus interacts with the body's disease-fighting immune system. The strength of our defenses is largely determined by genetic make-up—what we inherit from our mother and father.

There are a number of genetically determined cancers, all rather rare. One is cancer of the eye; others are multiple polyps of the colon that become cancerous, and xeroderma pigmentosum, a skin disease that develops into cancer. Some families experience aggregations of cancers. Women whose close female relatives have had breast cancer represent one such higher risk group.

Cancer cells require nutrients just as normal cells do. Therefore, diet must play a role in the development of cancer. In experimental animals, restricting food to levels that keep them lean but nutritionally well-fed not only reduces the occurrence of cancers, but lengthens the life span. Excess calories probably stimulate cancerous growth in human beings as well, so limiting one's food intake is sound advice, and it may protect against heart disease as well as cancer.

The body's immune system plays a role against cancer, as it does against any invader recognized as foreign. Individuals in whom the immune system is deficient or depressed are especially prone to develop cancers, as is seen in AIDS patients, who may fall victim to Kaposi's sarcoma.

CAN WE PREVENT CANCER?

A significant proportion of cancers can be prevented. Cancer of the lung is now the No. 1 cancer killer among both men and women. More than three-fourths of the cases of lung cancer are caused by smoking cigarettes.

Tobacco smoking also is involved in cancers of the mouth, pharynx, and esophagus, especially when combined with alcohol consumption and poor nutrition. And smoking is involved in cancer of the bladder. Alcohol, although not considered a primary carcinogen, is related to cancer of the liver. The elimination of tobacco smoking and of alcohol consumption, combined with proper nutrition, could reduce cancer cases by 30 percent.

Avoidance of unnecessary X-ray exposure and of too much sun are preventive steps individuals may take. Cancer prevention is best practiced as part of general health protection, as discussed in Chapter 1, "A Preventive Approach to Health."

Secondary Prevention

Recognizing cancer depends on being alert to certain signs and symptoms that may or may not mean that the disease is present. The American Cancer Society lists these seven warning signals:
- Change in bowel or bladder habits.
- A sore that does not heal.
- Unusual bleeding or discharge.
- Thickening or lump in a breast or elsewhere.
- Indigestion or difficulty in swallowing.
- Obvious change in a wart or mole.
- Nagging cough or hoarseness.

If these or other signs of abnormality or illness persist or progress for a few weeks, seek medical advice immediately.

The American Cancer Society recommends that women over age 40 should have a breast examination by a physician annually. They should examine their own breasts for lumps or changes every month, as illustrated in Chapter 27, "Cancer of the Breast," and have a baseline mammogram between ages 35 and 40. The cancer society also recommends a pelvic examination for uterine cancer every three years (and for sexually active teenagers) and regular "Pap" tests for cervical cancer—two initial tests a year apart, then a test at least every three years. The society recommends that both sexes should have annual rectal and stool tests for colon-rectal cancer after age 50, and visual examination by proctoscope every three to five years. Persons in high-risk groups, such as women with a family history of breast cancer, should have more frequent examinations.

TREATING CANCER

Doctors recognize three effective forms of cancer treatment:
- Surgery, removal of all or as much as possible of a cancer, and often of lymphatic structures through which cancer might spread.
- X ray and other controlled forms of radiation to destroy malignant cells.
- Chemotherapy, which is treatment with drugs or combinations of drugs.

Choice of treatment requires expert medical evaluation of a particular form of cancer in a particular patient. Specialists in cancer treatment (oncologists) often make this judgment. Some cancers are treatable by X rays; other forms are not, at least not in doses that can be tolerated by the patient. Forms of treatments may be combined or given in sequence. Radiation or chemotherapy may precede or follow breast cancer surgery.

Surgical techniques used in cancer treatment are described in Chapter 33, "Understanding Your Operation." Radiotherapy is described in Chapter 2, "Tests and Procedures," and in Chapter 27, "Cancer of the Breast."

Chemotherapy alone is used only for a few widely disseminated cancers that cannot be reached by other means. It has a high success rate in choriocarcinoma, a rare cancer in women; in acute lymphocytic leukemia, a blood cancer of children; and in testicular cancer. In combination with radiation, it has greatly improved the cure rate for Hodgkin's disease, a once fatal cancer of the lymphatic system.

Some prostate and breast cancers depend on hormones for growth. Antagonistic hormones may help in treatment of these cancers.

The Cure Rate for Cancer

For every type of cancer, the outlook, or prognosis, is much better if the tumor is removed or treated while still localized. The outlook becomes less favorable when the cancer has spread.

Doctors consider a cancer "cured" when the patient survives five years or longer after treatment, without recurrence of the disease. The cure rate by these standards is best for Hodgkin's disease, where the figure stands at 75 percent; childhood leukemia, 60 to 70 percent; and testicular cancer, 80 percent. Cancers of the uterus, cervix, and breast have a cure rate greater than 50 percent. For cancer of the colon and rectum, prostate, and bladder, the survival rate is between 30 and 50 percent. When the disease is treated while still localized, these figures can be nearly doubled. But for cancer of the esophagus, pancreas, and lungs, the percentage of cures is dismally low.

Effective treatment of cancer is, unfortunately, strenuous. Cancer surgery usually is radical, meaning that extensive tissue must be removed. Radiation treatment delivers doses that are lethal to cancer cells yet tolerable to the patient. Drugs used against cancer often have serious side effects.

More than half of all cancer patients die of or with their disease. The care of terminally ill patients is another serious medical and social problem. Hospices attempt to combine such care with emphasis on spiritual support and death with dignity. Increasingly, terminally ill cancer patients are allowed to live out their lives at home in familiar surroundings with loved ones nearby.

CHAPTER 32

INFECTIOUS DISEASES

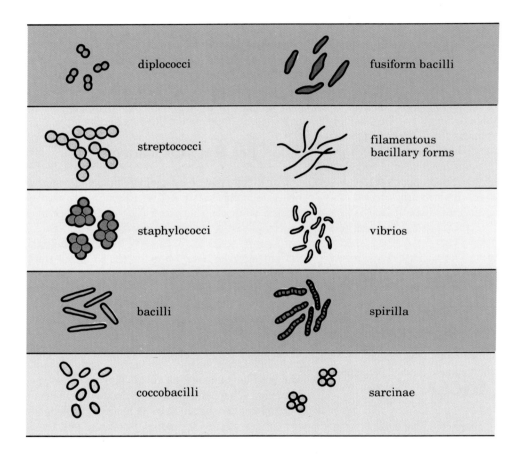

diplococci	fusiform bacilli
streptococci	filamentous bacillary forms
staphylococci	vibrios
bacilli	spirilla
coccobacilli	sarcinae

ONE FAMILY OF GERMS
Bacteria are among the most common disease-producing organisms, although the vast majority of bacteria are not harmful. They are found in many sizes, shapes, and configurations, 10 of which are shown here. The distinctive shape apparently is related to the organism's way of multiplying. The shapes enable microbiologists to identify which organisms are causing illness and to devise ways of treating them.

Infectious diseases are illnesses caused by germs. Germs are tiny living cells, so small they can be seen only with high-powered microscopes. Germs invade the tissues of our bodies, where they grow, multiply, and interfere with the normal functions of cells. Some of these germs manufacture and release poisons.

In general, infectious diseases target a particular organ or organ system, although the symptoms may be felt throughout the body.

Only a small minority of germs (or microbes) cause disease. They are divided into several categories, including bacteria, protozoa, and viruses. Bacteria are small, about $1/25{,}000$ of an inch long, and can be seen only with the highest magnifications of the ordinary light microscope. Bacteria normally are found in the body, especially in areas in contact with the environment, such as the skin, the mouth and nose, the intestinal tract, and the openings to the ears and to the genital organs. Streptococci and other unwanted bacteria inhabit the noses and throats of many persons without producing disease, and are spread via droplets of moisture exhaled in breathing. Therefore, certain disease-producing bacteria are carried in people who are apparently healthy, yet the bacteria are able to produce disease in them or in others, particularly if resistance is lowered.

Identification of bacteria—which indicates the best means of killing them—is the purpose of the bacteriological culture that is often taken during an illness, as described in Chapter 2, "Tests and Procedures."

Certain bacteria are known as higher bacteria because they tend to form branching cells and to appear as multicellular groups instead of single cells. Some of these become much like the smallest and simplest plants in their appearance. Some of these more complex bacteria also cause disease. Still larger and more complex are certain primitive plants known as fungi, the name given to common mushrooms and molds. Certain fungi also cause disease under certain circumstances. On the other hand, many of the higher bacteria and the fungi manufacture substances that kill off other bacteria. In recent years these substances have proven useful as medicines (antibiotics) to kill disease-producing bacteria.

Other types of microbes that are larger than bacteria are the protozoa, the smallest animal cells. Protozoa are found in soil, in ponds, on plants, in the body, and elsewhere. Some protozoa can produce disease. Still larger organisms that can produce disease are certain worms that become parasites. Parasites draw all of their nutrition from the host and live in or on the host. The ideal parasite does not kill the host so it can continue to live there. This is true of many worms.

Biological scientists discovered early in their research that there are materials that produce disease even when passed through filters so fine that they hold back all bacteria. This suggested that there was something in the filtered material that could produce disease, yet was too small to be seen by the ordinary microscope. Scientists called these mysterious organisms filterable viruses. In time, filterable viruses were detected using more advanced microscopes, and it now is clear that the diversity among viruses is as great as among bacteria. In contrast to most bacteria, viruses cannot multiply outside a living cell. Scientists who work with viruses either must pass them through a suitable host or must grow them in a tissue culture. The knowledge of how to grow viruses in tissue cultures played a major role in the study of viruses and the development of more and better vaccines.

Infectious diseases occur when these tiny microbes invade the tissues of a host or release poisons. Some microbes such as viruses multiply

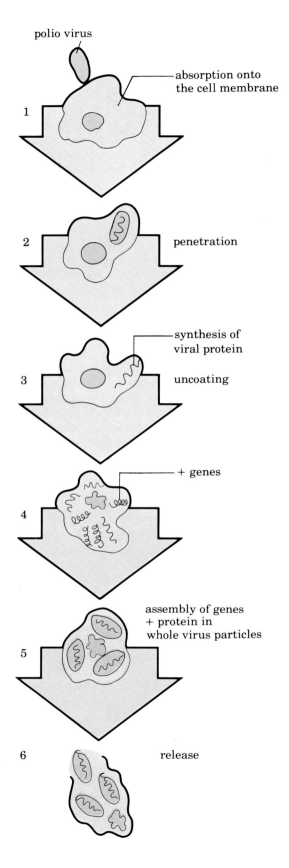

polio virus

1 — absorption onto the cell membrane

2 — penetration

3 — synthesis of viral protein / uncoating

4 — + genes

5 — assembly of genes + protein in whole virus particles

6 — release

INVADING A CELL

The six steps in the multiplication of a virus are charted here, with the polio virus used as an example. In step No. 1 the virus attaches itself to a living cell. Step No. 2 is penetration: the virus passes through the cell membrane into the cell body. The virus then sheds its outer covering, the capsid (step No. 3). In step No. 4 it uses the protein of the living cell to form new viruses containing the genes for further multiplication (step No. 5). In step No. 6 the new organisms pass back through the cell membrane to penetrate other cells. Unlike bacteria, viruses are not able to replicate themselves outside living cells. In the process, the cell may be altered or destroyed.

within a cell and destroy that cell. The polio (poliomyelitis) virus destroys certain cells of the brain or spinal cord, producing the paralysis that is polio's frightening feature.

Certain bacteria, such as those that cause tetanus or diphtheria, produce and secrete powerful poisons (toxins) that spread throughout the body. Botulism, on the other hand, is a disease produced not by bacteria but by eating poisons that have been secreted into food by bacteria.

Still another way that bacteria produce disease is by interfering with normal body functions. The bacteria that cause diarrhea disturb the functions of the intestinal tract so that large amounts of water and salts escape without being reabsorbed. Other bacteria can destroy tissue and cause vital organs to function improperly.

When bacteria or viruses are present in a susceptible host, certain steps must take place before disease occurs. In most cases, the organisms must attach themselves to host cells. Viruses then must penetrate into the cell and be able to multiply. Certain bacteria have attachment preferences for certain cells of the body. The body then tries to defend itself. One way is through inflammation. Blood vessels enlarge and more blood flows to the area, bringing antibodies, protective cells, and other substances, including cells called phagocytes that can "eat" (ingest) the bacteria.

Phagocytes are more efficient at ingesting if the bacteria are first coated with antibodies, proteins made by the body in response to foreign substances. When bacteria have been attacked by antibiotics, the bacteria stop multiplying and are more easily killed. Even tiny amounts of antibiotics can injure bacteria enough to make them susceptible to the protective activities of the body.

Everyone has experienced inflammation and has noticed that an inflamed area becomes reddened, swollen, and painful. The best way to reduce inflammation is to treat its cause. Occasionally, however, the degree of inflammation becomes so severe that it becomes a threat in itself. Some bacteria kill so many cells in a small area that the dead cells and tissue fluids accumulate and become pus. Often the pus also contains the bacteria that caused the inflammation. Judging when the bacteria have been killed, when the pus is safe to remove, and when removing it will spread the infection are aspects of medicine that require understanding and skill.

HOW THE BODY REACTS TO INFECTION

The first feelings of illness are headache, body ache, weakness, fatigue, listlessness, and poor appetite. As the illness worsens, more severe symptoms develop. The face becomes flushed, the skin and mouth become dry, and confusion and even delirium can develop. Prolonged illness can cause weight loss.

Fever. The body's internal temperature is normally kept within a very narrow range of 97° to 99° Fahrenheit (36.5° to 37.5° Celsius) with 98.6° considered "normal." The infectious agent triggers the release of certain substances that act on the temperature-regulating centers in the brain and allow this set point to rise. The body then takes steps to generate heat (which is why we shiver), apparently because bacteria cannot multiply at higher temperatures. It also withdraws iron from the blood, another essential for bacterial multiplication (which is why we may become anemic).

Fever thus is beneficial, and harmful only if it rises above 106° Fahrenheit. Reducing fever may make a person more comfortable, but it also may prolong the illness, and interfere with efforts to identify its cause or assess the results of treatment.

When infection subsides, the set point lowers and the body acts to cool itself: the fever "breaks." Sweating and heat loss through the skin are among the most useful ways the body can lose excess heat.

HOW INFECTION SPREADS

Infections spread in many ways. Respiratory spread occurs when people cough or sneeze, sending infected particles into the air. Inhaled infectious particles also may come from soil, as in coccidioidomycosis, or from bacteria-contaminated fluids such as cooling tower and air-conditioning water.

Another method of spread has to do with close contact. A person with a cold can transfer the virus by touching another person with hands that have rubbed the nose or eyes. The virus that causes infectious mononucleosis does not spread readily from one individual to another except by quite close contact. That is why the disease has sometimes been nicknamed "the kissing disease."

Sexual contact is another method of transmission, as has been dramatized by the spread of acquired immune deficiency syndrome (AIDS), discussed elsewhere in this chapter, and other venereal diseases. Infection also has been spread via blood transfusions, although more stringent screening methods have sharply reduced this risk.

Infectious agents also can be transmitted by the bites of insects. Mosquitoes transmit malaria, viral encephalitis, and yellow fever. Ticks transmit several diseases.

Water-borne infections occur primarily in areas of poor sanitation, when bacteria leave the body and enter the water supply. Infections spread by food occur relatively infrequently in industrialized countries, except when contaminated food is improperly prepared or stored before being eaten.

Common rules of hygiene are among the most important ways to prevent the spread of infections. Careful hand washing, thorough cooking, and proper refrigeration are important in preventing the spread of disease by food. Water supplies must be protected against sewage and body excretions. Isolation of persons with highly contagious or dangerous diseases sometimes is necessary. The use of a condom during sexual contact reduces the risk of infection.

Vaccination is a method of producing immunity against a specific organism. Most vaccines use the germ itself to give a mild dose of infection that then produces immunity that may last several years to life. Other vaccines use nonliving materials to produce the same effect. Many childhood diseases, including measles, mumps, German measles (rubella), diphtheria, whooping cough (pertus-

can be prevented by vaccination. Smallpox, once a major cause of death and serious illness, has been eradicated by vaccination.

RESPIRATORY INFECTIONS

The symptoms and signs for the common upper respiratory infections are well known: runny nose, stuffiness, headache, sneezing, general feeling of illness, occasional cough, and fever. These usually last five to seven days, but in more severe infections caused by certain viruses, symptoms are likely to persist for two or three weeks.

Respiratory infections also are discussed in Chapter 10, "The Lungs"; Chapter 15, "Ear, Nose, and Throat"; and Chapter 29, "Taking Care of Your Child."

The Common Cold

The common cold is caused by a variety of viruses. Thus, the same person may have many different attacks, with symptoms a bit different each time.

Colds are contagious. Most colds in families occur because schoolchildren come into close contact with one another, allowing an infection to spread rapidly and to be brought home. Viruses also can be transmitted by touching objects that have been handled by infected persons.

At the first sign of a cold, try to avoid contact with others. Colds are most contagious when the cold is developing and during the first day or two after symptoms have appeared. Aspirin or acetaminophen often is used to relieve the fever and general feeling of ill health. Other drugs can help to dry the nasal congestion. These measures do not hasten recovery, however.

The most important complications of common colds are secondary bacterial infections, such as sinusitis, pneumonia or bronchitis, and tonsillitis. In general, if a cold is not getting better, or becomes abruptly worse after appearing to improve, medical attention should be sought.

Influenza

Many respiratory infections are labeled "flu," but true influenza is caused by a specific group of viruses. The illness comes on suddenly, with fever, chills, muscle aches (particularly in the back), fatigue, and weakness. In contrast to the common cold, there is a dry nose and dry cough, and the eyes can be quite red. The disease is particularly severe in the elderly.

The influenza virus has a tendency to change (mutate) every few years, as described in Chapter 10, "The Lungs." Even those who have experienced previous "flu" attacks may not be immune to the new variety. These changes have produced the worldwide influenza epidemics of history and led public health authorities to establish laboratories in various parts of the world to try to isolate the responsible virus whenever an outbreak occurs. Influenza vaccines then are developed for persons at increased risk, such as pregnant women, infants, and the elderly.

Influenza usually is spread by infectious virus particles that have been coughed or sneezed into the air. Once an outbreak has begun, individuals should avoid crowded places. The drug amantadine is the mainstay of therapy for all strains of influenza. Bed rest, fluids, and aspirin or related compounds for comfort also are part of treatment. Persistent fever or worsening of symptoms may herald the onset of pneumonia, the most feared complication.

Sinusitis

The sinuses are air-filled spaces within the facial bones. The most important sinuses are illustrated in Chapter 15, "Ear, Nose, and Throat." They are connected through small passages to the nose or mouth, and the linings of the sinuses secrete a mucous substance that drains through these passages. Bacteria and viruses enter the sinuses through these connections, usually from a common upper respiratory infection. If the connecting ducts become inflamed, the sinuses will fail to drain, become painful, and swell. In rare instances the infection spreads from the sinus to surrounding bone. Acute sinusitis must be recognized and treated promptly. Antibiotics kill or inhibit the microbes. Drainage can be restored by drugs that shrink the tissues of the connecting ducts.

Sore Throat

Most sore throats stem from common respiratory viruses. A minority are caused by the common bacterium *hemolytic streptococcus.*

Bacterial sore throats can be difficult to distinguish from viral sore throats. Viral sore throats tend to get better within a few days without treatment. However, a "strep" throat, usually identified by culturing substances from the throat, should be treated with antibiotics to help prevent spread and to prevent the complication of rheumatic fever, described in Chapter 5, "The Heart and Circulation," which can lead to permanent scarring of the heart valves. Streptococcal infections should be treated for a minimum of 10 days.

Tonsil infection. Occasionally streptococci invade the tonsils and surrounding tissues, producing acute tonsillitis or abscesses around the tonsils or in the throat. These complications are characterized by persistent high fever, severe sore throat, and difficulty in swallowing. Usually an enlarged tonsil can be seen in the area of inflammation. Antibiotics are effective if administered early. A tonsillectomy sometimes is recommended for repeated infections.

Diphtheria. Diphtheria is uncommon in the United States now that most children are immunized. Occasionally it strikes adults who were immunized in childhood, but whose immunization no longer protects them.

In its mild form, diphtheria can look like other sore throats. In its severe form, the throat is covered with a gray inflammation that can interfere with breathing. Treatment for diphtheria involves antitoxin to neutralize the bacterial toxin and antibiotics to kill the bacteria so they cannot produce more toxin.

Laryngitis

Inflammations of the larynx, including the vocal cords, are common and often associated with acute respiratory illnesses, or with irritation caused by shouting. However, the hoarseness occasionally becomes more severe, particularly in children. The cough may become deep and barking, and worsen at night.

When laryngitis is caused by bacteria, antibiotics are helpful, but for viral laryngitis there is no treatment except rest, fluids, and analgesics. If the person has difficulty breathing, prompt medical attention is essential.

A common form of laryngitis in young children is called croup. It often comes on suddenly during upper respiratory illness, usually signaled by a barking cough and hoarse voice. Inflammation and swelling of the larynx narrow the airway and can impair breathing, making croup a serious disease. Croup and its treatment are discussed in Chapter 29, "Taking Care of Your Child."

Bacterial epiglottitis is an infection of the upper larynx, above the vocal cords. In children, it may be life-threatening because, as in croup, tissue swelling may completely block the epiglottal opening. Emergency treatment may be necessary. Antibiotics combat the infection. Epiglottitis also is discussed in Chapter 10, "The Lungs."

Pertussis (Whooping Cough)

Because of widespread immunization, this infection had virtually disappeared. As a result of controversy over the effects of pertussis vaccine, it has reappeared among the unvaccinated. Victims, primarily children under 2 years of age, experience long episodes of coughing so severe that they must take a huge inward breath which produces the characteristic whoop. The mucus in the bronchi is thick, sticky, and difficult to cough up, so the coughs come in paroxysms. The most life-threatening complication is pneumonia. The pneumonia usually can be treated with antibiotics, as can pertussis itself. Pertussis is also discussed in Chapter 29, "Taking Care of Your Child."

Pneumonia

Pneumonia is an infection of the lungs whose symptoms and treatment are described in detail in Chapter 10, "The Lungs."

The pneumococcus or *Streptococcus pneumoniae* is the most common cause of bacterial pneumonia. The disease begins when these germs are inhaled into the lung tissue. Often a viral respiratory infection has previously lowered resistance.

Other bacteria besides pneumococcus cause pneumonia. Different species require different treatments. Most forms of bacterial pneumonia respond to the proper antibiotic, usually in about two weeks. No antibiotic cures the viral form, which usually is less severe.

A pneumococcal vaccine has been developed to prevent certain kinds of pneumonia. The vaccine consists of bacterial products isolated from 23 types of pneumococci that are the most common causes of pneumonia. The value of the vaccine is still under investigation.

Legionnaires' Disease

The identification of Legionnaires' disease, a remarkable story of a previously unknown infectious disease caused by a previously unknown organism, is described in Chapter 10, "The Lungs."

Two major forms of Legionnaires Disease are known. The most severe causes a rapidly progressive pneumonia with dry cough, fever, muscle pains, and diarrhea, beginning one to three weeks after exposure. This form sometimes has been traced to bacteria-contaminated sprays from water towers and air-conditioning units.

A less severe influenzalike illness lasting two or three days, marked by fever but without cough or pneumonia, also has been identified. This type has occurred primarily in hospitals among individuals whose immunity is depressed. Antibiotic treatment is successful against both forms if the treatment is begun early.

Tuberculosis

Tuberculosis, described in detail in Chapter 10, "The Lungs," is no longer a major health threat in the U.S. However, it still is a scourge of third-world populations, and occurs in American slums and on tribal reservations. The disease also attacks AIDS victims, whose immune systems have been weakened by their disease.

Except in AIDS patients, tuberculosis is a completely treatable disease, with several effective drugs. However, drugs must be given for months or years.

GASTROINTESTINAL INFECTIONS

Gastrointestinal infections affect either the stomach or the intestines. When the stomach is irritated, there usually is nausea and vomiting (gastritis). When the intestines are irritated, there usually is diarrhea and cramping pains (enteritis). The two often occur together (gastroenteritis).

Gastroenteritis

Gastroenteritis usually lasts only one or two days. There can be many causes, but the most common causes are bacteria and viruses.

The most common toxin comes from food contaminated with staphylococci. Suspect foods are those containing dairy products, such as salad dressings and cream-filled desserts. Eating the food triggers illness within a few hours. The person may notice increased amounts of saliva, nausea,

vomiting, abdominal cramps, and mild diarrhea. If vomiting is severe, particularly in a small child, dehydration can occur.

A large number of viruses also cause gastroenteritis. The virus-caused variety sometimes is called "winter vomiting disease" or "intestinal flu." Usually, there is diarrhea with nausea and vomiting. The illness lasts a few days, then slowly goes away. There is no specific treatment except to correct dehydration. The virus probably is spread hand to mouth, or hand to food to mouth, via contact with infected people. Those who have symptoms should not prepare food for others.

Diarrhea

Diarrhea is best described as more and looser bowel movements than usual. The true definition is based on individual habits.

Diarrhea usually lasts only a short time. However, for infants, small children, elderly people, or those already dehydrated or sick from another cause, medical attention should be sought promptly. Medical help also is required if the diarrhea continues for more than one to two days, if it is accompanied by fever and severe abdominal cramps, if it is accompanied by blood, pus, or mucus in the stools, or if it is accompanied by rashes, jaundice (yellowing of the skin or whites of the eyes), or extreme weakness.

Cholera is the most severe form of diarrhea. It now is largely limited to tropical and subtropical countries. Victims may put out a huge amount of fluid from the intestinal tract—as many as 10 gallons a day. It is easy to see how they may become terribly dehydrated. However, with rapid replacement of the excreted water and salts, the person recovers quickly.

The major complication of diarrhea is dehydration. To offset it, persons who are not vomiting a great deal can drink fluids. Fluids that contain salts and small amounts of sugar are particularly beneficial. A good homemade mixture is a quart of water with a teaspoon of sugar and a pinch of salt. Rehydration therapy, described in Chapter 29, "Taking Care of Your Child," sometimes is used in children.

Typhoid Fever

Typhoid fever is a particularly severe form of salmonella infection caused by the species known as *Salmonella typhosa*. The disease spreads through water supplies contaminated by sewage. Because water supplies are now safe in most industrialized countries, typhoid has become rare. An occasional outbreak occurs because persons who have recently recovered from the disease continue to shed the infecting bacillus for days, weeks, or even a lifetime. If they move to a new environment, they then may infect others.

Typhoid fever can be treated with antibacterial drugs, and a vaccine is available.

Hepatitis

Type A hepatitis. "Infectious hepatitis," or Type A hepatitis, is caused by a virus ingested through food, then spread by bowel movements. Within two to five weeks, susceptible persons who have acquired the virus will develop nausea, vomiting, and loss of appetite, as well as fatigue and muscle and joint aches. The urine may become dark, the color of the stools more like clay, and jaundice (yellowing of the skin and whites of the eyes) may appear. Sometimes there is mild fever. Children often have a milder illness, but still may spread the virus.

Type A hepatitis usually clears up within a week or two. Rarely, the disease progresses to cause severe scarring of the liver, known as cirrhosis. The illness sometimes reappears, although generally in a milder form. A rare complication of Type A hepatitis is infection so severe that the liver is destroyed, causing death in less than a week.

Type B hepatitis often is more severe than Type A. The virus is most commonly spread from the blood of an infected individual to others. Type B hepatitis is a particular problem among homosexuals because it is spread by certain forms of sexual contact, and in drug users who exchange needles. Type B hepatitis also is slower to heal than type A, and more likely to cause scarring of the liver. A few persons retain Type B virus in the blood for many years. There is no specific treatment except bed rest.

Both types of hepatitis shed virus in feces, saliva, tears, and blood. Untreated sewage often contains hepatitis virus. Hepatitis outbreaks have been traced to shellfish taken from waters contaminated by untreated sewage.

Protection against Type A hepatitis can be achieved by injections of human gamma globulin, a blood protein that carries antibodies against the virus and that can neutralize the infectious particles before they spread. A vaccine for Type B hepatitis is recommended for persons at risk, including homosexually active males and drug users.

Precautions to Prevent Gastroenteritis and Diarrhea

- Infected persons should not handle food others will eat.
- Wash hands after using the toilet and before preparation of food.
- Prepared food should be refrigerated if not eaten promptly.
- Meat and meat products should be cooked. Avoid rare and raw foods.
- Never eat pork and poultry when they are pink (not thoroughly cooked).
- A frozen turkey or large fowl should be completely thawed before being stuffed and roasted. If the interior of the turkey is not completely thawed, it may not cook thoroughly. Bacteria will multiply and gastroenteritis will spread.

Blood tests can distinguish Type A and Type B hepatitis. The tests also disclose other forms of hepatitis, including one that is transmitted by blood products and is neither A nor B. It has been termed "non-A, non-B hepatitis," but in fact may represent a group of infections.

URINARY INFECTIONS

Urinary infections occur in 10 to 20 percent of women and in about one-half of 1 percent of men at some time in their lives. They are particularly prevalent among elderly women, especially those who are bedfast. The infections often are classified as urethritis or cystitis, depending upon whether the urethra or bladder is involved; if the infection has migrated to the kidneys, the term is pyelonephritis. The symptoms and treatment are described in Chapter 24, "The Kidneys and Urinary System."

Infections of the urinary system usually are caused by the common bacteria found in the intestinal tract. These bacteria find their way to the urethra, the conduit from the bladder that leads outside the body. The female urethra is quite short, opening near the vagina. The bacteria ascend along the urethra into the bladder and multiply in urine. The cells lining the urethra inhibit bacteria to some degree, so the greater length of the urethra in males probably explains why infections in men are much less common.

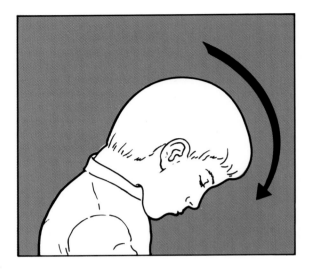

TEST FOR MENINGITIS
Life-threatening meningitis, or inflammation of the brain membranes, often resembles "flu" in its early stages, with sudden fever, chills, headache, and nausea and vomiting. One symptom of meningitis is severe aches in the back and neck, and neck stiffness. A quick test is to have the person try to touch chin to chest, as shown above. If the person cannot do so, meningitis may be indicated, and he or she should receive medical care immediately.

In older men urinary infections may result from enlargement of the prostate gland. The prostate is located just below the neck of the bladder. Enlargement can impede complete emptying of the bladder. Bacteria then can multiply within the bladder and spread to the kidney.

The diagnosis of urinary tract infection is made by finding numerous bacteria in the urine, often accompanied by pus or blood. The urine may look cloudy. Antimicrobial drugs usually relieve the discomfort in a day or two.

Drinking plenty of water probably helps prevent urinary infections by causing the bladder to be emptied often.

When a woman has repeated infections, or when infections occur in very young children, it is customary to X-ray the kidneys to be certain that there is no correctable anatomic defect and to assess the degree of damage. Many obstructions can be corrected surgically.

INFECTIONS OF THE NERVOUS SYSTEM

Meningitis

Meningitis, inflammation of the membranes that cover the brain and spinal cord, is a very serious infection when caused by bacteria. It usually is somewhat less serious when caused by viruses. Fortunately, bacterial meningitis is rare, and effective antibiotics are available.

Bacterial meningitis occurs in epidemics and as isolated single cases. The symptoms are fever, sleepiness to the point of inability to wake up, confusion, irritability, and stiffness and pain in the neck, with the person unable to put chin to chest. Often there is pain in the muscles of the back and legs. There also may be an associated rash, tiny dark red spots mainly on the trunk and buttocks. Because the brain and spinal cord are involved, muscle weakness or brain damage may occur afterward. The earlier and the more effective the treatment, the less the likelihood of severe damage.

The bacteria most often responsible are the meningococcus, pneumococcus, and *Hemophilus influenzae*. All are spread from person to person by cough or sneezing. The meningococcus is the most likely of the three to occur in outbreaks and most commonly affects children and young adults. Many people harbor the bacteria in the nose and throat without becoming ill, and appear immune to the meningococcus. It is not clear why a few people do not have this immunity. In susceptible persons, the organism is acquired through inhalation, resides in the nose and throat, and spreads through the bloodstream to the central nervous system. Small hemorrhages may occur in the skin, or in the joints, and small blood vessels tend to plug up. The organism can be identified by bacterial cultures.

The pneumococcus, the organism responsible for bacterial pneumonia, is the most common cause of meningitis in older persons. Often it will spread to the central nervous system through the bloodstream when a person already has lobar pneumonia, but sometimes may appear in the spinal fluid without an associated pneumonia.

The bacterial meningitis produced by *Hemophilus influenzae* is most common in children aged 18 months to 4 years. As children grow older, most develop antibody to hemophilus. Infants tend to be protected by the antibody passed from the mother during pregnancy. Thus, the period between the disappearance of this fetal immunity and the acquisition of new immunity is the period of highest risk. Fortunately, a vaccine now is available to protect children during the vulnerable 18-month-to-4-year period.

To determine which bacteria are producing meningitis, it is necessary to examine the spinal fluid. The sample usually is obtained by inserting a small needle between the vertebrae into the spinal cord. It is essential that the spinal tap be performed, because different antimicrobial drugs act differently on various bacteria. A drug that is effective against one type of meningitis does not always help against another.

Preventing the spread of meningitis is not critical except for the meningococcal form, in which it is customary to isolate ill persons and to examine members of the family and close contacts to determine whether they have acquired the bacteria.

Viral meningitis usually produces milder symptoms than those of bacterial meningitis. There is headache, pain in the neck muscles, fever, and sometimes a rash. The eyes may be sore, and the person often wants to avoid bright light. Most viral meningitis cases resolve spontaneously in a week to 10 days without treatment, and rarely cause nerve damage.

Encephalitis is an inflammation of the nerve cells of the brain. A variety of viruses can infect the brain, including herpes, measles, mumps, chickenpox, and the HIV virus of AIDS, but the spread of these viruses to the brain is rare.

Poliomyelitis

Until the mid-1960s, poliomyelitis was a dreaded disease that occurred in outbreaks each summer, affecting large numbers of children and often leaving a few of them with muscle paralysis. Since then, two types of vaccines have been developed, one using a killed virus and the other a live, weakened organism. Both vaccines have been effective, and their use has almost completely eradicated "polio" from the United States and from other countries in which they are widely used.

Poliomyelitis produces fever, headache, vomiting, sore throat, and later pain in the muscles, followed by paralysis. The virus probably is swallowed, and multiplies in the intestinal tract, spreading to the nervous system in a small percentage of persons. Before the vaccine, it was estimated that about 100 cases of mild and inapparent poliomyelitis occurred for each case of paralysis.

The most widely used vaccine is the live virus form. The attenuated virus then grows in the intestinal tract and induces immunity. The vaccine is easily swallowed in a liquid preparation. After a child has been immunized and the virus is multiplying in the body, persons in close contact with the child receive a certain amount of exposure, too, so their immunity may be boosted as well.

The killed virus vaccine appears to be slightly less protective and is not as widely used in the United States, although some countries continue to use it exclusively.

Rabies

Rabies is a viral disease of the central nervous system that many years ago was one of the most feared of all diseases. There are many "mad dog" stories describing how the animal acts irrationally, has jerking movements, and runs wildly in circles with saliva dripping from the mouth and jaws. This saliva contains the virus. A bite introduces it under the skin of a susceptible person, and then it spreads to the central nervous system.

Once symptoms of rabies appears in human beings, recovery is exceedingly rare. Fortunately, however, the incubation period between the time of the bite and the time the disease begins to produce its severe effects is several weeks, so there is time to immunize the bite victim. Most cases of rabies now result from the bites of wild animals or bites of dogs that have been bitten by wild animals. Among the animals that have spread the viruses to humans are bats, skunks, foxes, and horses.

Treatment must begin promptly. The bitten area should be flushed with large amounts of soap and water and scrubbed briskly to wash out the virus. An antiserum also prevents spread of the virus to the nervous system, and vaccines can be given to build up antibodies.

Tetanus (Lockjaw)

The organism that causes tetanus or lockjaw, *Clostridium tetani*, produces spores that act as tiny seeds. They can be found in the soil and in the intestinal tracts of man and animals. The spores transform themselves into multiplying bacteria only if little or no oxygen is present. Spores commonly enter all of our bodies through cuts, burns, scratches, and other wounds. If tissue has closed over a wound and excludes oxygen, the microorganisms develop and produce tetanus toxin, a powerful nerve poison that travels along the nerves to produce damage to the central nervous system.

The interval between the time of a wound and the appearance of symptoms ranges from a few days to months. Severe cases usually appear quickly. Symptoms include restlessness, irritability, stiffness of some muscle groups, and sometimes difficulty in swallowing. A muscle spasm in a limb or jaws sometimes is the first evidence of the disease, hence the name "lockjaw."

Treatment of tetanus consists of giving victims oxygen and assisting their breathing if the paralysis has affected the muscles of respiration. Although antibiotics kill the bacteria, they do not neutralize the toxin that already has been released. Accordingly, antitoxin is widely used as a neutralizing agent.

Tetanus toxoid has been even more useful in preventing the disease. This material has been produced from tetanus toxin by chemically changing it to make it nonpoisonous but still able to cause the body to produce antitoxin. Such toxoid, given to children at monthly intervals for three injections, will confer immunity for 10 years or longer. In adults it is customary after injury to give another dose of toxoid that immediately restimulates the immunity.

Botulism

Botulism results from eating canned foods that have been inadequately sterilized, allowing the organism *Clostridium botulinum*, common in soil and in feces, to multiply and produce its toxin. As in tetanus, the organism multiplies only in the absence of oxygen. The toxin is one of the most powerful poisons known. Even tiny traces can be fatal. Thus, if there is the slightest suspicion about home-canned foods, they should be boiled for at least 30 minutes before use and should not be tasted before boiling.

Persons who develop botulism usually complain first of blurred or double vision. The mouth becomes dry, the eyes are dilated, and there may be difficulty in speaking and ultimately in breathing. These symptoms sometimes appear within hours.

Antitoxins counter the lethal effect and are valuable in protecting persons in whom symptoms have not yet appeared.

EAR INFECTIONS (OTITIS)

Infections of the ear are called otitis. An infection of the outer ear is called external otitis, and infection of the middle ear is otitis media. These are described in Chapter 15, "Ear, Nose, and Throat."

BONE AND JOINT INFECTIONS

Osteomyelitis. Bones can become infected after an accident in which a bone breaks and fragments pierce the skin, when a wound infection spreads to the bone beneath, or when bacteria are carried to the bone through the blood. The staphylococci usually are responsible. Bone infections can be painful, and have the potential to cause scarring and chronic infection. They must be treated promptly and vigorously with antibiotics.

Septic arthritis, or joint infection, can develop after an accident in which the joint is opened and bacteria are introduced, or when bacteria from the blood spread to the joint. Gonococcus, the organism of gonorrhea, often attacks joints. Other organisms, such as staphylococci, also infect joints.

Infected joints become hot, painful, swollen, and tender. Sometimes the joint must be drained surgically. Prompt treatment with antibiotics is necessary to prevent scarring and lasting damage.

Both osteomyelitis and septic arthritis are discussed in Chapter 16, "The Bones and Muscles."

SKIN DISEASES

Boils and Carbuncles

Boils (furuncles) are areas of inflammation with pus in the center. They occur on the skin and in surrounding tissues. The infection usually originates in a hair follicle. Sometimes many boils come together to form a carbuncle, which represents a kind of "super boil." These in turn may extend deeper into surrounding tissues.

Boils and carbuncles usually are caused by staphylococcus organisms and occur most commonly in areas of the body that the hand can reach and scratch, such as the face, back of the neck, buttocks, chest, armpits, and other places with hair and sweat glands. Furuncles and carbuncles also follow minor scratches brought about by irritation from clothes, straps, and belts.

The treatment for most boils is conservative. Warm packs help the body fight the bacteria. The pus that forms represents the breakdown of body tissues, bacterial cells, and white blood cells that gather around the bacteria to destroy them. Boils should not be squeezed or lanced. If the boils are broken, the bacteria can spread throughout the skin. In addition, bacteria can enter the bloodstream and cause abscesses.

Chicken Pox and Shingles

Chicken pox (varicella) and herpes zoster, commonly called shingles, are caused by closely related or perhaps identical viruses. Chicken pox is one of the most common of childhood diseases, striking four out of five preschool children. Symptoms and treatment are described in Chapter 29, "Taking Care of Your Child."

Childhood infection usually lasts about two weeks. After the rash heals, the varicella virus apparently is able to persist in nerve cells for many years and reappear decades later as "shingles." Under these conditions, the virus multiplies in nerve cells involving a particular area of the spinal cord. The virus spreads along the nerve pathways and becomes distributed along that specific nerve.

In contrast to chicken pox, shingles produces pain. The pain may persist for months after the rash has cleared. Occasionally the muscles in the affected area remain weak.

Acyclovir, an antiviral drug, is useful in treating chicken pox and shingles in persons with impaired immune systems. Acyclovir also is used for elderly persons with shingles.

Herpes Simplex (Fever Blisters)

The herpes simplex virus causes an infection that is well known as cold sores or fever blisters. These sores occur particularly often at the junction between the lips and the skin. They also occur in the mouth and throat and on the genital organs. Occasionally, the virus spreads to scratches in the skin and causes typical lesions on the fingers and hands, similar to those caused by chicken pox or herpes zoster. Herpes occasionally spreads to the eye, where it can produce a severe eye infection (see Chapter 14, "The Eyes"). Drugs can be instilled into the eye to prevent growth of the virus, but these drugs have little effect on skin rashes.

Leprosy

Leprosy also is known as Hansen's disease, after the Norwegian scientist who first identified the bacteria that cause it. Leprosy bacilli look somewhat like the bacteria that cause tuberculosis. Leprosy probably infects many more people than those who develop its characteristic skin rash or nerve disorders. Because leprosy bacilli invade and damage the nervous tissues, certain areas of the body can lose the ability to feel temperature or pain. Mutilations and deformity may appear on the skin, arms, legs, or face because of injury caused by the lack of sensation.

Certain drugs cure leprosy, but successful treatment can take years. The disease is not highly communicable, and it takes prolonged contact to acquire it. Even spouses of persons with leprosy remain healthy after living together for years.

VENEREAL DISEASE

Of the infections that are spread by sexual contact, the most common have been syphilis and gonorrhea. Recently, it has been demonstrated that infectious agents such as Chlamydia, mycoplasma, *Herpes hominis*, Trichomonas, and others can be spread by sexual activity. Acquired immune deficiency syndrome (AIDS) can be transmitted by either homosexual or heterosexual contact. A section on AIDS is included in this chapter.

Chlamydia

A tiny bacterium called *Chlamydia*, almost a virus in size, now is recognized as the leading cause of venereal infection. It is described in Chapter 26, "The Female Reproductive System."

Chlamydia produces pain on urination and often a watery or mucous discharge from the penis or the vagina. Women often have fewer symptoms than men and may feel well until the infection reaches the uterus or adjacent structures, when pain develops. Internally, the infection can cause pelvic inflammatory disease.

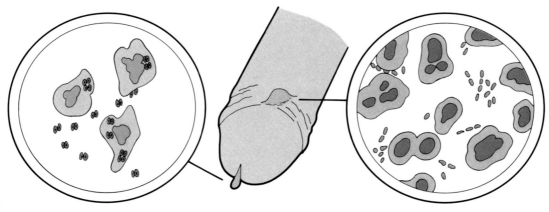

N. gonorrhoeae   Hemophilus ducreyi

VENEREAL DISEASE

A common form of disease spread by sexual contact is gonorrhea, caused by the gonococcus bacterium, shown in the circle at left. Male symptoms are painful urination and discharge from the penis (center drawing), which occur one to seven days after exposure. Females sometimes have no symptoms, but repeated or continued infection can cause sterility. The circle at right shows **Hemophilus ducreyi** *bacilli, which cause the venereal disease chancroid. Less common in the U.S. than in other areas, its first symptom is a small red lump on the genitals (as shown in center drawing) that may break down and form a painful ulcer. Another disease, nonspecific urethritis, also causes discharge and painful urination, but the organisms causing it are too small to be seen with a microscope.*

Antibiotics have been successful in treating these infections. It is important to treat all sexual partners and to refrain from sexual activity until the infection is cured.

Still other tiny bacteria called *Ureaplasma urealyticum* have been suggested as causes for some of these cases, and a protozoan, Trichomonas, also has been implicated. Certain common bacteria invading the urethra also have been suspected of causing the symptoms, so urethritis can stem from a variety of microorganisms.

Gonorrhea

Gonorrhea is caused by small round bacteria that come in pairs: *Neisseria gonorrhoeae*. Acquisition of the disease by nonvenereal sources is rare, although newborn infants can be infected by passing through the birth canal of an infected mother. Repeated episodes of gonorrhea can scar the fe-

male pelvic organs, sometimes leaving the woman sterile. In the male, local scarring leads to sterility and difficulty in urination. In newborns, the organism can enter the eyes and lead to blindness. Most states require that antibacterial drops be put into the eyes of all newborns as a precaution.

Initial symptoms of gonorrhea occur within a week after exposure. The male has a burning sensation on urination, soon followed by a discharge from the penis that drips small amounts of pus. On the other hand, many infected women notice no symptoms except slightly painful urination or a slight increase in discharge.

Gonorrhea usually can be treated with antimicrobial drugs. It is important in preventing the spread of gonorrhea that sexual partners be treated simultaneously.

Syphilis

Syphilis is caused by a spiral-shaped microorganism called *Treponema pallidum*. The disease is spread by direct contact, usually of a sexual nature. If a pregnant woman is syphilitic, the infection can spread to her infant. The organisms that cause syphilis initially produce a hard painless sore called a chancre at the site where the germs have entered. Chancres usually appear on the genitals and occasionally on the lips, but they can appear anywhere on the body.

The chancre represents the primary stage of syphilis. It usually disappears even without treatment. In the secondary stage weeks or months later, the organism spreads throughout the body and a generalized rash typically appears, often accompanied by ulcers in the mouth that are infectious. The rash itself is full of microorganisms. The infected person may have swollen lymph nodes. In the third stage, which may appear after many years, a variety of effects occurs. Among them are general paresis, which leads to severe mental illness; tabes dorsalis, in which there may be loss of feeling and movement difficulties affecting the legs; and aortic aneurysm, in which the body's main artery can become dilated and may rupture, causing immediate death. Disease of the heart valves also occurs.

With proper treatment, an infectious person can be made noninfectious to others in one or two days. Treatment is so effective that the tertiary forms of syphilis now are seen only rarely.

Genital Herpes

Herpes simplex. *Herpes genitalis, Herpes hominis B,* and *Herpes hominis type 2* are all names for the same common virus, which is spread by sexual activity. Within a few days after contact, small exceedingly painful blisters occur on the genitals or on other areas of contact. After a few days the blisters dry and ulcerate, with crusts forming on the surfaces, and then healing follows in a week or two. After healing, the virus may become latent, which means that it remains in cells in the area but produces no symptoms. Weeks, months, or even years later the sores may return again. The antiviral drug acyclovir now is used to treat genital herpes infections. It lessens the painful symptoms of the initial attack and can shorten the duration of later attacks. It also may be used to prevent recurrent attacks.

FEMALE GENITAL INFECTIONS

Vaginitis is a general term that describes a secretion of pus or excess mucus from the vagina. Several kinds of bacteria are present in the vagina and do not produce disease. However, bacteria occasionally are acquired, sometimes through sexual contact, that produce local infection. The vagina becomes painful, the amount of discharge increases, and bacterial cultures demonstrate the presence of bacteria.

Candida albicans is a yeastlike microorganism that can produce vaginitis. A small number of yeast cells are normally present in the vagina, but occasionally the numbers increase and produce inflammation. Overgrowth of the yeasts occurs by the elimination of normal bacteria through the use of antibiotics, and by changes in hormones during the menstrual cycle. Women who use oral contraceptives seem to have more yeasts than other women. Yeast infections are not sexually transmitted as a rule.

Trichomonas vaginalis is a small protozoan microorganism that produces vaginitis. The yellowish-green discharge has a distinct odor. The infection can pass from male to female sexual partners and back again. These organisms, which can be controlled by drugs, rarely produce any discomfort in males, only in females.

MISCELLANEOUS DISEASES

Infectious Mononucleosis

Persons who become ill with infectious mononucleosis (glandular fever) usually develop mild fever, sore throat, and headache. Lymph glands in the armpits, groin, elbows, and around the neck become swollen and somewhat tender. Occasionally, the liver is involved and jaundice develops. Most commonly, however, the disease makes people feel quite ill for a few days, then recovery occurs within days or weeks. The virus that causes "mono" is found in saliva and respiratory secretions but does not readily spread from one individual to another without close contact. It is for this reason that the disease has been incorrectly called the "kissing disease."

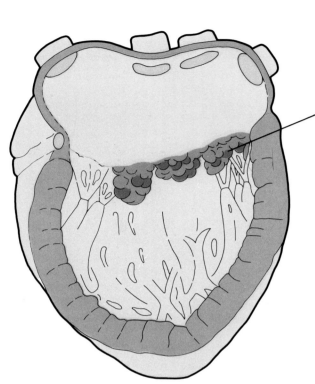

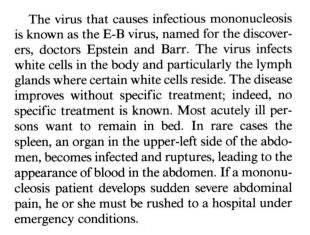

BACTERIAL ENDOCARDITIS
When bacteria infect the lining membrane of the heart and its valves, the condition is called bacterial endocarditis. Carried to the heart by the blood, the infecting bacteria cause inflammatory changes and growth of vegetation on the surface of the heart valves (yellow area). The organisms particularly attack congenitally deformed valves, or those injured by previous diseases, such as rheumatic fever. The disease also occurs in drug users because of contaminated needles. In many cases the infection is caused by **Streptococcus viridans** *(circle).*

The virus that causes infectious mononucleosis is known as the E-B virus, named for the discoverers, doctors Epstein and Barr. The virus infects white cells in the body and particularly the lymph glands where certain white cells reside. The disease improves without specific treatment; indeed, no specific treatment is known. Most acutely ill persons want to remain in bed. In rare cases the spleen, an organ in the upper-left side of the abdomen, becomes infected and ruptures, leading to the appearance of blood in the abdomen. If a mononucleosis patient develops sudden severe abdominal pain, he or she must be rushed to a hospital under emergency conditions.

Bacterial Endocarditis

Bacterial infection of the heart lining, bacterial endocarditis, occurs primarily among narcotics users who inject themselves using contaminated needles. Symptoms and treatment are described in Chapter 5, "The Heart and Circulation."

Toxoplasmosis

Toxoplasmosis is caused by a small protozoan known as *Toxoplasma gondii*. Toxoplasmas are common in the environment and can be isolated from virtually all domestic and farm animals. About one-fourth to one-half of American adults carry antibodies to toxoplasma, indicating that at some time they were infected. In adults the disease usually is mild, with swelling of the lymph nodes and minimal discomfort. However, if a pregnant woman acquires toxoplasmosis, the organism can spread to the developing fetus and cause serious defects involving the brain, heart, eyes, and other organs.

Toxoplasmas are spread among humans through infected raw meat, but heat kills the organisms quickly. However, the infection also is transmitted by the feces of young cats. Because of a peculiarity in the digestive system of cats, the parasites can survive in their intestinal tracts for long periods. This discovery alarmed many cat lovers, but it is not necessary to sacrifice the cat if sensible precautions are taken. A blood test for toxoplasmosis can be taken from any pregnant woman. If she has protective antibodies, there is no danger. If not, she should observe safeguards, such as eating only well-cooked meats (no rare food). Young kittens should not be allowed in the household. An expectant mother should not have contact with the litter box, and litter boxes should be emptied daily. The litter should be incinerated or disposed of carefully. If it is buried in the garden, a pregnant woman should not dig in the same area. In general, it is wise for a pregnant woman to avoid close contact with cats unless it is known that the cats are free of toxoplasma.

Drugs have been developed to treat toxoplasmosis, but there is no treatment after the fetus becomes infected.

Cat Scratch Disease

The organism responsible for cat scratch disease is not known, but it is assumed to be a virus carried by cats. Following a scratch or a bite by a cat, the individual develops a scaly ulcer at the site. The ulcer heals slowly and then the lymph nodes nearest the ulcer begin to swell without producing pain. The lymph nodes sometimes swell to the point at which they drain and heal spontaneously, but it may take many weeks to reach this point. When there is a suspiciously enlarged lymph node, doctors often recommend that the node be removed surgically and examined to be sure that the swelling stems from cat scratch disease rather than from a tumor. There is no treatment for cat scratch disease.

Kawasaki Disease

This disease, also known as mucotaneous lymph node syndrome, is named for the Japanese physician who first described it. It usually affects children under 5 years of age, causing fever, red eyes, red mouth and throat, rash, swollen legs or arms, and swollen glands in the neck. The cause is unknown. Some young victims develop abnormalities of the blood vessels of the heart, with serious complications.

The fever and rash usually last seven to 10 days, then gradually resolve. Hospitalization rarely is necessary. The rash occasionally is mistaken for measles, scarlet fever, or rubella.

Reye Syndrome

Reye syndrome is a serious complication that on rare occasions follows an upper respiratory infection or chicken pox in children. Several days after onset of the infection, the child may become sleepy or delirious, or suffer convulsions or coma. Some children have died.

Research has indicated that the complication has been more common among children who have been given aspirin in the early stages of the illness. The American Academy of Pediatrics has recommended that aspirin not be given to children with chicken pox or flu-like symptoms. Since the warning and since doctors have become more aware of the condition, the incidence of Reye syndrome has declined sharply.

ACTINOMYCOSIS
AND NOCARDIOSIS

Higher bacteria that cause disease include the organisms *Actinomyces bovis* and *Nocardia asteroides*. Actinomycosis is a chronic infection that is most common around the mouth and jaws, but sometimes occurs in the lymph nodes of the neck and occasionally spreads to the lungs and elsewhere. The organisms are common in soils and hay, and often are introduced into the tissues by a puncture wound. Many cases have occurred when people chew on hay and have punctured the gums with a sharp fragment.

Treatment is effective with antibiotics, but surgery sometimes is necessary.

Nocardial infections are particularly common in individuals whose immunity has been suppressed. Nocardia can produce fevers, pneumonia, pleurisy, and other changes. These infections usually are susceptible to sulfonamids.

Pneumocystis carinii is a small organism that is common in nature and rarely produces disease. However, in people who are receiving drugs for treatment of tumors or to suppress tissue rejection after organ transplant, pneumocystis may cause fever and pneumonia. The infection is a common cause of death among AIDS patients, whose immune defenses have been destroyed by the HIV virus.

FUNGAL INFECTIONS

In addition to *Candida albicans*, also known as Monilia, other pathogenic yeasts occasionally are associated with a variety of disease states. A yeast-like organism called *Blastomyces* can produce ulcers of the skin and mucous membranes, particularly in diabetics. Antibiotics often are effective in controlling infections caused by these organisms.

Histoplasma, coccidioidomycosis, and blastomyces are three fungi that cause lung infections in certain parts of the United States. They are discussed in Chapter 10, "The Lungs."

WORMS

Worms are the largest organisms that infect humans. Tapeworms can grow to a length of 10 feet. Worms are a problem in warm climates and where hygiene and sanitation are poor. Worldwide, hundreds of millions of people are infected with hookworm, roundworm, whipworm, and a variety of other parasites. Pinworm is the most common in the United States. It spreads rapidly among small children in play groups and at school.

Most worms reside in the intestine or in the blood vessels around the intestine. A few types are found in other areas of the body. For example, the worm that causes trichinosis burrows into muscles, and the longworm into the lung. Pinworms sometimes leave the intestine and burrow into the skin around the anus, where they deposit eggs that a child might pick up under the fingernails. Worms can live for many years inside the body. Most commonly the person carrying them shows no symptoms unless the infection is severe.

Intestinal worms, such as tapeworms, whipworms, roundworms, hookworms, and threadworms, produce mild abdominal cramping and diarrhea if the infection is severe enough. In more severe forms there is anemia, bowel obstruction, and possible malnutrition. Schistosomas, also known as Bilharzia, are worms that live in the bloodstream around the intestines. They sometimes spread to the liver, producing jaundice, or to the kidneys, producing blood in the urine. Although rare in the United States, schistosomiasis is a common infestation in much of the world.

Worms spread from person to person by several methods. One source is eating poorly washed or uncooked foods or foods that have been washed with contaminated water or contaminated with feces. Another source is eating beef or pork that has been inadequately cooked. In a few instances, an individual who walks barefoot on ground contaminated with human feces may pick up worms that hatch in the ground. These migrate through the skin, move throughout the body, and finally pass into the intestine.

Pinworm infection is acquired by another means. The worms spread to the anus, producing itching in the adjoining skin. The person, usually a child, scratches the area and picks up the eggs on his or her fingers. The eggs then are transferred to other people if the hands and fingernails are not clean. Usually, if there is pinworm infection in a family, it is advisable to treat all family members.

Trichinosis, named for the worm *Trichinella spiralis*, lives for a short time in the human intestines, then spreads throughout the body. It invades the muscles and forms small cysts. The worms produce the same cysts in pork, which may be ingested unless the pork is thoroughly cooked or kept frozen for at least 48 hours. Trichinosis usually produces no symptoms, but severe infestation causes diarrhea, muscle pains, weakness, fever, puffiness around the eyes, and sometimes evidence of kidney disorder.

All of the common worms can be eliminated with drugs.

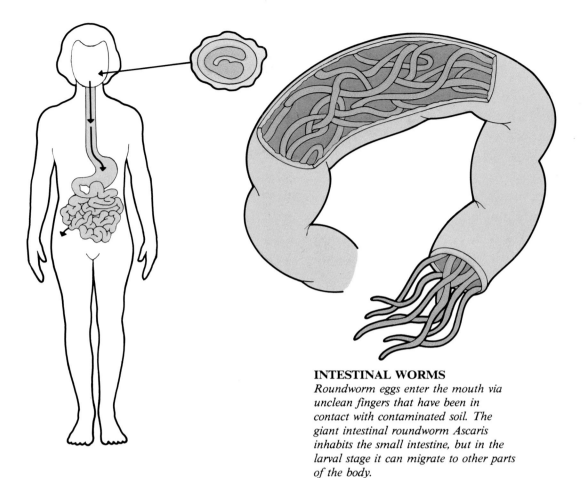

INTESTINAL WORMS
Roundworm eggs enter the mouth via unclean fingers that have been in contact with contaminated soil. The giant intestinal roundworm Ascaris inhabits the small intestine, but in the larval stage it can migrate to other parts of the body.

INSECT-BORNE INFECTIONS

Infections transmitted by insects are particularly common in countries with warm and moist climates. They are less common in the United States because of successful programs to control mosquitoes and other disease-carrying insects.

Viral Encephalitis

Viral encephalitis is an inflammation of brain tissue. The illness is caused by a virus spread by the bite of a mosquito. The mosquito first bites an animal that carries the virus, then transfers it when biting a human. Therefore, most encephalitis occurs during the mosquito season, from late spring until frost. A person who develops encephalitis may become confused, feverish, and sleepy; may develop a headache, vomiting, staggered walk, or difficulty in talking or talk nonsense; or may seem to be in a perpetual state of nightmare. Some of the viruses that cause viral encephalitis can destroy parts of the brain. Depending on the amount of invasion, the infected person might recover completely or might be left with brain damage. There is no specific treatment for mosquito-borne viral encephalitis.

Effective preventive measures include spraying, quarantine of infected animals, and use of household screens and insect repellents.

Varieties of encephalitis found in the United States include western equine encephalitis and eastern equine encephalitis, both spread from horses, and St. Louis encephalitis.

Plague

Throughout history plague, spread by the bites of fleas, has been one of the worst killers of all known infections. The disease is now rare in the United States, occurring primarily in the West, where flea-carrying ground squirrels and other small rodents are still a reservoir of the infection. Fleas spread from rodents (usually as they are dying of the plague) to the human host. Most people who develop plague have recently handled a dead or dying rodent. The bite of the infected flea injects the plague bacteria into the human tissues. Symptoms are high fever and swollen, enlarged lymph glands near the bite. These enlarged glands were known as buboes, accounting for the term bubonic plague. Because the flea bites most commonly occur in the legs, the glands of the groin are most likely to show buboes.

The germ of plague can spread to the lungs, causing pneumonia. This form, commonly known as pneumonic plague, is dangerous because coughing can spread the germ to others and the infection itself can be severe and life threatening. This germ was responsible for the great plagues of history. Several antibiotics now are effective in treating plague, and vaccines have been developed for persons in high-risk situations. Prevention primarily involves decreasing the rodent population near populated areas.

Rocky Mountain Spotted Fever

Rocky Mountain spotted fever is caused by a species of rickettsia, one-celled microbes that fall between viruses and bacteria, and that usually grow only in living cells. The disease gets its name from the Rocky Mountain area, where it is most common. However, cases have been found in fairly large numbers throughout the New England states and on islands such as Martha's Vineyard and Nantucket. The disease probably can be found throughout the United States. Rickettsias are carried by ticks, apparently picked up by the insects in biting common rodents. The tick then transmits the rickettsia to its descendants.

The disease generally occurs in late spring and summer, when ticks are abundant. Victims frequently are children who play in woods or wet grass. The child develops chills, fever, severe pains in bones and muscles, and a spotted rash that may become bloody after a few days. The rash appears first on the wrists, ankles, and back, then spreads over the body. Fortunately, antibiotics are completely effective, if the disease is recognized early and if the child or parents recall that it was preceded by a tick bite. If the disease is exceedingly severe or goes unrecognized, however, it may be fatal.

All wood ticks and dog ticks are potential carriers, so it is advisable to inspect your body or that of your child for ticks after walking in tick-infested areas or in woods or tall grass. A tick should be removed with a piece of tissue to avoid touching it directly and to avoid crushing. The animal should then be flushed down a toilet (see Chapter 35, "Emergency"). Parents who examine children should remember that ticks can crawl into the ear canals or hide in the hair.

Lyme Disease

Lyme disease is a recently identified tick-borne disease that gets its name from Old Lyme, Connecticut, where it was first reported in children in 1975. It has since been detected in other parts of the country, Europe, and Australia, and has been found in adults as well as children. The infectious agent is now known to be a spirochete, *Borrelia burgdorferi*, transmitted to the human by the tick's bite. The initial symptom is a characteristic reddish skin lesion, usually accompanied by fever, headache, stiff neck, fatigue, and swollen lymph glands. Weeks or months later, the patient may develop heart abnormalities and later yet, swollen joints and recurrent bouts of arthritis. (The disease originally was called "Lyme arthritis.") Treatment with penicillin or tetracycline when the skin lesion appears prevents or reduces the later complications, and more recent research indicates it is effective against established arthritis as well. As with the precautions for Rocky Mountain spotted fever, children who play in tick-infested areas should be inspected regularly for presence of ticks, and ticks removed and disposed of in the same manner.

Acquired Immune Deficiency Syndrome

As recently as 1981, acquired immune deficiency syndrome (AIDS) was virtually unknown in the United States. Since then, AIDS has become a major public health concern worldwide. The disease is believed to have originated in Africa, but now has spread to every major continent. Tens of thousands have died, millions are believed infected, and there is no known cure, despite a massive international research effort.

AIDS is caused by a virus that attacks the T-cell lymphocytes of the immune system, leaving the body vulnerable to several serious illnesses that would not be life threatening if the immune system were functioning normally. The two major "opportunistic" infections are pneumocystis carinii pneumonia, a parasitic infection of the lungs, and a cancer known as Kaposi's sarcoma. Cytomegalovirus (CMV) may attack the eye, causing severe visual impairment and even blindness. In addition, the infection may invade the brain and cause neurological complications leading to death.

The virus, isolated by American and French researchers, has been named human immunodeficiency virus (HIV) and resembles the virus that causes hepatitis B. The virus is transmitted through the blood and body fluids. It has been found in semen, saliva, and tears, although there are no known cases of AIDS being contracted through tears or saliva. However, health professionals and those who might provide emergency treatment to infected persons, such as police and paramedics, usually are instructed to take hygienic precautions.

No person has been known to have contracted AIDS through casual contact, such as a handshake or even an embrace with an infected person. Despite fears, there have been no known cases of the disease being transmitted by an insect bite.

Most AIDS patients belong to a few high-risk groups: promiscuous homosexual and bisexual men, intravenous drug users who share needles, hemophiliacs who receive transfusions of blood products, others who have received transfusions in the past, and sex partners of AIDS victims. The disease also has been transmitted to infants at birth by infected mothers.

The disease has been infrequent and slow to spread through the heterosexual population in the U.S., but is more common among heterosexuals elsewhere. For reasons unknown, AIDS appears to be more prevalent among minority groups.

There are no clear-cut symptoms. The first signs may be enlarged lymph nodes, tiredness, fever, loss of appetite or weight, and "night sweats." The early symptoms of pneumocystis carinii resemble other forms of pneumonia, including cough, fever, and breathing difficulty. Kaposi's sarcoma may begin with a bluish or brown spot resembling a bruise. Eye involvement may appear first as a loss of peripheral vision or inflammation of the retina. A less severe form of AIDS, AIDS-related complex (ARC), produces milder symptoms but eventually may develop into the full-fledged disease.

The progress of the disease varies widely. Some persons are symptom-free five years after known exposure. Once symptoms appear, the fatal outcome may be swift or prolonged. A few drugs appear to inhibit the virus and prolong life, but do not restore the immune system. Other treatments combat, but do not cure, the opportunistic infections. Some drugs can forestall visual impairment but carry severe side effects.

A major public-education campaign has been conducted to prevent the spread of AIDS. Persons are urged to practice "safe sex," by using a condom during intercourse, and to be cautious in choosing sexual partners. Authorities also have distributed "clean needles" to drug users to contain the epidemic in the drug-using population.

A test has been developed to identify HIV antibodies in the blood, indicating that a person is infected, even though symptom-free. The test has not been generally used except for certain populations, such as military recruits or prison inmates. However, the test is widely employed by blood banks and has succeeded in keeping donated blood supplies free of contamination.

CHAPTER 33

UNDERSTANDING YOUR OPERATION

Surgery is defined as the science of medicine in which operations are used as part of the treatment. But the term "surgery" refers not merely to the operative event but to the entire care of the patient.

Operations are classified as elective, urgent, or emergency procedures. An elective operation is one carried out for a disease or abnormality that is not life threatening or one in which a delay would not harm the patient. An example is a patient with gallstones who has had several attacks but does not have symptoms now. The operation could be performed this week, this month, or later. Speed is not the primary consideration. An urgent operation is one in which delay could produce serious problems or life-threatening complications if not carried out in a few days or weeks. An example is a cancer in which the malignancy could spread to other organs if not removed promptly. An emergency operation is one required immediately, within minutes or hours. In a ruptured abdominal aortic aneurysm, a defect in the main blood vessel in the abdomen, an operation may have to be carried out within a few minutes to save the patient's life.

BEFORE THE OPERATION

After an abnormality has been diagnosed and an operation recommended, the surgeon usually carries out an overall evaluation of the patient. This requires a detailed history of previous illnesses, operations, and family history. Of particular importance is information about allergies to certain drugs and medications, and about prior problems of bleeding. Previous illnesses, particularly of the heart and lungs, must be recognized. Basic laboratory studies will be necessary before or shortly after admission to the hospital. An electrocardiogram usually is recommended for patients over age 40 having a major operation.

From these findings, the surgeon can make a reasonable estimate of the risk of an operation. Any operative procedure requiring an anesthetic carries some degree of risk. Untoward and unpredicted events can occur that may be beyond the control of the surgeon and the operating team.

Obviously, before any operation the patient should be told the details of the procedure, the hazards, and possible complications. For example, a 35-year-old woman who is to have her gallbladder removed has a better than 99 percent chance of surviving and being well afterward. If, however, the woman were 65, had had two coronary attacks, and was diabetic, the risk of the same operation would rise to about 5 percent.

ANESTHESIA

Anesthesia is basic to virtually all surgery and the anesthesiologist is a key member of the surgical team. As described in Chapter 3, "Pain," anesthesias are divided into two types: general, which anesthetizes the entire body; and local, which blocks sensation of pain in one part of the body. General anesthesias may be inhaled or injected; local anesthesias are injected. The decision on the type used and how it is to be administered depends on the procedure and the patient's condition.

THE OPERATION

The operating room is a special environment in which absolute cleanliness and protection of the patient are the guiding principles. The "OR" is designed to be clean and easy to keep that way. An operating room requires constant airflow, with the air filtered to remove bacteria. Medical personnel must wear special clothing. This means "scrub suits," masks, head coverings, gloves, and coverings for shoes.

We sometimes speak of an operation as performed by a surgeon, as though he or she were working alone, but in fact, most operations require a surgical team. The surgeon usually will be aided by one or more assistant surgeons, plus corps of trained operating-room nurses and technicians.

During the operation, the anesthesiologist is responsible (with the surgeon) for supporting and maintaining the vital processes of the patient. While the surgeon is busy with the operation itself, the anesthesiologist maintains anesthesia and supports and assists breathing, often by way of a tube into the trachea—an endotracheal tube. He or she monitors heart action, blood pressure, adequacy of ventilation, kidney function in some patients, and the general state of the patient, and gives intravenous fluids to maintain the circulation and blood transfusion if necessary.

After the Operation

Following completion of the operative procedure, the incision is closed by sutures ("stitches") or surgical staples in each layer of tissue. Then a dressing is applied, anesthesia is stopped, and the patient is allowed to awaken.

The patient usually is taken from the operating room to a recovery room for close observation and care as he or she awakens from the anesthetic. If the patient has had a potentially life-threatening operation such as open-heart surgery, he or she may be taken directly to a surgical intensive-care unit and remain there for several days or longer. When a patient can breathe satisfactorily without assistance, when the circulation is stable, when kidneys are functioning normally, and if there are no other immediate threats to life, the patient may be discharged from intensive care to a regular hospital room for further convalescence.

Convalescence

Postsurgical convalescence has changed considerably in recent years. Hospital stays after most procedures have been shortened, and many procedures once requiring hospitalization now are done on an outpatient basis. In many cases the patient is sent home with medication or long-lasting anesthesia to recuperate there.

Healing after surgery occurs in four phases. The initial phase lasts two or three days, in which the person prefers to remain quiet, is not concerned about his surroundings, and may experience pain. Fortunately, much of it is relieved by medication. After about three to five days, the injury phase ends and the patient begins to feel more like himself or herself again. The third phase may cover about six weeks, during which the patient slowly regains strength and makes up the losses incurred in the injury phase. The fourth or final phase is that in which weight lost during the injury or operation is replaced. It may cover several months.

Complications

Complications after an operation can be classified into two categories: general complications that may follow any operation and specific complications after a particular operation.

Bleeding can occur after any operation, but is more common after those on the vascular system. Pulmonary problems may produce atelectasis, the collapse of portions of the lung. Clots can develop in the legs, particularly in the veins of the calves. If the clots break off and travel to the lungs, they can produce pulmonary emboli. These, on rare occasions, can be fatal.

If an organ has been damaged or diseased before an operation, the stress may overwhelm it and cause it to fail. Thus, a heavy smoker who has chronic lung disease may have lung failure.

Fortunately, complications usually can be kept to a minimum.

ABDOMINAL OPERATIONS

The abdominal cavity contains the organs of digestion (see Chapter 22, "The Digestive System"). It is separated from the chest cavity above by the diaphragm and at the lower boundary by the pelvis. The abdominal organs are illustrated in Chapter 22.

Any operation within the abdomen requires cutting through the skin, through a layer of fat under the skin called the subcutaneous tissue, and through a thick fibrous band overlying the muscles of the abdominal wall called the fascia. Under these three layers, forming an envelope or sac for the contents of the abdomen, is the thin shiny membrane called the peritoneum.

The incision itself depends on the operation and the location of the organ to be removed or repaired. The incision must be long enough to reveal the organs inside clearly, and to allow room to insert instruments or hands through the incision to carry out the procedure.

After the operation is completed, the incision must be closed. Several techniques are used. The basic principle is to close each layer with sutures or stitches. The peritoneum often is closed with a running suture of a material called chromic catgut, which will dissolve after two to three weeks. The muscles and fascia then are brought together, usually with a nonabsorbable suture of silk, cotton, plastic, or nylon, which will remain in place permanently. The subcutaneous tissue is brought together next, often with sutures that will be absorbed later. Finally, the wound in the skin is closed, using fine sutures of silk or other nonabsorbable material, metal clips, or staples. Depending on the location of the incision, skin sutures are left in place for a week to 10 days before being removed. During the first few weeks after an operation, the incision is held together by the sutures. After four to six weeks, the scar tissue is strong enough that the sutures are no longer relied on.

An infection in a healing incision usually is not evident until about the fifth day after an operation. It may produce a result as simple as slight redness around the sutures, or an abscess may form, requiring removal of the skin sutures and drainage. Rarely, an incision will fail to heal and will break open, a condition called wound dehiscence. If the entire wound separates, it is necessary to return the patient to the operating room for resuturing.

Operations on the Stomach And Duodenum

Hiatus hernia. Protrusions or bulges of abdominal organs through the diaphragm are called diaphragmatic hernias. The most common in an adult is through the esophageal hiatus, the oval opening through which the esophagus passes into the stomach. When this opening becomes stretched or enlarged, a portion of the stomach pushes up into the chest behind the heart. The abnormality interferes with the valve mechanism, which normally prevents stomach acid from refluxing up into the esophagus. Refluxing acid produces a burning sensation, the typical heartburn of indigestion. Frequent acid reflux will cause esophagitis, or inflammation of the esophageal lining, and if it continues, the esophageal wall will become scarred and thickened, interfering with swallowing.

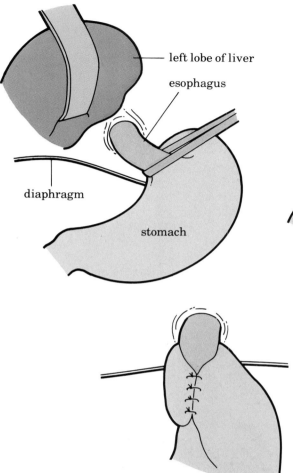

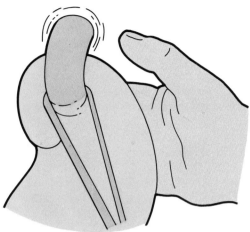

left lobe of liver

esophagus

diaphragm

stomach

HIATUS HERNIA

Repair of a hiatus hernia, which occurs when a portion of the stomach moves up through an enlarged opening in the diaphragm, takes place in three stages. At top left, the liver is moved aside and the stomach and esophagus are returned to their proper position. At top right, the stomach is wrapped around the esophagus. At left, the stomach is sutured into place. The operation prevents the condition from recurring and provides a new valve mechanism to prevent reflux of the stomach contents into the esophagus, the cause of heartburn. Most symptoms of hiatus hernia can be overcome without surgery.

The use of a group of acid-blocking drugs called Hz blockers has markedly reduced symptoms of hiatus hernia, and thus the need for surgery. When premalignant changes are detected in the affected tissue, however, repair usually is required. This procedure includes restoring the stomach to its normal position and strengthening the valve mechanism by wrapping a portion of the stomach around the esophagus and suturing it into place. Reflux of acid is prevented, but the patient can swallow normally.

Ulcer disease. The most common site of ulcers is the duodenum, the portion of small intestine just below the pylorus or outlet of the stomach. Basically, the cause is excess gastric acid production.

Ulcer surgery once was one of the most common operations, but ulcer's incidence, too, has declined markedly with the advent of acid-blocking drugs. Dietary changes also may have played a part.

Although most ulcers respond to medical treatment, certain problems may require surgical intervention. They include bleeding, perforation, obstruction, and "intractable" ulcers.

Most bleeding ulcers may be treated by inserting an endoscope, as described in Chapter 2, "Tests and Procedures," and coagulating the blood flow by a laser burn. Sometimes clotting agents may be injected via catheter. Both of these techniques avoid the risks of abdominal surgery.

When an ulcer perforates, causing an opening in the stomach wall, the first requirement is to close the perforation by suturing or stapling or by bringing a portion of the fatty tissue called the omentum over the hole and suturing or stapling it into place, to allow the opening to seal.

For obstruction caused by scar tissue, it is necessary either to remove the scarred area, eliminating that portion of the stomach and closing it off, or to bypass it by building a connection (anastomosis) around the obstruction to the intestine below it.

For intractable ulcers that do not heal or do not stay healed, the objective is to reduce acid formation and prevent recurrence. One approach is to remove the acid-producing lower two-thirds of the stomach (gastrectomy). The upper third of the stomach then is connected directly to the intestinal tract. This usually is done by bringing a loop of the jejunum, the part of the small intestine just beyond the duodenum, up over the colon and suturing or stapling to form an anastomosis of the stomach. The duodenum is closed into a blind pouch.

A second major approach is to cut the vagus nerves (vagotomy), which stimulate the stomach to produce acid. These nerves, which regulate many internal functions, pass along the esophagus to the stomach and other sections of the gastrointestinal tract.

Because vagotomy reduces the tone of the stomach so that it does not empty well, a procedure to promote drainage often is performed. The thickened muscle of the pylorus or the entire wall is divided and sutured to increase the pyloric opening. Another procedure, which removes the lower third of the stomach, including the outlet of the stomach and the pylorus, is called an antrectomy.

The most common operation for ulcer disease is a vagotomy plus gastrectomy or antrectomy. In this operation the ulcer is removed, particularly if it lies in the first portion of the duodenum. If the ulcer occurs farther down in the duodenum, it becomes impossible to remove because it lies close to where the common bile duct or the ducts from the pancreas come in. Then the ulcer is left in place, and the duodenum is closed above it.

Ulcers in the stomach (gastric ulcers) account for about one in five cases of ulcer disease. A benign gastric ulcer may heal without surgery. If it does not, the ulcer and the affected portion of the stomach usually are removed in a procedure similar to that for duodenal ulcers.

Tumors. Cancer of the stomach, which is much less common than in the past, may begin as an ulcer. If a cancer is confirmed by biopsy or gastros-

copy, the affected portion of the stomach is removed, along with a portion of normal stomach surrounding it, plus the adjoining lymph nodes. The remaining portion of the stomach is joined with the small intestine. It seldom is necessary to remove the entire stomach.

A major function of the stomach is to serve as a reservoir for food. If the upper one-third to one-fourth of the stomach can be left in place, patients can eat fairly normally.

Operations on the Small Intestine

The small intestine usually is classified as having three sections: the duodenum (just beyond the stomach), the lengthy jejunum, and the ileum, which joins the small intestine to the colon. Intimately associated with the small intestine is an apronlike skirt called the mesentery, which provides the intestine's blood supply.

Surgery on the small intestine frequently is performed because disease usually affects only a portion of the organ. The diseased section can be removed, and the severed ends joined together. A smooth union is possible because the intestine is of uniform diameter, and its great length allows for removal without the section being missed. When the section is cut out, a pie-shaped piece of the mesentery usually is removed with it. The usual procedure is to clamp off the target area, remove it, then suture the ends and mesentery back together. The blood vessels of the mesentery are tied off.

Most intestinal complaints, whether of the small or large intestine, that bring a person to a surgeon produce a similar group of symptoms. These include blood in the stool, abdominal pain that is sometimes sharp and severe, nausea and vomiting, bloating, and the inability to pass gas or stool. It is not always easy to determine the cause of the complaint, so exploratory surgery may be necessary.

Adhesions are the most common surgical problem involving the small intestine. Adhesions are fibrous connections or bonds between segments of intestine, abdominal wall, or omentum. Adhesions develop when segments of intestine adhere to one another or to the under surface of the incision. The resulting kinks or twists can cause partial or complete obstruction. Symptoms include crampy abdominal pain and bloating, followed by nausea and vomiting, with inability to pass gas or stool. The twists or kinks may cut off the blood supply to the intestine, producing life-threatening infarction or gangrene.

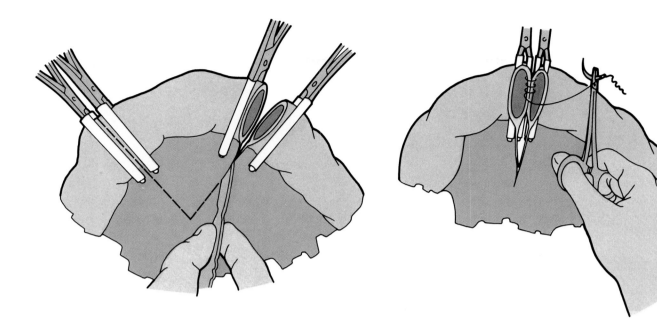

THE SMALL INTESTINE
A common operation for disorders of the small intestine is to remove the diseased section and shorten the bowel's length, as shown in these drawings. At left, the portion of bowel has been clamped off on both sides of the diseased area. The surgeon then cuts across the bowel *between the clamps and removes a wedge from the mesentery, the apronlike sheet of tissue that provides blood to the intestine. The blood vessels are divided and tied off, and the two ends of the bowel are sewn together (right) to restore continuity.*

To correct adhesions, it is necessary to open the abdomen, find the site of the adhesions and obstruction, and divide the adhesions, a procedure called lysis of adhesions. If a portion of the intestine is twisted and infarcted or gangrenous, that portion must be removed and the divided ends above and below the gangrenous segment sutured.

Tumors of the small intestine, both benign and malignant, various inflammatory diseases such as Crohn's disease or regional enteritis, and diseases of the blood supply to the small intestine also may require removal of a portion of the intestine and anastomosis.

Appendectomy

The appendix is a short, hollow blind tube of intestine attached to the cecum, the first portion of the large intestine lying just below its junction with the small intestine. Inflammation of the appendix (appendicitis) occurs when fecal material gets into the lumen or hollow channel of the appendix and obstructs it. The appendix cannot rid itself of this obstruction, and it contracts and becomes inflamed. At first a localized phenomenon, the infec-tious process moves through the wall of the appendix to adjoining organs. If the appendix perforates or becomes gangrenous, fecal material may leak into the peritoneal cavity.

Removal of an inflamed appendix (appendectomy) generally is uneventful. The procedure requires a small diagonal or oblique incision in the lower right portion of the abdomen. A few small blood vessels and the base of the appendix itself are divided, then tied off by a suture. The stump of the appendix may be tied or buried in the cecal wall.

Appendicitis is a great mimic of other diseases. Normally the appendix is only about 3 inches long, but may be far longer in some persons and extend into the pelvis alongside the colon or uterus or even into the left side. Thus, early diagnosis of appendicitis can be extremely difficult. For this reason, it is important to seek medical aid when abdominal pain does not subside rapidly.

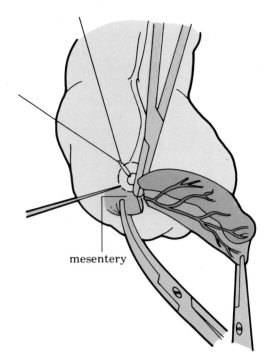

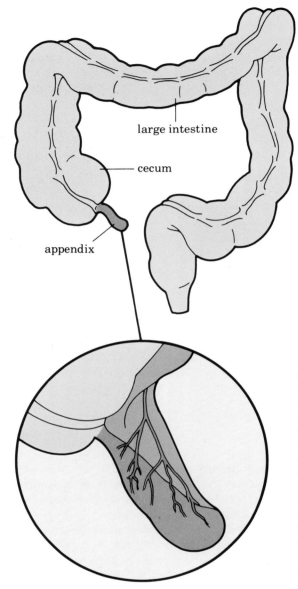

large intestine

cecum

appendix

mesentery

APPENDECTOMY

Surgery to remove a diseased appendix is very common. The drawing at top left shows the appendix in its normal location, attached to the cecum. The drawing at bottom left shows the link between the appendix and the mesentery, its normal source of blood supply. In an appendectomy, the vessels in the mesentery are clamped or tied off. In the drawing above, the appendix has been cut off from its blood supply and a clamp has been placed across its base. The organ will be amputated at the clamp, the remaining portion ligated, and a purse-string suture tied, inverting the stump.

Operations of the Colon

The primary disease processes involving the colon (large intestine) that may require an operation include cancer, diverticulitis, ulcerative colitis, and inflammatory bowel disease or granulomatous colitis. Polyps of the colon and bleeding from blood vessel abnormalities within the colon walls also may call for surgical care.

Cancer. Cancer of the colon usually announces itself by a change in bowel habits. The warning signs are increasing constipation, blood in the stool, crampy abdominal pain, weight loss, feeling poorly, loss of appetite, and anemia. If a person has one or more of these signs, diagnostic studies usually will be ordered. The first step usually is a test of the stool to see whether blood is present. The inside of the colon then may be inspected either by a sigmoidoscope, which allows inspection of the lower 10 inches of the intestine, where most cancers develop, or by the flexible colonoscope, which permits examination of the entire length of the colon.

If cancer is found, the type of surgery performed will depend on the site of the cancer. Regardless of its location, however, it always is necessary to remove the cancerous portion of the bowel surgically. A segment of colon above and below the tumor also is cut out to ensure that the cancer has been removed completely. The surgeon also removes the mesentery.

Sometimes, the first clue to a colon cancer is bowel obstruction or perforation. An emergency operation then is necessary. It may include a colostomy, in which a portion of the colon is brought through the abdominal wall outside the body. This artificially created sac allows contents of the colon to collect outside the body so they do not produce obstruction or contamination. The arrangement may be temporary or permanent. If it is permanent, the patient may be fitted with a collecting bag. The bag's contents may be disposed of at the patient's convenience, or the patient may be taught to irrigate the colostomy each day with a catheter.

If a cancer of the colon is located in the rectum or close to the anus, it may be necessary to remove the entire rectum and anus. The colon above the site of the tumor then is brought out through an incision in the abdominal wall to form a permanent-end colostomy. The operation also requires a bag for colon contents. Surgical stapling devices allow much lower anastamoses in rectal cancer than in the past, so colostomy is less often necessary. Radiation therapy also may be prescribed if the cancer has spread to local lymph nodes.

Polyps, which are small outpouchings on stalks, may develop in the lining of the walls of the colon. Polyps generally are benign, but may become malignant. Formerly it was necessary to remove polyps by an abdominal operation, but polyps now can be removed by colonoscopy. The lighted sighting device is fitted with tiny retractable blades or with an electric cautery that can seal off the growths.

Diverticulitis. A diverticulum is an outpouching in the wall of the colon. The most common location is in the sigmoid colon on the left side, just above the rectum. The outpouchings in themselves do not produce difficulty, but they may start an inflammatory process called diverticulitis. Diverticulitis can lead to swelling, obstruction, or perforation, producing peritonitis or bleeding. Pain may be intense.

Operation for diverticulitis depends on the stage and extent of the disease. If a person has had recurrent attacks of abdominal pain due to diverticulitis, an elective operation may be carried out to remove the affected segment.

Ulcerative colitis and inflammatory bowel disease (granulomatous colitis) produce somewhat similar symptoms, including inflammation of the lining of the intestine, diarrhea, weight loss, crampy abdominal pain, and bleeding. Both diseases may be treated by medication for long periods. However, many patients ultimately have repeated or acute attacks. In addition, ulcerative colitis that persists for a number of years increases the risk of cancer. Ultimately, it may become necessary to remove the affected portion of the colon, or even the entire colon, rectum, and anus. Removal of the entire colon (total colectomy) is followed by creation of an opening for the small intestine (ileostomy) to come out through the abdominal wall. A method of stripping the rectal segment to form a small bowel pouch, however, allows surgeons to preserve the rectum and avoid an ileostomy in many cases.

The Biliary Tract, Bile Ducts, And Gallbladder

The biliary tree or tract drains bile from the liver into the intestine. Small bile ducts within the liver merge into the two hepatic ducts from the right and left lobes of the liver, which then come together to form the common bile duct. The common bile duct runs down to and enters the duodenum, along with ducts bringing secretions from the pancreas. Coming off the common bile duct is the gallbladder, a reservoir for the storage of bile that fills between meals, then empties bile after eating to aid in digestion.

Gallstones (cholelithiasis) are the most common disease of the biliary system. The stones may produce symptoms in themselves, cause inflammation of the gallbladder (cholecystitis), obstruct the gallbladder, or pass through the cystic duct leading from the gallbladder and obstruct the common bile duct, so that bile backs up into the liver. The stones may be disintegrated without surgery by beaming shock waves at the body, a process called lithotripsy and described in Chapter 2, "Tests and Procedures." Lithotripsy has become the recommended treatment for gallstones (and kidney and bladder stones as well). Because stones may recur, however, removal of the gallbladder may be preferred. An incision is made on the right side of the abdomen and the gallbladder is removed from the enveloping capsule that holds it to the underside of the liver. The cystic duct is divided and tied off. If stones have passed into the common bile duct, it

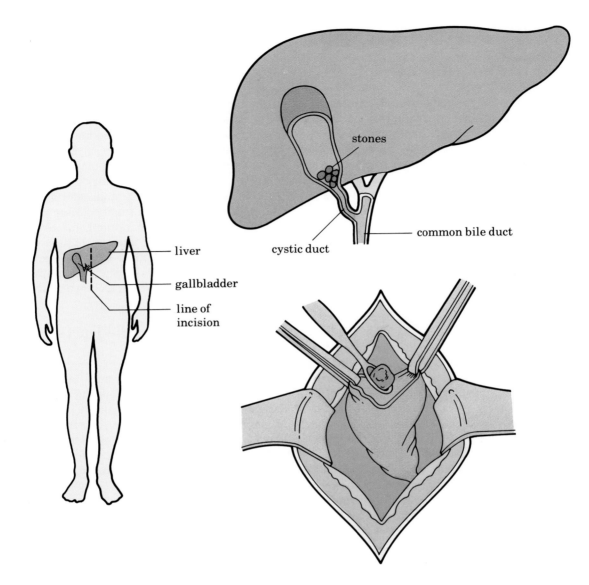

stones

common bile duct

cystic duct

liver

gallbladder

line of
incision

GALLBLADDER REMOVAL

When stones repeatedly form in the gallbladder, the organ often is removed. The drawing at left shows the gallbladder's normal location hanging from the liver just beneath the margin of the ribs in the right upper abdomen. The dotted line represents one common incision. Stones at the outlet to the cystic duct can obstruct the gallbladder or cause inflammation and severe pain.

A stone that passes into the duct may lodge farther down and block the common bile duct, causing bile to back up in the liver. At bottom right, the gallbladder has been opened and stones are being removed. More commonly, the gallbladder is removed and the cystic duct is tied off at its junction with the common bile duct. Lithotripsy allows stones to be dissolved without surgery.

may be necessary to remove the stones. Subsequently, surgeons commonly leave a small T-shaped tube in the common bile duct for about a week to prevent scarring, which might produce a narrowing that would obstruct bile.

Loss of the gallbladder is not a serious handicap. Most persons can live normal lives (and eat normal diets) without it.

Operations on the Pancreas

The pancreas is affected by two primary types of disease: pancreatitis and cancer.

Pancreatitis, or inflammation of the pancreas, sometimes is produced by obstructive gallstones. The condition also is associated with heavy drinking, and can be so extensive that it extends through the wall of the pancreas to liquefy or digest tissue. Acute pancreatitis usually is treated by medication and abstinence from alcohol. When pancreatitis becomes chronic, however, an operation may be recommended to drain the obstructed pancreatic duct. The pancreas also may be removed. Pancreatic hormones and insulin, which is produced in the pancreas, are given afterward.

Cancer of the pancreas most commonly occurs in the head of the pancreas. Such a tumor may block the confluence of the pancreatic duct and the common bile duct and produce jaundice as an early symptom. If the tumor has not spread, removal of a portion of the pancreas and the adjoining duodenum is required. The entire pancreas often is removed because of the possible microscopic extension of the cancer. Pancreatic enzymes and insulin may be given afterward.

The Liver

Injury is the most common reason for operations on the liver. It usually is caused by a vehicular accident or by a fall. The impact cracks or ruptures the liver, and the normally firm tissue breaks up, producing severe hemorrhage. An immediate operation is needed to control the bleeding, either by suturing the liver or by removing the portion that has been destroyed. A large portion of the liver can be removed because the remaining liver will increase in size to carry on the functions required.

Tumors of the liver, either benign or malignant, are rare. One type, the hepatic adenoma, has been associated with the use of birth control pills. These benign tumors cause discomfort mainly because of their large size. The liver is a common target organ for spread of cancer from other parts of the body,

but malignant tumors occasionally originate in the liver. If the tumor is limited to one lobe, it may be possible to remove the cancerous lobe.

Cirrhosis is a common disease of the liver, sometimes caused by chronic hepatitis, but more often by alcoholism. The disease causes the production of fibrous tissue that gradually destroys liver cells and interferes with the flow of blood.

A primary target is the veins of the lower esophagus, where the portal venous system of the liver connects with the systemic venous system returning blood to the heart. Large dilated veins in this area are called esophageal varices. They are thin-walled, and under high pressure they may break and produce severe hemorrhage. The bleeding, however, may be checked by sealing off the varices by endoscopic laser treatment. In rare cases, an immediate operation may be required to stop the bleeding and obliterate the veins or reduce the pressure so that they do not bleed again.

The Spleen

The spleen lies beneath the diaphragm on the left side of the abdomen, and helps remove various materials from the blood, including broken-down or old red blood cells, debris, and bacteria. It also contributes to the immune system. Direct injury to the left chest and left flank may tear or rupture the spleen or its capsule, producing hemorrhage. Formerly, any sign of rupture or injury to the spleen led to immediate operation and removal of the spleen (splenectomy). Recently, it has been recognized that the possibility of infection is increased after splenectomy, particularly in young children. Therefore, surgeons try to repair the spleen if the injury is not extensive.

Tumors of the spleen also may require splenectomy, as may several diseases producing abnormalities of the blood or lymphatic systems. The spleen also is removed for Hodgkin's disease, a cancer of the lymph nodes.

HERNIA

A hernia is a protrusion of the contents of a body cavity through its enveloping wall.

Inguinal hernia in the male is the most common hernia. Indirect inguinal hernia occurs frequently in newborn or young males. At birth the testicle, with its attached blood vessels and the spermatic cord, migrates through an opening in the abdominal wall (the internal inguinal ring) down a canal and into the scrotum. If the opening

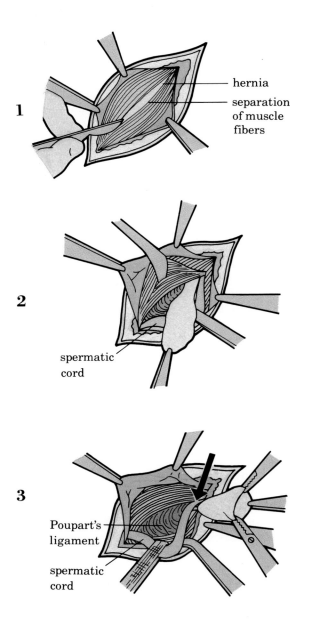

1   hernia
separation
of muscle
fibers

2   spermatic
cord

3   Poupart's
ligament
spermatic
cord

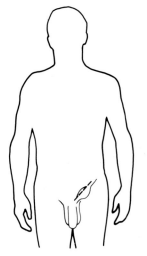

INGUINAL HERNIA

The common hernia of males occurs when the inguinal ring opening to the scrotum weakens and enlarges, allowing a portion of intestine to push through the opening and producing a bulge in the groin, as shown above. Stages of hernia repair are shown at left. (1) An incision is made, and the fasciae overlying the inguinal canal are separated, showing the hernia beneath. (2) The hernia sac is freed from surrounding tissue. The spermatic cord carrying blood to the testicles and sperm from the testicles can be seen below it. (3) The hernia sac is opened, inspected, and emptied. Fat or bowel is pushed back into the peritoneal cavity and the base of the hernia sac is sutured, closing off the weakened area behind the spermatic cord and narrowing the opening through which the cord passes. The muscle, fascia, and back wall of the inguinal canal are closed, but the cord is allowed to pass through the canal.

is somewhat large, or if a portion of the lining of the peritoneal cavity descends with the testicle, a sac of the lining tissue is formed. A portion of the wall or a loop of small intestine may be pushed into this sac, creating a painful bulge in the groin.

Direct inguinal hernia occurs in adult men. The stresses of life, particularly coughing, sneezing, straining during bowel movements, physical exercise, and lifting may combine with age-related relaxation of the tissues to produce a weakness that

allows the abdominal contents to push through the back of the inguinal canal. Direct inguinal hernia, too, produces an uncomfortable bulge and may press on other organs.

Inguinal hernias are much less frequent in the female. A hernia can occur in females, however, in which the protrusion and the sac are below the groin itself and extend into the upper portion of the thigh alongside the blood vessels supplying the leg (the femoral vessels), a condition called a femoral hernia.

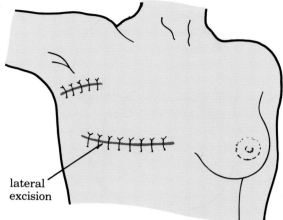

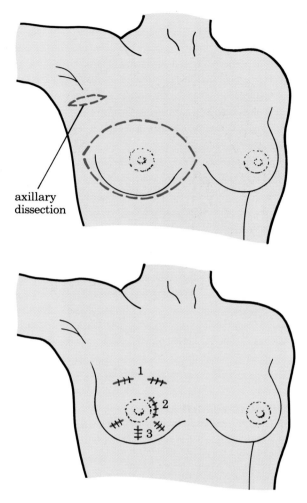

axillary
dissection

lateral
excision

BREAST SURGERY
Total mastectomy (top left), removal of the cancerous breast, is the most common surgical treatment for breast cancer. Less drastic than earlier operations, it spares underlying muscles. Underarm excision allows examination of axillary lymph nodes to determine if the cancer has spread. Excisions (top right) reduce the amount of scarring. Lumpectomy (bottom left) removes the cancer and bordering tissue but preserves the breast. Three common locations for tumor excision are shown. Lumpectomy normally is followed by radiation therapy.

The presence of either an inguinal or a femoral hernia requires an operation. When segments of large or small intestine enter the sac and cannot be pushed back into the abdomen, an urgent operation is recommended, because the ring through which the bowel has herniated may constrict the intestine, blocking its blood supply and producing gangrene. The intestine may be obstructed, too. It then is necessary to remove the strangulated portion of the intestine.

The repair of an ordinary inguinal hernia requires elimination of the emptied hernia sac by dissecting it free from the adjoining tissues, closing the neck of the sac where it protrudes from the abdomen, then repairing the tissues of the inguinal canal. The fascia or fibrous tissue and the muscles are brought together over the defect to close it permanently as illustrated in this chapter. However, in the young male, the spermatic cord still must come through the orifice in the abdominal wall

and run in the inguinal canal to the testicle. Thus, the orifice or internal ring cannot be closed so tightly that it obstructs the blood supply or blocks the flow of sperm.

Thanks to long-acting local anesthetics, hernia repair in an otherwise healthy male almost always is an outpatient procedure. The period of recuperation has been shortened, too, and most patients return to work within a week. However, the patient usually is told to refrain from heavy lifting for about six weeks.

BREAST OPERATIONS

Few areas of medicine have undergone such dramatic change in recent times as treatment, including surgery, for breast cancer. This disease, no longer the most common but still the most feared cancer among women, is discussed in detail in Chapter 27, "Cancer of the Breast."

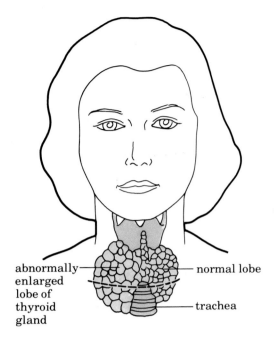

abnormally enlarged lobe of thyroid gland

normal lobe

trachea

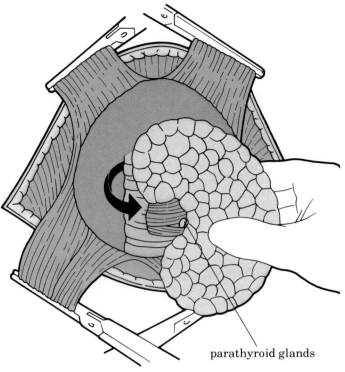

parathyroid glands

THYROID REMOVAL
An enlarged thyroid gland in the neck may require surgical removal. The drawing at top left shows enlargement of the patient's right thyroid lobe compared to the normal left lobe. The dotted line is where the usual incision is made. After the incision, the strap muscles of the neck are separated at the midline (bottom left) to expose the thyroid. The lobe is cut free from surrounding tissue. It then is pulled forward (top right) to divide and ligate the blood supply, and to expose and preserve the parathyroid glands adjacent to the thyroid.

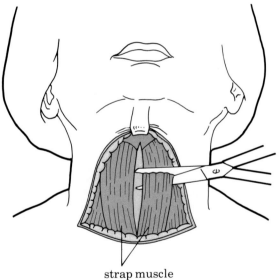

strap muscle

OPERATIONS ON THE
HEAD AND NECK

The thyroid gland. A nodule or lump within the thyroid gland may be a cyst, a benign tumor, or cancer. Needle biopsy often reveals whether the lump is benign or malignant, but sometimes it is necessary to remove the nodule and adjoining thyroid tissue to make the determination.

The normal thyroid gland has two lobes that lie on each side of the windpipe. They are joined across the middle. To operate on the thyroid gland, a transverse incision is made in the neck just above the clavicles or collarbones. The overlying neck muscles then are divided in the middle and held to the sides to expose the thyroid gland. Usually a nodule is found on only one side of the gland and that lobe is removed (lobectomy). With a benign tumor and certain forms of cancer, lobectomy

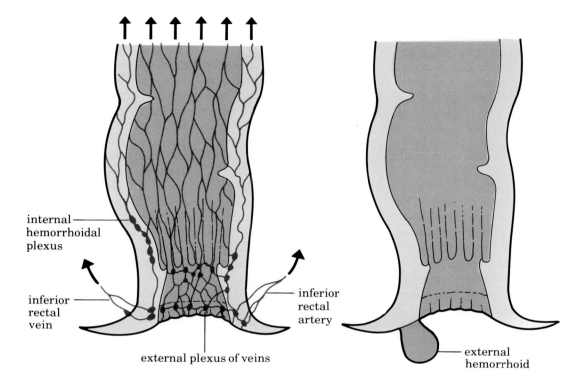

internal hemorrhoidal plexus

inferior rectal vein

inferior rectal artery

external plexus of veins

external hemorrhoid

HEMORRHOIDS
The usual sites for development of hemorrhoids are the internal plexus (just inside the anal sphincter muscle) and the external plexus (outside the anus). The arrows show the direction of blood flow in the area of the anus and rectum. At right, a clot (thrombosis) has formed in an external hemorrhoid. A thrombosed hemorrhoid may have to be treated surgically.

may be sufficient. For other forms of cancer it may be necessary to remove the thyroid totally (thyroidectomy). Afterward, the patient must take thyroid hormone by mouth.

Goiter is enlargement of the thyroid gland, often to massive size. The extraordinary growth usually is caused by lack of iodine in the diet. Although it is relatively painless, the bulge on the neck can become so huge that it is unsightly and uncomfortable, and hampers breathing. The goiter then must be removed surgically. A small portion of the thyroid tissue is left to provide thyroid hormone.

The parathyroid glands. The parathyroids, small endocrine organs adjoining the thyroid gland, secrete a hormone that influences calcium metabolism. Overactivity of the parathyroid glands produces a disorder of calcium metabolism. Stones may form in the kidneys, or the amount of calcium in the bones may decrease. This overactivity may stem from enlargement of the parathyroid glands, called hyperplasia, or from a benign

tumor of one gland. Either calls for an exploratory operation to inspect the glands and perhaps to perform a biopsy. It may be necessary to remove one or more of the glands.

Tumors in the mouth or on the tongue, throat, or lip are most commonly squamous-cell carcinomas, a form of skin cancer arising from the surface of the mucous membrane of the mouth (see Chapter 9, "The Skin"). Many are readily visible, and usually are detected and removed promptly. However, some tumors of the tongue and mouth require more extensive removal. If the tumor has spread to the lymph nodes in the neck, removal of the primary tumor must be followed by a radical neck dissection. An incision is made in the neck. The subcutaneous tissue, the sternocleidomastoid muscle (one of the major muscles in the neck), and all of the lymph nodes overlying the main blood vessels are removed.

OPERATIONS ON THE RECTUM AND ANUS

The rectal area just above the anus is a series of pockets, pleats, and tucks, the natural result of the gathering effects of the purse-string muscle that closes the natural opening. Inflammation, swelling, and infection can occur, and surgery may be necessary.

An anal fissure is a tear in the lining of the anal canal or its mucous membrane. The result is bleeding and pain during a bowel movement. Such a fissure usually is caused by constipation or straining. The doctor usually tries first to treat a fissure with stool softeners, changes in diet, medication to stimulate regular bowel movements, or sitz baths. If the fissure does not heal, it may be necessary to operate and remove it.

A fistula occurs when one of the glandular crevices of the anus, called a crypt, becomes inflamed or infected. The infection may burrow through the soft flesh and produce an abnormal opening to the outside, a tiny distance from the natural opening. The initial treatment is the same as for a fissure, but if preliminary treatment is not successful, an operation may be necessary. The procedure opens the fistula or excises it and dilates the anal sphincter to allow healing.

Hemorrhoids are dilated veins covered by folds of skin just within or outside the anal canal. They result from inflammation in the anal canal, aggravated by pressure such as straining during a bowel movement. Hemorrhoids frequently exist without symptoms, but occasionally they may bleed or cause pain during bowel movements.

Hemorrhoids should be treated initially by exactly the same approach as for a fistula or fissure. Medication applied externally also may be helpful. Sometimes a blood clot may form in a hemorrhoid, or a ring of hemorrhoids around the anus may become so large and bulky that they cause painful bowel movements. Laser treatment frequently is used to seal off the hemorrhoid, so surgery seldom is necessary.

AMPUTATIONS

Amputations of injured limbs and appendages have been one of the historical roles of surgeons. In the past it often was necessary to remove an arm, a leg, a finger, or a toe because it had been so badly damaged or crushed in a farm or industrial accident that repair was impossible. In addition, the injury threatened to spread infection to the rest of the body. The development of antibiotics has lessened the risks of infection, and improved surgical techniques have enabled surgeons to save many limbs that previously might have been lost. Indeed, it now sometimes is possible to restore a limb that has been cleanly severed.

Reimplantation surgery is the name given to the reattachment of a severed body part. Much of the work must be done under magnification, using tiny instruments. The first step is to reconnect the severed blood vessels by anastomosis. The major arteries and veins are brought together using suture material finer than a human hair. Severed muscles and tendons must be reattached, then the bony structures attached, where possible. Nerves may be reunited during the initial operation, or nerve repair may be delayed until the skin has been closed and allowed to heal. Functional results for reimplantation of fingers and hands have been better than for entire arms and legs.

Amputation itself still is necessary for particularly extensive or crushing injuries and for the effects of certain diseases. Tumors of the bone, tendon, soft tissue, or skin may force amputation as may arteriosclerosis or diabetes.

In most cases of amputation, the entire damaged area of bone is cut away, the blood vessels and nerves tied off, and a flap of skin sewn over the stump. Artificial limbs now may be applied immediately following amputation, greatly facilitating convalescence. Afterward, many persons walk without a limp and even engage in sports.

OPERATIONS ON BLOOD VESSELS

Arteriosclerosis, or hardening of the arteries, and its consequences are a frequent cause for surgery on the blood vessels. Blood pressure may be elevated, causing a blood vessel wall to become thin and bulge. This outpouching, or aneurysm, may rupture and bleed. Although an aneurysm can occur anywhere, the most common site is the abdominal aorta, the main artery below the diaphragm. The aneurysm may form a large pulsating mass. As it expands, it may cause pain in the back, the abdomen, or the flanks. Severe pain usually means that the aneurysm is expanding rapidly or beginning to rupture.

A ruptured aneurysm, even when treated promptly, is associated with a high mortality rate because so much blood is lost before the hemorrhage can be stopped. If the aneurysm is discovered before it ruptures, however, it can be treated quite satisfactorily by an operation. The ballooned portion of the vessel is removed. The section of the artery is replaced with a synthetic or plastic graft.

Narrowing and occlusion of blood vessels occur most commonly where blood vessels branch. A common site is in the carotid arteries in the neck, which supply blood to the brain. Narrowing in the internal carotid branch may result initially in attacks of dizziness, light-headedness, loss of memory, and other symptoms that together are called transient ischemic attacks. A stroke may occur at the onset or with persistence of symptoms. If transient ischemic attacks bring attention to the narrowing before a stroke occurs, an operation can be performed to remove the inner lining of the thickened portion of the artery and restore normal blood flow to the brain.

The next most common site for arteriosclerotic narrowing is in the blood vessels supplying the legs. This condition, described in detail in Chapter 6, "Blood Vessel Disorders," causes pain in the calf muscles while walking, a condition termed intermittent claudication. If the process becomes even more extensive, it may lead to gangrene of the foot, ankle, and lower leg, requiring amputation.

As described in Chapter 6, the use of balloon angioplasty, lasers, or cutting devices inserted via a leg artery allows these blockages to be removed and has revolutionized their treatment. Rarely, it becomes necessary to perform a bypass graft, in which a conduit is brought from above the block in the artery to a vessel below it. If the block or narrowing is in the abdominal aorta or its major branches coming down to the groin, the bypass is made with a plastic prosthetic graft. When a bypass graft is to be carried out from the femoral artery at the groin down to the popliteal artery entering the lower leg behind the knee, the surgeon usually will use one of the patient's veins.

OPERATIONS ON THE LUNGS AND ESOPHAGUS

The Lungs

Pneumothorax occurs when air finds its way outside the lung and into the thoracic cavity, compressing the lung, interfering with breathing, and producing chest pain. This most commonly is caused by rupture of a bleb, a small ballooned area at the top of the lung. To treat pneumothorax, a tube is inserted into the chest or pleural cavity, usually as an outpatient procedure. The tube is connected to a drain that terminates under water. As the patient breathes in, water rises in the tube; as the patient exhales, air is forced out of the pleural space and bubbles through the water as it is released. This water seal allows the ruptured area eventually to seal, the lung to expand, and the air to be eliminated from the chest space.

Tumors of the lung may be benign or malignant (see Chapter 10, "The Lungs"). There are a number of different types of lung cancers, each requiring individual and separate approaches. Commonly, the suspicion of tumor is raised when the patient begins to cough up blood (hemoptysis), leading to a chest X ray, or has a routine screening examination in which a mass is detected. Diagnostic tests then are undertaken to determine whether the mass or shadow is an inflammatory process, such as pneumonia, or a tumor.

An early step usually is bronchoscopy, visual inspection of the trachea and bronchi. Fiber-optic instruments allow the physician to look down into very small bronchi and obtain tissue or scrapings. Often the exact nature of the lesion can be determined by this technique. Needle biopsy guided by CT scan also helps in diagnosis, so exploratory surgery seldom is needed.

If the tumor is confirmed by these diagnostic techniques but is confined to one lobe of the lung, that lobe will be removed. If it is extensive or involves the origin of the main bronchus to a lung, it may be necessary to remove the entire lung. The pulmonary artery, which runs from the heart to the lungs, is ligated and divided, as are the pulmonary veins, which run from the lungs to the heart. Then the bronchus is divided close to the trachea, and the lung is removed. The stump of the bronchus is closed by sutures or a stapling device. The cavity in the chest gradually fills with fluid and later becomes fibrous tissue. Removal of a lung can be well tolerated if the other lung is healthy enough. Patients live normally for many years.

Esophagus

In addition to hiatus hernia, described earlier in this chapter, the esophagus also may develop benign tumors, which can be removed easily, or abnormalities of motion such as achalasia, which can be treated by an operation.

Cancer may develop in any portion of the esophagus, but is most common in the lower third, nearest the stomach. Unfortunately, many esophageal cancers are quite extensive when discovered, because the cancer must be large before it interferes with swallowing, the usual initial symptom. Removal requires an incision in the abdomen to free the stomach from its attachments, after which an incision is made in the chest. The tumor and much of the esophagus then are removed. Continuity usually is restored by joining the esophagus above the tumor to the stomach below the tumor.

HEART OPERATIONS

Abnormalities within the heart can be treated directly only by what is called an open-heart procedure. The heart-lung machine then is used to take over the work of the heart and the lungs temporarily, allowing the surgeon to work inside the heart without the heart beating.

Congenital heart defects usually are discovered in infancy or early childhood. These abnormalities, which are described in Chapter 5, "The Heart and Circulation," may be as simple as a "hole" in the heart (an atrial or ventricular septal defect in which a partition has failed to close) or failure of a valve to develop and open properly, producing a narrowing or stenosis.

Some of the simpler and more straightforward congenital problems can be corrected shortly after birth or during early years of childhood. Patent ductus arteriosus, in which an opening necessary in fetal life fails to close at birth, can be eliminated by ligation or division of the ductus. Before birth, the lungs do not function and the ductus arteriosus allows blood to bypass them. If it does not close at birth, it must be closed surgically so that aortic blood does not pass into the lungs and increase pressure.

Coarctation of the aorta, failure of a major blood vessel to develop properly, is corrected by cutting out the narrowed section of this important blood vessel and bringing the severed ends together. It sometimes is necessary to insert a graft.

In the past, some severe congenital cardiac defects required preliminary procedures shortly after birth to help the infant survive until a total correction could be carried out later. In recent years, however, even newborns have been operated on using the heart-lung machine. The procedure has been made safer by hypothermia, which means lowering the infant's temperature so organs will better tolerate a period without blood.

Valvular heart disease in an adult usually occurs as the aftermath of rheumatic fever and rheumatic heart disease (see Chapter 5, "The Heart and Circulation"). It primarily involves the mitral valve between the heart's two left chambers, the left atrium and the left ventricle, or the aortic valve at the outlet of the left ventricle to the aorta, where blood enters the general circulation. Sometimes aortic valve disease results from a birth defect. The valve normally has three leaflets, but some persons are born with a two-leaflet aortic valve. Later in life, calcium deposits or other abnormalities may form in the defective valve, producing narrowing (stenosis) or leakage.

Coronary artery disease also may produce abnormalities of the cardiac valves. And, as part of the aging process, the fibrous bands that hold the mitral valve (chordae tendineae) can rupture.

The first operation to be performed on heart valves was a mitral commissurotomy, or mitral valvotomy, in which, with the heart beating, the surgeon inserted a finger into the narrowed valve to push it open. The valve often would function satisfactorily thereafter. Gradually surgeons learned to use instruments for this purpose. But today when valve disease causes symptoms or problems, the valve simply is replaced.

The two basic types of artificial valves are a ball-and-cage valve and a flat or disk valve. Commonly, the replacement for an aortic valve is taken from the heart of a pig. The tissue is processed and preserved by fixing solutions, then attached to a ring, sterilized, and sewn into the heart. Porcine valves have been in place for up to seven years, and usually are more successful than plastic valves.

Valve replacement requires an open-heart procedure using a heart-lung machine. The incision is made in the midline of the chest, dividing the sternum and approaching the forward surface of the heart. The silent heart is opened, and the diseased valve is removed. The replacement valve is

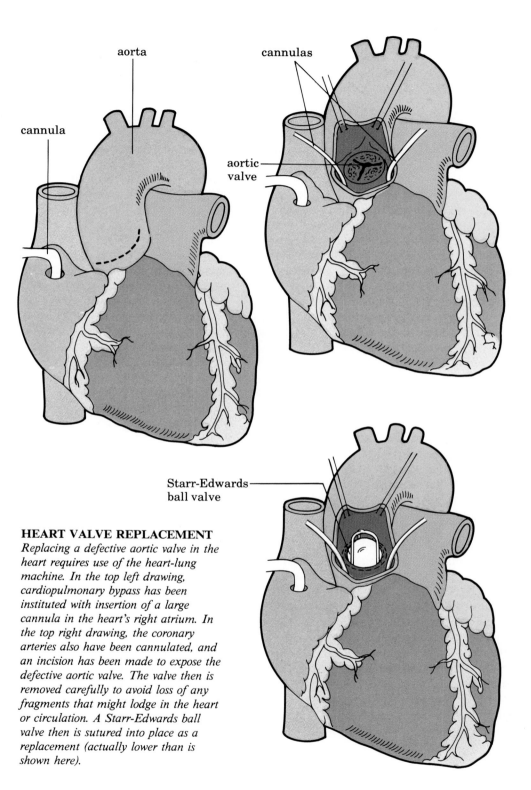

aorta

cannula

cannulas

aortic valve

Starr-Edwards ball valve

HEART VALVE REPLACEMENT

Replacing a defective aortic valve in the heart requires use of the heart-lung machine. In the top left drawing, cardiopulmonary bypass has been instituted with insertion of a large cannula in the heart's right atrium. In the top right drawing, the coronary arteries also have been cannulated, and an incision has been made to expose the defective aortic valve. The valve then is removed carefully to avoid loss of any fragments that might lodge in the heart or circulation. A Starr-Edwards ball valve then is sutured into place as a replacement (actually lower than is shown here).

sewn in place, using strong nonabsorbable sutures. Afterward, the edges of the divided sternum are held together with wires, allowing it to heal.

Coronary artery disease, the leading cause of death in developed countries, refers to narrowing of the small arteries that bring blood from the aorta to the heart muscle. Blockages in these vital arteries can trigger myocardial infarction ("heart attack") or death of a portion of the heart muscle by cutting off the blood supply. The lucky patient recovers. Many die.

A great step forward was taken when it became possible to study obstructed coronary blood vessels by coronary arteriography. In this technique, a small tube (catheter) is inserted into the femoral artery in the groin or into the brachial artery at the elbow, threaded up into the aorta, and then into each of the coronary arteries. A dye is injected that can be seen on an X ray. A moving picture is taken before, during, and after injection of the dye to watch the blood flow in the coronary arteries and identify the areas of narrowing.

Arteriography led to the coronary bypass graft, now performed hundreds of thousands of times a year. This procedure uses the large superficial veins of the thighs and legs, the saphenous veins, to build a conduit around the obstruction in an artery. The bypass graft comes from the ascending aorta just above the heart and runs with an anastomosis to the small coronary artery beyond the point of narrowing or obstruction. The internal mammary artery lying along the chest wall also may be used for a conduit.

Bypass grafts usually are carried out around any vessel more than 50 percent obstructed. As many as six grafts may be carried out in an individual.

Coronary balloon angioplasty, illustrated and explained in Chapter 5, "The Heart and Circulation," is used increasingly for opening narrowed coronary arteries. In this procedure, a catheter carrying a tiny balloon at its tip is guided to the point of narrowing by techniques of arteriography. The balloon then is inflated under pressure, opening the artery. In most cases the artery remains open. Angioplasty usually is reserved for cases in which only one artery is narrowed.

OPERATIONS ON THE FEMALE ORGANS

Disorders of the female reproductive system (uterus, ovaries, fallopian tubes, and vagina) may involve only one organ, or the entire system, as described in Chapter 26, "The Female Reproductive System." The most common symptom is abnormal bleeding, which, if persistent, may be investigated by the operation dilatation and curettage, or "D and C." Dilatation opens the mouth of the uterus, the cervix, and the cervical canal with gradually larger dilators; the interior of the uterus or womb then is scraped with a long-handled, spoonlike instrument. The tissue obtained is submitted for pathological examination.

A common abnormality of the uterus is development of a benign tumor called a fibroid. Fibroids seldom present great difficulty. They may be left in place or removed in an operation called myomectomy. Occasionally, total removal of the uterus (hysterectomy) may be necessary.

Hysterectomy (which may be performed for reasons other than tumors) sometimes is carried out vaginally, more commonly through an incision in the lower abdomen. The uterus is freed from surrounding tissues. The ovaries of a young woman may be left in place to avoid producing immediate menopause, but the fallopian tubes usually are removed along with the cervix.

In an older woman, the uterus sometimes tends to fall from its normal position (prolapse of the uterus). The uterus then may be removed by vaginal hysterectomy. Sometimes the bladder, too, may protrude into the vagina, producing a bulge called a cystocele, or into the rectum, a rectocele. It may be difficult to control urine, especially during straining or coughing. The bladder can be restored surgically to its normal position to prevent leakage of urine.

Cysts of the ovary are common and often benign. Some cystic tumors of the ovary, however, are malignant. A mass in the area of the ovary that does not subside over a full menstrual cycle may require an exploratory laparotomy and possibly removal. Some ovarian tumors produce hormones and are discovered by their abnormal hormonal effects. Others interfere with fertility or normal female development, and require an operation for biopsy and incisions within the ovary to improve function.

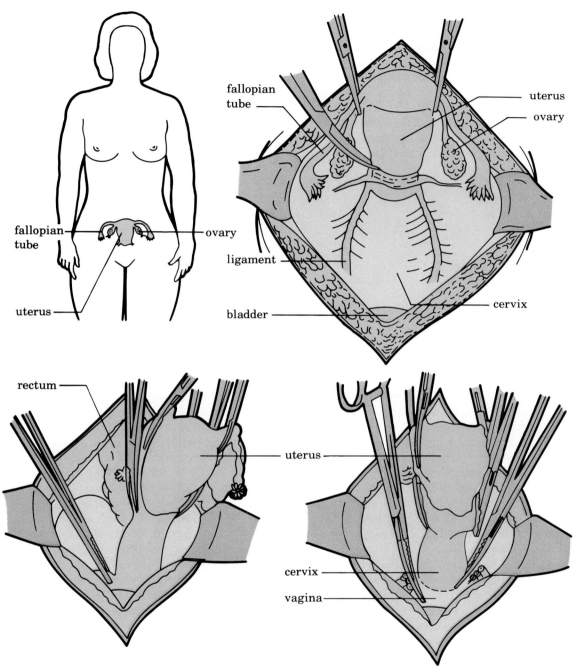

fallopian tube

ovary

fallopian tube

uterus

uterus

ovary

ligament

bladder

cervix

rectum

uterus

cervix

vagina

HYSTERECTOMY

Removal of the female uterus may be undertaken for many reasons. The top left drawing shows the location of the uterus, ovaries, and fallopian tubes. In the top right drawing, the uterus, tubes, and ovaries are being held up by two clamps. The body of the uterus is being separated from the broad ligament by which it is suspended. The cervix, or mouth of the uterus, also is removed. In the bottom left drawing, the ligament

has been dissected and the blood vessels of the uterus have been divided and ligated. The rectum can be seen behind the uterus. In the bottom right drawing, the vagina is being cut across at the base of the uterus. The vagina will be closed at its upper end to preserve its length. Hysterectomy also is sometimes carried out through the vagina, without opening the abdomen.

Endometriosis is an abnormality in which tissue ordinarily lining the uterus is found outside the uterus. The woman usually has pain and difficulty conceiving. Nodules or masses of endometrial tissue may be found on pelvic examination. An exploratory operation may be necessary, followed by surgery to remove the tissue.

Diagnosis of abnormalities of the fallopian tubes and ovaries has been advanced through use of the laparoscope, described in Chapter 2, "Tests and Procedures."

OPERATIONS ON KIDNEYS, BLADDER, AND MALE ORGANS

Although the kidneys normally are well protected, an auto accident or other crushing force can damage them. Either a kidney is ruptured or it is torn loose from its blood supply. The kidney then must be removed. An incision is made in the flank or abdominal wall. The renal artery and vein are ligated and divided where they join the aorta and vena cava, the body's main artery and main vein. The kidney is separated from the surrounding tissue and from the adrenal gland that lies on top of it. The ureter then is divided, and the kidney is removed. Fortunately, the remaining kidney takes over the function of the lost organ.

Malignant tumors of the kidney, such as the rare Wilms' tumor in children or renal-cell carcinoma in adults, also may require kidney removal.

Kidney stones, while painful, frequently are small and may pass down the urinary system to the outside. Sometimes, however, a stone obstructs the ureter, causing urine to back up in the kidney. Then an operation is necessary to extract the stone. Stones that develop within the kidney, nicknamed "staghorn" calculi for the shape they take, require that the kidney be gently split open and the stone lifted out. The two halves of the organ then can be reunited.

The blood supply on which the kidney depends can be compromised by arteriosclerosis or a disease called fibromuscular hyperplasia. Either narrows the renal artery. The narrowed portion can be bypassed, using a synthetic graft. Or angioplasty, described in Chapter 5, "The Heart and Circulation," may be used to force open the narrowed artery.

Bladder problems requiring a surgeon's attention include stones, tumors, and infection. A removal technique called fulguration allows tumors to be burned off with a miniature electric cautery fitted on the end of the scope. Sometimes, however, a bladder tumor is not detected until it is so large that the entire organ must be removed.

When the bladder is removed, a way must be provided for the collection and disposal of urine. The Bricker or ileal pouch uses a section of small intestine to construct a conduit and reservoir. A length of the intestine is removed, and the divided ends are rejoined by anastomosis. The segment then is sewn closed at one end, and the two ureters are attached. The open end of the intestinal segment is brought out through the abdominal wall, and a bag is worn for collection of urine.

Prostate trouble is the most common abnormality of the male urogenital system. As described in Chapter 25, "The Male Reproductive System," the prostate gland, which surrounds the urethra and provides seminal fluids, often enlarges in older men, and squeezes the urethra. Early symptoms are slowing of the stream during urination and necessity to get up frequently at night to urinate. Eventually, complete obstruction can occur, and it may be necessary to remove part or all of the prostate. Operation through the bladder or around the base of the bladder (suprapubic prostatectomy or retropubic prostatectomy) removes the entire prostate gland by "shelling" it out of its capsule. A transurethral resection, which does not remove the entire gland, is performed by insertion through the urethra of an instrument called a resectoscope. Diathermy or cautery is used to cut out the inside of the prostate gland, thus opening the outlet of the bladder and allowing for freer flow of urine.

Cancer of the prostate gland, described in detail in Chapter 25, "The Male Reproductive System," is said to occur in more than 60,000 men annually, most of them past age 60. Treatment consists of irradiation, orchiectomy, or a radical perineal prostatectomy. Hormone therapy is used to suppress the prostate gland and spread of the cancer. A radical operation is done only if the tumor is small and confined to the prostate gland.

ORTHOPEDIC SURGERY

The most publicized orthopedic surgery is that performed on athletes. But as more and more people take up sports, an increasing number of athletic injuries come to the orthopedist's attention.

Fractures do not always require surgery, although they do require medical attention. A displaced fracture, in which the broken ends of bone are out of alignment, often requires an open operation to bring the fracture edges together. Sometimes it becomes necessary to insert a screw into a broken segment of bone to hold it in place, or to fasten a metal plate across the fracture site. Or a metal rod may be fitted into a bone such as the femur, the large bone of the thigh.

Severe or recurrent dislocations may require surgery because the tissues around the joint have become so lax that the joint can slip in and out with minimal cause. Other injuries include the tearing of structures around a joint, such as the four ligaments supporting the knee and the cartilage (meniscus) cushioning its two bones. These injuries, common among football players and other athletes, are illustrated in Chapter 16, "The Bones and Muscles." Ligament repair or removal of torn cartilage may be performed by arthroscopy, also illustrated in Chapter 16.

Arthritis is treated by medical means, but the arthritic changes in the joints, which produce pain, disability, and limited motion, may be treated much more satisfactorily by an operation—usually a joint replacement, as illustrated in Chapter 17, "Arthritis and Related Diseases." Total replacement of the hip joint has become a widely performed and highly successful procedure, allowing almost complete rehabilitation.

Malignant tumors of the bone once were almost always treated by radical amputation of the limb, but today chemotherapy may be used. For benign tumors or locally malignant tumors involving large amounts of bone, it is possible to replace the damaged area with a large bone graft.

NEUROSURGERY

The use of magnetic resonance imaging (MRI), described in Chapter 2, "Tests and Procedures," has greatly enhanced the neurosurgeon's ability to localize and swiftly remove or treat lesions or damaged areas of the brain and spinal cord.

Hydrocephalus, an abnormality of formation and removal of fluids of the central nervous system, is present in some children at birth. The fluid collects in the brain, causing pressure, enlargement of the skull, and stretching of the brain tissue. This abnormality may be treated surgically by attaching a valved conduit from the brain to the abdomen or kidney to allow removal of the fluid.

Brain injury usually results from a fall or auto accident. If the skull is fractured, an operation may be required to remove pressure. If not, blood collects under the skull and compresses the brain. An incision is made in the skull directly over the site. Then a small burr hole is drilled through the bone, or a small circle of bone is removed, allowing the clot to be lifted from the brain lining.

Benign brain tumors often develop within an enclosed capsule and can be removed in their entirety if near the surface. As illustrated here, a portion of the cranium or skull is removed to expose the tumor, after which the tumor is removed. Tumors deeper in the brain, even when benign, are more difficult to remove. These may occur in young people. The highly malignant tumor called glioblastoma multiforme may require an operation for diagnosis, but treatment is difficult because it is difficult to remove the entire tumor.

As described in Chapter 13, "Stroke," an aneurysm, or a bulge in the wall, may develop in the small blood vessels of the brain. These cerebral aneurysms may blow out, causing hemorrhage, sudden loss of consciousness, and death. If the aneurysm can be detected before symptoms occur, a tiny clip can seal off the aneurysm.

Arteriosclerosis and hypertension also may cause narrowing or obstructions of small blood vessels. A bypass graft can route blood around the blockage. Vessels in the neck are joined through the skull to the small vessels in the brain beyond the obstruction.

Spinal cord injury, most commonly due to fracture of the cervical spine (broken neck), may cause total paralysis below the point of injury. It usually is irreversible because the spinal cord does not regenerate. Partial injury, however, may be helped by surgery to take the pressure off the cord.

A ruptured intervertebral disk is a common problem of the spine. Disks, small elliptical sections of fibrous cartilaginous tissue, serve as cushions between the vertebral bodies of the spine. By degeneration of tissues, by pressure, and perhaps by forward bending of the spine, the tissues may give way, allowing a disk to be pushed out from between the vertebrae, causing pressure on the nerves or nerve roots, and severe pain in the back extending down the legs.

Bed rest is the initial treatment for a ruptured disk. But if it is unsuccessful and MRI discloses the location of the rupture, the disk may be re-

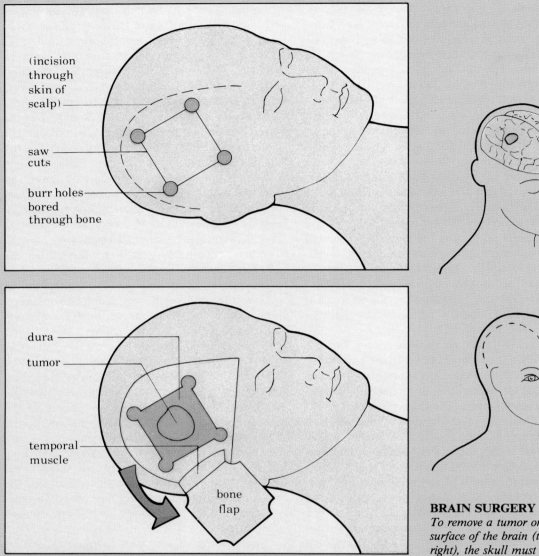

(incision through skin of scalp)

saw cuts

burr holes bored through bone

dura

tumor

temporal muscle

bone flap

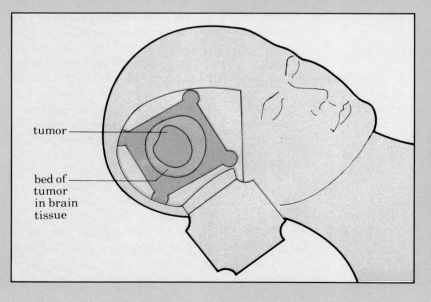

tumor

bed of tumor in brain tissue

BRAIN SURGERY

To remove a tumor on the surface of the brain (top right), the skull must be opened, a procedure called craniotomy. The usual incision is marked by the dotted line in the top left drawing. Four holes are drilled as shown, connected, and the flap of bone turned back, exposing the tumor and the brain covering (dura). The tumor is lifted from its bed in the brain tissue, keeping the tissue itself intact. The bone and skin flaps are replaced and the incision closed, as shown in the bottom right drawing.

moved in a procedure called a laminectomy. An incision is made over the back and a portion of bone is removed over the spinal cord and its distal nerves. These then are retracted gently and the disk pulled from its site behind the nerve roots.

The primary problem involving nerves of the arms and legs is injury by laceration or amputation. This may require suturing the nerves together carefully. A divided nerve will degenerate all the way back to the spinal cord to its parent nerve cell. A sutured nerve gradually may regenerate itself, with sensation and muscular function returning, although this may take many months.

OPERATIONS ON THE EARS, NOSE, AND THROAT

Tonsillectomy continues to be an extremely common operation, as explained in Chapter 29, "Taking Care of Your Child." It often is combined with an adenoidectomy, removal of the adenoid tissue at the back of the nose. At one time it was felt that a combined operation should be done routinely on all children to decrease likelihood of throat infections, tonsillitis, and, particularly, streptococcal infections, which later could lead to rheumatic fever and rheumatic heart disease. It has been increasingly recognized, however, that routine removal of tonsils and adenoids is not necessary and may be inadvisable for some children, because the tonsils are a part of the immune system. A tonsillectomy should be carried out only if the child's tonsils are so enlarged that he or she has shortness of breath, difficulty swallowing, repeated severe bouts of tonsillitis, ear infections, abscesses, or serious enlargement of lymph nodes.

A tonsillectomy should be done with the child admitted to the hospital. The tonsils are dissected from the surrounding throat tissue and a snare or ligature or cautery applied at the base of the tonsil, where the blood supply enters. With careful dissection and control of bleeding, there should be a minimal risk of hemorrhage later. The adenoids are hidden above the palate and therefore are hard to visualize without general anesthesia. Whether they should be removed at the same time depends on the amount of enlargement.

The larynx. Benign polyps or papillomas on the vocal cords can be removed with a laryngoscope, inserted down the throat under local anesthesia. Laryngeal cancer, if confined to the midportion of one vocal cord, can be treated best by radiotherapy, which leaves the patient with a good voice. If a cancer is more extensive, reaching the junction of the cords, it is best treated by removing a portion of the larynx (hemilaryngectomy). An even more extensive tumor calls for a total laryngectomy, removal of the entire larynx. The trachea or windpipe then must be brought out through the skin and sutured to the neck. The patient must learn substitute methods of speech, as explained in Chapter 15, "Ear, Nose, and Throat."

Tracheostomy is illustrated in Chapter 10, "The Lungs." This operation is performed when injuries, obstruction, or other problems block the trachea, or windpipe, below the larynx. A small incision is made in the skin of the neck. The muscles are separated in the midline. The isthmus or connecting portion of the thyroid gland is pulled upward. An incision then is made in the larynx, usually removing a small circle of one of the tracheal rings. A cannula, or tracheostomy tube, then can be inserted to allow breathing. A small cuff around the tracheostomy tube seals it, so that a breathing-assistance device can push air into the patient's lungs. A tracheostomy usually is temporary. After the tube is removed, the hole will close and heal within a few days.

The ear. Middle ear infection in children, called serous otitis media, may require an operation to drain fluid collected behind the eardrum. This is called myringotomy, an office procedure done with local anesthesia. For chronic infections, it may be necessary to leave a tiny drainage tube in place through the eardrum. The placement of tubes, called tympanotomy, usually is temporary and usually requires hospitalization.

A common cause of hearing loss, otosclerosis, produces fixation and immobility of the small bones of the middle ear, which transmit sound from the eardrum through the middle ear. The operation to replace the ossified stapes bone is illustrated and explained in Chapter 15, "Ear, Nose, and Throat."

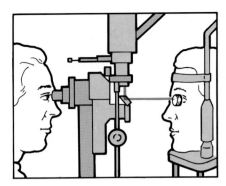

LASER EYE SURGERY
Open-angle glaucoma, or chronic glaucoma, causes damaging buildup of fluids in the eye and can result in blindness if not treated. Beta-blocking drugs in eye drop form or beta-blockers combined with a drug to reduce production of aqueous fluid are used to treat the condition.

If drug treatment does not work, laser surgery to open the drainage canal may be performed. As illustrated above, this office procedure uses a laser beam to "burn" open the canal.

If this surgery is unsuccessful, the laser may be used to burn a series of small holes in the eye's trabecular meshwork, or a small opening may be made, allowing fluid to flow directly under the conjunctiva.

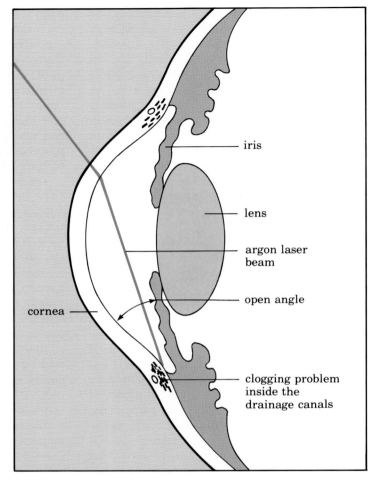

iris

lens

argon laser beam

open angle

cornea

clogging problem inside the drainage canals

OPERATIONS ON THE EYE

As illustrated and explained in Chapter 14, "The Eyes," a cataract is clouding of the normally transparent lens of the eye. The hardening interferes with the transmission of light through the lens onto the retina at the back of the eye.

In the past, it was necessary to delay an operation to remove cataracts until the entire lens had hardened. This no longer is necessary, and cataract surgery, as discussed in Chapter 14, has become one of the most commonly performed operations and has restored sight to millions of people. The operation now is performed on an outpatient basis, under local anesthesia. The entire lens and capsule is removed and replaced with a lens implant. Restoration of vision is immediate.

The cornea of the eye can become cloudy as a result of injury, infection, or genetic predisposition to progressive deterioration. Light is blocked from passing through the lens to the retina. The condition is treated by transplanting a healthy cornea from a human donor, one of the most successful of transplant operations.

Other eye problems that may be corrected surgically, often with the use of lasers, also are discussed in detail in Chapter 14, "The Eyes." These include detachment of the retina, the light-receptive tissue at the back of the eye, which can be "spot-welded" by laser; diabetic retinopathy, proliferation of blood vessels on the retina as a consequence of diabetes; and certain forms of glaucoma, the leading cause of blindness in the United States.

Transplant Surgery

Human organ transplant has developed rapidly in recent years. Surgeons now successfully transplant hearts, livers, lungs, kidneys, pancreas, and combinations of those organs. Even brain tissue has been transplanted experimentally.

Many of the early transplants failed because the body's immune system identified the transplanted organ as foreign and rejected it. When the immune system was suppressed by drugs then available, the body was left defenseless against infection. Introduction of the drug cyclosporin overcame the problem of organ rejection and ushered in the age of transplantation. Cyclosporin combats rejection while still maintaining the defenses against infection.

Kidney transplant has been the most successful and widely performed transplant operation, and is the treatment of choice for end-stage kidney disease. Experienced surgical transplant teams achieve a success rate greater than 90 percent when the donor is a living relative, and over 80 percent when the kidney is received from a person who has died of other causes. Even if a kidney transplant fails, the patient can be returned to kidney dialysis ("artificial kidney") until a second kidney is available.

Liver transplant is much less common but is performed in an increasing number of hospitals, with good success. Leading candidates for transplants have been children with congenital liver problems and adults with certain rare liver diseases. Transplants of the pancreas (and of pancreatic cells, especially those producing insulin) have been less frequently performed and still are considered experimental.

Heart transplants are now performed in the thousands every year. At one time they were reserved for young, otherwise healthy adults for whom a new heart was the only hope. More recently, infants and even men and women in their 70s have been transplanted. As many as 80 percent of new-heart recipients survive at least a year after transplant and as many as 60 percent, at least five years. Because the heart and lungs work together, lungs are sometimes damaged by heart problems so the organs often are transplanted together with good success.

Transplant of cells into the brain, either from the recipient's own adrenal gland or from fetal donors, as a treatment for Parkinson's disease has achieved only modest success. But many neurologists are convinced the technique will improve and better overcome the disease's debilitating symptoms.

Even with cyclosporin, transplant is a delicate procedure. Tissue must be carefully matched between donor and recipient; and where possible, the two should be of approximately the same body size—a child recipient requires another child's donated organ. Immunosuppressive drugs must be continued lifelong to prevent rejection. (In some cases, however, a second transplant has been successfully performed after a first heart has failed after several years.) The main problem with a transplant has been a shortage of organs. Many states now append consent forms to driver's licenses so that organs may be donated in the event of accidental death. A national network has been established to recover organs and speed them to potential recipients, and elaborate methods are used to preserve the organs en route. In the hands of an experienced team, however, the transplant surgery itself is fairly straightforward and smoothly accomplished.

CHAPTER 34

CARING FOR THE ILL PATIENT AT HOME

Not too many years ago, persons who were ill or injured remained in their homes and doctors came to them. Later, it became customary to hospitalize the ill, because resources were concentrated in one place, and to keep them there until full recovery. Now, home care has achieved renewed importance because of the prevalence of chronic disease, especially among the elderly, and because persons are being discharged from hospitals much more quickly than in the recent past.

There is one additional reason for the reemphasis on home care: people fare better and are more comfortable in familiar surroundings.

CARE OF THE ELDERLY

Home care is especially important for older people. Home health care programs for the aged serve two major purposes: The wishes of the older people themselves are fulfilled, and the interest of the public is served as well, because care at home is significantly less costly than nursing home care.

Many agencies offer services designed to help the aged stay at home, living either independently or with relatives. These include visiting nurse agencies, which provide professional and homemaker staffs, plus meals-on-wheels programs, friendly visitor programs, and telephone reassurance programs. Local offices for the aging are good sources of information about these programs.

For older people who are seriously disabled, hospital-based teams of doctor, nurse, and social worker often work with them in their own homes.

Elderly persons should understand that they need not be manipulated into a nursing home or other chronic care institution. When a patient has no family, it is the responsibility of community agencies to create a network of services for care at home. When relatives or friends are available, they can help.

ILL PEOPLE AT HOME

When people of any age are ill or recovering from surgery or injury at home, paying attention to the practical details of their care makes the difference between comfort and misery, success and failure of treatment. If care will continue for a long time, it might be wise for one or more members of the family to take a course in home nursing. Such courses are offered by local Red Cross chapters and other community agencies.

Other agencies provide advice and support for home care givers, and often will relieve the care giver of duties temporarily, providing a much-needed "breather." You usually can find out about such help from a city or county department of health or social services. The Visiting Nurse Association, the local senior center, or hospital charitable agencies and church groups provide advice and support, too.

Whatever your program, it should stress independence, not dependence. Remember, the basic goal of all treatment is to return the patient to active life as quickly as possible. Patients should be encouraged to carry out some normal activities of daily living, such as washing, eating, combing hair, or brushing teeth. Muscles should be used as soon as possible. Stretching in bed, moving arms and legs deliberately, graduating from bed to chair and from chair to walking all should be urged.

Good Nursing Habits

Regardless of the nature or duration of the patient's illness, certain nursing practices always should be followed.

Hand washing. Wash your hands with soap and running water before and after attending the patient. Keep your fingernails trimmed closely. Wash above your wrists. Rinse well. Rinse the bar of soap after each use. Dry your hands with a clean towel or paper towel.

Waste disposal. Flush away the patient's bowel and bladder wastes immediately. Provide a covered container for soiled tissues and bandages. Line it with a paper or plastic bag that can be closed without touching the contents. Keep paper tissues within the patient's reach.

Dishes. Depending on the illness, it may be a good idea for the patient to have separate dishes and eating utensils—possibly disposable ones. However, hot water and detergent, plus hot water rinsing and drying, remove or destroy most infectious agents. A dishwasher is ideal because it uses a water temperature higher than human hands can tolerate.

Linen. Collect soiled sickroom linens in a bag or newspaper and wash separately from other laundry.

Medications

Follow the doctor's directions in giving medicines to a patient cared for at home. It is particularly important that prescription medicines be given at the proper time and in the proper dosage. Some medicines should be given before meals on an empty stomach, some should be taken with food, and others should follow a meal.

Certain drugs, such as antibiotics, are commonly used only during the illness. Others must be taken for prolonged periods, even a lifetime.

Be sparing with pain medication. No one likes to see a loved one in pain, but improper use of painkillers can be dangerous. Use caution with nonprescription drugs.

If the Patient Has A Communicable Disease

Illnesses that spread from person to person require extra precautions. Widespread immunization has substantially decreased many of these. But chicken pox, influenza, the common cold, and hepatitis are still with us.

The AIDS epidemic has reemphasized the need for such precautions. Those dealing with AIDS patients must be especially cautious with body fluids and secretions, particularly blood. Although the disease is not spread by casual contact, infection is possible via breaks in the skin.

If the patient has a respiratory disease that can be spread by coughing or sneezing, both patient and home nurse may wish to wear a mask covering nose and mouth. These can be bought at a pharmacy or fashioned from gauze or cloth.

For a disease such as hepatitis, which is transmitted through blood, stool, and bodily secretions, care must be taken in disposing of the patient's wastes. If the person is bedfast and requires a bedpan, the wastes should be flushed away immediately and the utensil thoroughly rinsed. The helper should scrub his or her hands thoroughly afterward, or use rubber gloves.

The "Sickroom"

The ideal location for a patient is a cheery, well-lighted room. It should be quiet, well-ventilated, and preferably on the first floor near the bathroom. It should be arranged for efficiency, but not stripped down like a hospital ward. The basics are the patient's bed, a night table that he or she can easily reach, chairs for the patient and visitors, a waste can lined with a paper or plastic bag, and a table for supplies. A bed table for meals or reading is handy, too. You'll probably want a television and radio and perhaps a videocassette player.

If the room is near the living quarters of the house, the patient can call you when needed. But if the only available room is upstairs or isolated from the mainstream of the household, he or she will need a way to attract attention. A bell or buzzer is suitable, or even a tin pan.

Keep medicines and other supplies together and easy to reach. Clean the room with a damp cloth and use a vacuum sweeper so that you do not stir up dust.

The Patient's Bed

For a brief confinement, the patient's own bed is usually satisfactory. For extended home care, choose a bed that saves the nurse's energy. A single or twin bed is easier to make than a double bed, and the patient is more accessible. If the patient is completely bedridden and likely to require care for a long time, it may be wise to rent a hospital bed. Equipment also is loaned by community agencies.

The mattress should be firm and resilient. If the bedspring sags, a piece of plywood between mattress and spring will give support. Position the bed so that neither the foot nor the sides are against the wall.

It is convenient to use a fitted sheet as the bottom sheet. It fits snugly at the corners of the mattress and leaves few wrinkles. The top sheet should be wide and long enough to be tucked under the mattress to hold the sheet smoothly and firmly, yet allow the patient to move freely and to accommodate pillows, footrest, or other appliances under the covers. Use enough blankets for comfort.

If the patient needs bedpan care, is incontinent, or perspires profusely, a pad of moisture-resistant material may be needed under him or her. Washable waterproof materials with a cloth covering can be purchased. Oilcloth or old shower curtains are serviceable substitutes. You may even use a large plastic garbage bag.

Use pillows and backrests imaginatively and in quantity for patient comfort. Besides providing support in the sitting position, pillows can hold people on their sides, elevate the feet, or keep the knees flexed. An upholstered backrest with arms is worthwhile.

Footrests are used to keep bedclothes from pressing on the toes and to give a firm surface to exercise against.

Moving the Patient in Bed

Urge the patient to move himself or herself, if possible. Otherwise, explain what you are going to do before you do it. Remove or pull down top bedding for freedom of movement. Roll and slide the patient gently; do not lift unnecessarily. Think of the hips and shoulders as "pivots." The patient

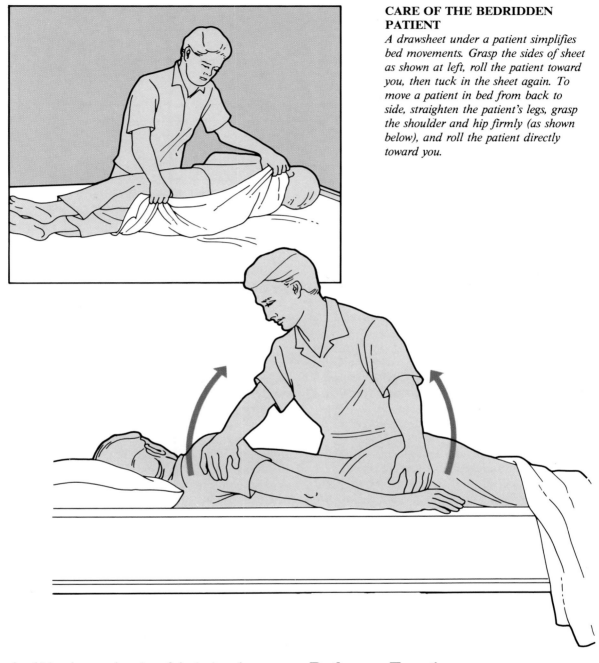

CARE OF THE BEDRIDDEN PATIENT
A drawsheet under a patient simplifies bed movements. Grasp the sides of sheet as shown at left, roll the patient toward you, then tuck in the sheet again. To move a patient in bed from back to side, straighten the patient's legs, grasp the shoulder and hip firmly (as shown below), and roll the patient directly toward you.

should be close to the edge of the bed so the nurse doesn't have to bend awkwardly.

If the patient is to get into a chair brought to the bedside, help him or her sit up and provide support while you swing the legs around. A patient's chair should be sturdy, with arms that can be grasped to help himself or herself out of bed.

Bathroom Functions

A bedpan is an uncomfortable, inefficient device in which people are expected to urinate and defecate. However, if a patient cannot get out of bed, there may be no alternative. Obtain a lightweight plastic bedpan of the smallest useful size. The larger it is, the more difficult for the patient to use.

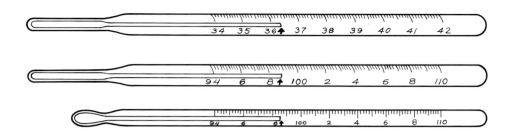

CLINICAL THERMOMETERS

Two types of mercury thermometers are used to measure body temperature. Oral thermometers (top two drawings) have a relatively long bulb that holds the red or silver measuring material. The rectal type, most commonly used in infants and certain older patients, has a shorter, fatter bulb. It also may be used in the axilla or armpit. Thermometers are graduated in either Fahrenheit (bottom two drawings) or Celsius (top drawing) scales. Normal rectal temperature is about one degree Fahrenheit higher than oral temperature.

Graduate the patient to a bedside commode as quickly as possible. This is a chair with a hole in the seat and a bucket or pan underneath that can be withdrawn for cleaning.

Finally, allowing the patient to go into the bathroom and use the toilet, when the doctor permits, often is a moment of great joy, with important psychological benefits in addition to physical ease.

Always remember that patients value privacy, especially in these circumstances, and respect this need when possible.

For persons who are incontinent, disposable, moistureproof undergarments are available.

Skin Care

Basic cleanliness of the patient is of high importance. It is common sense, good hygiene, important for morale, and necessary to avoid complications such as inflammations and infections of the skin. If patients who are incontinent soil themselves, careful and prompt cleaning is required. Permitting the patient to lie in wet sheets is undignified, uncomfortable, and leads to skin breakdown.

Bedsores (decubitus ulcers) are skin sores that, when not dealt with aggressively, lead to destruction of underlying tissue such as muscles and tendons, extending down to bone. These ulcers tend to occur over areas where pressure is applied to the skin by the body's position in bed. The heels, lower back, elbows, shoulder blades, and back of the skull are vulnerable.

The earliest sign of a bedsore is tender, warm, and slightly reddened skin. In later stages, the skin is purplish, broken, and raw; circulation is impaired; and treatment is difficult.

Moisture from discharges predisposes to skin breakdown. Keep the patient's skin dry. In washing, don't rub reddened, tender skin areas vigorously. Wash gently with warm soapy water, rinse, pat dry, sponge with rubbing alcohol (unless the skin is broken), and cover with large cotton pads unless the doctor advises other measures.

Patients who face the highest likelihood of bedsores are those who cannot move freely in bed. Frequent turning of the patient is essential, as is the use of foam rubber "doughnuts" to keep skin away from sheets.

Bathing the Patient

A quick bath stimulates circulation and is refreshing and cleansing. A daily bath for the patient is customary. More frequent baths may be necessary if there is too much soiling. On the other hand, frequent or prolonged baths can be fatiguing and may cause softening of the skin.

For bed baths, protect bedding with towels or blankets. Wash each part of the body quickly. Rinse off the soap, dry thoroughly, cover, and proceed to the next area. Dry skin creases and folds particularly well. A light dusting of talcum powder, especially in the armpits, back, and genital and buttocks areas, promotes drying and makes the person comfortable.

Measuring Pulse and Respiratory Rates

The doctor may ask you to count the patient's pulse and respiratory rate. If so, keep a written record of the reading, the date, and the hour. You will need a watch or clock graduated in seconds.

The pulse usually is counted at the wrist. A little below the base of the thumb, just inside the point where a projection of the wristbone can be felt on the thumb side, an artery runs under the skin of the inner surface of the wrist. Place your fingertips (not your thumb) on this part of the patient's wrist. Press just hard enough for pulsations to be felt. Count for 60 seconds.

The average adult has a pulse rate of 70 to 72 per minute, but this can vary considerably in either direction and still be normal.

Respiration (the breathing rate) is best counted when the patient is not aware, because mere observation may change the rate. The breathing rate of adults at rest ranges between 14 and 18 per minute. It is faster in children and faster still in infants.

Use of Heat and Cold

The use of heat and cold is important for the patient's comfort and in some cases is part of treatment. However, too much heat or cold can cause injury or make the person's disease worse.

Heat is soothing, eases muscle spasms, and decreases some forms of pain. Heat may be applied dry (by electric pad, hot water bottle, or lamp) or moist (by compresses).

Too much heat can burn. Don't apply anything to the patient's body that is too hot to hold in your hands, or that feels too warm to the skin of your inner forearm. Never apply heat for more than one hour at a time without a doctor's advice.

Remember that a comatose or disoriented patient or a baby can't tell you that a heating pad is too hot. Be careful when applying heat to an infant or to a patient who is sedated. Also, be careful with those who have diabetes mellitus or circulatory or neurological problems, which decrease sensation.

A hot compress furnishes moist heat. Use folded gauze, flannel, or soft woolen fabrics. Dip into water, then squeeze out excess moisture. Test the compress on your own skin. Apply loosely to the affected part. A strip of plastic sheeting can be laid over the compress to keep moisture in. Cover with a towel or soft cloth, or use a hot water bag to maintain heat and hold the compress in place. Replace the compress with a warm one when the first begins to cool.

Steam inhalation is soothing to congested breathing passages. Inhaled steam helps to soften thick secretions, and eases coughing, hoarseness, and sore throat.

An electric vaporizer is a worthwhile investment. Satisfactory steam inhalation also can be obtained from simple household equipment. Pour steaming water into a broad-mouthed pitcher or container placed in a pan on a table low enough for the seated patient to lean over it. Drape a blanket or towel over the patient's head and shoulders and above the pitcher in such a way that steamy vapor is concentrated for inhalation.

Cold compresses or soaks are used for comfort, to reduce swelling or bruises, and for other purposes. Soak folded gauze, flannel, or soft cloth in a basin of ice water. Wring thoroughly so water doesn't drip. Apply to the affected part. Replace with a freshly wrung compress when the first becomes warm.

If you can fit the part of the body to be soaked into a tub or basin of cold water, do so. Soaking is more efficient than a compress.

Equipment

Some items of sickroom equipment make it easier to give care or make the patient more comfortable and contented.

A bed table is a flat surface on which meals are served and which the patient can use for writing, drawing, and other activities while sitting or propped up in bed. Simple U-shaped tables with long feet that slide under the bed and a top that projects above the bedclothes can be bought or rented. The tops can be tilted and adjusted for height. An ironing board also can be used.

CHAPTER 35

EMERGENCY

In an emergency, time counts. It is important for anyone suddenly taken ill, injured, poisoned, burned, or otherwise hurt to receive skilled medical attention as quickly as possible. Fortunately, most communities today have trained paramedics or emergency crews who can respond quickly when summoned. The first step in any family first-aid program is to know how to call for aid and to memorize the emergency phone number or post it near the telephone. In most communities, the phone number is 911.

Second, you should know when immediate first-aid care—care *you* must provide—is essential and potentially lifesaving. The checklist below helps you to quickly size up the needs and to carry out first-aid measures when necessary. However, in some cases the best thing you can do is keep the injured person calm, comfortable, and safe from further injury until trained help arrives.

Many minor injuries do not require professional care but call for immediate treatment at home. These are covered later in this chapter.

Finally, the most important step is to keep injuries from happening. Safety precautions are described at the end of this chapter.

PREPARING
FOR EMERGENCIES

Every family member should be prepared to provide first aid. A good beginning is for one or more family members to take a first-aid course, as well as one in cardiopulmonary resuscitation (CPR), the technique for maintaining or restoring a victim's heartbeat and respiration. Both types of courses are offered by local Red Cross chapters, American Heart Association chapters, YMCAs, Boy Scout troops, and other community groups. It is important to keep your skills, too. CPR requires yearly certification because with lack of practice, one quickly forgets the technique.

Having your own physician (or a relationship with a clinic, group practice, or local hospital) is part of emergency preparation, too. Then your medical history will be recorded in one place. That makes it easier for a physician on the scene during an emergency to learn about your previous illnesses, drug allergies, and medications, and thus provide better care.

Besides the emergency number, another important telephone number is that of the local poison control center. These centers provide immediate information about how to deal with the effects of almost every known drug or chemical that people may take either accidentally or intentionally. In some communities, you may call the central emergency number and the dispatcher will put you in touch with the poison control center, or provide the necessary information.

A list of first-aid supplies that should be in every home is provided in this chapter. But don't limit them just to the home medicine chest. Be sure to carry a similar first-aid kit in your car, recreational vehicle, boat, and anywhere else you might need it in an emergency.

WHAT TO DO
IN AN EMERGENCY

● Don't get hurt yourself. You can't help the victim if you're injured in a foolhardy attempt at rescue. If you cannot reach an injured person without risking injury, wait for assistance.
● Do not move the victim unless the victim is at risk of further injury, because spinal cord damage can result.

● If the patient appears unconscious, make sure that he or she is breathing. If not, open the airway and give mouth-to-mouth resuscitation, if necessary (see below).
● Make sure that the mouth and throat are free of blood, secretions, or vomit. Wipe them out with a finger or a handkerchief.
● If the patient has suffered a fall, try to avoid moving the neck. Attempt to open the airway to ease breathing by lifting the jaw. This is done by putting your hands on each side of the jaw and lifting the jaw up and away from the back of the throat.
● Check for a pulse by feeling in the neck over the carotid artery, or in infants, in the armpit.
● If no pulse is present, begin external cardiac compression (cardiac massage).
● Stop serious bleeding. Apply pressure directly on the wound with any clean cloth, gauze, or handkerchief. Push hard. If bleeding is from an arm or leg wound, elevate the limb above the level of the body.
● Treat shock (see below).
● If the person appears cold, pale, and clammy, lay the person down, cover him or her with a light blanket, and provide reassurance. Avoid giving anything by mouth if the person is unconscious or semiconscious. A good rule of thumb is to give water only if the patient can hold the container and does not have chest or abdominal wounds.

THE TWO-MINUTE
PATIENT EVALUATION

Sometimes you do not actually witness an accident, but simply come upon a person who has been involved in one or who appears seriously ill. You need to make quick assessment of the condition. Do this in two steps: the primary survey and the secondary survey.

Primary Survey. First, check the person's airway, breathing, and circulation ("ABC" is a good way to remember it). Look for obvious bleeding. Immediately take care of the airway, breathing, and circulation if obstructed, as outlined in this chapter and following what you have learned in a CPR course. Stop any significant bleeding by direct pressure.

Secondary survey. If the person is conscious, start at the wrist by checking the pulse. Talk to the person and establish how the brain is functioning by asking simple questions about the victim and the surroundings, or ask the victim to follow simple commands. In an unconscious person, check the head first.

● Quickly look at the person's eyes to see whether the pupils are equal and respond to light. A difference in pupil size may indicate head injury or brain damage. Feel the scalp and the sides of the head and the neck for evidence of blood, injuries, or pain. Be careful about moving the head and neck. Protect the neck with rolled towels or clothing to immobilize it if moving is necessary. Note whether the person is bleeding from the ears or nose, and whether a clear fluid resembling water is draining from the ears or nose, which indicates a skull fracture. Examine the mouth for injuries. Remove any dentures or loose teeth if the patient is not fully conscious, or if he or she appears likely to become unconscious.

● Check the neck for tenderness, and gently palpate (feel with your hands) the shoulders from both sides, checking for tenderness that could indicate fracture of the shoulder girdle and collarbones. Compress the chest by pushing inward on both sides and then from front to back. If you produce pain, a fracture somewhere in the chest is possible. Ask a conscious person to take a deep breath.

● Remove enough clothing to look at the chest and abdomen. Seat belt marks, bruises, or tire tread imprints and similar marks may indicate possible internal bleeding.

● Compress the pelvis from side to side. Pain or tenderness may suggest pelvic fractures. Check the legs and thighs for pain, tenderness, or blood. Ask the person to move his or her feet and check whether the person can feel your touch. Do the same for the arms and hands.

● Always remember to examine the back of the patient, including the buttocks and upper thighs. Often, because patients are lying on their backs or because they are clothed, important injuries are overlooked. If there is a possible neck injury, do not move the patient, but feel underneath for tenderness or blood.

MOUTH-TO-MOUTH RESUSCITATION

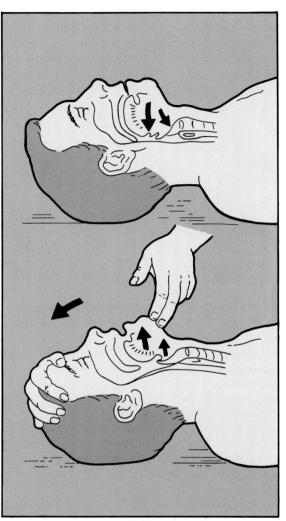

1 *Before attempting mouth-to-mouth resuscitation,* **call or send for help.** *Then place the victim on his or her back and attempt to open the airway, which is blocked in the top drawing, above. Clean any visible foreign matter from the mouth with your fingers or with a cloth wrapped around your fingers. Open the airway as shown in the lower drawing, by lifting the chin and pressing back on the forehead. The chin should point directly upward.*

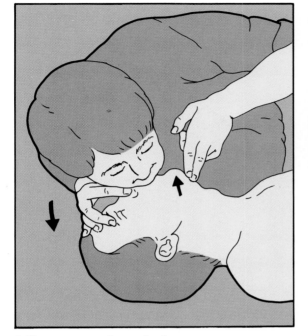

2 *Place your mouth completely over the victim's mouth. Keep your hands on the forehead and under the chin to maintain a straight airway. Breathe into an adult victim's mouth at a rate of 12 breaths per minute, one every five seconds.*

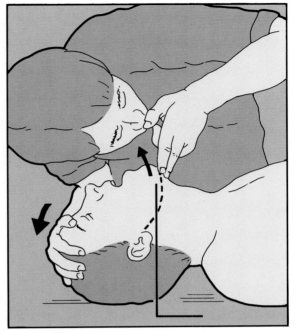

3 *After four quick breaths, remove your mouth and listen for outflow from the victim's lungs; look to see if the chest is moving. If you do not feel the person exhale, or see the chest rise and fall, or if you feel resistance to your own breath, recheck the head and mouth positions.*

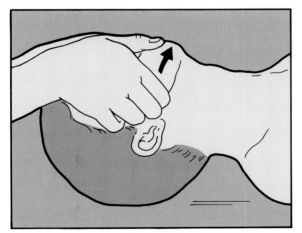

4 *If air does not move in and out of the victim's chest easily, pull or push the victim's jaw from behind into a jutting-out position, to prevent the tongue from falling back into the victim's throat. If breathing still does not occur, use the Heimlich maneuver (page 449) to open the airway.*

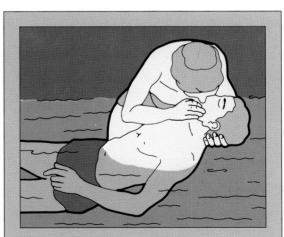

DROWNING
In a suspected drowning, start artificial respiration while still in the water (as soon as you can support the victim's head and shoulders). Continue as you wade toward shore.

MOUTH-TO-MOUTH RESUSCITATION OF SMALL CHILDREN

An infant or small child who has stopped breathing requires a mouth-to-mouth resuscitative technique that is different from the technique used for an adult.

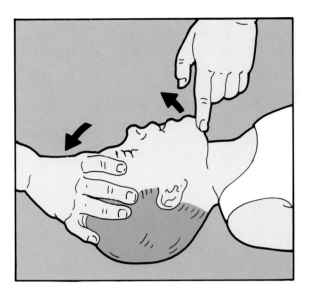

1 *Place the child on his or her back, and lift the child's chin to provide a straight airway, as with adults.*

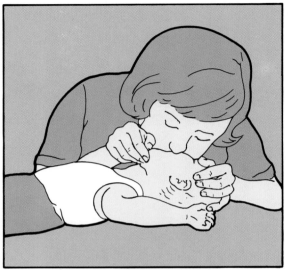

2 *Put your mouth over both mouth and nose to make a leakproof seal. Breathe at a rate of about 20 breaths per minute—about once every three seconds—for an infant, and about 15 per minute for a young child.*

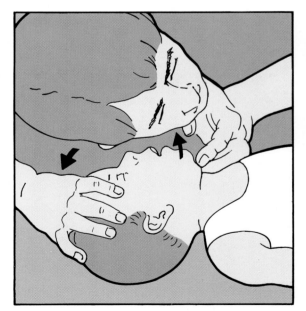

3 *Check to see if you are getting an air exchange. If not, check the jaw position to be sure the airway is clear.*

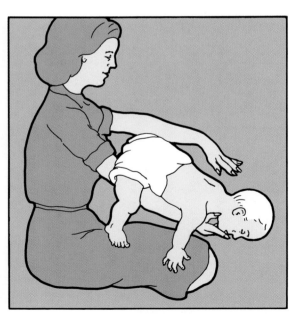

4 *Hold an infant headdown over your arm, as shown, and whack between the shoulder blades, as shown. For an older child, use the Heimlich maneuver to open the airway.*

ARTIFICIAL CIRCULATION (CARDIAC COMPRESSION)

If a person has stopped breathing, the heart also may have stopped. If no pulse can be felt, emergency measures must be taken to stimulate the heart and restore circulation. Compressing the victim's chest can start the heart beating as follows.

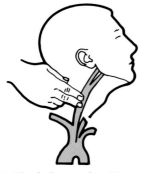

1 *Check for a pulse. The most sensitive pulse is in the carotid artery of the neck, between the windpipe and the neck muscle. It often can be felt when other pulse beats have ceased. Feel gently with your fingers to avoid damage to the windpipe.*

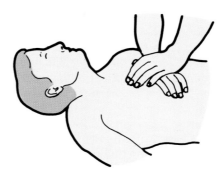

2 *If you feel no pulse, place both hands on the breastbone, 2 inches above the "V" of the ribs and compress the chest at a rate of 80 to 100 per minute (100 per minute for a child). The area of compression should be 1½ to 2 inches in an adult, half that in a child. For an infant, compress with your thumbs only.*

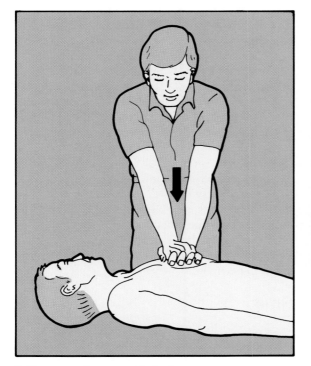

3 *If you are alone, provide both artificial breathing and cardiac compression. Give two quick breaths and compress the chest 15 times (a rate of 80 to 100 per minute). Then give two more quick breaths, followed by 15 more compressions.*

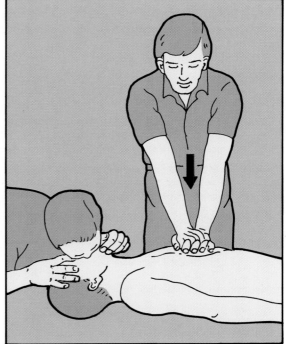

4 *If two persons are present, one can provide breathing; the other, chest compression. Take positions on either side of the victim, and change off, if you like. Compress the chest 80 to 100 times a minute. For every five compressions, there should be one breath.*

CARDIOPULMONARY RESUSCITATION

Any time an adult or child stops breathing, artificial respiration, or mouth-to-mouth resuscitation, may become necessary. This is a method of breathing for the victim by blowing your breath into his or her lungs. It can be lifesaving, and it has the advantage of needing no special equipment or preparation time. Speed is important, because irreversible brain damage can occur if breathing stops for more than four to six minutes. CPR cannot be learned on a crash basis, with the victim in front of you. You should take instruction beforehand and keep your skills up to date. The drawings on pages 444 – 446 illustrate the basic technique, and should be reviewed regularly.

CHOKING

Adults or children can choke to death on small objects that become lodged in the windpipe. In adults, the offending object often is a bit of food. With children, toys, parts of toys, or other small objects more often are responsible. Choking on food often occurs in a restaurant and happens so suddenly that it may be mistaken for a heart attack, hence the nickname "café coronary."

The best way to rid oneself of an obstruction in the windpipe is by coughing it out. In a choking incident, one should not jump too soon. If a person is choking but appears able to talk (or to cry normally, in the case of an infant), it probably is unnecessary to do anything initially. A person who can talk has an adequate airway and should generate enough pressure to push out the obstruction.

If a person cannot talk, if the cry sounds as if the airway is partially obstructed, or if the person loses consciousness, emergency steps must be taken immediately. These procedures are known as the obstructed airway maneuver, the abdominal thrust, or the Heimlich maneuver. They are illustrated on these pages. Like CPR, they should be learned in a training course.

MEDICAL EMERGENCIES

Heart Attack and Chest Pain

A heart attack occurs when the blood supply to the heart muscles has been blocked or abruptly reduced. The usual cause is a clot obstructing one or more of the coronary arteries. In some persons, the result may be sudden, severe chest pain and almost immediate collapse. Victims need instant CPR and emergency treatment in order to survive. They should be brought immediately to a hospital emergency department (with CPR administered en route) or have CPR administered until emergency equipment can be brought to them. Medications to dissolve the clot often can reverse the attack if administered within six to eight hours of initial symptoms. Sometimes these medications can be administered by paramedic personnel even before the hospital is reached.

A second group of heart attack victims develops chest pain following exercise, although sometimes it occurs while doing nothing very active. The pain often is in the center of the chest behind the breastbone and sometimes radiates down the left arm. It may be accompanied by nausea, vomiting, and sweating.

If the person already is under care for a cardiac condition, and pain is more severe than usual or does not respond to prescribed medication (usually nitroglycerin tablets), it is most important that the physician be notified and the emergency ambulance summoned. Medication should be administered if the physician so directs. In such patients, this chest pain indicates a condition called angina pectoris due to a temporary decrease in blood to the heart. It usually will go away quickly with medication or rest without serious aftermath. When the pain does not disappear soon after onset, or if the patient has never been treated for such pain before, he or she must be taken to an emergency department.

Stroke

Stroke usually occurs in persons over age 50 and is caused by sudden bleeding in the brain, or by a blockage in a blood vessel that cuts off the blood supply to a portion of the brain. The person usually complains of weakness, loss of sensation, or inability to use one side of the body. Sometimes speech is slurred, or the person has difficulty speaking, even though conscious. He may seem

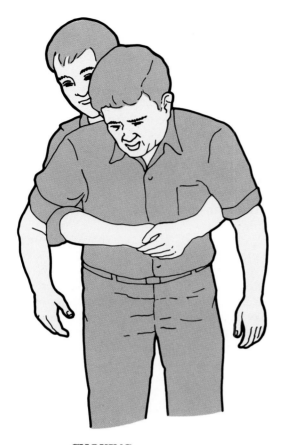

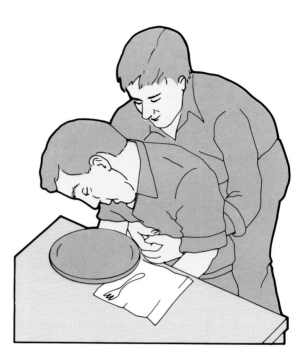

CHOKING

If a choking victim is conscious and gets to his or her feet, stand behind the person, slip your arms around his or her waist, lock your hands under the ribs in the solar plexus area, and rapidly squeeze the abdomen four times. Air will be forced out of the victim's lungs against the obstruction, propelling it into the mouth. Continue until the victim's airway is clear.

If the victim is sitting, go behind the person's chair and lean him or her forward. Encircle the victim's body with your arms. Locking your hands under the ribs as above, squeeze the abdomen.

UNCONSCIOUS CHOKING VICTIM

Place an unconscious victim on his or her back, jaw jutting upward to provide an airway. Kneel on one side of the victim. Compress the lower part of the person's chest four times to force air out of the lungs and into the windpipe. Immediately turn the victim's head to one side and clear the mouth of secretions, then repeat the maneuver.

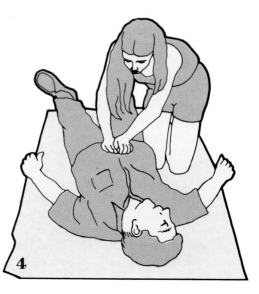

confused and unable to understand what is said. The face may be paralyzed on the same side of the body and the corner of the mouth may droop.

Keep the person quiet and reassured; do not give anything by mouth. An ambulance should be summoned and the patient should be transported to a hospital emergency department.

Unconsciousness

A person who is breathing but is hard to rouse or appears unable to respond to simple commands may be stuporous or unconscious. Whatever the cause, unconsciousness is a serious condition calling for immediate measures. The first and most important step is to make sure that the person can breathe properly. If the person is lying on his or her back and you are not sure whether there is head or neck injury, leave the person in that position but perform the jaw lift shown earlier to ensure an adequate airway. If the head or neck seems unhurt, turn the person on the side with head slightly downward. If vomiting occurs, the material then will run out of the mouth rather than being sucked into the lungs. Look for a tag, bracelet, or other information identifying the person as a diabetic, an epileptic, or a victim of another condition explaining the loss of consciousness. Do not give anything by mouth.

Shock

Shock is the medical condition that occurs when body tissues do not receive enough oxygen-carrying blood. It can arise from a number of causes. The basic components of the system involved in preventing shock are the heart, which pumps blood to the tissues; the blood vessels through which the blood flows; and the blood inside the vessels, which contains red cells that carry oxygen, as well as proteins, white blood cells, and nutrients for the tissues.

Conditions that affect the pump are heart attacks, or injuries to the chest that damage the heart and prevent it from working properly. Conditions that affect the amount of blood flow are injuries (such as stab wounds or bullet wounds) that damage blood vessels and allow blood to pour out, either externally or internally. A third way in which this system can break down is when the vessels themselves are damaged because of allergy (including insect bite) or infection. The vessels dilate, enlarge, and develop tiny holes. Fluid leaks through the vessel walls into the tissues, causing severe swelling. The swelling can occur in such important areas as the tongue, the back of the throat, or the windpipe, and can interfere with breathing.

Any of these conditions can cause a catastrophic drop in blood pressure, the chief indication of shock. In mild shock, the pulse becomes very fast, the skin becomes pale, cold, and clammy, and the patient often is slightly confused and unable to respond to simple questions. In severe shock, the patient may become unconscious and the pulse may be barely detectable. In allergic (anaphylactic) shock, the pulse is fast but the skin is warm and flushed.

Shock can be fatal and should be treated promptly. The first step is to check airway, breathing, and circulation. Start mouth-to-mouth resuscitation if the patient is not breathing properly, and cardiac compression if the pulse cannot be felt.

The patient should be placed flat if conscious, or on his or her side if unconscious. The head should be level, or lower than the rest of the body. External bleeding should be stopped immediately by direct pressure. The legs may be elevated by flexing them at the hips. Nothing should be given by mouth. In cases of anaphylaxis (allergic reaction) resulting from insect stings, persons known to be at risk often carry emergency kits, including directions for use.

Fainting

Fainting usually is caused by temporary insufficiency of the blood supply to the brain.

If you feel faint or about to "pass out," lie down or bend forward at the waist from a sitting position and put your head between your knees. If you can't lie or sit, kneel on one knee as if tying a shoe, to position your head lower than your heart.

In a crowded place, if someone feels faint, don't try to walk the person out. Bend the person's head forward between his or her knees until the person feels better. Keep the patient lying down, with head lowered or legs and hips elevated. Sprinkle cold water on the person's face.

After the person regains consciousness, coffee or tea may be given. Recovery should be rapid—within five minutes. If unconsciousness is prolonged or fainting spells recur, call a physician or an ambulance.

BLEEDING

Internal Bleeding

Internal bleeding is extremely dangerous because the blood loss cannot be seen. Sometimes the person may appear uninjured, or believe he or she has suffered only minor superficial injuries, and may lose large volumes of blood before the internal bleeding is recognized. The bleeding may occur in the abdomen following injury to the spleen, the liver, or the kidneys; in the pelvis following fractures or damage to the bladder or the large blood vessels; in the thigh following fracture to the thighbone; or in the chest following damage to the heart, the lungs, or the large vessels. Often the first indication of internal bleeding occurs when the patient starts going into shock.

Internal bleeding always should be suspected when a person has been involved in a major fall or accident with a violent impact. A driver who is thrown against the steering wheel, or a passenger who is thrown from a car is a possible victim.

A careful examination may show certain telltale signs of possible internal bleeding, such as bruising and abrasions of the skin over the chest. The victim may complain of pain and tenderness over the chest. Similarly, tenderness over the upper abdomen may indicate damage and bleeding of the internal organs. Abrasions, bruises, or even the imprint of a seat belt over the upper abdomen also may be clues. Other signs can be:
- In a stomach injury, vomited material is black-brown, resembling coffee grounds.
- In an injury to the upper intestine, the stools may be black and tarry.
- An injury to the lungs and chest may produce coughed-up blood that is frothy or contains dark lumps of blood.

If there are signs of internal bleeding, do not move the person. Do *not* give any liquids or anything by mouth. Treat the person for shock, and keep the person covered with a light blanket. Summon an emergency ambulance.

Visible Bleeding

Serious bleeding. For deep cuts, severed blood vessels, and spurting or oozing blood, press a clean cloth firmly against the wound.

Remove enough clothing to see the wound clearly. Cover the wound with a sterile compress and apply firm hand pressure directly over the wound. Exert steady, not intermittent, pressure using your finger, hand, or heel of your hand. Continue until the bleeding stops.

Use clean materials, such as sterile gauze, folded clean handkerchiefs, freshly laundered towels, or strips from sheets, to cover the bleeding point.

If no sterile items are available, do not hesitate to use clothing, soiled materials, or your bare hand. Blood loss is more dangerous than an immediate risk of infection.

Bleeding from legs and arms. If a wound is in an arm or leg, elevate the limb and support it with pillows or similar padding. The wound should be higher than the level of the heart. Do not elevate the limb if bones are broken or if a fracture is suspected.

Pressure dressing. When bleeding stops, apply a pressure dressing. Put a gauze compress or folded layers of clean cloth over the bleeding point (do not use fluffy absorbent cotton in direct contact with the wound). Press the compress with your fingers and apply a suitable bandage to fix the dressing in place.

General measures. Do not apply salves, ointments, or medicines to deep wounds. Covering a wound with sterile gauze or clean cloth protects against further contamination.

Do not try to cleanse a deep or seriously bleeding wound (bleeding cleanses it internally) unless medical help is long delayed or there is gross contamination. Then cleanse the skin around the wound with clean (tap or boiled) water stirred with soap to make a sudsy solution. Cover the wound and a small area of surrounding skin with sterile gauze. Dip sterile absorbent cotton into the soapy solution and apply it gently to the exposed skin, stroking away from the wound. Use a fresh cotton tuft for each stroke. Greases and oils may be removed with kerosene, naphtha, or rubbing alcohol.

Puncture Wounds

Penetrating, perforating injuries are inflicted by relatively small objects driven under the skin, sometimes deeply, or entirely through the body, leaving entrance and exit wounds (perforating wounds). They may be caused by stepping on a nail; bullets or shot; wood, glass, or metal splinters; and particles driven by firecrackers, firearms, or other types of explosions.

A small puncture wound may be washed with soap and water and rinsed under running water. Cover with a dressing or adhesive bandage. The entrance point of a puncture wound usually is small and bleeds little. It cannot be cleaned in depth, so it is useless to try to force antiseptics into the wound.

Treat punctures like other wounds, according to the immediate emergency. If you are sure it will not cause further injury, encourage bleeding to "wash out" the wound by pressing gently around its edges.

Always see a doctor for treatment of puncture wounds. There is danger of serious infection, including tetanus (lockjaw), from organisms that may be carried into the body.

BURNS

First-degree burns cause only redness of the skin. Sunburn is a first-degree burn. Widespread sunburn, which can be accompanied by swelling and fluid collection under the skin, often is called sunstroke. It may be accompanied by heatstroke (below), a much more serious condition.

Second-degree burns result in redness of the skin plus blistering. These areas can be large as well, and the blistered areas can become infected and result in serious scar formation.

Third-degree burns are those in which the superficial skin and fat are burned and deep structures such as muscle, nerves, and blood vessels are visible or even damaged. These are the most serious burns, although they may not be painful because nerve endings have been destroyed.

Another way of classifying burns is by calling them partial- or complete-thickness burns.

Partial-thickness burns are those in which only the skin and part of the underlying tissue are red and blistered and damage goes no deeper. These are very painful because the nerve endings are not destroyed.

Full-thickness burns involve the whole skin and subcutaneous tissue down to muscle or fat. They often are not painful because the nerve endings have been destroyed.

Burns acquired in a closed space, such as a room with little ventilation, are dangerous because hot smoke containing chemicals may have been inhaled. Often these burns do not show their dangerous effects for 12 to 24 hours. Anyone who has burns around the mouth or inside the mouth or who coughs up sooty sputum should be examined by a doctor or an emergency department for burns of the lungs. Burns of the airway can result in the swelling and eventual narrowing of the airway, causing breathing difficulty.

In major burns involving more than 20 percent of the body surface, shock can occur because the injury "burns off" water from the body, and the body oozes fluids through the burn. The victim needs intravenous fluids to replace those lost through the burn site.

Treatment of Burns

Severe burns that cover more than 5 percent of the skin area and burns of the face and hands require prompt medical attention. The larger the burn, the greater the need. Meanwhile, immediate treatment can be given by placing the burned area under cold running water, or by covering it with cloths soaked in cold water. Cover the area with a dry, clean dressing before transporting the patient.

Chemical burns. Drench the burned area with clean water immediately. Place the victim in a shower, if one is available, and forcefully spray the burned areas. Remove the victim's clothing while he or she is under the shower. Summon an ambulance, or transport the patient to an emergency department.

Treatment of minor burns is described under "Home Treatment."

FALLS AND ACCIDENTS

Head Injuries

Assume that any severe blow to the head sufficient to stun the patient, even if he or she does not become unconscious, is a concussion (a bruise of the brain). Any person—especially a child—who has suffered a head injury should be kept quiet and receive medical attention as soon as possible, even if he or she seems to have "recovered." More severe symptoms may be delayed.

For immediate first aid, keep the person lying down and warm. Do not let the person sit up or walk. Observe the person closely. Ask simple questions or give simple directions. It is important to note the person's responses so you will be aware of any change later.

A very important sign of serious brain damage may be found by directing a flashlight beam at the eyes. Normally the pupils will react to light by constricting. Both pupils should react equally. If one pupil is large and fails to respond to light, and the other is smaller and constricts normally, the person may be bleeding around the brain or into the brain and should be seen at an emergency department as quickly as possible.

Watch, too, for a change in the level of consciousness. If a head-injury patient becomes stuporous or sleepy, or if he develops slurred speech, cannot carry on a simple conversation, or cannot follow simple commands, this may indicate bleeding inside the skull and possibly in the brain. This is especially important if the patient appeared fine after the accident or injury, but later begins to have difficulty with speech, memory, or simple tasks.

If the person loses consciousness, turn the person on his or her side, watch for vomiting, and be sure the airway is open. Be prepared to do mouth-to-mouth resuscitation and cardiac compression, if it should become necessary.

Neck or Back Injuries

The best first-aid advice is to do nothing until medical help arrives. Tragedy can result if the victim of a spinal injury is moved by well-intentioned but uninformed persons. Even a slight movement of the head or back may sever nerves and cause paralysis or death. What you don't do in the first few minutes is more important than what you do.

What to do. Suspect a broken back or neck and treat it as a fracture if the patient has had a bad fall, a "whiplash" neck injury, or a crushing or impact injury, or has been involved in any accident in which the back or neck is badly bent or struck.

If the person is conscious, ask him or her to move a hand or fingers. If the patient cannot, suspect a neck fracture. If the person can move arms and hands but not legs, feet, and toes, suspect a back fracture. The person may complain of pain in the neck or back. There may be no other sign.

Summon medical help at once. Advise the person not to move. Place rolled newspaper or folded blankets next to the head to immobilize the head and neck. While waiting, keep the patient warm and covered.

Abdominal Injuries

In addition to internal bleeding, injuries to the pelvis (the basin-shaped structure between the spine and lower limbs) can be very serious. Broken bones may damage important abdominal organs. Automobile accidents and squeezing, crushing hip injuries are among the causes. Watch for great pain in the lower abdomen and possible difficulty in urination or blood in the urine. Be extremely careful in handling a person with a possible fractured pelvis. Do not move the person unless absolutely essential.

Arm and Leg Injuries

Most injuries to upper and lower limbs require medical evaluation. Severe swelling or pain often indicates a fracture. An X ray often is required.

If the injury is to an arm, hand, shoulder, or collarbone, the person usually can be transported to an emergency department unless other injuries are apparent.

Facial Injuries

Fractured jaw (lower). A broken lower jaw is indicated by severe pain at the site or loosened or damaged teeth. There may be bleeding from the mouth. Raise the lower jaw gently to a normal position, and support it with a broad bandage under the chin tied at the top of the head.

Fractured nose. A broken nose may result from an athletic event, a bicycle accident, or a hard fall. Misalignment and swelling are the chief clues. If the nose bleeds, press the nostrils together between the thumb and index finger for several minutes. Press cold cloths over the nose. A broken nose is not a dire emergency, but get prompt medical attention for the patient to prevent deformity. Occasionally the person vomits swallowed blood, which is frightening but not very dangerous.

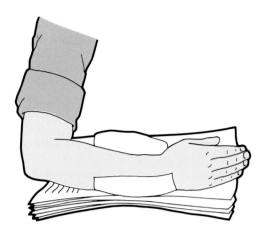

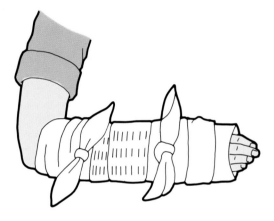

EMERGENCY SPLINT

Any rigid material will immobilize a broken limb during an emergency. Rolled newspapers are often handiest. Place a pad inside the folded paper, then tie as shown. If the fingers turn blue, the splint is too tight and should be loosened.

Fractures

A fracture seldom is an emergency. Call paramedics or other assistance (the ski patrol if the injured person is a skier, for example) and wait for help.

You should suspect a broken bone if:
● The victim can't move the injured part.
● The part is deformed, or appears to be out of shape.
● Movement is painful.
● Sensation is lacking.
● The skin is swollen or blue.

A simple fracture exists under unbroken skin and may not be obvious. A compound fracture shows bone protruding from the skin, or an open wound at the fracture site; frequently there is severe bleeding from the wound.

Principles of first aid for fractures. Any of the body's 206 bones can be fractured, but certain principles of care apply regardless of location.
● Do not move the person unless he or she is at risk of further injury. Great harm can be done if the patient is moved hastily, pulled, bundled into the back seat of a car, or allowed to stand or sit up, or to move the injured part.
● If moving is absolutely necessary, pull at the legs or armpits along the axis of the body.
● Examine the person first for other injuries. Stop serious bleeding by hand pressure or a gauze dressing over the wound.
● Check the victim's mouth and throat for possible obstruction of breathing.
● Keep the patient warm and lying down.
● Do not put a pillow under the person's head if the neck is injured. Instead, block the head with padding to prevent neck movement.

If medical help will be delayed and the patient must be transported:
● Do not try to set bones.
● Always apply splints before moving or transporting the patient. Splint the patient where he or she is.
● Apply a clean dressing and bandage (no antiseptic) if a bone protrudes through the skin. Do not attempt to push the bone back into place.

Dislocations

A blow, fall, or sudden twist may force a bone out of place at a joint, causing a dislocation. Some persons are prone to repeated dislocation of certain joints.

An indication of a dislocation is that the joint looks out of shape compared to a similar joint. Swelling usually is rapid, and there is pain and tenderness at the injury site. The patient can't move the joint, or motion is limited.

Immediate first aid. Call an ambulance or transport the person to a hospital emergency department if it can be done without risk.

Do not try to straighten the joint or force the bone back into place (except for a knee, jaw, finger, or toe dislocation; see below).

Suspect that bones may be fractured.

Put the patient in a comfortable position. Keep weight off the injured part. Give gentle support to the injured part.

Apply an ice bag or cloths wrung out of very cold water to the injured part to ease pain and minimize swelling.

Dislocation of the knee. Athletic injury is the usual cause of a dislocation of the knee. The dislocation usually is evident because the lower leg is out of alignment at the knee, displaced either forward or backward. The injury requires immediate attention because of the danger that the artery supplying blood to the lower leg may be stretched or trapped and the flow interrupted. Treatment requires two persons. One holds the victim at the shoulders, and the other grasps the foot on the dislocated leg and pulls down as hard as possible to relocate the knee in a normal position. Call for emergency help.

Finger or toe dislocation. With one hand on each side of the dislocated joint, slowly pull the free end of the finger or toe in a straight line until it snaps in place. Do not use great force. If one or two attempts fail, wait for medical help. Do not try to reduce the large joint at the base of the thumb or the great toe joint.

Jaw dislocation. Suspect a dislocated jaw if the lower jaw sags and the patient cannot close his or her mouth.

Wrap your thumbs with cloth to protect them. Face the patient, and put your thumbs in his or her mouth on the lower back teeth and your fingers under his or her chin. Press down firmly and back with your thumbs, and upward with your fingers under the chin. Remove your thumbs quickly to prevent injury when the jaw snaps back in place.

Shoulder dislocation. The awake patient experiences pain and complains of being unable to move the arm. Examination of the shoulder reveals that the normal shape of the shoulder is changed, and in certain kinds of dislocations the head of the humerus (the upper arm bone) can be felt below the collarbone. The shoulder tip is not rounded, and drops off sharply.

Shoulder dislocation is not a true emergency unless the patient complains of tingling or numbness in the hand on the injured side, or unless it is difficult to feel the pulse at the elbow or in the wrist. Absence of pulse means that the injury may have interfered with circulation, and the patient should be seen by a physician immediately.

HOME TREATMENT

Wounds, Cuts, and Bruises

Abrasions. Skinned knees, scraped elbows, and other children's injuries can bleed or ooze blood. Extract coarse bits of dirt from the wound with small tweezers, sterilized by passing them through a match or a gas flame. Rub the wound gently with a bar of plain mild soap under running water, or wash lavishly with soap and water and a clean cloth or pieces of sterile gauze or cotton (use a fresh piece for each swabbing). Rinse under running tap water. Cover with sterile dressing or an adhesive bandage. If dirt is ground into the wound, get medical attention.

Blisters. If a water or blood blister is small and unbroken, wash it gently with soap and water, and cover it with sterile gauze or an adhesive bandage. Leave the blister undisturbed until fluids are absorbed naturally.

A large blister is likely to be bumped and broken, or to rupture spontaneously. If blistered skin has been rubbed off, exposing the raw skin surface, clean the area with warm soap and water and sterile cotton swabs. Cover with a sterile dressing. Watch for signs of infection (spreading redness, radiating red lines, or pus).

Bleeding from bruises. Bruises, or contusions, are caused by blows or falls that break small vessels under the skin without breaking the skin surface. The injury is first red, then discolored (a "black eye" is a typical bruise). Most bruises are minor, but internal bleeding may accompany bruises of the abdomen. Other severe bruises may involve broken bones. For minor bruises, ice, an ice bag, or cloths wrung out in very cold water will relieve pain and limit discoloration.

Cuts and scratches. Minor wounds seldom require antiseptics. The area around the wound may be cleansed with warm water, mild soap, and a clean cloth, or with cotton swabs dipped into warm soapy water. Rinse under running water. Cover the wound with an adhesive bandage or sterile gauze held in place by adhesive tape.

For deep or extensive cuts, control bleeding by hand pressure over a gauze pad, clean cloth, or handkerchief. Tie a bandage over sterile dressing. Deep cuts may need stitches to minimize scars. Always get medical aid.

Splinters. If one end of a splinter or thorn protrudes above the surface of the skin, it may be grasped with tweezers or the fingers and pulled out at the same angle at which it entered. Wash afterward with warm, soapy water, and apply an antiseptic. If the splinter is completely embedded in the skin, sterilize a needle or knife blade in an open flame. Probe the splinter until it can be removed with tweezers. Apply an antiseptic and cover with an adhesive bandage.

If the splinter is large or too deeply embedded to remove without damaging the surrounding flesh, medical treatment may be required. A tetanus injection also may be needed.

Minor burns. Minor common burns from touching a stove or other hot surface can be treated at home. When in doubt, call your doctor or go to an emergency department.

Immediate care is to place the burn under cold running water to relieve pain. Then cover it with a clean, dry dressing. Gauze impregnated with petroleum jelly sometimes can be used if the burn is small. Cover the burn with a clean dressing, and change the dressing daily. The burn can be washed with soap and water while healing. If signs of infection occur, such as an increase in pain, swelling, fever, or the appearance of pus, the patient should see a physician.

For superficial burns that cover 5 to 10 percent of the body and do not involve the face or hands, follow these simple steps.
- Don't open intact blisters.
- If blisters are ruptured, carefully trim the edges of the broken flesh.
- Wash burns with soap and water.
- Keep burns covered with a dry, clean dressing.
- Watch carefully for signs of infection, such as increased redness, pain, swelling, or draining.

Bites

Poisonous snakebites. Not everyone who claims to have been bitten by a snake actually has been bitten. Often, simply seeing a snake nearby convinces a frightened person that he or she has been bitten. When a bite does occur, the skin is not always broken. Even if it is broken, the snake's venom may not have been injected into the wound. Thus, only a minority of snakebite victims are in danger of poisoning. (Remember, however, that venom may enter the body through an existing break in the skin.) For a true bite, hospital emergency care is required. Meanwhile, cover the bite with a clean dry dressing. Keep the limb elevated. Do not apply ice, cut the wound, or apply a tourniquet, all of which can cause tissue damage.

Insect bites. For relief of pain and itching from mosquito, flea, or other insect bites, apply ice or wet dressings; hold under cold water. Apply a paste of baking soda moistened with water, or apply diluted household ammonia to the bite and surrounding skin. Calamine lotion and rubbing alcohol or lotions containing alcohol also help to relieve itching. Do not scratch an insect bite. Scratching may result in infection.

Tick bites. Ticks are small insects that burrow into the skin and can cause such serious diseases as Lyme disease and Rocky Mountain spotted fever. A tick often can be felt before it starts to burrow under the skin, but usually not after it begins to suck. Ticks often are picked up in areas of damp grass or woodlands, but they sometimes are brought indoors by domestic animals, or may be found in suburban gardens. Children are especially vulnerable. Examine their clothing, skin, and hair after playing in "tick territory," especially in the spring.

The head of a tick tenaciously resists removal from skin. Don't try to remove ticks with unprotected fingers or allow crushed parts or juices to contact the skin. It may help to make ticks "let go" if you coat them with nail polish, petroleum jelly, or grease, or smother them with kerosene, turpentine, or gasoline. Remove them carefully with tweezers. Afterward, wash the site thoroughly with soap and water.

Wear high-top shoes with trouser ends tied around the tops when hiking in tick country.

Stings. Bee, wasp, hornet, or yellow jacket stings may be relieved by cold packs containing baking soda. Ice bags also give comfort.

If you upset a nest of insects and suffer a "massive dose" of many separate stings, get into a tepid tub bath with a package or more of baking soda stirred into it.

Bees often leave their "stinger" in the center of the sting. The stinging apparatus can be seen as a tiny dark object. It continues to pump venom into the wound after the bee is gone. Pinch the stinger between two fingernails or grasp it with tweezers and remove it gently. Do not remove the stinger with a scraping motion of a fingernail.

Spider bites. Two common American spiders can inflict serious bites: the small brown (recluse) spider and the black widow. The latter is a coalblack spider with a pea-size abdomen marked with a reddish hourglass design; the brown recluse is about an inch long and ranges in color from tan to dark brown, with a darker spot on the underparts.

The black widow's bite causes intense pain, muscle spasm, and weak pulse. The pain moves gradually from the wound and concentrates in the abdomen. The brown spider's bite may not be immediately painful, but if not treated it causes tissue breakdown in the area of the wound. The effects are more marked in children, and may include swelling around the bite, fever, chills, nausea, vomiting, and weakness.

Get to a doctor or hospital emergency department immediately. Save the dead spider for identification, if possible. Meanwhile, wash the wound with soapy water and watch for signs of shock.

Animal bites. Immediate first-aid treatment of animal bites is the same as for other common wounds, except for the possibility of rabies. Bite injuries range from barely perceptible tooth marks to severe, major wounds. An unprovoked bite by a domestic animal calls for evaluation for rabies at an emergency department. The animal may need to be quarantined.

Most bites inflicted by dogs, cats, squirrels, rats, mice, and small animals are local soft-tissue injuries. Immediate first aid aims to prevent infection and promote healing.

Cleanse the wound thoroughly with soap and water. Preferably, wash it under running water with soap. Paint with antiseptic. Cover the bite wound with a sterile dressing and bandage. Always see a doctor if the bite, no matter how trivial, is on the face, hands, head, or neck area. Cat bites over a joint, such as fingers or knuckles, are potentially dangerous. The long sharp teeth may penetrate into the joint.

Human bites. A human bite may be a real bite or it may be inflicted by teeth that stop the blow of a fist. The human mouth commonly contains varied and virulent bacteria, and serious, undermining, spreading infections can follow human bite wounds.

Give first aid as for an animal bite, then get medical attention.

Lodged, Inhaled, Or Swallowed Objects

Ear. Children may insert small objects into the ear canal. Peas, beans, and popcorn swell when wet and are hard to remove.

Do not dig at the object with a toothpick, hairpin, or wire, which risks grave danger of injuring the ear canal or eardrum, and may push the object further inside. If the object appears loose, gently pull the earlobe backward and tilt the child's head so the object can fall out. If the object is a bean or seed, a little olive oil or mineral oil can be dropped in the child's ear to lessen the swelling. If this fails, take the child to a doctor or emergency department with instruments to remove the foreign body.

Insect in the ear. Turn the person's head to one side and drop in some warm olive oil, mineral oil, or warm water to suffocate the insect. Or turn out the lights and shine a flashlight into the person's ear to attract the insect.

Nose. Children sometimes slip beans, grains, or small objects into the nose. The object itself usually is not dangerous, but great harm can be done trying to remove it with crude instruments. Drop olive oil into the nostril to soothe tissues and prevent swelling. The child may blow the nose gently (both nostrils open), never forcibly, after oil is instilled. If this does not dislodge the object, take the child to a doctor.

Stomach. Tacks, open safety pins, needles, and other small sharp objects frequently are swallowed by children. Do not administer a laxative. Seek emergency help. Most foreign objects that reach the stomach pass through the bowel harmlessly, but a doctor may intervene if the object becomes lodged or penetrates tissues. Never force a child who has swallowed a sharp object to vomit.

Sprains and Strains

Sprains result from tearing or stretching ligaments that link the bones at joints and allow movement. They have become increasingly common because of weekend athletics. It may be difficult to distinguish between a severe sprain and a fracture—both may result from the same injury. X rays usually are necessary to make the distinction.

The symptoms of a sprain are: pain in the joint that increases on movement, tenderness to the touch, difficulty in using the joint without pain, rapid swelling, and black and blue discoloration (that might not appear for several hours or days).

Immediate aid. Sprains are not emergencies. Except for minor injuries, have the injury examined by a doctor within six to 12 hours. In skiing injuries, summon the ski patrol.

Treatment is summed up in the acronym ICE: ice, compression, elevation. For the first few hours after injury, apply an ice bag or cold compresses. This contracts vessels, minimizes swelling, and eases pain. Do not apply heat immediately after the injury.

Compress the injured area by direct pressure or preferably by elastic bandage to reduce swelling. The bandage also may hold the ice bag in place.

Elevate the sprained joint higher than the rest of the body so it gets less blood and therefore will have less swelling. Support it with a pillow or padded clothing.

Bandage the joint to prevent unnecessary motion if the accident occurs far from medical help. Loosen the bandage if swelling increases.

Sprained ankle. If the injury occurs far from help or if it is absolutely essential for a sprained ankle to bear weight, a snug ankle bandage gives support for walking. Never walk with a sprained ankle (it might be broken) unless it's a serious emergency.

To support a sprained ankle, leave the shoe on, but loosen laces. Place a long bandage under the shoe in front of the heel. Bring bandage ends behind and above the heel, cross, bring them forward, and cross them over the instep. On each side of the foot, tuck the ends under the loops formed by the first step of bandaging. Pull the ends together and tie over the instep. For a sprained knee, wrist, or elbow, wrap well with an elastic bandage. Use a sling for a sprain of the wrist or elbow.

Strains. A strain is caused by overstretching or "pulling" muscles or tendons. Back strain ("crick in the back") is common.

Symptoms include a sharp pain or "stitch" at the time of injury, stiffness and soreness that get worse in a few hours, and pain on movement.

How to help. Put the injured part at rest. Sit or lie in the most comfortable position.

Apply heat in any form—hot water bottle, lamp, or heating pad. Give a gentle massage with warm rubbing alcohol. If the pain eases sufficiently, rub more forcefully or knead gently to help loosen stiffened muscles. Aspirin or acetaminophen can relieve pain.

See a doctor if back strain is severe. Back strains frequently need strapping.

POISONING

Poisons can enter the body in different ways. These include swallowing, breathing (inhalation), smoking, absorption through the skin, and injection or envenomation. Injected poisons include abused drugs such as heroin and "speed" (amphetamines); envenomation refers to bites by snakes or insects. Cocaine may be smoked in its "crack" form and cause poisoning symptoms.

To treat a poisoning victim, follow these steps:
● Remove the patient from any further exposure to the poison.
● Ensure that the airway, breathing, and circulation are adequate.
● Reduce the chance of further absorption of the poison. Depending on how the poison was taken in, this may be done by washing the skin with water, by giving a lot of water to drink, by causing vomiting, by giving a laxative or cathartic, or in rare cases, by using a specific antidote.
● Phone your local poison control center, and provide the following information:
   Your name.
   Your address.
   Your telephone number.
   The patient's name and age.
   What the poison is.
   When it was taken.
   What symptoms have occurred.
   What steps you have taken to treat it.
● Follow the instructions given to you by the poison control center.

Swallowed Poisons

If you are unable to contact the poison control center or other emergency facility for instructions, take these steps:
● If the patient is conscious and can talk to you or hold a glass, give as much water as he or she can drink. Large amounts of fluids may cause vomiting, and vomiting should be encouraged for all swallowed poisons except caustics. This usually is easy to determine because caustic substances burn the mouth, tongue, and throat. Or, information on the poison's container may state that the contents are caustic.
● Give the victim syrup of ipecac—two tablespoons for an adult, one tablespoon for a child. As noted in the list on page 463, ipecac, available without prescription, should be part of every family's first-aid supplies. Have the victim drink six to

eight glasses of water. If vomiting has not occurred in 20 to 30 minutes, ipecac may be repeated in the same quantity. Do not repeat more than once.

Ipecac should *not* be given and vomiting should *not* be induced if the offending substance is caustic or corrosive, such as lye, disinfectant, ammonia, or toilet-bowl cleaner, because substances that burn on the way down also may burn on the way up. Look for burns around the lips or in the mouth. Nor should ipecac be used for swallowed kerosene, gasoline, or turpentine.

A so-called universal antidote for swallowed poisons, available in some drugstores, should *not* be used. Follow directions from the poison control center.

After the person has vomited and if he or she appears wide awake, alert, and unharmed, you may give activated charcoal, also available in drugstores, in a quantity of about one teaspoon to a glass of water. Follow the charcoal with a large dose of Epsom salts or any other common laxative.

Transport the patient to a hospital emergency department. Take the bottle, box, or container from which the poison came, including the remaining liquids, tablets, powders, or particles, and the label if it contains information. For prescription drugs, take the container with the pharmacist's name and the prescription number.

Poisoned unconscious victims. If the patient is not fully conscious and is unable to hold a glass of water, lay the patient on his or her stomach or side. Keep the patient's mouth free of secretions by wiping it with a handkerchief or finger. Keep the airway open by using the techniques described earlier. Call an ambulance.

If breathing appears inadequate, start mouth-to-mouth resuscitation, and if the pulse disappears, start cardiac compression.

Keep the patient warm. Do not give stimulants of any kind. Give nothing by mouth.

Food Poisoning

Do not assume that all severe intestinal upsets after eating are caused by food poisoning. Appendicitis and other illnesses may cause similar symptoms. The chief clue to food poisoning is when more than one person becomes ill after eating the same foods.

Staphylococcal food poisoning may cause symptoms almost immediately, commonly within two to four hours after eating. Symptoms of salmonella poisoning usually are longer delayed—from six hours after eating to a day or even two days later.

Nausea, vomiting, diarrhea, and cramps are the primary symptoms of food poisoning. There also may be considerable abdominal pain and distress; the abdomen feels soft, rather than rigid. Salmonella poisoning may cause chills and fever, too. A doctor should be consulted promptly.

Do not give laxatives, cathartics, or anything by mouth as long as there is persistent nausea and vomiting. Put the patient to bed and keep him or her warm. After nausea and vomiting subside, give large quantities of water or soft drinks.

Botulinum Poisoning

Botulinum poisoning is caused by powerful toxins of organisms that may be in improperly home-canned foods, especially low-acid foods. Commercially canned foods and home-canned foods canned by the pressure method are safe. Boil home-canned foods for 30 minutes before eating to ensure their safety.

Symptoms commonly begin 18 to 24 hours after eating contaminated food, but may not appear for several days. Nausea and vomiting may not occur. More common symptoms include: great fatigue; dizziness; headache; blurred or double vision; difficulty in breathing, swallowing, or speaking; and muscular weakness. The body temperature may be subnormal.

Botulinum poisoning can be fatal. Medical attention should be obtained *at once*.

Mushroom Poisoning

The best first aid is prevention. No test can prove unknown mushrooms safe to eat. Avoid all wild mushrooms.

If mushroom poisoning occurs, call an ambulance immediately. Keep the person quiet and lying down. If symptoms occur in the woods or far from medical aid, get the person to a hospital emergency department immediately.

Symptoms of mushroom poisoning may appear within a few minutes to two to three hours after eating, but some varieties do not cause symptoms for up to 48 hours.

Common symptoms include abdominal pain, diarrhea, dizziness, blurred or double vision, cold sweating, and cramps in the arms or legs.

If possible, keep a sample of the mushroom for identification.

Weed and Plant Poisoning

Leaves, roots, berries, seeds, and other parts of many weeds, wild plants, and garden plants (foxglove, monkshood, rhubarb leaves, lilies, and others) may be toxic if eaten. Teach children not to eat strange berries, fruits, or plant parts; avoid them yourself. Check your garden for poisonous plants. Ask your local nursery for advice. Symptoms of plant poisoning vary. They usually include abdominal pain, cramps, nausea, and vomiting. Stains may be visible around the mouth.

Give large amounts of water or milk, as well as the standard dose of ipecac. After the person has vomited, give activated charcoal. Call the poison control center and an ambulance.

ANAPHYLAXIS (ALLERGIC REACTION)

Anaphylaxis results from an allergy to a foreign substance such as pollen, fish, penicillin, or bee or wasp stings. It is described in detail in Chapter 23, "Allergy and the Immune System."

Usually the reaction begins soon after exposure. The major serious effects are breathing difficulty and shock. Early signs include skin rashes, blebs on the skin, swelling of the tongue, and itching in the back of the throat. These may progress to severe wheezing, difficulty with breathing, confusion, and collapse. Swelling of the face, eyelids, and extremities may occur, and the person may collapse, or, in some cases, suffer cardiac arrest.

Call emergency help immediately. Pay careful attention to the airway and be prepared to give CPR, if necessary. Persons known to be vulnerable to serious allergic reactions should receive an epinephrine injection. Often these people carry epinephrine in their purses or pockets, and wear an identification "Medic-Alert" tag. It may be necessary for you to administer the epinephrine (adrenaline) if they are not able to do so.

HEAT AND FREEZING

Heat Cramps

Heat cramps are painful spasms of abdominal, leg, or arm muscles caused by loss of body salt through profuse, prolonged sweating. They are most common in persons who do very hard physical labor in extremely hot surroundings for long periods. Cramps usually respond to firm hand pressure, warm wet towels, or a hot water bottle. Give the patient sips of slightly salted water.

Heat Exhaustion

Heat exhaustion occurs because body fluids and the salts they contain have been passed off from the body. The person's skin is pallid, clammy, and moist; he or she may sweat profusely. Body temperature may be about normal, or slightly lowered or slightly elevated. The patient may exhibit nausea, scant urine, and dizziness, and may faint.

Remove the patient to circulating air. Have the patient lie down and rest. Loosen his or her clothing. Give sips of slightly salted water (one teaspoonful of salt to each pint of water) or coffee or tea as stimulants.

If symptoms do not subside readily, call a physician or emergency assistance.

Heatstroke

Heatstroke is a grave emergency and can be fatal. Symptoms include very hot, absolutely dry skin and no sweating. Body temperature is very high, up to an incredible 110 degrees. The victim may exhibit weakness, dizziness, rapid breathing, nausea, unconsciousness, and sometimes mental confusion. Onset is often dramatically sudden.

Cool the victim rapidly. Apply an ice bag, crushed ice wrapped in a cloth, or cold cloths to the head. If the victim can't be moved to shelter, drench the person's clothes with warm water, poured on or sprayed from a hose.

Preferably, strip the victim's clothing, wrap the person in a sheet, and keep the sheet wet with cold water. Place electric fans to blow on the cold sheet, and keep cloths or ice on the victim's head. At the same time, rub the victim's arms and legs toward the heart through the sheet.

Check body temperature every 10 minutes. Repeat the cooling procedures until body temperature drops to between 101 and 102 degrees.

Frostbite

Skiers, snowmobilers, children who play outdoors in cold weather, and those who work outdoors are all susceptible to frostbite. Exposed parts of the body, especially the face or ears and the extremities, may appear bluish, or white with grayish-yellow cast, and feel numb.

Do not rub the frozen part with snow or anything else. Frozen tissue is fragile and easily damaged. Do not expose to intense direct heat, such as that from a hot stove, radiator, or heat lamp.

If outdoors, thaw the frozen part by using the patient's body or the body of another as a warmer. Place a frozen hand under an armpit or between the thighs. Place a warm hand over a frozen ear or nose.

Indoors, immerse the frozen part in water warmed to about 100 degrees. Or, cover the part with warmed (not hot) towels or blankets. If the part is deeply frozen, the condition requires immediate medical aid.

Prolonged Exposure

Chilling of the entire body, from mild chilling to numbness, can be serious. Drowsiness can be a symptom and death can result.

For a mild chill, put the patient to bed in a warm room, cover well, and give hot drinks.

For serious freezing exposure, get the victim to a warm place. If this is not possible, two or three persons may warm the victim with their bodies, under blankets, or in a sleeping bag. If breathing is imperceptible or stopped, give mouth-to-mouth resuscitation.

Rewarm the victim rapidly by immersing in a tub of water at 78 to 82 degrees. Then wrap the victim in warm blankets and put him or her to bed. Give warm drinks, and summon help.

EYES

Chemical Burns

When dangerous chemicals get into the eyes, wash the eyes immediately with large amounts of cool water. Immediate flushing of the chemical minimizes eye damage and may prevent it entirely.

Hold the head under a faucet with the eye in the running stream. The stream should have good flushing force but not high pressure. Turn the head so the stream flows over the affected eye and away from the unaffected eye. If both eyes are contaminated, direct water on both eyes simultaneously or in rapid alternation. Continue irrigating the eyes

with water for 5 or 10 minutes or until you are very sure that all dangerous chemical material has been washed out. Remember, powder particles may be trapped under the eyelids. Separate the lids gently so water can reach all parts.

If there is no faucet handy, seize any source of water or any bland fluid—a carton of milk will serve in an emergency. Put the person on the floor, flat on his or her back, and pour the liquid into the corner of the eyes next to the nose so the fluid streams over the eyeballs and under the eyelids. Or, the eyes may be held in a stream of water bubbling from a drinking fountain. Or, the eyes may be submerged in a bowl of water while the patient repeatedly blinks them.

What you do in the first few seconds and the next few minutes to wash acids or alkalis from the eyes is more important than anything the doctor can do later. Cover both eyes with a sterile gauze compress (even if only one has been affected) and take the patient to a doctor, or call for emergency assistance.

Contusions of the Eyeball

Hard blows that do not cut or penetrate the eye may "bruise" it internally and can be serious, even though the injury may not "look bad." Delayed damage may result from slow hemorrhage or injury to internal eye structures. Apply cold (never hot) compresses and arrange for prompt medical examination.

Foreign Bodies in the Eye

Simple first-aid measures will remove cinders, eyelashes, or specks that rest loosely on the surface of the eyelid or eyeball. Do not attempt to remove embedded particles. Never rub or scratch an eye that "has something in it," especially if you have felt something strike the eye. This may cause scars or drive particles farther into the eyeball. Always wash your hands before touching the eyes.

Pull the upper eyelid out and down over the lower lid, or shut both eyes for a few minutes to cause a flow of tears.

If this does not succeed, fill a clean medicine dropper with warm water or a boric acid solution to "flood" the eye and flush out the foreign body.

If the speck is visible, gently pull the lower eyelid out and downward for inspection. Use a moistened cotton applicator or the corner of a clean

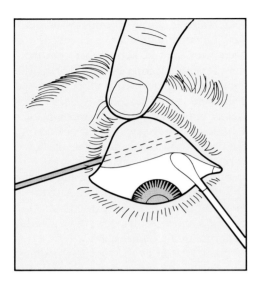

SPECK IN THE EYE
A dust particle or small object, seen when the upper eyelid is turned back over a stick, may be removed with a moistened cotton-tipped applicator. Do not rub a speck embedded in the eye because you may scratch the eyeball.

cotton cloth to lift out the speck. If the speck is not visible, lift the upper lid and look for it. Remove with an applicator or a clean cloth.

For embedded particles, cover with a sterile gauze compress held or gently taped in place, and see a doctor immediately.

Penetrating Eye Wounds

All perforating wounds of the eye are serious, no matter how small, and call for immediate medical help. A tiny speck buried deep inside the eye may leave little outward trace. Do not apply oils or ointments. Instead, cover both eyes with a sterile compress (to lessen harmful eye movements) and bandage lightly in place. Seek medical aid at once.

Some penetrating eye wounds, such as stabs from pointed objects, are obvious and terrifying, but equally serious injuries may look less frightening. A tiny piece of steel hurled off from tool-grinding or nail-pounding may be lodged in an eye that looks normal. Anyone who has felt something strike his eye should be examined by a doctor promptly.

Black Eye

An "ordinary" black eye is a bruise. For immediate first aid, apply pressure to the involved area, preferably with cold compresses or cloths wrung out in cold water. If done at once, this helps to minimize discoloration. A severe black eye may involve deeper injury and need more intensive attention. If the eyes do not move equally well, the "black eye" may be more seriously damaged.

MISCELLANEOUS

Gas Poisoning

First and most important, get the victim to fresh air. Be sure to protect yourself when entering the gas-filled area. Use an efficient mask if you can; crawl or remain near the floor. After removing the victim from the gas area, start mouth-to-mouth resuscitation, if necessary. Immediately call for an ambulance, or paramedics, who usually are equipped to provide oxygen.

Electric Shock

Serious electric shock paralyzes breathing centers and causes unconsciousness. Ordinary house current can cause a fatal electrical shock under some circumstances.

Don't touch the victim until the current is turned off or the victim is free of contact with the current. Insulate yourself from the earth and from the victim with dry, nonconducting materials. Stand on dry newspapers, a dry board, the dry rubber floor mat of your car, or a dry folded coat.

Use a dry stick, a dry board, dry rolled newspapers, or a dry floor mat to pull or push the wire from contact with the victim. Insulate your hands with dry gloves, cloth, or newspapers. If your hand is insulated, you may with caution grasp a dry part of the patient's clothing and drag him away.

After contact is broken, give immediate mouth-to-mouth resuscitation and continue until help arrives. Breathing centers paralyzed by electric shock take a long time to recover—victims have recovered after eight hours of artificial respiration.

Lightning

Use the same first aid as for electric shock, except that you may touch the victim immediately and begin artificial respiration at once.

FIRST-AID SUPPLIES

You can buy a fairly complete first-aid kit at a pharmacy or department store, but a prepared kit isn't necessary. Your own medicine cabinet already may be amply stocked. Always keep your supplies together, so you won't have to hunt for them in an emergency. Check them regularly to see whether they need to be replenished. Never keep them locked, because you don't want to be forced to search for a key in an emergency.

You may wish to store the supplies in a moistureproof container so they can be taken along on family outings. Better yet, keep a duplicate kit in the family car. There should be a complete kit in every car, boat, or recreational vehicle.

Quantity	Item
20	Paper cups, for giving fluids.
1	Flashlight and spare batteries.
1	Blanket.
1	Pillow (or inflatable cushion).
	Newspapers (to place under the person on cold or wet ground or for use as emergency splint).
10 of each	Individual adhesive bandages in ½-inch, ¾-inch, 1-inch, and "round" spot sizes.
Box of 12	2x2-inch sterile first-aid dressings, individually packaged.
Box of 12	4x4-inch sterile first-aid dressings.
1 roll	Roller gauze bandage, 1 inch by 5 yards.
1 roll	Roller gauze bandage, 2 inches by 5 yards.
1 roll each	Adhesive tape, 1- and 2-inch widths.
2	Triangular bandages, 36x36 inches, folded diagonally, for use as a sling.
6	Safety pins, 1½-inch size.
1 bar	Mild white soap, for cleaning wounds and scratches.
1 pair	Scissors with blunt tips, for cutting bandages and tape.
1 pair	Tweezers, for removing splinters.
1 container	Syrup of ipecac, for use in cases of suspected poisoning.
1 bottle	Rubbing alcohol.
1 pair	Nail clippers.
2 containers	acetaminophen (one, adult strength; one, children's strength).
1 bottle	Calamine lotion, for insect bites.
1 bottle	activated charcoal, for use in poisoning.
1	2-inch elastic bandage.
1	razor blade (single edge).
1 bottle	PhisoHex.
1 bottle	Diphenhydramine (Benadryl).

PREVENTING ACCIDENTS

Preventing Burns

Keep handles of pots and frying pans turned away from the edge of the kitchen range.

Don't put hot tea, coffee, or other liquids on a tablecloth or scarf hanging over the sides of a table. A child may pull the cloth or run into it and tip over steaming liquids.

Never leave a small child alone in a bathtub. He or she may turn on the hot water faucet. Place the child in the tub facing the faucet so he or she won't back into the hot metal.

Don't hold a child in your lap while you drink or pass hot beverages.

Cover hot pipes and radiators.

Keep matches and cigarette lighters out of reach until a child is old enough to be taught their safe use.

Never leave children alone around a bonfire, outdoor grill, fireplace, glowing coals, or an open flame.

Preventing Poisonings

Keep household chemicals out of reach of small children. A high shelf or locked cabinet should be used for disinfectants, lye, ammonia, flammable and nonflammable cleaning fluids, insecticides, bleaches, rat poisons, moth balls, paint thinners, turpentine, kerosene, and gasoline.

Never put chemicals into a soft drink bottle or a container associated with food—a sip can be swallowed before it can be spit out.

Never put anything on food shelves except food. Keep drugs, both prescription and nonprescription, locked up.

Do not leave pills in a purse, pocket, or bedside table where children may find them.

Never tell a child that a pill is candy or "tastes like candy."

Never take a medicine until you have read the label. If the label is gone or is illegible, discard the bottle.

Preventing Asphyxiation And Drowning

Keep beans, peanuts, fruit pits, buttons, pins, beads, and coins out of reach of small children. Permit no toy smaller than a child's fist. Check toys for small loose parts that may be taken into the windpipe.

Never leave a small child alone in a bathtub, even for a second.

Fence your swimming pool; do not allow children to use it without adult supervision.

Have gas heaters, ranges, appliances, and home furnaces checked regularly by trained servicemen.

Never run your car engine with the garage door closed. Have your car exhaust system checked regularly.

Preventing Electrical Accidents

Locate all switches and appliances where they can't be touched from the bath, shower, or sink.

Don't touch electrical appliances or outlets while standing on wet floors or in puddles.

Use three-prong grounding plugs or have equipment permanently grounded.

Shut off electricity at the fuse box or circuit breaker before making electrical repairs.

Replace all frayed electric cords. Cover unused wall sockets with protective plates, adhesive tape, or blank plugs. Never touch a dangling wire; call the utility company. Don't use metal ladders close to electricity.

Preventing Swallowing Accidents

Never give popcorn, candy, nuts, or cookies that contain nuts to infants who can't chew them and may inhale them.

Don't let small children play with dry beans, peas, buttons, coins, nails, or screws. Check stuffed animals and other toys for easily removable small parts that a child may remove and swallow or stuff into body openings.

Make a habit of closing safety pins. Don't hold tacks, pins, or nails in your mouth while doing chores, or let children see you doing so.

Be sure that all bone fragments are removed from foods for small children.

Preventing Back Strain

Low back strain is most often caused by improper lifting technique, or attempting to lift objects that are too heavy. The most important lifting rule is never to let the lower back arch forward. Do not bend from the waist, stiff-legged, to lift an object from the floor. Place your feet close to the object, crouch with your back straight and feet flat on the floor, and grasp the object firmly; lift slowly, using your thigh muscles.

Don't lean over a projection such as a radiator to lift a stuck window. Don't reach to pick up something when one arm is loaded with packages. Get help if the object to be lifted is heavy.

Don't lift if your footing is insecure—a slip or twist may wrench your back.

Sudden, quick lifting of heavy objects is dangerous, especially if you are unaccustomed to it. Do not continue trying to lift an object if you feel a slight discomfort in your back. Rest frequently when carrying heavy objects.

Preventing Food Poisoning

In sanitary food handling, lack of refrigeration (keeping foods at room temperature or warmer for several hours) underlies most cases of food poisoning. Food handlers with cut fingers, colds, and boils may introduce germs that can multiply rapidly in foods that are not thoroughly cooked or that are heated very little, such as salads, meringues, salad dressings, creamed dishes, custard fillings, and cold cuts.

Refrigeration retards growth of germs. If no refrigeration is available, consume foods soon after preparation; discard leftovers. On picnics, car trips, and camping trips, keep food in a portable icebox.

Preventing Bites and Stings

Teach children not to maul or torment pets and not to approach stray animals.

Wear calf-high boots in snake country; watch your step in the woods; probe the underbrush with a stick before trampling on it (75 percent of snakebites occur near the ankle; most of the rest in wrist or hand areas).

Tie shut the open ends of sleeves and trouser legs when strolling through tick-infested grasses and weeds.

Wear light-colored clothing. Bees and stinging insects are attracted to dark colors, tweeds, flannels, sweaty clothing, hair oils, and perfumes. If "attacked" by a hostile bee, move slowly, don't make jerky movements, slap, or run, unless a whole hive is after you.

Wear gloves when cleaning out a garage to protect against a possible bite from a black widow spider.

INDEX

Page numbers in **boldface** refer to illustrations or illustrated text.

If you would like to order any additional copies of our books, call 1-800-678-2803 or check with your local bookstore.